PROBLEMS IN

HEALTH CARE LAW

NINTH EDITION

ROBERT D. MILLER, JD, MS HYG

ASSOCIATE GENERAL COUNSEL
UNIVERSITY OF WISCONSIN HOSPITALS AND
CLINICS AUTHORITY
MADISON, WISCONSIN

JONES AND BARTLETT PUBLISHERS
Sudbury, Massachusetts
BOSTON   TORONTO   LONDON   SINGAPORE

World Headquarters

Jones and Bartlett Publishers
40 Tall Pine Drive
Sudbury, MA 01776
978-443-5000
info@jbpub.com
www.jbpub.com

Jones and Bartlett Publishers
Canada
6339 Ormindale Way
Mississauga, Ontario
L5V 1J2
CANADA

Jones and Bartlett Publishers
International
Barb House, Barb Mews
London W6 7PA
UK

Jones and Bartlett's books and products are available through most bookstores and online booksellers. To contact Jones and Bartlett Publishers directly, call 800-832-0034, fax 978-443-8000, or visit our website www.jbpub.com. Substantial discounts on bulk quantities of Jones and Bartlett's publications are available to corporations, professional associations, and other qualified organizations. For details and specific discount information, contact the special sales department at Jones and Bartlett via the above contact information or send an email to specialsales@jbpub.com.

Library of Congress Cataloging-in-Publication Data

Miller, Robert D. (Robert Desle), 1947-
   Problems in health care law / Robert D. Miller. — 9th ed.
      p. cm.
   Includes bibliographic references and index.
   ISBN-13 978-0-7637-4555-4 (pbk.)
   ISBN-10 0-7637-4555-3 (pbk.)
   1. Hospitals—Law and legislation—United States. 2. Medical care—Law and legislation—United States. I. Title.
   [DNLM: 1. Legislation, Hospital—United States. 2. Hospital Administration—legislation & jurisprudence—United States. 3. Economics, Hospital—legislation & jurisprudence—United States. 4. Delivery of Health Care—legislation & jurisprudence—United States. WX 33 AA1 M6pa 2206]
   KF3825.M53 2004
   344.7303'21—dc22

                                             2005021194

   6048

Production Credits
Publisher: Michael Brown
Production Director: Amy Rose
Associate Editor: Kylah Goodfellow McNeill
Production Assistant: Rachel Rossi
Associate Marketing Manager: Marissa Hederson
Manufacturing Buyer: Therese Connell
Composition: Paw Print Media
Cover Design: Timothy Dziewit
Printing and Binding: Malloy, Inc.
Cover Printing: Malloy, Inc.

Printed in the United States of America
10 09 08 07 06   10 9 8 7 6 5 4 3 2

Contents

Preface

We are pleased to present this new edition of *Problems in Health Care Law*. This edition has been restructured into a format that emphasizes the problems of health care law by heading most of the sections with a question. The chapters have been reorganized and regrouped and new material has been added throughout the book.

Chapter 1 provides an overview of legal system and contract principles. Chapters 2 through 5 address the major organizational, physical, and staffing resources that are necessary to deliver health care. Chapters 6 through 8 address the relationship with the patient, including medical decisionmaking and the handling of medical information. Chapters 9 and 10 address the financing of health care services, including payment of providers and coverage of individual patients. Chapters 11 through 13 deal with liability issues, including civil liability, criminal liability, and antitrust issues. Chapter 14 addresses reproductive issues and Chapter 15 addresses the determination of death and the handling of dead bodies.

The restructuring and additions have been assisted by the recommendations of users of prior editions. Our goal has been for *Problems in Health Care Law* to continue to provide the helpful, one-volume overview of health care law that it and its predecessor *Problems in Hospital Law* have provided since 1968.

Acknowledgments

Many individuals and organizations assisted in the preparation of this book. Students at the University of Wisconsin, the University of Iowa, and the University of Miami and others who have used the book have helped to establish the structure. Hospital administrative staff, physicians, nurses, other health professionals, and health care clients have taught me the practical aspects of applying law to the day-to-day provision of health care services. They have also presented the questions that have given me the opportunity to address many of the problems of health care law discussed in this book.

Many people have reviewed and commented on chapters of this book. I would like to thank my colleagues in the administration of the University of Wisconsin Hospitals and Clinics Authority for their assistance.

The strong support from the Jones and Bartlett staff has again made the preparation of this book an enjoyable experience.

I wish to thank my wife, Jill, and daughter, Katie. They have again provided support and encouragement during the many hours devoted to revising this book.

CHAPTER ONE

Introduction to the American Legal System

Objectives

The objective of this chapter is to provide an overview of the framework of the legal system. All the remainder of the book fits into this framework. The reader should learn some of the ways government entities interact in creating and changing the law; the major sources of the law; how the court system functions; and how private entities can create their own private law through contracts. This should help the reader to assess what the laws are that need to be followed, which laws are likely to change, and some of the ways that laws are changed. The reader should understand the nature of legal advice and some of the ways to use it.

Health care services are among the most highly regulated industries. Those who provide, receive, pay for, and regulate health care services make many decisions that are affected by legal principles and have potential for legal consequences. Legal advice cannot be obtained before each decision; so it is useful to develop a general understanding of the law to help identify problems requiring legal counsel and to assist in making alternate decisions consistent with applicable legal principles.

This chapter includes general information about law, including the workings of the legal system and the roles of the branches of government in creating, administering, and enforcing the law. The chapter is divided into sections on the nature of the law (1-1), governmental organization and functions (1-2), sources of law (1-3), and organization of the court system (1-4).

One very important aspect of the law is the way that it facilitates private ordering of relationships through contracts. An overview of contracts is provided in 1-5.

1-1 The Nature of the Law

Law is a system of principles and processes by which people who live in a society attempt to control human conduct, to facilitate cooperative enterprise, and to minimize the use of force in resolving conflicting interests. Through law, society specifies standards of behavior and means to enforce those standards. The purpose of law is to create an infrastructure within which cooperative enterprise can flourish and to avoid conflict between individuals and between government and individuals. Since conflicting interests are inevitable, law also provides ways to resolve disputes.

Like medicine, law is not an exact science. Lawyers are frequently unable to provide a precise answer to a legal question or to predict with certainty the outcome of a legal conflict because much of the law is uncertain. Many questions have never been precisely addressed by the legal system. Even when questions have been addressed and answered through the law, the legal system can change those answers in response to changing conditions. The ability of the law to adjust to individual situations is one of its strengths. Legal uncertainty is similar to the uncertainty encountered in making medical and nursing diagnostic and treatment decisions. When dealing with systems as complicated as the human body or human society, uncertainty is inevitable. A lawyer's advice is always valuable, just as a physician's advice is valuable, because an attorney can use knowledge of how the law has addressed similar questions in the past to predict the most probable answer in the present. After a dispute has arisen, a lawyer plays the role of an advocate who can assure legal dispute resolution mechanisms are used to the client's advantage.

In daily life, law is a guide to conduct. Most disputes or controversies between persons or organizations are resolved without lawyers or courts. In many situations, the existence of the legal system is a stimulus to orderly private dispute resolution. Legal principles reinforce those settlements. The likelihood of success in court affects the willingness of parties to negotiate private settlements. So, it is advantageous to have a basic knowledge of legalities when faced with a dispute.

Laws govern relationships of private individuals and entities with each other and with government. Laws are divided into civil law and criminal law. Civil law can be divided further into contract law, tort law, and other governmental statutes and regulations. Contract law concerns enforcement of agreements and payment of compensation for failure to fulfill those agreements. Tort law defines duties that are not based on contractual agreement and imposes liability for injuries that are caused by breaches of those duties.

A third area of civil law includes the governmental statutes and regulations that require individuals and organizations to act in specified ways. Many of the areas addressed by these statutes affect heath care institutions and professionals, including health care quality, medical device safety, hazardous waste disposal, labor relations, employment policies, facility safety, and other important topics. The primary goal of many of these regulations is to attain compliance, not to punish offenders.

Criminal law forbids conduct deemed injurious to public order and imposes punishment for those who engage in the forbidden conduct. Criminal law has become a more significant concern for hospitals since the government has expanded its use of the criminal law to restructure the health care system. Some traditional conduct in the health care system has been redefined as criminal, and criminal penalties are exacted for violations of new regulations.

1-2 Governmental Organization and Functions

Government is divided into three branches: legislative, executive, and judicial. Their primary functions are as follows. The legislature makes laws, the executive enforces laws, and the judiciary interprets laws. Actual functions of the branches overlap in practice.

Separation of Powers
Separation of powers means that none of the branches is clearly dominant over the other two; each branch can affect and limit the functions of the others. Thus, the process for enacting legislation is

a system of checks and balances. On the federal level, statutes are enacted by Congress; however, usually they do not become the law until they are approved by the president. When the president refuses to approve the law, it is called a veto. Congress has the option to override the president's veto by a two-thirds vote. In addition, when the president fails to issue a veto or approval within a given time limit, a statute can become law. A bill that has become law can ultimately be overturned by the United States Supreme Court or by another court in the judicial branch if it is decided that the law violates the Constitution.

The executive and legislative branches affect the composition of the judicial branch. The president's nominees for federal judges, including Supreme Court justices, must be approved by the Senate. The Supreme Court's decision is final unless Congress and the president enact revised legislation to change the law. Another method of overriding a Supreme Court decision, while complex and often time consuming, is to amend the Constitution.

Following is a discussion of the primary functions of each branch.

Legislative. The function of the legislative branch is to enact new laws and amend existing laws. The legislature determines the need for new laws and for changes in existing laws. Legislatures generally assign legislative proposals to committees charged with oversight of the areas addressed by the proposals. The committees investigate and hold hearings at which interested persons may present their views. These hearings provide information to assist the committees in considering the bills. Hearings are often used to publicize issues to develop public support for action. Some bills eventually are released from the committees and reach the full legislative body, where after consideration and debate, the bills can be either approved or rejected. Congress and every state legislature, with the exception of Nebraska, consist of two houses. (Nebraska has only one house.) Both houses must pass identical versions of a bill before it can be presented to the chief executive. Differences in the versions passed by the two houses are sometimes resolved by a joint conference committee composed of leaders from both houses, and their compromise is then voted on by both houses.

Executive. The primary function of the executive branch is to enforce and administer laws. The chief executive, state governor, or United States president also has a role in law creation through the power to approve or veto bills passed by legislatures. Until 1996, North Carolina was the only state without a governor's veto power, but in that year, the state constitution was amended. If the chief executive approves a passed bill, it becomes law. If the chief executive vetoes the bill, it can become law if the legislature overrides the veto.

The executive branch is organized into departments. The departments are assigned responsibility for specific areas of public affairs and enforce the law within their assigned areas. Much of the federal law affecting hospitals is administered by the Department of Health and Human Services. In most states, there is a department assigned the responsibility for health and welfare matters, including the administration and enforcement of most laws affecting hospitals. Other departments and governmental agencies also affect hospital affairs. On the federal level, for example, laws concerning wages and hours of employment are enforced by the Department of Labor.

Judicial. The function of the judicial branch is adjudication — deciding disputes in accordance with law. For example, courts decide suits brought against hospitals by patients seeking compensation for harm they feel was caused by the wrongful conduct of hospital personnel. News of malpractice suits and suits by the government against hospitals frequently receives the greatest attention, but less well known is the fact that hospitals also sue to enforce rights or to protect legally protected interests. For example, hospitals initiate suits to challenge acts by governmental agencies; to have legislation concerning hospitals declared invalid; to collect unpaid hospital bills; and to enforce contracts.

Many disputes are resolved by negotiation or arbitration without resort to courts. However, sometimes a controversy cannot be ended without submitting to the adjudicative process of courts. When a dispute is brought before a court, the judicial process decides the meaning of agreements and laws, decides what the facts are, and applies the law. This application of law to determine facts is the essence of the judicial process.

1-3 Sources of Law

Four primary sources of law are constitutions (1-3.1); statutes (1-3.2); decisions and rules of administrative agencies (1-3.3); and court decisions (1-3.4). International law embodied in treaties

(1-3.5) is a fifth source of law, but it rarely has a direct affect on health care providers. Private agreements can be viewed as a sixth source of law. In many contexts, the legal constraints that are self-imposed through the private ordering of contracts has more direct impact on day-to-day decision-making than the other governmental sources of law.

1-3.1 Constitutions

The Constitution of the United States is the supreme law of the land. It establishes the general organization of the federal government, grants powers to the federal government, and places limits on what the federal and state governments can do. The Constitution establishes the three branches of the federal government and grants them powers.

The Constitution is a grant of power from the states to the federal government. The federal government has only the powers that the Constitution grants expressly or by implication. Express powers include, for example, the power to collect taxes, declare war, and regulate interstate commerce. The federal government is also granted broad implied powers to enact laws "necessary and proper" for exercising its other powers. However, federal courts do enforce limits on how expansively Congress can define its powers by sometimes declaring laws to be outside the authorized powers.[1] When the federal government establishes law within the scope of its powers, that law is supreme. All conflicting state and local laws are invalid.

The Constitution also limits what the federal and state governments can do. Many limits on federal power appear in the first ten amendments to the Constitution, called the Bill of Rights. The Bill of Rights protects the right to free speech; free exercise of religion; freedom from unreasonable searches and seizures; trial by jury; and no deprivation of life, liberty, or property without due process of law. Some of the most frequently applied limits on state power are stated in the Fourteenth Amendment: "...nor shall any State deprive any person of life, liberty, or property, without due process of law; nor deny to any person within its jurisdiction the equal protection

---

[1] *E.g.,* Brzonkala v. Virginia Polytechnic Inst., 169 F.3d 820 (4th Cir. 1999) (*en banc*) [law making rape a federal crime exceed interstate commerce power]; *Civil rights law on rape victims is unconstitutional, court says,* N.Y. Times, Mar. 6, 1999, A8.

of the laws." These clauses are frequently referred to as the *due process clause* and the *equal protection clause*.

DUE PROCESS OF LAW. The due process clause restricts state action, not private action. Actions by state and local governmental agencies, including public hospitals, are state actions and must comply with due process requirements. Actions by private individuals at the behest of the state can also be subject to these requirements. In the past, private hospitals were sometimes considered to be engaged in state action when they were regulated or partially funded by governmental agencies. As discussed in Chapter 8, it is now rare for private hospitals to be engaged in state action.

The due process clause applies to state actions that deprive a person of "life, liberty, or property." Liberty and property interests can include a physician's appointment to the medical staff of a public hospital and a hospital's institutional license. Thus, in some situations public hospitals must provide due process, and in other situations, hospitals are entitled to due process. The process that is due varies depending on the situation. The two primary elements of due process are (1) rules must be reasonable and not vague and (2) fair procedures must be followed in enforcing rules. Rules that are too arbitrary or vague violate the due process clause and are not enforceable. The primary elements of a fair procedure are notice of the proposed action and an opportunity to present information as to why the action should not be taken. The phrase "due process" in the Fourteenth Amendment also has been interpreted by the Supreme Court to include nearly all of the rights in the Bill of Rights. Thus, state governments cannot infringe on those rights.

EQUAL PROTECTION OF THE LAWS. The equal protection clause also restricts state action, not private action. Equal protection means that like persons must be dealt with in a like fashion. The equal protection clause addresses the classifications used to distinguish persons for various legal purposes. When a classification is challenged, the court must determine whether a difference between persons justifies the particular difference in rules or procedures. Courts generally require governmental agencies to justify differences with a "rational reason." The major exceptions to this standard are the strict scrutiny courts apply to distinctions based on "suspect classifications," such as race, and the intermediate level of scrutiny applied to sex-based classifications.

Courts have ruled that the equal protection clause imposes a constitutional right of interstate travel that has been applied to strike down state limitations on welfare benefits for new residents.[2]

The equal protection clause of the Fourteenth Amendment includes an express grant of enforcement powers to the Congress. This supercedes the Eleventh Amendment that otherwise bars most suits against states seeking money, unless the state consents. Congress can authorize suits against states to enforce equal protection.[3] Other federal powers, such as the Commerce Power, generally do not permit Congress to abrogate Eleventh Amendment immunity.[4]

STATE CONSTITUTIONS. Each state has a constitution. The state constitution establishes the organization of state government; grants powers to state government; and places limits on what state government can do. Many of these documents contain rights similar to the rights in the United States Constitution, and some provide additional rights.

1-3.2 Statutes

Another major source of law is statutory law, which is law enacted by a legislature. Legislative bodies include the United States Congress, state legislatures, and local legislative bodies, such as city councils and county boards of supervisors. Congress has only the powers delegated by the Constitution, but those powers have been broadly interpreted. A state legislature has all powers not denied by the United States Constitution, valid federal laws, or the state constitution. A local legislative body has only those powers granted by the state. Some states have granted local governments broad powers through either statutes or constitutional amendments authorizing "home rule."

---

[2] Shapiro v. Thompson, 394 U.S. 618 (1960) [state cannot require year residency for welfare benefits]; Memorial Hosp. v. Maricopa County, 415 U.S. 250 (1974); Bethesda Lutheran Homes & Servs. v. Leean, 122 F.3d 443 (7th Cir. 1997) [state Medicaid residency rule for coverage of intermediate care struck down]; Maldonado v. Houstoun, 157 F.3d 179 (3d Cir. 1998) [striking down state law limiting welfare benefits to new residents for one year to lesser of state's benefits or prior state's benefits]; *but see* Jones v. Helms, 452 U.S. 412 (1981) [state may impose additional penalty for leaving state after abandoning child]; McCarthy v. Philadelphia Civil Serv. Comm'n, 424 U.S. 645 (1976) [city may require city employees to be residents of city].

[3] Fitzpatrick v. Bitzer, 427 U.S. 445 (1976).

[4] Seminole Tribe of Fla. v. Florida, 517 U.S. 44 (1996); Abril v. Virginia, 145 F.3d 182 (4th Cir. 1998) [cannot authorize private suits against states under Fair Labor Standards Act].

PREEMPTION. When state or local law conflicts with federal law, valid federal law supersedes. Federal law *preempts* some areas of law, and in those areas state law is superseded even when it is not in direct conflict. Some laws, such as bankruptcy laws and the Employee Retirement and Income Security Act (ERISA),[5] explicitly forbid dual state regulation. In other laws, courts find that preemption is implied from the aim and pervasiveness of the federal scheme, the need for uniformity, and the likelihood that state regulation would obstruct the full goals of the federal law. Courts tend not to find implied preemption when the state is exercising its police power to protect public health. For example, in 1960 the Supreme Court ruled that the extensive federal regulation of shipping did not preempt a city ordinance concerning smoke emissions; so a federally licensed vessel could be prosecuted for violating the pollution ordinance.[6] In 1985, the Supreme Court ruled that county ordinances regulating blood plasma collection were not preempted by federal regulation of drugs.[7] Some federal laws preempt only some aspects of an area, leaving others to state regulation. For example, the Minnesota Supreme Court ruled in 1986 that federal law preempted state licensure of air ambulances, but that the state could enforce staffing, equipment, and sanitary requirements.[8]

When local laws conflict with state laws, valid state laws supersede. State law can preempt an entire area of law; so local law is superseded even when it is not in direct conflict.[9]

PRIVATE RIGHT OF ACTION. When a statute does not specifically authorize private individuals to bring a lawsuit to enforce the statute, the courts have to determine whether there is a private right of action implied.[10] If there is no private right of action, then only the government can enforce the statute.

---

[5] 29 U.S.C. § 1144 [ERISA preemption]. ERISA preemption is discussed in Chapters 9 and 10.

[6] Huron Portland Cement Co. v. Detroit, 362 U.S. 440 (1960).

[7] Hillsborough County v. Automated Med. Labs., 471 U.S. 707 (1985).

[8] Hiawatha Aviation of Rochester, Inc. v. Minnesota Dep't of Health, 389 N.W. 2d 507 (Minn. 1986).

[9] *E.g.*, Robin v. Incorporated Village of Hempstead, 30 N.Y.2d 347, 285 N.E.2d 285 (1972).

[10] *E.g.*, Suter v. Artist M., 503 U.S. 347 (1992) [child beneficiaries of Adoption Act cannot enforce requirement of reasonable state efforts to keep children in their homes]; Gentry v. Department of Pub. Health, 190 Mich. App. 102, 475 N.W.2d 849 (1991) [no private right of action to enforce nursing home patient bill of rights]; Evelyn V. v. Kings County Hosp. Ctr., 819 F. Supp. 183 (E.D.N.Y. 1993) [Medicaid recipients have no statutory right to enforce Medicaid regulations against provider]; *but see* Wilder v. Virginia Hosp. Ass'n, 496 U.S. 498 (1990) [providers can enforce Medicaid "reasonable rates" requirement]; Fulkerson v. Comm'r, Maine Dep't of Human Servs., 802 F. Supp. 529 (D. Me. 1992) [Medicaid recipients may enforce equal access to care provision].

1-3.3 Decisions and Rules of Administrative Agencies

The decisions and rules of administrative agencies are another source of law. Legislatures have delegated to administrative agencies the responsibility and power to implement various laws. These delegated powers include the quasi-legislative power to adopt regulations and the quasi-judicial power to decide how the statutes and regulations apply to individual situations. These powers are delegated because the legislature does not have the time or expertise to address the complex issues concerning many regulated areas. Examples of federal administrative agencies include the Centers for Medicare and Medicaid Services (CMS); Food and Drug Administration (FDA); National Labor Relations Board (NLRB); and Internal Revenue Service (IRS). CMS administers the Medicare program and the federal aspects of the Medicaid program. The FDA promulgates regulations and applies them to individual determinations concerning manufacturing, marketing, and advertising foods, drugs, cosmetics, and medical devices. The NLRB decides how national labor laws apply to individual disputes. The IRS promulgates regulations and applies them to individual disputes concerning federal taxation. Many administrative agencies seek to achieve some consistency in their decisions by following the position they adopted in previous cases involving similar matters.[11] This is similar to the way courts develop the common law discussed later in this chapter. When dealing with these agencies, previous decisions, as well as rules, should be reviewed.

Administrative regulations are valid only to the extent they are within the authority validly granted by legislation to the agency. Delegation can be invalid when it violates the constitutional requirement of separation of powers by not sufficiently specifying what regulations the administrative body can make. Delegations by Congress have seldom been found to be invalid. Broad delegation, specifying the general area of law, has been permitted.[12] In the past, state courts often have declared delegations to be unconstitutional unless there was considerable specificity. Today state courts also permit much broader delegation.

---

[11] *E.g.,* Citrosuco Paulista, S.A. v. United States, 704 F. Supp. 1075, 1088 (Ct. Int'l Trade 1988).
[12] Yakus v. United States, 321 U.S. 414 (1994) [broad price control delegation during World War II upheld].

The Congress and many state legislatures have passed administrative procedure acts. These laws specify the procedure for administrative agencies to adopt rules and to reach decisions in individual cases when no other law specifies different procedures for the agency. Generally, these laws require proposed rules to be published so that individuals have an opportunity to comment before finalization. Many federal agencies must publish both proposed and final rules in the *Federal Register*. Some changes do not have to be published.[13] Many states have similar publications that include proposed and final rules of state agencies. Health care providers should monitor proposed and final rules through these publications and publications of professional or institutional associations or other sources. Despite their expertise, administrative agencies do not know all the implications of their proposals. They rely on the public and those regulated to alert them to potential problems through the comment process.

Some administrative agencies use negotiated rule-making, giving those regulated and other interested parties more input in the developmental of regulations.[14]

Agency enforcement of statutes and regulations is constrained by the resources of the agency. Sometimes when legislators are opposed to a law or regulation that politically or procedurally they cannot repeal directly, they curtail or eliminate the funding for enforcement.[15] Even when an agency is not targeted in this fashion, its funding generally is limited for budgetary reasons. Enforcement funds and practices often define the practical meaning of the regulations. When approvals from the government are required, this can lead to delays in approvals.[16]

---

[13] *E.g.*, National Med. Enterprises v. Shalala, 43 F.3d 691 (D.C. Cir. 1995) [reclassification of labor costs to different cost center for Medicare payment purposes was not substantive rule requiring notice and comment]; Association of Am. R.R. v. Dep't of Transportation, 309 U.S. App. D.C. 7, 38 F.3d 582 (D.C. Cir. 1994) [when final rule differs from proposed rule, agency not required to give separate notice if final rule is "logical outgrowth" of rule-making proceeding].

[14] *E.g., Negotiated rulemaking panel reaches consensus; sends outline of rule to HCFA*, 7 HEALTH L. RPTR. (BNA) 425 (1998) [hereinafter HEALTH L. RPTR. (BNA) will be cited as H.L.R.]; *Advisory group gives seal of approval to managed care anti-kickback safe harbor*, 7 H.L.R. 155 (1998); S. Martin, *Reinventing rule-making*, AM. MED. NEWS, Feb. 23, 1998, 7.

[15] *See House GOP hopes to cut funding used to enforce dozens of U.S. regulations*, WALL St. J., June 1, 1995, at A16.

[16] *E.g., Lack of funds forces HCFA to revise survey priorities*, 4 H.L.R. 407 (1995) [HCFA could not complete survey and certification of home health agencies (HHAs), which threatened moratorium on new HHAs].

1-3.4 Court Decisions

Judicial decisions are a fourth source of law. The role of courts is to resolve disputes. In deciding individual cases, courts interpret statutes and regulations; determine whether specific statutes and regulations are permitted by the state or federal constitution; and create the common law when deciding cases not controlled by statutes, regulations, or a constitution.

INTERPRETING STATUTES AND RULES. There is frequently disagreement over the application of statutes or regulations to specific situations. Often an administrative agency has the initial authority to decide how they will be applied. Under the doctrine of *primary jurisdiction*, courts generally will refuse to accept a suit until the administrative remedies have been pursued.[17] This is sometimes referred to the requirement of *exhaustion of remedies*. The final administrative decision can usually be appealed to courts. Courts generally defer to decisions of administrative agencies in discretionary matters. While there is some deference to the agency interpretation of the law concerning the agency, there is no presumption that the agency conclusions of law are correct.[18] Courts review whether the delegation to the agency was constitutional and whether the agency acted within its authority, followed proper procedures, had a substantial basis for its decision, and acted without arbitrariness or discrimination. The court might have to interpret a statute or regulation or decide which of several conflicting statutes or regulations applies. Courts have developed rules for interpreting statutes. Some states also have a statute specifying interpretation rules. These rules or statutes are designed to help determine the intent of the legislature.

CONSTITUTIONALITY OF STATUTES AND RULES. Courts also determine whether statutes or regulations violate the Constitution. All legislation and regulations must be consistent with the Constitution. Courts can declare a law invalid when it is unconstitutional.[19] Laws can be unconstitutional because of their content or because of how they are enacted. For example, in Florida, like in some other states, an appropriation bill cannot change the law that says how the money will be spent; so in 1995, the Florida Supreme Court

---

[17] *E.g.*, Johnson v. Nyack Hosp., 964 F.2d 116 (2d Cir. 1992) [physician must first pursue N.Y. state administrative remedies before suit challenging privilege termination].

[18] *E.g.*, Keeton v. D.H.H.S., 21 F.3d 1064 (11th Cir. 1994).

[19] Marbury v. Madison, 5 U.S. (1 Cranch) 137 (1803).

ruled that a provision of the Medicaid appropriation bill that purported to reinstate pharmacy copayments was unconstitutional.[20] The legislature had to make the change in a nonappropriation bill.

COMMON LAW. Many legal principles and rules applied by courts are the product of the common law developed in England and the United States. The term *common law* refers to principles that evolve from court decisions. Common law is continually being adapted and expanded. During the colonial period in North America, English common law applied. After the American Revolution, each state adopted part or all of the existing common law. Subsequent common law has been developed by each state, and so common law differs from state to state. The federal courts have also developed a federal common law. Statutory laws have been enacted to restate many legal principles that initially were established by courts as part of the common law. Many cases, especially disputes among private entities, are decided according to the common law. The common law can be changed by statutes that modify the principles or by court decisions that establish different common law principles.

1-3.5 International Law

International law expressed in the treaties between the United States and other nations is a fifth source of law. International law has rarely had an impact on health care providers except when they enter business transactions with businesses in other countries. Such transactions are increasingly likely to occur.

International law can have an impact on domestic policy and practices. For example, the European Union adopted strict requirements for privacy of medical information, which some American businesses had to address in order to engage in business involving European medical information.[21] This has been less of a problem because U.S. standards were strengthened under the federal Health Insurance Portability and Accountability Act (HIPAA) in 2003. Another example is the use of the North American Free Trade Agreement (NAFTA) to challenge a large liability award by an American court.[22]

---

[20] Moreau v. Lewis, 648 So.2d 124 (Fla. 1995).
[21] *European Union directive may not impact health care, other business operations*, 7 H.L.R. 1705 (1998).
[22] T. Carlisle, *Loewen seeks $725 million from U.S.*, WALL ST. J., Jan. 13, 1999, B11 [notice of claim filed with United States Dep't of State under North American Free Trade Agreement, claiming bias and seeking damages for state jury verdict].

1-4 Organization of the Court System

The structure of the court system determines which court decisions serve as precedents in a geographic area. There are over fifty court systems in the United States, including the federal system, each state's system, the District of Columbia's system, and the systems of Puerto Rico and the territories. These courts do not all reach the same decisions concerning specific issues. Frequently a majority approach and several minority approaches exist on an issue. Careful review is necessary to find the court decisions applicable to an individual hospital and, if there are no such court decisions, to predict which approach courts are likely to adopt.

Some of the variation in outcome is due to different approaches to the law. In some cases, courts consider subsequent social developments when interpreting constitutional and statutory language and common law principles, taking a more active role in the development of the law. In some cases, courts seek to interpret constitutional and statutory law more strictly, leaving development of the law to other branches of government. While some courts tend to use one approach more than the other, many courts use both approaches depending on the issue presented.

The federal court system and many state court systems have three levels of courts: trial courts, intermediate courts of appeal, and a supreme court. Some states do not have intermediate courts of appeal.

This section is divided into discussions of trial courts (1-4.1), the state court system (1-4.2), and the federal court system (1-4.3). This is followed by discussions of two legal principles that determine the effect of court decisions — *stare decisis* (1-4.4) and *res judicata* (1-4.5) — and determine who may take cases to court — standing (1-4.6).

1-4.1 Trial Courts

In both the state and federal trial courts, the applicable law is determined, and the evidence is assessed to determine what the "facts" are. The applicable law is then applied to those facts. The judge determines what the law is. If there is a jury, the judge instructs the jury as to what the law is, and the jury determines the facts and applies the law. If there is no jury, the judge also determines the facts. In some cases, everyone agrees on the facts, and the court is asked only to determine what the law is. In other cases, everyone agrees what the law is, but there is disagreement over the facts. Many cases involve both questions of law and questions of fact.

The determination of facts must be based on evidence properly admitted during trial; so "facts" are not necessarily what actually happened. To determine facts for purposes of deciding a case, the credibility of witnesses and the weight to be given to other evidence must be determined.

The judge has significant control over the trial even when a jury is involved. If the judge finds that insufficient evidence has been presented to establish a factual issue for the jury to resolve, the judge can dismiss the case or, in civil cases, direct the jury to decide the case in a specific way. In civil cases, after the jury has come to a decision, the judge can decide in favor of the other side.

DEFAULT OUTCOME AND BURDEN OF PROOF. When analyzing any statute or legal principle, it is helpful to identify the default outcome, that is, what happens if no one can prove that something else should happen. If that default outcome is not desired, the next step is to identify what must be done to convince the judge or jury to determine that the default outcome should not occur. The person who wants a different outcome has the *burden of proof*. Much of legal planning is to make the default outcome favorable or at least to design documentation to meet the burden of proof for the desired outcome.

Generally, in a trial the plaintiff who brings the suit has the initial burden of proof, but when that initial burden is met, frequently the burden shifts to the defendant to prove that an exception applies.

An example of this analysis is a Florida case in which a hospital sought to collect from a guarantor the balance of the bill that had not been paid by insurance. The trial court placed the burden of proof on the hospital to demonstrate that the services beyond those paid by insurance were medically necessary; so the default position was no payment from the guarantor. The hospital lost. The appellate court ruled that the burden of proof should have been on the guarantor to prove lack of medical necessity; so the default position was payment by the guarantor. A new trial was ordered to give the guarantor an opportunity to meet the burden of proof.[23]

---

[23] Public Health Trust v. Holmes, 646 So.2d 266 (Fla. 3d DCA 1994).

Courts often distinguish three aspects of the burden of proof. First, the plaintiff generally has to demonstrate a *prima facie* case before the defendant is obligated to do anything. A prima facie case is demonstrated by providing some evidence that all of the elements necessary for the claim are present. Failure to submit a prima facie case can lead to dismissal. Second, when a prima facie case has been demonstrated, there is usually a burden of going forward, frequently called a *burden of production*. In some types of cases, the burden of production requires the defendant to explain why some defenses apply. For example, after a prima facie case of employment disability discrimination is made, the employer has the burden of production to articulate a legitimate, nondiscriminatory reason for the adverse action against the plaintiff. Third, there is the ultimate *burden of persuasion*. This is the burden to convince the court that based on the evidence the court should rule in a particular way. If the burden of persuasion is not met, then the court should rule for the default position. The burden of persuasion generally remains with the plaintiff. [24]

1-4.2 State Court System

The trial courts in some states are divided into separate courts for specific issues, such as family courts, juvenile courts, probate courts, courts limited to lesser crimes, or courts limited to civil cases involving limited amounts of money. Some states have created specific courts with new functions.[25] Each state has trial courts of general jurisdiction that can decide all disputes that are not assigned to other courts or barred by valid federal or state law.

Most state court systems have intermediate appellate courts. Usually, these courts decide only appeals from trial court decisions. Some states permit a few issues to be taken directly to an intermediate appellate court. When an appellate court is deciding an appeal, additional evidence is not accepted. Only evidence in the trial court record is used. An appellate court almost always accepts determinations of fact from the trial court because the jury and

---

[24] *E.g.,* Brenneman v. Medcentral Health Sys., 366 F.3d 412 (6th Cir. 2004); St. Mary's Honor Ctr. v. Hicks, 509 U.S. 502 (1993).

[25] L. Eaton & L. Kaufman, *In problem-solving court, judges turn therapist*, N.Y. Times, Apr. 26, 2005, A1.

judge see witnesses and can better judge their credibility. Usually, the appellate court bases its decision on whether proper procedures were followed in the trial court and whether the trial court properly interpreted the law. However, an appellate court will occasionally find that a jury or trial judge verdict is so clearly contrary to the evidence that it will either reverse the decision or order a new trial.

Each state has a single highest court, usually called the *supreme court*. In some states, the name is different. For example, in New York the highest court is called the Court of Appeals, while trial courts are called supreme courts. The highest court decides appeals from intermediate appellate courts and some direct appeals from trial courts. The highest court usually also has other duties, including adopting procedural rules for the state court system, determining who can practice law in the state, and disciplining lawyers and other judges for improper conduct.

In most states, there is no right to review by the highest state court. The highest court has discretion whether or not to grant review. Thus, the intermediate appellate court decision is the final decision in many cases.

1-4.3 Federal Court System

The federal court system has a structure similar to that of state court systems. The trial courts are the United States District Courts and special purpose courts, such as the Court of Claims, which determines certain claims against the United States.

LIMITED JURISDICTION. Federal trial courts are fundamentally different from a state trial court because they all have limited jurisdiction. A suit must either present a federal question or be between citizens of different states. In many types of cases, the controversy must involve at least $75,000. Federal question cases include those involving applications of federal statutes and regulations and those involving possible violations of rights under the United States Constitution. When a federal trial court decides a controversy between citizens of different states that does not involve a federal question, it is acting under what is called its *diversity jurisdiction*. In diversity cases, federal court procedures are used, but the law of the applicable state is used, rather than federal law.

ABSTENTION. Sometimes federal trial courts will decline to decide state law questions until they have been decided by a state court. This is called *abstention*.[26] It is designed to leave state issues for state courts and minimize the federal court workload. Federal courts generally do not abstain when important federal questions are affected by the state law question. Some states have procedures by which federal courts can ask the highest state court to decide a question of state law.

FEDERAL CIRCUIT COURTS OF APPEAL. An appeal from a federal trial court goes to a United States Circuit Court of Appeals. The United States is divided into twelve circuits, geographic areas numbered one through eleven plus the District of Columbia Circuit and a nongeographic Federal Circuit.

UNITED STATES SUPREME COURT. The highest court is the United States Supreme Court. It decides appeals from courts of appeals. Decisions of the highest state courts can also be appealed to the Supreme Court if they involve federal laws or the United States Constitution. Sometimes when the court of appeals or the highest state court declines to review a lower court decision, a lower court decision can be reviewed by the Supreme Court.

The Supreme Court has the authority to decline to review most cases. With few exceptions, a request for review is made by filing a petition for a *writ of certiorari*. If the Court grants the writ, the lower court record is transmitted to the Supreme Court for review. In most cases, the Court denies the writ, which is indicated by "*cert denied*, [vol.] U.S. [page] [year]" at the end of the case citation. Denial of a writ of certiorari does not indicate approval of the lower court decision; it merely means the Court declined to review the decision.

1-4.4 Stare Decisis

Courts generally adhere to the doctrine of *stare decisis*, which is frequently described as "following *precedent*." By applying principles developed in previous, similar cases, the court arrives at the same ruling in the current case as it did in the preceding one. Slight differences in circumstances can provide a reason for the court not to apply the previous rule to the current case. Even when such differences are absent, a court may conclude that a common law principle is no longer appropriate and may depart from precedent. An

---

[26] *E.g.*, Trent v. Dial Med. of Fla., Inc., 33 F.3d 217 (3d Cir. 1994).

example of this overruling of precedent is the reconsideration and elimination of the common law principle of charitable immunity, which for many decades provided nonprofit hospitals with virtual freedom from liability for harm to patients.[27] Courts in nearly every state overruled precedent that had provided immunity; so now nonprofit hospitals can generally be sued[28] except in the few states that have reestablished charitable immunity by statute.[29]

When a court is presented with an issue, it is bound by the doctrine of *stare decisis* to follow the precedents of higher courts in the same court system that have jurisdiction over the geographic area where the court is located. Each appellate court, including the highest court, is also generally bound to follow the precedents of its own decisions unless it decides to overrule such precedent due to changing conditions. However, many courts issue some opinions that are not published and cannot be used as precedent.[30] Another reason that a court can change its prior position is that controlling statutes or regulations have changed. Most decisions by a federal circuit court of appeals are made by a panel of three judges. There is a special procedure, called *en banc* review, by which all the active judges in the circuit can review the decision of a panel and overrule the decision.[31]

Decisions from equal or lower courts do not have to be followed. Federal circuit courts consider but do not defer to decisions of other circuits.[32] Usually, decisions from courts in other court systems do not have to be followed. One exception is when a federal court is deciding a controversy between citizens of different states and must follow state law as determined by the highest court of that state. Another exception is when a state court is deciding a controversy involving a federal law or constitutional question and must follow the decisions of the United States Supreme Court. State courts do not have to follow decisions of other federal courts, even when deciding federal law questions.

---

27 *E.g.,* Mikota v. Sisters of Mercy, 183 Iowa 1378, 168 N.W. 219 (1918) [established charitable immunity].
28 *E.g.,* Haynes v. Presbyterian Hosp. Ass'n, 241 Iowa 1269, 45 N.W.2d 151 (1950) [overruled charitable immunity].
29 *E.g.,* Marsella v. Monmouth Med. Ctr., 224 N.J. Super. 336, 540 A.2d 865 (1988).
30 *See* Hart v. Massanari, 266 F.3d 1155 (9th Cir. 2001) [constitutional to forbid use of unpublished decisions].
31 *E.g.,* Atchison, Topeka and Santa Fe Ry. Co. v. Pena, 44 F.3d 437 (7th Cir. 1994) (en banc), *aff'd,* 516 U.S. 152 (1996).
32 *Id.*

A third exception occurs when a court determines that the law of another jurisdiction governs some aspect of the case. The court must then follow the decisions of the highest court in the state or country whose law governs. With the growth of interstate and international transactions and travel, courts are frequently confronted with issues of *choice of law*, having to decide what law governs. It is not unusual for the law of another state or country to govern some or all aspects of a case, especially in contract disputes, where the contract will often specify that the law of another jurisdiction governs. Many courts will not research foreign law. They place the burden of proof on the person who is relying on the foreign law to prove what that law is and adopt the default outcome of assuming that the other law is no different than the forum state's laws.

When a court is presented with a question that is not answered by statutes or regulations and that has not been addressed by the applicable court system, the court will often examine judicial solutions in other systems to help decide the new issue. Judicial decisions from other systems are also examined when a court reexamines an issue to decide whether to overrule precedent. Most court systems tend toward some consistency. A trend across the country provides a basis for a reasonable legal assessment of how to act even when courts in a hospital's area have not decided the issue. However, a court is not bound by decisions from other systems, and it may reach a different conclusion.

There can be a majority approach to an issue that many state court systems follow and one or more minority approaches that other state courts follow. State courts show more consistency on some issues than others. For example, nearly all state courts have completely eliminated charitable immunity. However, while nearly all states require informed consent to medical procedures, some states determine the information that must be provided to patients by reference to what a patient needs to know, while other states make the determination by reference to what other physicians would disclose.

Courts can reach different conclusions because state statutes and regulations differ. For example, Georgia had a statute that specified that a physician need only disclose "in general terms the treatment or course of treatment" to obtain informed consent.[33] In 1975,

---

[33] GA. CODE ANN. § 31-9-6(d) (1985).

a Georgia court interpreted that statute to eliminate the requirement that risks be disclosed to obtain informed consent.[34] As a
result, Georgia courts stopped basing liability on failure to disclose
risks[35] until 1989, when a state statute again required risk disclosure for most surgery and some other procedures.[36] Courts in other
states are unlikely to consider Georgia court decisions concerning
this issue because these decisions are based on Georgia statutes,
not on a change in Georgia common law.

In summary, while it is important to be aware of trends in court
decisions across the country, legal advice should be sought before
taking actions based on decisions from court systems that do not
have jurisdiction over the geographic area in which the hospital is
located.

1-4.5 Res Judicata

Another doctrine that courts follow to avoid duplicative litigation
and conflicting decisions is *res judicata*, which means "a thing or
matter settled by judgment." When a legal controversy has been
decided by a court and no more appeals are available, those
involved in the suit cannot take the same matters to court again.[37]
This is different from *stare decisis* in that *res judicata* applies only
to the parties involved in the prior suit and to issues decided in that
suit. The application of *res judicata* can be complicated by disagreements over whether specific matters were actually decided in
the prior case.

1-4.6 Standing

Another important requirement is that the person bringing the suit
must have *standing*. Courts can only decide actual controversies,
and the person bringing the suit must have an actual stake in the
controversy. Persons with such a stake are said to have standing.

---

[34] Young v. Yarn, 136 Ga. App. 737, 222 S.E.2d 113 (1975).

[35] *E.g.*, Padgett v. Ferrier, 172 Ga. App. 335, 323 S.E.2d 166 (1984). The Georgia Supreme Court
has interpreted a similar statute concerning consent to sterilization as limiting the applicability of the informed consent doctrine, Robinson v. Parrish, 251 Ga. 496, 306 S.E.2d 922 (1983).

[36] GA. CODE ANN. § 31-9-6.1(1988 Supp.).

[37] *E.g.*, Lim v. Central DuPage Hosp., 972 F.2d 758 (7th Cir. 1992), *cert. denied*, 507 U.S. 987
(1993) [physician's second antitrust suit barred by *res judicata*].

Sometimes parties with a stake do not have standing for other reasons. For example, in some states governmental entities do not have standing to challenge the constitutionality of state statutes and regulations.[38]

1-5 Contracts

A contract is a legally enforceable agreement. Health care providers have many contracts involving all areas of operations, including employment contracts; contracts to purchase supplies and equipment; construction contracts; sales contracts; contracts to purchase services; and contracts involving leases, loans, and other matters. The primary purpose of a written contract is to set forth the agreement to facilitate compliance, not to prepare for litigation. All elements of contracts should be carefully thought through and clearly articulated. This section outlines some of the legal problems associated with contracts. The law of contracts is complex, and there are exceptions to these general rules. Contracts should be reviewed with the assistance of legal counsel. Health care administrators are expected to be sophisticated in business matters and will find themselves bound by contracts, even when they are not in the organization's best interest or even harmful to the organization.

WHEN IS THERE A CONTRACT? Usually, agreements to agree in the future are not enforceable. Generally, there is no contract until the agreement itself is reached. However, sometimes courts find that a contract exists before the formal contract is signed; so administrators should be circumspect with promises, negotiations, correspondence, and letters of intent.

Agreement can sometimes be inferred from conduct. Thus, it is prudent to state intent clearly and in writing. For example, when a contract between a Pennsylvania hospital and a managed care company expired, the hospital sent the company a written rejection of the company's offer to extend the contract. When the hospital continued to submit claims and accept payments, the company asserted that the hospital had accepted the offer of extension by its

---

[38] *E.g.*, Trustees of Worcester State Hosp. v. Governor, 395 Mass. 377, 480 N.E.2d 291 (1985) [statutes]; Palomar Pomerado Health System v. Belsh, 180 F.3d 1104 (9th Cir. 1999) [regulations].

conduct. A Pennsylvania court rejected this assertion, ruling that the express written rejection barred implied assent by conduct.[39]

CONSIDERATION. Courts usually require all participants, often called *parties*, to pay a price in order for a contract to exist and be binding. This price, called the *consideration* for the contract, can be an act, forbearance, change of legal relationship, or promise. When one party has not provided any consideration, the courts usually will not let that party enforce the contract. One exception is that most written sales contracts are enforceable against merchants without consideration because of state laws called the *Uniform Commercial Code* (UCC).

UNENFORCEABLE CONTRACTS. Courts will not enforce many other contracts, such as illegal contracts,[40] contracts that are viewed by the court as against public policy,[41] oral contracts of the type the law requires to be written, and unconscionable contracts. The public policy rule was applied by a federal appellate court to declare that a contract with an unlicensed nursing agency was unenforceable.[42] The agency could not sue to enforce the contract because it did not have the license required by state law. The *statute of frauds* requires contracts of certain types (e.g., conveyances of land, leases for over a year, and certain employment contracts) be in writing to be enforceable, unless an exception applies.[43] *Unconscionable contracts* are contracts that shock the conscience of the court, usually by being extortionate. Because courts usually apply the unconscionability doctrine only to consumer contracts, health care providers are seldom protected by the doctrine in dealings with other businesses. However, some contracts with patients, such as exculpatory contracts purporting to limit the patient's right to sue, could be found to be unconscionable and thus unenforceable.

---

[39] Temple Univ. Hosp., Inc. v. Healthcare Management Alternatives, Inc., 764 A.2d 587 (Pa. Super. 2000).

[40] *E.g.,* Nursing Home Consultants Inc. v. Quantum Health Srvcs., 112 F.3d 514 (*without op.*). 1997 U.S. App. LEXIS 10544 (8th Cir. 1997) [contract violating anti-kickback provisions is void].

[41] *E.g.,* Swafford v. Harris, 967 S.W.2d 319 (Tenn. 1998) [contingency fee contract with physician expert witness void as against public policy].

[42] United States Nursing Corp. v. Saint Joseph Med. Ctr., 39 F.3d 790 (7th Cir. 1994).

[43] *E.g.,* Preventive Med. Inst. v. Weill Med. College (N.Y. Sur. Ct.), N.Y.L.J., July 19, 2002, 17 [alleged oral agreement concerning name on clinic sign barred by statute of frauds]; Americare Health Alliance of Ga. LLC v. America's Health Plan Inc., No. (N.D. Ga. Mar. 3, 1998) *as discussed in* 7 H.L.R. 473 (1998) [alleged contract between health plan, provider group unenforceable under statute of frauds which requires such contracts to be in writing].

Courts occasionally refuse to enforce part of an agreement. For example, courts will generally not enforce penalty provisions. Another example is that in many circumstances courts will not enforce agreements not to compete.[44] Many contracts specify that if the agreement is found partly invalid that the remainder is still enforceable. This provision can create problems when the invalid portion was of central importance, but it can also save advantageous arrangements when the invalid portion is less significant.

PAROLE EVIDENCE RULE. Courts tend to review only the words in the written contract by applying the *parole evidence rule*, under which oral promises made during negotiations that are not included in the final written agreement are assumed to have been negotiated away.[45] Health care providers cannot rely on oral statements made prior to signing a written contract. If these statements are important to the agreement, they should be in the written contract.

COURT-ADDED TERMS. In some circumstances, a court will add terms to contracts.

Ambiguous or missing elements. When a written contract is ambiguous or does not have critical elements, the court will sometimes consider testimony concerning oral understandings. The court will try to avoid this, but sometimes oral understandings must be considered. The court then must sift through the usually conflicting recollections of the parties and decide what to believe.

Lack of agreement. Sometimes it is clear that no agreement, written or oral, was reached concerning critical elements, such as the delivery date. The court will sometimes fill these gaps with a provision the court considers to be reasonable. However, courts will not always fill the gaps forcing the parties to solve the problem on their own.

Implied elements. The law routinely implies some elements in contracts if the element is not otherwise addressed. For example, the UCC specifies that certain sales contracts will be interpreted as having certain provisions unless the contract provides otherwise. One such provision specified by the UCC is an *implied warranty of merchantability*, which means that the goods are fit for the ordi-

---

[44] *E.g.,* Meadox Meds., Inc. v. Life Sys., Inc., 3 F. Supp. 2d 549 (D. N.J. 1998) [medical products manufacturer granted two-year exclusive distribution agreement that included a non-competition covenant for term plus one year, court refused to enforce one year non-competition after non-renewal, lack of proprietary relationship in information manufacturer sought to protect].

[45] *E.g.,* Coram Healthcare Corp. v. Aetna U.S. Healthcare Inc., 94 F. Supp. 2d 589 (E.D. Pa. 1999); International Business Mach. Corp. v. Medlantic Healthcare Group, 708 F. Supp. 417 (D. D.C. 1989).

nary purposes for which such goods are normally used. In addition, another provision is an *implied warranty of fitness for a particular use*, meaning that the goods are fit for the specific use the seller has reason to know the buyer intends for the goods. There are many exceptions to these warranties. One of the clearest is when the contract explicitly disclaims warranties.

Some states recognize an implied covenant of good faith and fair dealing in every contract.[46] However, some of these states restrict the scope of this covenant so that it cannot be used to override the express terms of the agreement and can only be used when an express term of the contract has been breached.[47] Where the covenant is restricted in this manner, it cannot be used to add a term that the parties did not address in the agreement.

Courts will sometimes imply additional elements — for example, that the person signing the contract has the authority to do so. Administrators should be cautious about making promises or concessions, especially in writing. Other employees should be instructed not to sign documents without proper authority and review.

BREACH OF CONTRACT. The purpose of the contract is to document plans for completing the agreement and for dealing with contingencies that preclude completion. As a last resort, litigation can be required to deal with breach of contract. The courts will compel performance of some contracts, such as contracts to transfer land or unique goods. Courts will also sometimes issue an injunction prohibiting another party from violating a restrictive covenant, such as an agreement not to compete or not to disclose a trade secret. However, in most situations the only remedy the court will award is money, called *damages*. When it is difficult to calculate the damages from breach of a contract, the parties sometimes agree in advance what the amount of damages will be. This agreed amount is called *liquidated damages*. Although courts usually do not enforce contract provisions that are considered penalties, courts frequently enforce liquidated damages provisions when the amounts are reasonable.

DISPUTE RESOLUTION. Contracts can address other issues concerning dispute resolution. They can specify which state's law

---

[46] *E.g.*, Maglione v. Aegis Family Health Ctrs., 607 S.E.2d 286 (N.C. App. 2005); County of Brevard v. Miorelli Eng'g, Inc., 703 So.2d 1049 (Fla. 1997).

[47] *E.g.*, Insurance Concepts & Design, Inc. v. HealthPlan Servs., Inc., 785 So.2d 1232 (Fla. 4th DCA 2001).

governs the contract and where litigation can be brought.[48] Some contracts specify that disputes will be resolved by arbitration, rather than by court litigation.

DEFENSES TO CONTRACT SUITS. There are several defenses to contract suits, including waiver and default. Sometimes courts interpret conduct of the parties, such as regular acceptance of late delivery without complaint, as implying a modification to the agreement, waiving rights under the agreement. The defense of default arises from the recognition that some promises are dependent on others and that some events must occur in a sequence. A party that fails to perform an earlier step in the sequence can be found to be in default, excusing the other parties from carrying out subsequent steps. Vendors sometimes claim that their delay is due to failure of the hospital to provide needed data or material. Sequences should be carefully structured so that this defense is available only when it is appropriate.

THIRD PARTY BENEFICIARIES. Sometimes courts will permit persons, called *third party beneficiaries*, who are not parties to contracts to enforce the part of the contract that affects them.[49] Sometimes this is intended. For example, where a contract between a hospital and health maintenance organization (HMO) states that the hospital will not bill the patient even if the HMO does not pay, the patient generally can use that contract to oppose billing efforts by the hospital. Generally, a third party beneficiary must take the limitations in the contract along with the benefits. In a Colorado case, a physician claimed to be a third party beneficiary to a hospital purchase contract. The court ruled that the claim had to be arbitrated under the arbitration clause in the contract because third party beneficiaries have to take the burdens with the benefits.[50]

CONTRACTS WITH GOVERNMENT AGENCIES. One ambiguous area of the law is the extent to which relationships with governmental agencies are governed by contract law principles. In some areas, contract law principles are applied. In other areas, the government retains the power to make unilateral changes which a

---

[48] *See* Hyland Lakes Spuds, Inc. v. Schmieding Produce Co., Inc., 25 F. Supp. 2d 941 (E.D. Wis. 1998) [contract construed to be consent to jurisdiction, not exclusive forum selection].

[49] Smith v. Chattanooga Med. Investors, Inc., 62 S.W.3d 178 (Tenn. App. 2001) [Medicaid-eligible person was third party beneficiary of Medicaid contract between nursing and state which was breached by refusal to readmit after hospitalization]; *but see* Kirkpatrick v. Merit Behavioral Care Corp., 99 F. Supp. 2d 458 (D. Vt. 2000) [beneficiaries of health plan not third party beneficiaries of plan contract with utilization review provider].

[50] Lee v. Gandcor Med. Sys., Inc., 702 F. Supp. 252 (D. Colo. 1988).

party to a private contract could not do. In some areas, the government claims that contract principles do not apply. For example, a federal appellate court ruled that the relationship between the federal government and a physician in the National Health Service Corps is a statutory relationship, not a contractual relationship; so no contractual defenses were available.[51]

MALPRACTICE SUITS BASED ON CONTRACT. Most malpractice suits against physicians, hospitals, and other health care providers are based on tort law, not on contract law. One type of malpractice case based on contract law is the claim that the physician promised a certain outcome that was not achieved. Absent a specific promise to cure, a physician is not an insurer of a particular outcome. However, if the physician is incautious enough to make a promise, the law will sometimes enforce it. One of the most publicized cases was *Guilmet v. Campbell*,[52] in which the Michigan Supreme Court upheld a jury finding that a physician had promised to cure a bleeding ulcer. On that basis, the court imposed liability for the unsuccessful outcome even though the physician was not negligent in providing the care. The Michigan legislature later passed a law[53] making promises to cure unenforceable unless they are in writing, in effect overruling *Guilmet*. In states that do not have these laws, a consent form that disavows any assurance of results can provide protection from these claims.[54]

A breach of contract suit can also arise from failure to use a promised procedure. In a Michigan case, the patient had been promised that her child would be delivered by a Cesarean operation.[55] The physician failed to arrange for the operation, and the baby was stillborn. The physician was found liable for breaking his promise to arrange for the operation. A New York appellate court ruled that when a physician orally agreed to deliver a baby for a Jehovah's Witness mother without using transfusions, obtaining a court order and giving a transfusion could constitute a breach of contract.[56]

---

51 United States v. Vanhorn, 20 F.3d 104 (4th Cir. 1994).
52 Guilmet v. Campbell, 385 Mich. 57, 188 N.W.2d 601 (1971); *see also* Bobrick v. Bravstein, 116 A.D.2d 682, 497 N.Y.S.2d 749 (2d Dept. 1986) [contract suit allowed against physician].
53 MICH. COMP. LAWS § 566.132. Some states have similar laws, *e.g.*, FLA. STAT. § 725.01; Flora v. Moses, 727 A.2d 596 (Pa. Super. 1999).
54 *E.g.*, Moore v. Averi, 534 So.2d 250 (Ala. 1988).
55 Stewart v. Rudner & Bunyan, 349 Mich. 459, 84 N.W.2d 816 (1957).
56 Nicoleau v. Brookhaven Mem. Hosp., 201 A.D.2d 544, 607 N.Y.S.2d 703 (2d Dept. 1994).

Cases based on oral promises are unusual, but they demonstrate that physicians and other health care providers should be careful in what they say to patients so that their efforts to reassure do not become promises they cannot fulfill.

With the summary of the legal system provided by this chapter as a framework, the remainder of this book will address a wide variety of the specific legal problems of health care law.

Discussion Points

1. What are some of the reasons that legal advisers cannot give precise answers?
2. What are the roles of the branches of government? How does the system of checks and balances function so that each limits the powers of the others?
3. What are the primary sources of law?
4. How do the Due Process Clause and Equal Protection Clause of the United States Constitution restrict the scope of permissible laws?
5. Which law should be followed when there are conflicts among laws?
6. On what grounds can the enforceability of laws be challenged? How does this differ when the law being challenged is a statute, regulation, or court decision?
7. How does the role of the courts as a source of law differ when it is interpreting statutes and regulations, determining the constitutionality of laws, or creating the common law?
8. What are the "facts" for the purpose of a trial?
9. Discuss the effect of the designation of the default outcome and the assignment of burden of proof in communicating priorities and determining the outcome of disputes.
10. What are some of the limits that are placed on who may take cases to court and the types of cases courts will consider? How does this differ between federal and state courts?
11. Discuss the extent to which precedent binds other courts.
12. When do private parties have a binding contract? What is necessary to create a contract? What types of contracts are unenforceable?
13. When will courts add terms to private contracts?
14. When does a contract create rights for persons who are not parties to the contract?

CHAPTER TWO

Organization of the Health Care Delivery System

Objectives

The objective of this chapter is to provide an overview of the organization of the health care delivery system. The reader should learn the importance of understanding the legal structure of any health care entity, some of the possible legal structures, and how that structure determines the organization and powers of the entities. The reader should understand the selection and role of the leadership of organization. Licensing and accreditation requirements for organizations are also covered. The reader should also learn some of the ways that organizations can be reorganized, changed, or closed.

Almost all health care is delivered within an organized system. Clinical and regulatory complexity requires an infrastructure that can be provided only by an well-ordered structure.

A hospital, practitioner office, or other health care organization is a legal entity that derives its powers and many limitations on its powers from its legal structure. Familiarity with the entity's legal structure is essential to understand its organization and powers. A hospital or other health care entity can be one of six types of organizations: governmental entity, nonprofit corporation, for-profit corporation, partnership (limited or general), limited liability company, or sole proprietorship. There are also special organizations that combine features of more than one of these types. In some cases, the hospital or health care organization is not a distinct entity but is an owned component or division of an entity that is one of these types.

The organization of most health care entities, regardless of their type, includes a governing body and a chief executive officer. The organization of most hospitals also includes an organized medical staff. The governing body has the ultimate responsibility and authority to establish goals and policies, select the chief executive officer, and appoint medical staff members. The governing body is usually called the "board," but it can have other names. The chief executive officer is delegated responsibility and authority to manage day-to-day business within policies established by the board. The organized medical staff is delegated responsibility and authority to maintain the quality of medical services, subject to ultimate board responsibility. The duties, authority, liability, selection, and rights of the board, chief executive officer, and medical staff are discussed in more detail in this chapter and in Chapter 5.

The hospital is a unique organization because many decisions concerning use of its staff, equipment, and supplies are made by physicians who are not employees or agents of the hospital. Physicians are often legally independent of the hospital and accountable primarily through the organized medical staff. Some physicians are employees of hospitals, medical groups, or other entities. Changes in the relationship between physicians and hospitals are occurring.

Changing utilization, payment, and other market conditions and changing government requirements and programs have lead health care organizations voluntarily or involuntarily to change their legal basis through conversions, mergers, consolidations, sales, and other restructuring or to go through other changes such as dissolution, closure, relocation, and bankruptcy.

This chapter focuses predominantly on hospitals, but the same principles generally apply to other health care entities.

The questions addressed in this chapter are:

2-1. What are the key characteristics of the six types of organizations?
2-2. How are governing bodies selected, and what is their role and responsibility?
2-3. How are CEOs selected, and what is their role and responsibility?
2-4. What are the licensing and accreditation requirements for health care organizations?

2-5. What are the issues when an organization is converted from one type into another?

2-6. What are the issues when an organization is merged, consolidated, sold, or dissolved?

2-7. What are the issues when an organization closes or relocates a hospital or other delivery location?

2-8. What is the impact of bankruptcy law?

2-1 What Are the Key Characteristics of the Six Types of Organizations?

The powers and governance structure of a health care organization are derived from its legal basis, which also imposes limitations on those powers. Some states do not permit certain forms of ownership. The Rhode Island Supreme Court ruled that the state could ban ownership of health care facilities by corporations with publicly traded stock.[1] The Arkansas Supreme Court ruled that ownership of retail pharmacies by nonprofit hospitals could be banned.[2]

While a health care organization's powers usually cannot be expanded without changing the underlying legal basis, many additional limitations are imposed by government regulations or by private actions, such as restrictions in accepted gifts and bequests, or in contracts entered by the organization.

The six basic types of organizations are governmental entity (2-1.1), nonprofit corporation (2-1.2), for-profit corporation (2-1.2), partnership (2-1.3), limited liability company (2-1.4), or sole proprietorship (2-1.5).

2-1.1 Governmental Entity

The legal basis of governmental hospitals is found in state and federal statutes and in local ordinances. Many governmental hospitals are not corporations. They are created by a special statute for the specific hospital or by a governmental unit, pursuant to a statute authorizing such units to create hospitals. For example, some counties and cities created hospitals under laws authorizing counties to

---

[1] *In re* Advisory Opinion to House of Representatives, 519 A.2d 578 (R.I. 1987).
[2] Arkansas Hosp. Ass'n v. Arkansas State Bd. of Pharmacy, 297 Ark. 454, 763 S.W.2d 73 (1989).

establish hospitals. Some governmental hospitals, such as some public hospital authorities, are also corporations, especially when they are not also governmental agencies.

These statutes often include specific duties or limitations. In some states, county hospitals are required to care for indigent residents. In 1997, a Colorado court ruled that hospital service districts in Colorado can only provide care directly; they cannot contract with other facilities to provide the services.[3] Some county hospital statutes prohibit purchases from board members and restrict how and to whom hospital property can be sold or leased. Illinois law gives county commissioners the power to establish a limit on expenditures by county hospitals regardless of the source of funds.[4] Asset transfers, facility leases, and joint ventures of public hospitals with private corporations have been challenged. In 2000, the Tennessee Supreme Court ruled that a county hospital was a quasi-governmental entity and the state constitutional restrictions on lending credit were not applicable to quasi-governmental facilities; so the hospital could enter a joint venture and guaranty financing for a building project without voter approval.[5]

When a governmental entity acts outside its authority, its actions are usually void. For example, a Missouri court ruled that a hospital district created for certain counties could not operate a home health agency outside those counties.[6] The North Carolina Supreme Court ruled that a three-year contract with a public hospital administrator was unenforceable. The board's authority to enter long-term contracts had been revoked by implication when it adopted a resolution of intent to transfer control to a nonprofit corporation.[7] The Missouri Supreme Court ruled that a bank could not collect on certain debts that a public hospital had endorsed because the hospital did not have authority to endorse them.[8]

In some states, governmental hospitals are subject to open meetings and open records laws. For example, a Minnesota appel-

---

[3] Haggerty v. Pudre Health Servs. Dist., 940 P.2d 1105 (Colo. Ct. App. 1997).
[4] County of Cook v. Ayala, 76 Ill. 2d 219, 390 N.E.2d 877 (1979).
[5] Cleveland Surgery Ctr. v. Bradley County Mem. Hosp., 30 S.W.3d 278 (Tenn. 2000).
[6] Professional Home Health & Hospice, Inc. v. Jackson-Madison County Gen. Hosp. Dist., 759 S.W.2d 416 (Tenn. Ct. App. 1988).
[7] Rowe v. Franklin County, 318 N.C. 344, 349 S.E.2d 65 (1986).
[8] Fulton Nat'l Bank v. Callaway Mem. Hosp., 465 S.W.2d 549 (Mo. 1971); *accord* Board of Trustees v. Peoples Bank, 538 So.2d 361 (Miss. 1989) [copier lease void because not approved by purchasing department].

late court ruled that a county hospital board could not give the chief executive officer a private performance evaluation because of the state open meetings law.[9] States vary as to whether open meetings and records laws apply to governmental hospitals that are leased to or operated by private entities.[10]

2-1.2 Corporations

A corporation is a separate legal entity distinct from the individuals who own and control it. In the past, each corporation was created by an individual act of the state legislature, granting articles of incorporation. In some states, nonprofit corporations were created under judicial petitions filed by citizens. Today states have general corporation laws that authorize a state official to create a corporation by issuing articles of incorporation. Legislatures in most states can still create some corporations, especially public corporations. So some corporations do not have articles of incorporation; their legal authority is the statute creating them.

One legal benefit of incorporation is that each owner's liability is generally limited to that owner's investment in the corporation. Usually, an owner is not individually liable beyond this investment except when the owner causes the injury by personal acts or omissions; fails to observe the corporate formalities; guarantees personally the corporation's debts; or is involved in situations where special statutory liabilities apply, such as environmental and pension laws. The corporation itself is liable to the extent of its resources, which include the owners' investments in that corporation.

To maintain corporate status and the attendant immunity from personal liability, there must be compliance with corporate formalities, such as filing required reports with the state, holding required meetings, and maintaining required records.

Another benefit is corporate perpetual life. Death of an owner does not terminate the corporation; only the ownership is changed.

---

[9] Itasca County Bd. of Comm'rs v. Olson, 372 N.W.2d 804 (Minn. Ct. App. 1985).
[10] *E.g.*, Memorial Hosp. Ass'n, Inc. v. Knutson, 239 Kan. 663, 722 P.2d 1093 (1986) [private lessee not subject to Kansas open meetings law]; State *ex rel.* Fostoria Daily Review Co. v. Fostoria Hosp. Ass'n, 40 Ohio St. 3d 10, 531 N.E.2d 313 (1988) [private lessee subject to Ohio open records law]; Memorial Hosp. - West Volusia Inc. v. News-Journal Corp., 729 So.2d 373 (Fla. 1999) [operator of public hospital subject to open meeting requirements].

Unless the corporation is tax exempt or elects another special tax status, the corporation must pay taxes on its earnings, but in most situations, the owners do not have to pay personal income tax on corporate earnings until the earnings are distributed to them.

Corporations can be nonprofit or for-profit.

NONPROFIT CORPORATIONS. The earnings of a *nonprofit corporation* cannot be distributed for the benefit of individuals.

Many nonprofit health care institutions are also a *charity,* and many have exemption from some taxes. However, these characteristics are not always linked. The corporation must engage in charitable activities as defined by state law in order to be considered a charity. Some tax exemption usually results from charitable status, but the two are not always linked. In some states, charities are subject to an implied charitable trust to carry out their purposes. This *charitable trust doctrine* has been the basis for state challenges to actions by the charity.

Nonprofit corporations are held to various standards of public accountability. In most states, the state attorney general or other officials can take steps to compel nonprofit corporations to meet these standards.[11] This issue arises most frequently when a nonprofit corporation seeks to sell or otherwise convert some or all its assets to a for-profit organization. Examples of challenges to these transactions are discussed later in this chapter. Some states require state approval before nonprofit corporations engage in some transactions.[12] In other cases, nonprofit corporations voluntarily seek prior approval to avoid the risk and delay involved in challenges. For example, in 2002, under state charity laws, the Massachusetts Attorney General approved a complex deal that was designed to continue the operation of a hospital through a transfer and lease arrangement.[13]

There are limits to a state's control over entities incorporated in other states. For example, in 2003, a Kansas judge ruled that the

---

[11] *E.g.*, Tauber v. Commonwealth, 255 Va. 445, 499 S.E.2d 839 (Va. 1998) ["This Court long ago recognized the common law authority of the Attorney General to act on behalf of the public in matters involving charitable assets."]; Hatch v. Allina Health Sys., No. MC 01-004160 (Minn. Dist. Ct. Aug. 14, 2004), *as discussed in* H.L.R., Aug. 21, 2004, 1303 [confirming authority of attorney general to oversee "corporate rehabilitation" of health plan].

[12] *E.g.*, Wis. Stat. § 165.40 [certain hospital acquisitions].

[13] J. Chesto, *AG approves Waltham Hospital deal*, Boston Herald, May 25, 2002, 20. Unfortunately, the plan did not succeed, and the hospital was closed about a year later. E. Sweeney, *Hospital draws last breath: The sad end of an era for patients and employees*, Boston Globe, July 27, 2003, 1.

Kansas Attorney General could not challenge how a Missouri non-profit corporation compensated its CEO in the sale of the corporation to a for-profit hospital.[14] However, when an out-of-state nonprofit corporation plans to sell assets located in a state, some states where the assets are located will exercise oversight of whether such sales can occur and how the proceeds are used. In 2003, the South Dakota Supreme Court ruled under the implied charitable trust doctrine that the state could restrict the transfer out of state of the proceeds from the sale of a hospital in South Dakota.[15] In 2004, a settlement was reached in which a $1.8 million payment was divided among five communities.[16]

FOR-PROFIT CORPORATIONS. A *for-profit corporation* is operated with the intention of earning a profit that can be distributed to its owners. A for-profit hospital is sometimes called an *investor-owned* or a *proprietary* hospital.

For-profit hospitals can be owned in various ways. Some are closely held by a small number of investors. Some are wholly owned by a multihospital system or other parent corporation. The parent can then have publicly traded stock that can be purchased through the stock market. The stock of some hospitals has been owned by their employee's pension plans through an Employee Stock Ownership Plan (ESOP). In some cases, the parent owns only part of the stock in the hospital, and other local investors, sometimes physicians, own the rest. Sometimes the ownership of a hospital is structured as a partnership, which is discussed later in this chapter.

Securities laws and shareholder rights. There is extensive federal and state regulation of the offering and sale of stock and partnership interests. The details of securities laws, shareholders rights, and other restrictions on for-profit corporate behavior are beyond the scope of this book. Shareholders have various rights, including access to corporate books and records[17] and the right to challenge the failure of a corporation to disclose important information that could affect the value of the shares.[18] Corporate officers and other insiders can be personally liable when they purchase or

---

[14] *Judge rules Kansas can't sue over Health Midwest CEO pay*, AP, Jan. 17, 2003.

[15] Banner Health System v. Long, 2003 SD 60, 2003 S.D. LEXIS 86.

[16] *State settles lawsuit with Banner Health*, AP, Mar. 18, 2004.

[17] *E.g.*, Estate of Purnell v. LH Radiologists, 90 N.Y.2d 524, 664 N.Y.S.2d 238, 686 N.E.2d 1332 (1997).

[18] *E.g.*, J. Jacob, *Shareholders file class-action lawsuit against United*, AM. MED. NEWS, Sept. 7, 1998, 18 [alleged withholding of information about Medicare HMO losses].

sell shares based on important information that they know but have not disclosed to other shareholders and the public.[19] Securities laws require that formal filing be made before certain transactions.[20]

Sarbanes-Oxley Act. The degree of public scrutiny and regulation of corporations increased substantially in 2002. After a series of corporate scandals, Congress enacted the Sarbanes-Oxley Act (SOA).[21] This law directly applies only to companies with publicly traded stock. Full compliance is very costly; so some smaller publicly traded companies elected to become private.[22] However, some companies — both nonprofit and private for-profit — who are not subject to the law have elected voluntarily to comply with some of the Act's provisions to achieve confidence of the public, lenders, bond holders, donors, and others who rely on the integrity of the governance and financial status of the institution.[23] A few states have passed laws extending to nonprofit corporations requirements similar to some of the Sarbanes-Oxley requirements.[24]

Section 101[25] of SOA establishes a Public Company Accounting Oversight Board to register, regulate, and inspect accounting firms. Section 107[26] provides that the Board functions under the oversight and authority of the Securities Exchange Commission (SEC). Section 103[27] establishes auditing, quality control, and independence standards for auditing firms. Section 104[28] requires inspections of auditing firms. Section 105[29] provides investigation and disciplinary procedures for auditing firms. Section 108[30] specifies when the SEC is authorized to recognize accounting standards.

---

[19] *E.g.*, *Oxford Health faces NY AG probe on top of shareholder class actions*, 6 HEALTH L. RPTR. [BNA] 1758 (1997) [alleged insider trading; alleged officers sold stock before announcing loss] [hereinafter HEALTH L. RPTR. [BNA] cited as H.L.R.].

[20] *E.g.*, *Columbia/HCA plan to spin off hospitals is outlined in filing*, WALL ST. J., Dec. 15, 1998, B8 [filing with Securities Exchange Commission discussed].

[21] Pub. L. No. 107-204, 116 Stat. 745 [codified at 15 U.S.C. §§ 7201 et seq. & scattered sections of the U.S.C.]

[22] A.R. Sorkin, *Kissing the public goodbye*, N.Y. TIMES, Aug. 8, 2004, 4BU [first year of Sarbanes-Oxley - 99 public companies became private; second year - 59].

[23] *See* A. Field, *Some private companies embrace tougher rules*, N.Y. TIMES, July 15, 2004, C6; *Nonprofits pressured to stay 'ahead of the curve' in governance*, H.L.R., Aug. 5, 2004, 1149; M.W. Peregrine, J.R. Schwartz & W.W. Horton, *Advising the nonprofit audit committee*, H.L.R., May 26, 2005, 726.

[24] *E.g.*, Uniform Supervision of Trustees for Charitable Purposes Act, CAL. GOV. CODE § 12581 et. seq.

[25] 15 U.S.C. § 7202.

[26] 15 U.S.C. § 7217.

[27] 15 U.S.C. § 7213.

[28] 15 U.S.C. § 7214.

[29] 15 U.S.C. § 7215.

[30] 15 U.S.C. § 7218.

Section 201[31] prohibits auditing firms from providing many nonauditing services contemporaneously with an audit, unless they are preapproved by the company's audit committee. Section 203[32] requires that the lead auditor must change at least every five years. Section 204[33] specifies certain items that auditors must report to the audit committee. Section 206[34] precludes the use of any auditing firm that key officers of the audited company were employed by in the past year.

Section 301[35] specifies the composition of the company's audit committee and requires that the committee members be independent, which means that they cannot be paid fees by the company other than a fee for being on the board and they cannot be an affiliated person of the company or any subsidiary. The audit committee must be responsible for the appointment, compensation, and oversight of the auditing firm. The audit committee must have authority to engage independent advisers. Section 906[36] requires the CEO and the CFO of the company to certify that financial statements comply with requirements and that each periodic report "fairly presents, in all material aspects, the financial condition and results of operations" of the company. A knowing and intentional violation gives rise to liability. Section 303[37] makes it a crime to fraudulently influence, coerce, manipulate, or mislead an auditor in an effort to make the financial statements materially misleading. Sections 304 and 305[38] impose various penalties for violations, including barring a violator from serving as an officer or director of any publicly traded company.

Section 401[39] specifies additional disclosures that must be made in financial reports, including off-balance sheet transactions and other relationships with consolidated entities that might have a material effect on the financial condition of the company. Section 402[40] prohibits nearly all personal loans to executives and directors.

---

[31] 15 U.S.C. § 78j-1(g)-(i).
[32] 15 U.S.C. § 78j-1(j).
[33] 15 U.S.C. § 78j-1(k).
[34] 15 U.S.C. § 78j-1(l).
[35] 15 U.S.C. § 78j-1(m).
[36] 18 U.S.C. § 1350.
[37] 15 U.S.C. § 7242.
[38] 15 U.S.C. §§ 77t, 78u, & 7243.
[39] 15 U.S.C. § 78m(j).
[40] 15 U.S.C. § 78m(k).

Section 403[41] requires reporting of certain transactions with officers, directors, or 10 percent owners. Section 404[42] requires each annual report to include an internal control report by the management and an attestation by the auditing firm. Companies are required to disclose their codes of ethics and any change or waiver of that code. Section 409[43] requires prompt public disclosure of information on material changes in the financial condition or operations of the company.

Title VIII extends whistle-blower protections to employees who lawfully disclose information.[44]

The details of the Sarbanes-Oxley Act and its implementing regulations are beyond the scope of this book.

Taxation. In standard for-profit corporations, there is so-called double taxation of income through the tax on the corporation and the tax on the individual shareholder when dividends are distributed to the shareholders. This double taxation does not apply to corporations that qualify as Subchapter S corporations; they are taxed similar to partnerships with their income being taxed to the individual owners.

MULTIHOSPITAL SYSTEMS. Many hospitals, both for-profit and nonprofit, are part of multihospital systems. For financial and liability reasons, each hospital is usually owned by a distinct entity, and those entities are owned or controlled by a parent corporation. The parent corporation generally retains control over many aspects of the hospital to take advantage of size efficiencies and to achieve other parental goals but usually leaves some aspects to local control by the individual hospital. Various structures are used to achieve the parental control. They limit the latitude of the local corporation in varying degrees.

The ultimate control of the parent is illustrated by when a parent company's board of directors ousted the board at one of its hospitals and substituted itself as the board for the local hospital. The local board had been opposing a merger that the parent favored.[45]

ARTICLES OF INCORPORATION. The powers of a corporation include only those powers expressed or implied in the articles of

---

[41] 15 U.S.C. § 78p.
[42] 15 U.S.C. § 7262.
[43] 15 U.S.C. § 78m(1).
[44] 18 U.S.C. § 1514A.
[45] P.A. McKay, *Health system trustees oust hospital's board*, WASHINGTON POST, Apr. 10, 1999, V3.

incorporation. Some corporations have articles that limit the type of business the corporation can conduct. When a hospital corporation plans to start a new line of business or abandon a present activity, the articles must be examined. Many modern corporations have articles that do not limit the scope of their activities; the articles authorize any business that a corporation can lawfully conduct. Other corporations might find it necessary to amend their articles before substantially changing their scope of business.

Some hospital corporations have articles of incorporation that limit them to hospital-related activities. Activities that provide services for patients, their families, and other visitors — such as gift shops and parking lots — are usually considered hospital-related. The scope of hospital-related activities has tended to expand.

EXPRESS CORPORATE AUTHORITY. Any corporation derives authority to act from the state that creates it. The articles of incorporation assert the corporation's purposes and create its express powers to carry out those purposes. State corporation laws also grant some express authority. Acts performed within the scope of this express authority are proper, while expressly prohibited acts are improper.

IMPLIED CORPORATE AUTHORITY. In addition to express authority, implied powers are inferred from corporate existence. Examples of implied authority include the power to have a corporate seal and perpetual existence; to enact corporate bylaws; and to purchase and hold property. For some corporations, these powers can be enumerated as express authority.

Corporations have implied authority to do any acts necessary to exercise their express authority and to accomplish corporate purposes. While the act need not be indispensably necessary, the act must tend to accomplish the corporate purpose in a manner not otherwise prohibited by law. Benefit or profit to the corporation alone is usually not sufficient.

CONSEQUENCES OF *ULTRA VIRES* ACTS. When a corporation acts outside its authority, the act is said to be *ultra vires*. In some states, an *ultra vires* contract cannot be enforced; so courts will not require the parties to do acts specified in the contract and will not order payments for injuries that result from noncompletion. In other states, the defense that an action was *ultra vires* has been abolished; so these contracts can be enforced, unless a corporate member or the state obtains an injunction to prevent performance of *ultra vires* acts. For example, a California appellate court ruled that the articles of incorporation required a nonprofit corporation to continue operating a hospital; so the board was barred from leasing the hospital and using the rent to operate clinics.[46] *Ultra vires* acts can also justify revocation of the articles of incorporation by the state, thus dissolving the corporation.

If an *ultra vires* act is already completed, courts will normally permit it to stand unless the state intervenes. The state may obtain an order for the corporation to erase the *ultra vires* act by disposing of property, discontinuing services, or taking other steps.

Some courts have imposed a stricter standard on nonprofit corporations because of the public interest in their charitable activities. For example, in New York, a nonprofit hospital is required to obtain judicial approval before selling the bulk of its assets. A New York City hospital entered a contract to sell its assets and agreed to pay the purchaser its out-of-pocket expenses of $800,000 if the court did not approve the sale. In 1999, the court found that the sale did not meet the statutory tests and denied approval.[47] When the purchaser sought to collect its out-of-pocket expenses, the hospital refused to pay, and the purchaser sued. The lower courts ruled that the court's disapproval of the transaction had rendered the entire agreement void; so no money was owed. The highest court reversed this decision and returned the case to the lower court to determine whether the agreement to pay the purchaser was fair, reasonable, and in furtherance of the not-for-profit's purpose.[48] If the lower court found this to be the case, then that provision of the agreement would be valid and the money would be owed. If the court found otherwise, the provision to pay the out-of-pocket expenses would be beyond the hospital's authority and invalid.

BYLAWS. Corporations adopt bylaws to define some key elements of their internal operations. Bylaws cannot expand the authority of the corporation. Bylaws can allocate how the authority will be exercised.

CHANGING CORPORATE DOCUMENTS. Articles of incorporation and bylaws are changed for many reasons, including (1) to authorize expansion into new activities, (2) to reorganize the cor-

---

[46] Queen of Angels Hosp. v. Younger, 66 Cal. App. 3d 359, 136 Cal. Rptr. 36 (2d Dist. 1977).
[47] *In re* Manhattan Eye, Ear & Throat Hosp., 186 Misc. 2d 126, 715 N.Y.S.2d 575 (Sup Ct. 1999).
[48] 64th Assocs., L.L.C. v. Manhattan Eye, Ear & Throat Hosp., 2 N.Y.3d 585, 813 N.E.2d 887, 780 N.Y.S.2d 746 (2004).

poration, and (3) to adapt to other environmental changes.[49] Corporate document changes can be made if proper legal procedures are followed and if other corporate members are treated fairly.

Articles of incorporation. When changing basic corporate documents, there is a duty to deal fairly with other members of the corporation. If this duty is violated, changes can be declared void. An Arizona court ruled that an amendment to the articles of incorporation was void because of the unfair way it was adopted.[50] A few hours before the vote on the amendment, the board designated 159 new corporate members from among their associates so that, together, they would have more votes than the sixty physicians who were the other corporate members. Though the board had authority to appoint new members, the court found the appointment of the new members, plus the way their proxy votes were used, to be unfair.

The legislature that creates the corporation reserves the power to amend corporation laws and the articles. The highest court of New York upheld a legislative amendment to the articles of a hospital requiring outgoing board members to be replaced by persons selected by the remaining board members, rather than by a vote of the corporation's membership.[51]

Bylaws. Corporations have broad powers to change their bylaws if they comply with the procedures and restrictions in their articles and in state corporation law. The Illinois Supreme Court ruled that, because the corporate articles did not forbid the change, a board could amend the bylaws to end elections of board members and to provide for the selection of replacement board members by present board members.[52]

Agreements not to change corporate documents. In some circumstances, hospitals can enter enforceable agreements not to change their corporate documents. In 1998, at the request of the state attorney general, a Rhode Island court issued a temporary

---

[49] *E.g.*, *Queen of Angels board amends bylaws to eliminate need for bishop's approval*, 7 H.L.R. 493 (1998); B. Japsen, *Baylor system blocked sale by bylaw change*, 27 MOD. HEALTHCARE, June 23, 1997, 3 [5 of 13 hospitals changed articles, barring university from appointing their boards].

[50] Hatch v. Emery, 1 Ariz. App. 142, 400 P.2d 349 (1965); *contra* Harris v. Board of Directors, 55 Ill. App. 3d 392, 370 N.E.2d 1121 (1st Dist. 1977) [board could unilaterally amend bylaws to become self-perpetuating despite desire of members to remove board].

[51] *In re* Mt. Sinai Hosp., 250 N.Y. 103, 164 N.E. 871 (1928).

[52] Westlake Hosp. Ass'n v. Blix, 13 Ill. 2d 183, 148 N.E.2d 471, *appeal dismissed*, 358 U.S. 43 (1958).

restraining order prohibiting a hospital from changing its corporate bylaws, allegedly contrary to promises made when the attorney general approved a prior hospital merger.[53]

2-1.3 Partnership

A business can be organized as a partnership of several individuals or organizations.

One benefit of a partnership is that income tax is paid only by the partners; no separate income tax is paid by the partnership, avoiding the double taxation that is applied to the income of most for-profit corporations. The limited liability company also addresses these tax issues (see 2-1.4).

It is sometimes more difficult to arrange partnership affairs to survive the death or withdrawal of a partner. Often partnerships are structured so that one or more partners have an option to buy out others or to require others to buy them out.[54]

One disadvantage of the partnership is that there is no limit on the potential liability of general partners.[55] The potential liability of some partners can be limited through a limited partnership. Limited partners are only liable to the extent of their investment, provided they do not participate in the management or operation of the business or interfere with control of the business.[56] Physicians and others who invest as limited partners in hospitals need to limit their involvement in control of the business, unless they are willing to accept the risk of unlimited liability beyond any insurance coverage that is provided. There must be at least one general partner whose liability is not limited. Usually, the general partner will be a corporation. In multihospital systems, the general partner is usually controlled by the parent corporation.

Liability of general partners can include criminal liability. A New York court ruled that, without any showing of individual culpability,

---

[53] Rhode Island v. Lifespan, No. 98-2801 (R.I. Super. Ct. June 16, 1998), *as discussed in* 7 H.L.R. 1103 (1998).

[54] *E.g.*, P. Limbacher, *Optioned in Fargo*, 27 MOD. HEALTHCARE, Sept. 1, 1997, 12 [one partner required to buy out another pursuant to option].

[55] *See, e.g.*, S. Harris, *Don't get stuck picking up your business partner's tab*, AM. MED. NEWS, Feb. 23, 1998, 16.

[56] *See* Annotation, *Liability of limited partner arising from taking part in control of business under Uniform Limited Partnership Act*, 79 A.L.R. 4TH 427.

the forty-two partners in a hospital could be charged in an indictment that alleged the hospital permitted an unauthorized person to participate in a surgical procedure and falsified records to conceal the crime.[57]

Partners owe duties to each other. For example, a Texas court ruled that a general partner had a fiduciary duty to notify a limited partner before selling partnership assets.[58]

Some states permit limited liability partnerships (LLPs) that permit partners to fully participate in management and operations, while limiting their individual liability for their partners' acts to their investment in the partnership.

2-1.4 Limited Liability Company

Some states have authorized the formation of limited liability companies (LLC) that function like partnerships, without personal liability of the participants for the acts of the company.[59] Some courts will intervene to require fair dealing among the participants. For example, in 2005, at the request of a participant, a Delaware court ordered the dissolution of a LLC when the corporate documents did not provide a fair exit mechanism.[60]

2-1.5 Sole Proprietorship

A business can also be organized as a sole proprietorship, which means it is owned by one individual who has not incorporated the business. All income of the business is taxed as personal income of the owner, and there is no limitation on the owner's potential liability. Hospitals are seldom operated as sole proprietorships. It is not unusual for small professional practices or consulting businesses to be sole proprietorships.

---

[57] People v. Smithtown Gen. Hosp., 92 Misc. 2d 144, 399 N.Y.S.2d 993 (Sup. Ct. 1977).

[58] Hughes v. St. David's Support Corp., No. 03-00197-CV (Tex. Ct. App. Mar. 6, 1997), *as discussed in* 6 H.L.R. 549 (1997).

[59] *E.g.,* WIS. STAT. ch. 183; IOWA CODE ch. 490A; *e.g.,* Jana L. v. West 129th Street Realty Co., LLC, 2005 NY Slip Op.50199U, 6 Misc. 3d 1026A (Sup. Ct. Feb. 22, 2005) (unpub.).

[60] Haley v. Talcott (Del. Ch. Dec. 16, 2004), 8 DEL. L. WEEKLY 4 (Jan. 26, 2005).

2-2 How Are Governing Bodies Selected and What Is Their Role and Responsibility?

Most health care entities have a governing board, which has the ultimate governance responsibility. The chief executive officer and the organized medical staff also have roles in governance.

The governing board has ultimate legal responsibility for operations. Active involvement of members is essential as communities, governmental agencies, and courts hold the board accountable for the organization's activities.

The same general duties of supervision and management are applicable to the boards of for-profit and nonprofit entities. Most governmental boards have similar duties. Each member has a duty to act as a reasonably prudent person would act under similar circumstances when faced with a similar problem.

In some multihospital systems, the local board might have only some of the powers and duties of the board of an independent hospital. Some powers and duties can be centralized in the board of the parent.

This section addresses the following questions:

2-2.1. What are the duties of board members?
2-2.2. When can board members be personally liable for their actions related to the health care organization?
2-2.3. How are board members selected and removed?

2-2.1 What Are the Duties of Board Members?

The duties of board members generally include the duty of care and the duty of loyalty. Board members have a duty to exercise reasonable care and skill in the management of the entity's affairs and to act at all times in good faith and with complete loyalty to the entity.

DUTY OF CARE. The duty of care generally requires that board members be informed and make good faith decisions intended to further the organization's purposes. Board members must exercise the degree of diligence, care, and skill that an ordinarily prudent person would in similar circumstances. The details of the standard vary among the states and can also differ somewhat between governmental, nonprofit, and for-profit boards.

Although board members are sometimes called trustees, they are usually not held to the strict standard of a trustee of a trust but instead are judged by the standard applicable to directors of other business corporations.[61] Trustees of trusts are generally liable for simple negligence. Directors of business corporations are generally not liable for mere negligence in exercising their judgment concerning corporate business; they are liable only for gross or willful negligence. This "business judgment" rule offers board members wide latitude for actions taken in good faith.[62] In 1985, the Delaware Supreme Court ruled that there was a presumption that directors acted with due care.[63]

In some settings, the business judgment rule might not apply. For example, in 2003, when the Maryland Insurance Administration Commissioner reviewed the proposed conversion of the nonprofit CareFirst health plan to a for-profit entity, followed by acquisition by another for-profit network, the Commissioner ruled that the business judgment did not apply in the regulatory review; so he did not have to show any deference to the board's judgment concerning the public interest. The board was vested with a public trust to address the economic value of the enterprise as a public asset. The Commissioner found that the process used by the board was deficient so that it had not used due diligence.[64] The reorganization was not approved. The state adopted legislation exerting more control over CareFirst. When the national Blue Cross organization sought to withdraw use of the Blue Cross trademark, the state reached a settlement modifying some of the state control.[65]

The duty of due care requires each board member to fulfill membership functions personally. The board member must attend meetings and participate in the consideration of matters before the

---

[61] *E.g.*, Stern v. Lucy Webb Hayes Nat'l Training School, 381 F. Supp. 10003 (D. D.C. 1974); *but see* People v. Larkin, 413 F. Supp. 978 (N.D. Cal. 1976) [trust principles applied].

[62] For discussion of cases concerning business judgment rule, *see* K. Christophe, *Recent developments in the law affecting professionals, officers, and directors*, 33 TORT & INS. L. J. 629, 644-47 (Wint. 1998).

[63] Aronson v. Lewis, 473 A.2d 805 (Del. 1985).

[64] T.K. Hyatt & E.S. Kornreich, *Legal ethics: Governance reforms for nonprofit organizations: Sarbanes-Oxley and beyond*, presented at Am. Health Lawyers Ass'n 2004 Annual Meeting; the text of the Commissioner's report is posted at http://www.mdinsurance.state.md.us/jsp/availPubInfo/Reports.jsp10?divisionName=Reports&pageName=/jsp/availPubInfo/Reports.jsp10 [accessed Sept. 11, 2004].

[65] P. Dickens, *Gov. Ehrlich signs CareFirst reform legislation, triggers lawsuit*, DAILY RECORD (Baltimore, Md.), May 23, 2003; MD. INS. CODE §§ 14-102 et seq.; T. Stuckey, *Settlement reached in state dispute with Blue Cross*, AP, June 6, 2003.

board. All board members assume responsibility for board decisions that they do not oppose.

Board members cannot bargain away their duties. A Minnesota case declared void an agreement by two individuals not to take part in hospital management if elected to the board.[66] A District of Columbia court found that delegation of investment decisions to a committee of board members without any supervision by the board was a failure to use due diligence.[67]

Board members can rely on information and data provided by others as long as it is reasonable under the circumstances.[68] When directors know that those presenting the information are not disclosing all relevant information or know that they have a conflict of interest, they have a duty to challenge the information.

The Sarbanes-Oxley Act discussed earlier in this chapter is placing more focus on board responsibility for assuring appropriate financial controls. The law directly places this responsibility on directors of publicly traded companies. The resulting focus on this issue is raising the level of expectation of directors of all corporations.

Preservation of assets. The general duty to act with due care requires reasonable steps to preserve assets from injury, destruction, and loss. Prudent judgment must be exercised to decide which property should be protected and how, which can include maintenance, adequate insurance, and other protections. The duty applies beyond land, buildings, equipment, and investments to include rights under contracts, wills, and other legal claims and protection against liability losses. In some circumstances, it becomes prudent to sell the organization's assets. Such sales are discussed later in this chapter.

Some health care organizations have complete or partial immunity from liability based on their governmental or charitable nature. In some states, liability insurance might not be necessary, but purchasing liability insurance is seldom considered beyond the board's authority. Sometimes purchasing insurance waives immunity to the extent of the insurance.

The board has a duty to pay taxes that are owed. The board should treat tax exemptions as corporate assets to be preserved

---

[66] Ray v. Homewood Hosp., 223 Minn. 440, 27 N.W.2d 409 (1947).
[67] Stern v. Lucy Webb Hayes Nat'l Training School, 381 F. Supp. 1003 (D. D.C. 1974).
[68] *E.g.,* N.Y. NOT-FOR-PROFIT CORP. LAW § 717(b).

and protected like other assets. There are circumstances where it can be prudent to relinquish deliberately this asset, like others.

The board should assure that the organization's rights are being enforced. This includes collection of bills for services and authorizing appropriate legal suits when justified. The board has a corollary duty to defend the organization from claims. The board must act reasonably under the circumstances. Some claims are not worth pursuing or should be settled out of court. The board's duty will generally be satisfied if the board conforms to sound business practices.

Basic management duties. The board has general authority to manage the organization's business. This authority is absolute when the board acts within the law. Questions of policy and internal management are usually left by courts wholly to board discretion. When departure from board duties is clear, courts will intervene.

Some of the basic management functions of the board include:

1. selection of corporate officers and other agents,
2. general control of compensation of such agents,
3. delegation of authority to the chief executive officer and subordinates,
4. establishment of policies,
5. exercise of businesslike control of expenditures,
6. providing for planning, and
7. supervision of and vigilance over the welfare of the whole corporation.

Authority to manage business can be delegated to the chief executive officer or to committees. In practice, much authority is expressly or implicitly delegated. If authority is not delegated or is not conferred on officers by statute or by the articles or bylaws, the board is generally the only body authorized to exercise that authority and to represent the organization. The board has no obligation to delegate any management functions. Any delegation of policy-making functions is subject to revocation by the board at any time. If revocation breaches a contract, the organization might have to pay for injuries the revocation causes.

The board cannot delegate its responsibility. The power to delegate authority is implied from the business necessities of managing corporations. To avoid abdicating its responsibility, the board should have some procedure to oversee the use of delegated authority.

The board has inherent authority to establish organizational policies. The board can directly exercise this authority by adopting rules, or it can delegate the authority. An example of this policy-making power is a Georgia Supreme Court decision upholding a hospital rule requiring all computerized tomography (CT) scans of hospital patients to be performed with the hospital machine, not with an external machine.[69] Similarly, the Arkansas Supreme Court upheld a hospital rule prohibiting megadose vitamin therapy for allergies.[70] A Florida appellate court upheld a board rule that the surgeon, not the anesthesiologist, makes the final decision on whether to attempt emergency surgery.[71] Hospital chief executive officers, their subordinates, or hospital committees are often permitted to make policies or formulate rules and regulations.

Duty to provide satisfactory patient care. The duty to provide satisfactory patient care is an essential element of the board's duty to operate the health care organization with due care, applying equally to for-profit and nonprofit organizations. Through fulfillment of this duty, the basic purpose of the organization is accomplished. Actions required by this duty extend from the purchase of suitable equipment for patient treatment (subject to the organization's financial ability) to the hiring of competent employees. Two important required actions are (1) selection and review of the performance of medical staff and (2) selection and supervision of a competent chief executive officer.

The board has the duty to select medical staff members as part of its duty to manage the organization and maintain a satisfactory standard of patient care. The board, while cognizant of the importance of medical staff membership to physicians, must meet its obligation to maintain standards of good medical practice in dealing with matters of staff appointment and discipline.

In 1965, the Illinois Supreme Court ruled in the famous *Darling* case, that a hospital board has a duty to establish procedures for the medical staff to evaluate, provide advice, and, where necessary, take action when an unreasonable risk of harm to a patient arises from the treatment being provided.[72]

---

[69] Cobb County-Kennestone Hosp. v. Prince, 242 Ga. 139, 249 S.E.2d 581 (1978).
[70] Brandt v. St. Vincent Infirmary, 287 Ark. 431, 701 S.W.2d 103 (1985).
[71] Martin Mem. Hosp. Ass'n, Inc. v. Noble, 496 So.2d 222 (Fla. 4th DCA 1986).
[72] Darling v. Charleston Comm. Mem. Hosp., 33 Ill. 2d 326, 211 N.E.2d 253 (1965), *cert. denied*, 383 U.S. 946 (1966).

In 1981, a Wisconsin hospital was found liable for failing to exercise due care in evaluating and checking the claimed credentials of an applicant for medical staff membership.[73] This has evolved into the corporate liability doctrine discussed in Chapter 11. Hospitals should have appropriate procedures for evaluating the competency of candidates for staff appointments and for determining privileges to be given to physicians. Hospital responsibilities and physician rights concerning medical staff matters are discussed further in Chapter 5.

DUTY OF LOYALTY. The board's duty of loyalty requires directors to act in good faith and in a way that they reasonably believe is in accordance with the best interests of the corporation. Good faith is generally a subjective requirement that looks at the person's motivation. Reasonable belief in the best interests of the corporation is both a subjective and objective test. The director must actually and honestly have the belief (subjective), and it must be a belief that a reasonable person could have in the circumstances (objective). Some of the ways that the duty of loyalty can be violated include seizing corporate opportunities, self-dealing, and not disclosing conflicts of interest.

Duty of obedience. Part of the duty of loyalty for nonprofit health care organizations is the duty of obedience to the purposes stated in the hospital's charter. It is not always sufficient that the assets continue to be used for any charitable purpose. They generally need to be used for the stated charitable purpose.[74]

Corporate opportunities. A board member who becomes aware of an opportunity for the corporation has a duty not to seize that opportunity for private gain unless the corporation elects not to pursue the opportunity. One example of such a seizure concerns a professional service corporation that contracted to provide services to a hospital in Illinois.[75] While the corporation was negotiating with the hospital to continue the contract, one of the two board members of the corporation created a competing corporation that contracted with the hospital to provide the services. The court found the new contract was an improper seizure of a corporate opportunity, violating the duty of loyalty to the first corporation.

---

[73] Johnson v. Misericordia Comm. Hosp., 99 Wis. 2d 708, 301 N.W.2d 156 (1981).

[74] *See* M.G. Tebo, *A matter of trust: Art and chocolate mix over the issue of who should benefit from an endowment,* 89 A.B.A.J. 24 (Jan. 2003); Commonwealth v. Barnes Found., 398 Pa. 158, 159 A.2d 500 (1960); *In re* Milton Hershey School Trust, 807 A.2d 324 (Pa. Commw. 2002).

[75] Patient Care Servs., S.C. v. Segal, 32 Ill. App. 3d 1021, 337 N.E.2d 471 (1st Dist. 1975).

Not all opportunities are subject to this rule. In 1996, the Delaware Supreme Court ruled that there was no duty to present an opportunity to a corporation when the corporation could not afford the opportunity.[76]

As health care organizations become involved in corporate ventures with competitors and place their officers on the boards of those corporations, they should structure the relationship so those corporations cannot claim a right to corporate opportunities that the health care organization identifies.

Self-dealing. Self-dealing is a contract between the corporation and an entity in which a board member has a financial interest. Statutes in some states specifically forbid some types of self-dealing transactions. One state makes it a crime for trustees or officers of a public hospital to own stock in any company that does business with the hospital.[77] Forbidding all self-dealing can be disadvantageous to the hospital because sometimes the most advantageous contract is with a board member or with a company in which a board member has an interest.[78] Unless there is a statutory prohibition, most health care organizations permit contracts between the corporation and a board member if (1) the contract is fair; (2) the interested board member does not speak or vote in favor of the contract; and (3) the board member makes full disclosure of all important facts concerning the interest, including both favorable and unfavorable facts. Courts generally believe the disinterested remainder of the board is able to protect corporate interests.

Courts have the power to declare any self-dealing contract void. In a South Carolina case, two board members challenged the sale of hospital land to another board member.[79] Although the purchaser did not participate in the final vote on the sale, a board member who was his business associate actively participated. The court declared the sale void because the board members did not meet the high standard of loyalty. If the fairness of the contract is questioned, the

---

[76] Broz v. Cellular Info. Sys., Inc., 673 A.2d 148 (Del. 1996); *see also* Robinson Leatham & Nelson, Inc. v. Nelson, 109 F.3d 1388 (9th Cir. 1997) [restructuring transaction not a corporate opportunity, so no violation for former director to relinquish interest in entity related to restructuring].

[77] N.C. GEN. STAT. § 14-234 (1986 Supp.); N.C. Att'y Gen. Op. Dec. 6, 1982.

[78] *See* V. Rouch, *Proposed policy change at Wilmington, N.C., hospital questioned by trustees*, MORNING STAR (Wilmington, N.C.), Mar. 22, 2003 [local debate over proposal to ban all business with companies owned in part by directors or senior staff].

[79] Gilbert v. McLeod Infirmary, 219 S.C. 174, 64 S.E.2d 524 (1951).

burden of proving fairness falls upon the board member with the financial interest. For example, the North Carolina Supreme Court required those involved to prove the fairness of a lease of an entire hospital to one board member.[80]

Courts sometimes adopt a strict view of the responsibility of board members of governmental entities. An Arkansas court held that a laundry service contract between a board member and a governmental hospital was improper although the board member's bid was the lowest bid.[81] The court allowed the hospital to pay the fair value of services already performed.

Membership on the board of a governmental hospital is a public office. Many courts consider the danger of conflicts of interest of public officers to justify holding all contracts between board members and governmental hospitals improper and invalid even when otherwise advantageous to the hospital. However, the Mississippi Supreme Court ruled that it was not a violation of ethics or the prohibition of contracts with state officers for a public hospital to grant a physician board member medical staff membership and clinical privileges.[82]

Conflict of interest. Conflict of interest is closely akin to self-dealing. While there might be no actual self-dealing involved, nondisclosure of conflicting interests can result in statutory penalties or breach of common law fiduciary duties. Boards should require periodic disclosure of all potentially conflicting interests.

One of the most extensive judicial discussions of duties of hospital board members concerning self-dealing and conflicts of interest arose out of Sibley Hospital, a nonprofit hospital in the District of Columbia.[83] The board had routinely approved financial arrangements made by two members, the treasurer and the chief executive officer. When the chief executive officer died, the other trustees discovered that substantial hospital assets were in bank accounts drawing inadequate or no interest and the banks were associated with several board members.

The court ruled that board members have a general financial responsibility and breach their duty to the hospital if they (1) fail to supervise actions of persons to whom responsibility for making

---

[80] Fowle Mem. Hosp. v. Nicholson, 189 N.C. 44, 126 S.E. 94 (1925).
[81] Warren v. Reed, 231 Ark. 714, 331 S.W.2d 847 (1960).
[82] State by Mississippi Ethics Comm'n v. Aseme, 583 So.2d 955 (Miss. 1991).
[83] Stern v. Lucy Webb Hayes Nat'l Training School, 381 F. Supp. 1003 (D. D.C. 1974).

those decisions has been delegated; (2) allow the hospital to conduct a transaction with a business in which they have a substantial interest or hold a significant position without disclosing their interest and any facts that would indicate such a transaction would not be in the hospital's best interest; (3) vote in favor of or actively participate in decisions concerning transactions with any business in which they have a substantial interest or hold a significant position; or (4) fail to perform their duties honestly, in good faith, and with a reasonable amount of care and diligence. Although the court found that the board members had breached their duty, it did not remove the members from their positions. Written financial procedures and policies were required, and board members were required to disclose their interests in financial institutions with which the hospital dealt. Written financial statements were to be issued to the board before each meeting. In addition, the court required newly elected board members to read the court's directions.

In 1999, a Delaware court ruled that the board of a health company be sued for failing to disclose the motives behind an asset sale that favored the majority shareholder. This breach of the duty of loyalty placed the action outside the immunity granted to the directors by the company charter.[84]

Board membership on health care entities can be an important service to the community and a rewarding experience, but the days are past when board membership can simply be an honor or a reward for past contributions to the organization. It is increasingly important for board members to be attentive to their duties.

2-2.2 When Can Board Members Be Personally Liable for Their Actions Related to the Health Care Organization?

CRIMINAL LIABILITY OF BOARD MEMBERS. Board members can be criminally liable. A federal court affirmed criminal convictions of several members of a county council, which served as the county hospital board, for soliciting and receiving kickbacks from architects in return for awarding contracts for a hospital project financed with federal funds. They were each sentenced to one year in prison.[85] Board members of for-profit corporations have been con-

---

[84] O'Reilly v. Transworld Healthcare, Inc., 745 A.2d 902 (Del. Ch. Ct. 1999).
[85] United States v. Thompson, 366 F.2d 167 (6th Cir.), *cert. denied*, 385 U.S. 973 (1966).

victed of violations of securities laws.[86] A Texas hospital board member was indicted for violating the state open meetings act, but charges were dropped when she agreed to probation.[87]

CIVIL LIABILITY. As discussed earlier, under the "business judgment" rule, board members are generally not liable for simple negligence in exercising their judgment concerning corporate business; they are liable only for gross or willful negligence. This "business judgment" rule offers board members wide latitude for actions taken in good faith. The business corporation standard was applied to hospital board members in the Sibley Hospital case.[88] Board members were not personally liable for the money lost while hospital funds were earning inadequate interest.

Board members are sometimes named as individual defendants in malpractice suits involving hospitals. A board member is generally not personally liable for medical malpractice unless the member participated in or directed the wrongful act that caused the injury. A South Carolina court ruled that board members could not be sued for a patient's death during an operation due to erroneous installation of a medical gas system in which the oxygen and nitrous oxide lines were crossed.[89] The court said that board members would not be personally liable even if the plaintiff's claims — that the board members failed to hold meetings, oversee hospital management, and confirm inspection of the medical gas unit — were correct. While the hospital could be liable for the consequences of the crossed lines, board members could not. However, when a corporate officer or director knows that the corporation is violating a standard of care and fails to take any action, the officer or director can be personally liable. A District of Columbia court ruled that a corporate officer of a clinic could be personally liable to a patient harmed by overnight treatment prohibited by local law when the officer knew of the practice and did nothing to stop it.[90]

Some federal laws impose personal liability on directors. Directors can be personally responsible for the costs of some environmental

---

[86] *E.g.*, F. McMorris, *Ex-chairman of Health Management is convicted of directing fraud scheme*, WALL ST. J., May 11, 1998, B4 [misstatements in financial results for two years].

[87] *Hospital board member could face fine, jail time*, HOUSTON CHRONICLE, Apr. 11, 2003, A36; *Hospital board member gets probation open meeting violation*, AP, Sept. 27, 2003.

[88] United States v. Thompson, 366 F.2d 167 (6th Cir.), *cert. denied*, 385 U.S. 973 (1966); *accord*, Beard v. Ackenbach Mem. Hosp. Ass'n, 170 F.2d 859 (10th Cir. 1948).

[89] Hunt v. Rabon, 275 S.C. 475, 272 S.E.2d 643 (1980).

[90] Vuitch v. Furr, 482 A.2d 811 (D.C. 1984).

cleanup of lands owned by the corporation.[91] Board members have been sued under federal law for alleged misuses of pension funds.[92] Sometimes shareholders bring suits against board members of for-profit corporations.[93]

LIABILITY LIMITS, INDEMNITY, AND INSURANCE. Some state laws limit the liability exposure of directors of nonprofit corporations for their actions as directors. For example, Illinois forbids suits against uncompensated directors unless their actions are willful or wanton.[94] Even though the liability exposure of board members is limited, defense of these suits can be costly. It is not reasonable to expect board members to serve unless the corporation protects them from defense costs and from liability for good faith actions. Corporations generally can indemnify directors for defense costs, judgments, fines, and other expenses resulting from civil or criminal actions if the directors acted in good faith and reasonably believed their actions to be lawful and in the corporation's best interests. Many hospitals purchase insurance to protect board members from these costs. This insurance is generally called directors and officers (D & O) liability insurance. However, some D & O insurance policies might not provide the protection they appear to provide. A federal district court ruled that one officer's misrepresentations in the insurance application invalidated the coverage for all directors and officers.[95]

One issue when providing defense is the selection of the defense attorney. The person being defended wants a good defense, and the entity wants the fees to be reasonable. In 1999, a Delaware court was confronted with a case where the entity paying the fees misused its power over attorney selection to try to force the involved executive to accept a weak defense. The Delaware Supreme Court found this to be a violation of the indemnity agreement.[96]

---

[91] 42 U.S.C. §§ 9601(20)(a), 9607(a); Sidney S. Arst Co. v. Pipefitters Welfare Educ. Fund, 25 F.3d 417 (7th Cir. 1994).

[92] *E.g.*, Herman v. Health Care Delivery Servs., Inc, No. 98-CV-06460 (C.D. Cal. filed Aug. 7, 1998), *as discussed in* 7 H.L.R. 1324 (1998) [Labor Dept. suit against health care organization, eight board members for allegedly transferring pension funds to business].

[93] Oran v. Stafford, 226 F. 3d 275 (3d Cir. 2000) [failure to show violation by directors].

[94] ILL. REV. STAT. ch. 32, § 108.70(a).

[95] Shapiro v. American Home Assur. Co., 584 F. Supp. 1245 (D. Mass. 1984); *but see* Shapiro v. American Home Assur. Co., 616 F. Supp. 900 (D. Mass. 1984) [due to severability provision in policy, Securities Act policy must provide coverage despite fraud of insureds].

[96] Chamison v. Healthust, Inc., 735 A.2d 912 (Del. Ch. 1999), *aff'd*, 748 A.2d 407 (Del. 2000).

2-2.3 How Are Board Members Selected and Removed?

SELECTION OF BOARD MEMBERS. Board members are selected in several ways. Many boards are self-perpetuating. Vacancies are filled by replacement members selected by the remaining board members. Some boards are elected by stockholders or corporate members. Board members for governmental hospitals are frequently elected by a vote of the people in a governmental subdivision or appointed by elected officials.[97] Usually terms of office are staggered so that all members are not replaced at the same time. Experienced members can provide continuity of governance.

If board members are not selected in accordance with applicable laws, articles of incorporation, and bylaws, courts can declare board actions void. In a Tennessee case, board members were not selected as specified in the articles, and several members did not satisfy membership qualifications.[98] As a result, the court declared a board vote to transfer ownership of the hospital to the county to be void. In 1997, a New York court ordered a new board elected through a committee established by the CEO not to act and authorized the existing board to act until the next annual meeting.[99]

The composition of the board is one of the factors that the Internal Revenue Service (IRS) uses in determining whether a nonprofit corporation is eligible for tax exemption; so nonprofit hospitals need to consider IRS guidelines in selecting board members.

At least one legislature has controlled the composition of boards. West Virginia requires 40 percent of the board of each nonprofit or local governmental hospital to be consumer representatives selected in equal proportions from small businesses, organized labor, elderly persons, and lower-income persons. Special consideration must also be given to women, racial minorities, and the disabled. Failure to comply can result in loss of the hospital's license, a fine, or imprisonment.[100] Federal courts have ruled that the statute is constitutional.[101]

---

[97] *E.g.*, State *ex rel.* Board of Trustees of City of North Kansas City Mem. Hosp. v. Russell, 843 S.W.2d 353 (Mo. 1992) [board members selected by mayor with approval of city council, could be removed by city government].

[98] Bedford County Hosp. v. County of Bedford, 42 Tenn. App. 569, 304 S.W.2d 697 (1957).

[99] *Court rules for board in Health Rite fight*, N.Y. TIMES, Dec. 27, 1997, B14.

[100] W. VA. CODE § 16-5B-6a; Christie v. Elkins Area Med. Ctr., Inc., 179 W.Va. 247, 366 S.E.2d 755 (1988).

[101] American Hosp. Ass'n v. Hansbarger, 594 F. Supp. 483 (N.D. W.Va. 1984), *aff'd*, 783 F.2d 1184 (4th Cir. 1986), *cert. denied*, 479 U.S. 820 (1986); *see also* Blue Cross v. Foudree, 606 F. Supp. 1574 (S.D. Iowa 1985) [upholding required subscriber majority on board].

Sometimes board composition becomes an issue in litigation or in state challenges to mergers or other corporate transactions.[102] In 1997, a settlement of a California challenge to alleged self-dealing by directors included an agreement that four directors would resign, the board size would be expanded, and more persons would be made eligible to participate in selection of new directors.[103] In 2003, the hospital chain, HCA, Inc., entered a settlement with state pension funds that included an agreement that at least two-thirds of its board would be independent directors.[104]

REMOVAL OF BOARD MEMBERS. Sometimes a board tries to remove a member. The procedure specified in the articles and bylaws must be followed. In New Jersey, a private hospital board member must be provided with notice of the reason for the action and an opportunity to be heard even if the articles and bylaws do not require these steps.[105] In an Oregon case, the court affirmed the removal of a public hospital board member by the board of county commissioners after he was provided with notice and opportunity to be heard.[106] The court ruled that substantial evidence supported the commissioners' decision that the member's lack of candor caused a lack of trust, which diminished his effectiveness as a board member, and that this was sufficient reason to remove him from the board.

Some board members are removed by public vote. In 2001, it was reported that the behavior of one board member of a California public hospital led to the hiring of a security guard for meetings, installation of a microphone cutoff system, and restrictions on her entering the hospital. In the 2002 election, she was voted out of office.[107]

---

[102] *See Activists named to board at Hardin County Hospital; Facility's ties to OhioHealth are still a concern for some*, COLUMBUS DISPATCH [Ohio], Dec. 7, 2002, 3B [two members of community group threatening to sue hospital were appointed to board]; *Detroit Medical Center restructures board*, AP, June 24, 2003 [part of effort to seek financial support from city, county & state]; K. Norris, *Six named to Detroit Medical Center funding panel*, DETROIT FREE PRESS, Aug. 21, 2003 [governor appointed an oversight committee to watch over public funding given to hospitals].

[103] Rhode Island v. Lifespan, No. 89-2801 (R.I. Super. Ct. settlement Jan. 5, 1999), *as discussed in* 8 H.L.R. 157 (1999).

[104] *HCA to overhaul corporate governance; Hospital chain agrees to changes under proposed settlement with state pension funds*, L.A. TIMES, Feb. 5, 2003, pt. 3, 13.

[105] State *ex rel.* Welch v. Passaic Hosp. Ass'n, 59 N.J.L. 142, 36 A. 702 (1897).

[106] Coldiron v. Board of Comm'rs, 39 Or. App. 495, 592 P.2d 1053 (1979).

[107] J. Behrman, *Hospital board member under fire*, SAN DIEGO UNION-TRIBUNE, July 1, 2001, N1; J. Behrman, *Tri-City Healthcare board hires guards to attend its meetings*, SAN DIEGO UNION-TRIBUNE, Apr. 26, 2002; J. Behrman, *Three sworn in as Tri-City Healthcare District board directors*, SAN DIEGO UNION-TRIBUNE, Dec. 4, 2002, NC-2.

There are many reasons why boards might want to remove members. Board members who do not attend meetings generally can be removed.[108] Sometimes medical staffs seek to remove board members.[109] In 1997, a California hospital removed two physicians from the board after the physicians filed suit to have the board dissolved.[110]

Sometimes the state attorney general or regulatory agencies seek to change board composition. For example, in 2003, the Minnesota attorney general sought to install additional members on the board of a health system. The system opposed the effort. A compromise was reached where the board agreed to accept an additional person as an adviser, rather than a board member.[111]

Sometimes competing groups seek to be recognized as the board of directors. Unless the matters can be settled, courts have to resolve the matter.[112] For example, in 2002, an Alabama judge had to determine who constituted the board of a health services company and appointed an overseer during the transition.[113] In 2003, a New York appellate court affirmed the appointment of a receiver by the court to run the hospital while the courts sorted out a power struggle over control.[114]

2-3 How Are CEOs Selected and What Is Their Role and Responsibility?

The chief executive officer (CEO) of the hospital is concerned with all the topics covered in this book. The CEO's personal intervention will probably be required when some legal problems arise. In this

---

[108] *See* J. Garofoli, *Hospital board ousts duo for missed meetings*, SAN FRANCISCO CHRONICLE, Aug. 16, 2000, A21.

[109] *E.g.*, *Doctors vote against hospital's president, board chairman*, AP, Oct. 17, 2002 [Owensboro, Ky.]; *Hospital chairman resigns*, AP, Oct. 30, 2002 [Owensboro]; S. Vied, *CEO of Owensboro, Ky., health system to resign in May 2004*, MESSENGER-INQUIRER, Oct. 31, 2003 [public board dissolved, new fourteen-member private board].

[110] *Queen of Angels board removes dissident physicians after suit*, 6 H.L.R. 1817 (1997).

[111] *HealthPartners vows to fight Hatch on board seats*, AP, Jan. 27, 2003; *Hatch, HealthPartners reach settlement on Glen Taylor's role*, AP, June 11, 2003.

[112] For a settlement, *see* C. Brown, *Hospital agreement reached*, ATLANTA JOURNAL-CONSTITUTION, Apr. 25, 2002, 3c [settlement of suit over control of hospital, board restructured].

[113] *Judge says 7 who refused to quit are health care group's board*, AP, Feb. 1, 2002; *Judge returns West Alabama Health Services control to board*, AP, Apr. 27, 2002 [court ends overseer].

[114] Singh v. Bruswick Hosp., 2 A.D.3d 433, 767 N.Y.S.2d 839 (2d Dept. 2003) [aff'g appointment of receiver]; B.J. Durkin, *Court enters hospital struggle*, NEWSDAY (New York, N.Y.), Dec. 8, 2001, A14 [appointment of receiver].

section, the CEO's duties, authority, qualifications, and personal liability will be covered.

DUTIES. The CEO is directly in charge of the organization and is generally responsible only to the governing board, but can be responsible to systems officers when the organization is part of a larger system. The CEO is the general supervisor of all operations, and the board delegates to the CEO the authority to fulfill this responsibility. Although areas of responsibility are usually delegated to subordinates, the CEO is primarily responsible for management. The CEO is the agent and usually the employee of the governing board and is subject to its superior authority. Even when the CEO is also a board member or a part owner, the CEO is a board agent and has a duty to carry out board policies.

Many health care facilities are part of a larger organization. Both for-profit and nonprofit organizations apply systemwide policies concerning many aspects of management. To promote efficiency, the organization often uses shared services, uniform accounting procedures, centralized support services, and other management methods made possible by the umbrella structure. A CEO in a larger system might or might not be an employee of the larger organization, but will be subject to its policies.

Chief executive officers of governmental organizations are usually appointed public officials. Whether they are public officials or hired supervisors, they are directly responsible to the governmental body that controls the organization. Their conditions of employment can fall within civil service laws or other statutory requirements.

The CEO has only the duties imposed by law, or delegated expressly, or by implication by the board. The CEO is usually charged with certain general management duties. By resolution, bylaw, order, or contract, the board can assign the CEO additional duties.

Chief executive officers sometimes have dual roles in which they also serve as board members.[115] When CEOs are nonvoting members, their positions do not present legal difficulties. When CEOs serve as voting members of a nonprofit hospital board, caution is required; CEOs cannot vote on any question concerning their personal status or compensation.

---

[115] *But see* A. Raghavan, *More CEOs say 'no thanks' to board seats*, WALL ST. J, Jan. 28, 2005, B1.

When a new CEO is appointed, there is usually a duty to abide by the contractual and other commitments of the predecessor until they are legally terminated. For example, at one hospital, a new president committed an unfair labor practice by refusing to bargain with a union the predecessor had voluntarily recognized.[116]

In addition to delegated duties, duties are imposed on CEOs by statutes and regulations.

As discussed in section 2-1 on the board of directors, there is increasing focus on the personal responsibilities of the CEO regarding financial controls. The Sarbanes-Oxley Act requires the CEO to personally certify financial statements of publicly traded companies. CEOs of all corporations are increasingly expected to focus attention on these areas and to make sure that there are appropriate financial controls in place. CEOs are expected to avoid conflicts of interest.

In addition, CEOs are expected to assure that their institutions maintain an environment that is committed to compliance with legal requirements. An effective compliance program as discussed in Chapter 12 can be one part of this effort.

AUTHORITY. The CEO's primary source of authority is the governing board, which normally delegates to the CEO the duty and responsibility of managing the hospital, together with the authority to accomplish this duty. Board resolutions or policies can specify the CEO's authority or grant special authority to deal with certain problems. Some authority can be granted in legal documents governing the hospital — such as hospital articles or bylaws — while some aspects of the CEO's authority can be covered in an employment contract. State statutes or regulations can provide for certain administrative powers.

Authority can be either express or implied. Express authority is a written or oral grant giving the CEO power to accomplish certain ends. The scope of the CEO's express authority can be as broad or as limited as the board desires. Implied authority consists of those powers that are conveyed along with express authority so that desired ends can be accomplished. The CEO can possess only those powers and duties that can be properly delegated. The board cannot delegate authority that it does not possess, and it cannot delegate certain responsibilities that are nondelegable. For example, in

---

[116] Exxel/Atmos, Inc. v. NLRB, 307 U.S. App. D.C. 376, 28 F.3d 1243 (1994).

most states, the board probably cannot delegate the power to grant appointments to the medical staff, except on a temporary basis. The scope of the CEO's power to enter into contracts is discussed later in the civil liability section.

The CEO can do many things that are not challenged, either because people are unaware of the actions or because people with the right to challenge or forbid them do not do so. A CEO acting beyond authority is subject to several possible legal consequences, including being dismissed by the board in accordance with its established rules; being sued by the hospital for breach of the employment contract and for any resultant financial damage to the hospital; being held liable by employees or other persons for damages resulting from negligence or intentional wrongdoing; and being subjected to prosecution for any specific criminal laws violated.

SELECTION, EVALUATION, AND TERMINATION. Governing boards are responsible for selecting CEOs to act as their agents in hospital management. Boards that try to run hospitals without CEOs are subject to extensive criticism and risk legal liability.[117] Some boards use interim CEOs while searching for permanent CEOs.[118] The board must select a competent CEO who will set and maintain satisfactory patient care standards. Minimum standards for CEOs are contained in some hospital licensing statutes and regulations and in some statutes creating governmental hospitals. Where legal requirements exist, the CEO must at least satisfy those requirements.

After appointing a CEO, the board must periodically evaluate the CEO's performance. The board can become liable if it fails to exercise proper oversight of the CEO's performance. When not satisfied with performance, the board should take appropriate action.

When the board is considering replacement of the CEO, it should follow the procedures in applicable law, the articles of incorporation, and the bylaws. However, some courts have declined to intervene when bylaws were not followed. For example, in a Louisiana case, a public hospital CEO was terminated without the warning and opportunity to correct deficiencies required by the bylaws. The Louisiana Supreme Court refused to order reinstate-

---

[117] *See Community hospital's questionable ethics*, and Barkholz, *Maryland system's board refutes allegations, promises improvements*, MOD. HEALTHCARE, June 7, 1985, 5, 44 [hospital operated eighteen months without CEO].

[118] *See* Droste, *Temporary CEOs take up the slack in hospitals*, 63 HOSPS., Sept. 20, 1989, 104.

ment because the CEO could not show that he had been harmed by the deviation from the bylaws.[119] Similarly, the Minnesota Supreme Court refused to intervene when a CEO was discharged.[120] The applicable law provided that the CEO served "at the pleasure of the county board," and he was not entitled to a hearing. In some circumstances, CEOs of public hospitals can be entitled to due process.[121]

Generally, courts will not order reinstatement of removed CEOs, but the hospital will generally be liable to pay damages when the removal breaches a contract[122] or is done in an improper manner.[123] On the other hand, in certain circumstances, some severance packages can be unenforceable.[124]

Under some state laws it can be possible for someone other than the board or a court to order removal of a CEO. A New York court ruled that the state's Department of Health had authority to order removal of a CEO for not being sufficiently qualified by education or experience.[125] In 2002, the board removed the four top administrators of an Arizona hospital when it received a petition signed by 138 hospital shareholders demanding the removal of the executives and threatening recall of the board if it did not act.[126] Nursing home administrators are another example because they are licensed under state law. This license can be revoked by the state for patient abuse or other violations of the licensing law.[127] Unlicensed persons must be removed.

LIABILITY. CEOs can be criminally or civilly liable for actions related to their employment in several circumstances.

---

[119] Lamm v. Board of Comm'rs, 378 So.2d 919 (La. 1979).

[120] State *ex rel.* Stubbin v. Board of County Comm'rs, 273 Minn. 361, 141 N.W.2d 499 (1966); *accord* Heath v. Rosebud Hosp. Dist., 620 F.2d 207 (9th Cir. 1980) [CEO not entitled to hearing before termination].

[121] *See* Heath v. Rosebud Hosp. Dist., 620 F.2d 207 (9th Cir. 1980) [42 U.S.C. § 1983 suit dismissed, due process was provided].

[122] *E.g.*, Browning v. Salem Mem. Dist. Hosp., 808 S.W.2d 943 (Mo. Ct. App. 1991).

[123] *E.g.*, American Medical Int'l, Inc. v. Giurintano, 821 S.W.2d 331 (Tex. Ct. App. 1991) [hospital, assistant administrator and individual physicians liable to prospective hospital administrator for intentional infliction of emotional distress for spreading rumors, other actions to prevent appointment].

[124] *E.g.*, A. Goldstein, *Judge denies severance to former hospital chief*, WASHINGTON POST, May 10, 2002, B3; R. Winslow, *Regulators stop Oxford ex-chairman's severance*, WALL ST. J., Apr. 3, 1998, B5.

[125] Harlem Hosp. Ctr. Med. Bd. v. Hoffman, 84 A.D.2d 272, 445 N.Y.S.2d 981 (1st Dept. 1982).

[126] M. Marizco, *Board fires top hospital execs in Winslow, Ariz.*, ARIZONA DAILY SUN (Flagstaff, Ariz.), Dec. 28, 2002.

[127] *E.g.*, Goldsmith v. DeBuono, 245 A.D.2d 627, 665 N.Y.S.2d 727 (3rd Dept. 1997).

Criminal liability. CEOs who become involved in fraudulent and other illegal schemes can be held criminally liable, similar to those in other industries.[128] For example, a Florida CEO who caused a hospital to issue twenty-one checks, fraudulently endorsed them, and appropriated the proceeds, which exceeded $850,000, was sentenced to twenty-five years in prison.[129] Embezzlement or bribery is also a federal crime when committed by an agent of an organization that received over $10,000 under a federal program in a one-year period that includes the offense.[130] A hospital CEO was convicted under this law.[131] In 2002, a federal appellate court upheld the conviction of a former West Virginia hospital administrator for misusing hospital funds on a shopping center and other ventures.[132]

Fraudulent schemes can also result in forfeiture of benefits. An Ohio court ruled that a CEO who had embezzled funds forfeited all compensation, including deferred compensation, during the period of faithlessness.[133]

Some prosecutors have pursued criminal charges against CEOs for treatment of patients. The Wisconsin Supreme Court upheld the conviction of a nursing home CEO for abuse of residents but reversed a conviction for reckless conduct causing death.[134] One resident had died of exposure after walking away from the facility. Other residents had lost weight and had developed bed sores. The state claimed this was due to understaffing by the CEO. Several other nursing home administrators have been convicted of patient abuse or neglect.[135]

---

[128] *E.g., Former hospital official pleads guilty to manipulating its finances*, AP, July 11, 2000 [Lee County Community Hosp., Virginia]; *Three convicted of bribery, extortion from medical center*, AP, Sept. 7, 2000 [LaFollett Med. Ctr., Tenn.].

[129] Bronstein v. State, 355 So.2d 817 (Fla. 3d DCA 1978); *see* Touche Ross & Co. v. SunBank, 366 So.2d 465 (Fla. 3d DCA), *cert. denied*, 378 So.2d 350 (Fla. 1979) [effort by hospital to recover losses due to CEO's crimes]; *see also Former Hermann Hospital exec released from prison*, Mod. Healthcare, Dec. 18, 1987, 21.

[130] 18 U.S.C. § 666.

[131] United States v. Stout, Crim. 1990 U.S. Dist. LEXIS 12343 (E.D. Pa.), *post conviction proceeding*, 1994 U.S. Dist. LEXIS 3182 (E.D. Pa.), *aff'd without op.*, 39 F.3d 1173, 1994 U.S. App. LEXIS 31128 (3d Cir. 1994); *see also* United States v. Sadlier, 649 F. Supp. 1560 (D. Mass. 1986) [denying dismissal of charges against respiratory therapist].

[132] United States v. Morrison, 2002 U.S. App. LEXIS 1948 (4th Cir.).

[133] Roberto v. Brown County Gen. Hosp., 59 Ohio App. 3d 84, 571 N.E.2d 467 (1989).

[134] State v. Serebin, 119 Wis. 2d 837, 350 N.W.2d 65 (1984).

[135] *E.g.*, State v. Boone Retirement Ctr., Inc., 26 S.W.3d 265 (Mo. App. 2000); State v. Cunningham, 493 N.W.2d 884 (Iowa Ct. App. 1992); State v. Springer, 585 N.E.2d 27 (Ind. Ct. App. 1992); Annotation, *Criminal liability under statutes penalizing abuse or neglect of the institutionalized infirm*, 60 A.L.R. 4TH 1153.

Civil liability. CEOs, like other members of society, can be individually liable for their own wrongful actions that injure others.

A CEO can be liable for injuries caused by a subordinate only when the CEO is at fault due to negligent supervision or careless hiring of the subordinate. A CEO who is not personally at fault is not liable for injuries caused by subordinates.[136] Employers are liable for the injuries wrongfully caused by their employees, but CEOs are not the employers of their subordinates. The organization is the employer. Because CEOs are employees of the organization, the organization can be liable for wrongful acts of CEOs. If the organization pays money to an injured person as the result of a lawsuit, it usually has the right to repayment from the employee who caused the injury. Health care organizations seldom exercise this right of indemnification beyond the employee's individual insurance coverage. Liability issues are discussed in Chapter 11.

CEOs are not personally liable for contracts they make on behalf of the organization when acting within their authority to contract. When CEOs enter contracts that exceed their authority, the organization is not always bound by the contract. CEOs can be personally liable to the other party to the contract for the loss resulting from the failure to bind the organization. CEOs are not liable if the organization ratifies the contract and adopts it as its own. CEOs are generally not liable for unauthorized acts if they innocently believe they have the power to make the contract and the organization clothe the CEO's position with such apparent authority that the other contracting parties reasonably believe the CEO has authority. If the organization creates this apparent authority so that innocent third parties are misled, the law imposes liability on the organization. If the other contracting parties should have suspected the CEO lacked authority, they are required to make appropriate inquiries. If the inquiries would have disclosed the lack of authority, no recovery is allowed against the organization.

The CEO can be liable to the other contracting parties even when the CEO has apparent authority but makes the contract with intent to defraud. In a Mississippi case, an insurance company sought to recover excessive amounts it had paid to a hospital

---

136 *E.g.*, Portlock v. Perry, 852 S.W.2d 578 (Tex. Ct. App. 1993) [investor/president of diagnostic radiology center not liable for death of child after technicians gave too much choral hydrate for sedation; claimed failure to have adequate policies and procedures not sufficient to impose personal liability].

because the CEO had padded bills.[137] The court found both the CEO and the hospital liable to repay overcharges.

CEOs can be liable civilly or criminally for breach of duties imposed on them by statute. For example, when a license or permit is required before the hospital performs certain acts, often the CEO is required to obtain the license or permit and failure to obtain it can lead to fine or imprisonment. CEOs can also be required to submit certain reports to the state. While hospital CEOs are seldom fined personally for failure to discharge such a statutory duty, the possibility exists. In a Mississippi Supreme Court case involving the same CEO and hospital as the case discussed here, a state auditor sought to force the CEO and the hospital board to repay county hospital funds that had been spent without authority.[138] The court analyzed each type of expenditure the state auditor claimed to be unauthorized and found several to be, in fact, unauthorized, which required personal repayment by the CEO and the board members.

Some laws impose personal liability on CEOs. For example, the CEO can be personally liable for unpaid wages under the Fair Labor Standards Act.[139] A New York federal court ruled that a new CEO could be personally sued for sex discrimination for excluding the vice president/chief nursing officer from vice presidential meetings, refusing to meet with her and firing her.[140]

The federal government and some states have provided some official immunity from personal civil liability for some public officials when following a legal mandate (i.e., performing a "ministerial duty") or when exercising administrative judgment (i.e., performing a "discretionary duty"). Rules vary considerably, and courts tend to restrict the application of immunity doctrines.

MANAGEMENT CONTRACTS. Some hospital boards have entered contracts with other corporations to manage their hospitals. The CEO is generally supplied by the management corporation. The board retains ultimate authority; so no change is required in the hospital's license in most states. The authority of the board and the contractor should be carefully defined. The board should preserve its authority to terminate the contract without prohibitively onerous penalties.

---

[137] Reserve Life Ins. Co. v. Salter, 152 F. Supp. 868, 870 (S.D. Miss. 1957).
[138] Golding v. Salter, 234 Miss. 567, 107 So.2d 348 (1958).
[139] Fegley v. Higgins, 19 F.3d 1126 (6th Cir.), *cert. denied*, 513 U.S. 875 (1994).
[140] Dirschel v. Speck, 1994 U.S. Dist. LEXIS 9257 (S.D.N.Y.).

These contracts are sometimes difficult to terminate. A Mississippi board tried to terminate a management contract after the management company increased hospital rates and revised the hospital budget without the board approval required in the contract. The court ruled that termination was not justified because the board had authority to nullify the breach without termination.[141]

Hospitals that have or plan to issue tax-exempt bonds need to consider the IRS requirements limiting the length and other features of such contracts.[142]

Often hospitals enter management contracts because of confidence in individuals who own or manage the management corporation. They do not want to be managed by others; so they restrict assignment of the contract. Restrictions on assignment of contracts with corporations can easily be avoided by sale of the management corporation's stock. Unless provided in the contract, the hospital will not be able to terminate the contract when these stock sales occur. An Alabama hospital sued when all the stock of a management company was sold to another company despite a prohibition of assignment of the management contract. The court upheld a temporary injunction of transfer of hospital funds, conversion of the hospital into an abuse facility, and movement of property out of the hospital.[143] Hospitals should not rely on courts to provide these protections. It is prudent to require the management corporation to inform the hospital of all substantial changes in stock ownership and to give the hospital the option to terminate the contract after such a change.

2-4 What Are the Licensing and Accreditation Requirements for Health Care Organizations?

Hospitals and other health care entities are among the most extensively regulated institutions. They are regulated by all levels of government and by numerous agencies within each level. They occasionally are confronted with conflicting mandates. Since this

---

141 UHS-Qualicare, Inc. v. Gulf Coast Comm. Hosp., 525 So.2d 746 (Miss. 1987), *pet. reh'g withdrawn*, 525 So.2d 758 (Miss. 1988) [settlement].

142 Rev. Proc. 93-17, 93-19; IRS issued proposed regulations on private activity bond restrictions, 59 FED. REG. 67658 (Dec. 30, 1994) [to replace Rev. Proc. 93-17, 93-19].

143 Ex parte Health Care Management Group, 522 So.2d 280 (Ala. 1988).

logistical problem has received more attention, relief has been provided in some areas. Conflicts still remain because of underlying conflicts in societal goals. There are also numerous private entities that develop standards and accredit institutions that satisfy their standards.

LICENSURE. Licensure is different from accreditation. *Licensure* is governmental regulation. For example, the state legislature grants an administrative agency authority to adopt standards hospitals must meet, grant licenses to complying institutions, and enforce continuing compliance. Hospitals are barred from operating without a license. Persons who operate hospitals that violate the standards can lose their licenses or be fined or penalized. Numerous other health care entities must obtain state and local licenses and comply with licensing standards. Some of the entities that are licensed include health maintenance organizations, nursing homes, ambulatory surgery centers, hospices, home health agencies, and clinical laboratories.

The discussion of licensure of institutions is divided into: authority to license (2-4.1), scope of regulations (2-4.2), inspections (2-4.3), and violations and sanctions (2-4.4).

ACCREDITATION. In contrast, *accreditation* is granted by private authorities and is not legally mandated. Accreditation is discussed in section 2-4.5.

MEDICARE CONDITIONS OF PARTICIPATION. Medicare also has standards called *conditions of participation*[144] that apply to health care organizations including hospitals; immediate care facilities for the mentally retarded; home health agencies, comprehensive outpatient rehabilitation facilities; organ procurement organizations; rural primary care hospitals; and providers of outpatient physical therapy and speech-language pathology services. They are not licensing standards, but health care organizations must comply to qualify for Medicare payment for most services for Medicare beneficiaries. The Medicare law provides that hospitals accredited by the JCAHO or AOA are *deemed* to meet most conditions of participation

---

[144] 42 U.S.C. § 1395x(e) [hospitals]; 42 C.F.R. pt. 482 [hospitals]; 42 C.F.R. §§ 483.400-483.480 [ICF/MR]; 42 C.F.R. pt. 483 [HHA]; 42 C.F.R. §§ 485.50-485.74 [CORF]; 42 C.F.R. §§ 485.301-485.308 [organ procurement]; 42 C.F.R. §§ 485.601-485.645 [rural primary care hospitals]; 42 C.F.R. §§ 485.701-485.729 [physical therapy, speech pathology]; 42 C.F.R. §§ 483.1-483.75 [long-term care facilities]. In 2005, HCFA proposed changes to the hospital conditions of participation, 70 FED. REG. 15266 (Mar. 25, 2005).

unless a special Medicare inspection finds noncompliance.[145] Institutions have mixed results in their efforts to use the courts to stop termination of Medicare participation.[146]

OTHER PRIVATE STANDARDS. Some institutions are subject to other private standards that they have voluntarily accepted. For example, hospitals operated by the Roman Catholic Church are subject to the rules of the Church, including canon law. Canon law has an important role in many decisions of these institutions.[147]

2-4.1 Authority to License

State governments have the *police power* which gives them authority to regulate health care institutions.

LEGISLATION. All states have enacted hospital and nursing home licensing statutes, and many have statutes that license other health care entities.

AGENCY ACTIONS. Licensing statutes usually grant an agency authority to adopt standards, grant licenses, and revoke licenses or impose other penalties when standards are violated. Licensing statutes and regulations must be a reasonable exercise of the police power and must not deny due process or equal protection of the laws.

Authority to adopt rules. To be enforceable, agency rules must be within authority properly delegated to the agency by statute. Rules must be adopted using the state procedure for administrative rule-making. This procedure usually includes public notice of proposed rules and an opportunity for public comment before they become final. In some circumstances, emergency rules are exempt from some requirements, but rules can be declared unenforceable

---

[145] 42 U.S.C. §§ 1395aa(c), 1395bb; 70 Fed. Reg. 15331 (Mar. 25, 2005) [JCAHO]; 70 Fed. Reg. 15333 (Mar. 25, 2005) [AOA]; *see also* Cospito v. Heckler, 742 F.2d 72 (3d Cir. 1984), *cert. denied*, 471 U.S. 1131 (1985) [not a constitutional violation for patients at psychiatric hospital to lose Medicare, Medicaid benefits when hospital lost JCAHO accreditation].

[146] *E.g.,* Mediplex of Mass., Inc. v. Shalala, 39 F. Supp. 2d 88 (D. Mass. 1999) [continued Medicare payments ordered for nursing home cited for public health deficiencies until showing of immediate harm to residents]; Northern Health Facilities, Inc. v. United States, 39 F. Supp. 2d 563 (D. Md. 1998) [denied injunction of HCFA termination of nursing home from Medicare/Medicaid, despite no immediate jeopardy violations, pact with DOJ to improve conditions; court noted this was "inequitable result"]; Ponce de Leon Healthcare Inc. v. Agency for Health Care Administration, 1997 U.S. Dist. LEXIS 10690 (S.D. Fla.) [nursing home cannot seek injunction of termination of Medicare and Medicaid provider agreements due to deficiencies found in survey until it exhausts administrative remedies].

[147] *E.g.,* Burda, *Abortion a business hurdle for nation's Catholic hospitals,* Mod. Healthcare, Aug. 25, 1989, 40.

when rules are not eligible for the emergency rule process.[148] Some states require additional steps, such as an economic impact statement, before a rule becomes enforceable.[149]

Rules are difficult to challenge if they are within the statutory authority of the agency, do not violate due process by being vague or arbitrary, and are adopted through proper procedures. For example, detailed hospital licensing rules were contested in Pennsylvania on the grounds that they were an attempt by the Department of Health to take away "management prerogatives" of hospital boards and administrators. The Pennsylvania Supreme Court decided that the department had statutory authority and upheld the rules even though they might supplant part of traditional management authority.[150]

When rules conflict with statutory law or exceed the rule-making authority granted to the agency, courts will invalidate the rules. For example, in 2004, a Florida appellate court struck down a rule that required supervision of nurse anesthetists in outpatient facilities because the agency had exceeded its delegated authority.[151]

Not a taking of private property. Most actions that states take under licensing laws have been interpreted not to constitute a taking of private property; so the constitutional requirement of just compensation for takings generally does not apply.[152]

2-4.2 Scope of Regulations

The scope of licensing regulations varies depending on the entity being regulated.

HOSPITALS. Hospital licensing regulations usually address hospital organization, requiring an organized governing body or some equivalent, an organized medical staff, and an administrator. The relationship among these elements usually is also addressed. Regulations can require general hospitals to provide certain basic services, including laboratory, radiology, pharmacy, and some emergency ser-

---

[148] *E.g,,* Florida Health Care Ass'n v. Agency for Health Care Admin., 1998 Fla. App. LEXIS 14400 (1st DCA) [quashing emergency nursing home rule].

[149] Department of Health & Rehabilitative Servs. v. Delray Hosp. Corp., 373 So.2d 75 (Fla. 1st DCA 1979).

[150] Hospital Ass'n of Pa. v. MacLeod, 487 Pa. 516, 410 A.2d 731 (1980).

[151] Ortiz v. Dep't of Health, 882 So.2d 402 (Fla. 4th DCA 2004).

[152] *E.g.,* Hospital Ass'n of N.Y.S. v. Axelrod, 164 A.D.2d 518, 565 N.Y.S.2d 243 (3d Dept. 1990); Village of Herkimer v. Axelrod, 88 A.D.2d 704, 451 N.Y.S.2d 303 (3d Dept. 1982), *aff'd,* 58 N.Y.2d 1069, 462 N.Y.S.2d 633, 449 N.E.2d 413 (1983).

vices. Regulations generally require use of adequate nursing personnel. They also can establish standards for facilities, equipment, and
personnel for specific services, such as obstetrics, pediatrics, and
surgery. Regulations can also address safety, sanitation, infection control, record preparation and retention, and other matters.

Objective versus subjective rules. All standards do not have to
be in objective numerical terms to satisfy due process requirements, but some courts are reluctant to uphold overly subjective
rules. A New York court found that several nursing home rules violated due process requirements because they were so subjective
that they did not provide adequate notice of the conduct
required.[153] The invalidated rules required sewage facilities, nursing staff, and linen laundering to meet the "approval" and "satisfaction" of the Commissioner of the Department of Health. No
objective standard was included in the rules. The court upheld
another rule that required nursing staffing be based on "needs of
the patients." The court considered this to be an objective standard
because it believed the needs would be "reasonably well identifiable
by all competent observers." Courts recognize that in some areas
objective standards either are impossible to develop or if developed
would be too arbitrary. Thus, courts have upheld enforcement of
some subjective standards if fairly applied. This is illustrated by
another New York nursing home case in which somewhat vague
standards were upheld because the actual violations clearly deviated from the rules' objective and the agency had provided written
explanations of violations to the owners.[154]

Building integrity. One focus of hospital licensure is the
integrity of hospital buildings. This is discussed in Chapter 3.

Exceptions and waivers. Often administrative agencies have
authority to permit exceptions to their rules by granting a waiver or
variance. Undue hardship can result from unbending application of
the rules, and the public's best interest might not be served by
inflexibility. For example, one state required all hospital rooms to
have showers for patients. When the rules were written, apparently
no one thought of intensive care units where patients could not use
showers; so it was necessary for hospitals to obtain waivers until the
rule could be changed. Waivers are sometimes needed because

---

153 Koelbl v. Whalen, 63 A.D.2d 408, 406 N.Y.S.2d 621 (3d Dept. 1978).
154 Eden Park Health Servs., Inc. v. Whalen, 73 A.D.2d 993, 424 N.Y.S.2d 33 (3d Dept. 1980).

some rules, especially building and fire codes, are so complex that individual rules contradict each other when applied to unusual situations. It might be necessary to obtain an official determination of which rule to follow and a waiver for conflicting rules. Waivers can also be necessary to implement innovative practices. Waivers are generally granted only when (1) there is a substantial need for relief from the rule, (2) the public purpose will be better served by the exception, and (3) the exception will not create a hazard to the health and well-being of patients or others that is excessive in light of the public purpose being served.

Bed count. Hospital licenses usually specify the number of beds the institution is permitted to operate. The license can specify that certain numbers of beds be approved for a specified use. In 1992, a Washington court ruled that a lessee/operator of a nursing home facility did not breach its lease or other agreements by entering into an agreement with the state agency to reduce its number of licensed beds.[155] States usually look to the licensed operator for issues related to licenses. Thus, owners and lenders need to clearly specify in their contracts with operators any limits on their authority to modify the license.

Have regulations gone too far? Sometimes questions are voiced concerning whether the state has gone too far in its regulation. Occasionally, courts will ask an agency to reconsider the scope of its regulations. In 1999, a California appellate court ordered a state agency to reconsider regulations that would have required friends of a paralyzed woman to obtain a state license before she could live with them.[156] The regulation required anyone other than a relative to obtain a license before caring for a disabled person.

When regulatory agencies act contrary to or beyond the scope of their statutory authority, courts will strike down the regulations. For example, see section 2-4.1.

2-4.3 Inspections

Generally, licensing agencies have a right to make unannounced inspections of complex licensed entities, like hospitals. Applying for the license is viewed as consent to reasonable inspections within the scope of the agency's authority. However, some inspections,

---

[155] Watkins v. Restorative Care Ctr., Inc., 66 Wash. App. 178, 831 P.2d 1085 (1992).
[156] Grimes v. Department of Social Servs., 70 Cal. App. 4th 1065, 83 Cal. Rptr. 2d 203 (2d Dist. 1999).

even with search warrants, can be conducted in such a manner as to violate the rights of those searched. Pursuant to a search warrant, an agency searched a birthing clinic at 2 A.M., rousting newborns and parents and photographing them. The basis for the search was suspected practice of medicine without a license. A federal appellate court ruled that those involved in the search could be sued for violating the civil rights of the newborns and parents.[157]

In most jurisdictions, licensing agencies have discretion whether or how to inspect. They cannot be held liable for either failure to inspect or failing to discover or correct deficiencies through inspections.[158]

2-4.4 Violations and Sanctions

DUE PROCESS. Two fundamental elements of due process are notice and an opportunity to be heard. Unless deficiencies immediately threaten life or health, the state can close a licensed institution or impose other penalties for licensing law violations only after giving adequate notice of violations and an opportunity to be heard. For example, a New York court ordered the hospital licensing agency to provide a hearing before deciding not to renew a hospital's license — even though the hospital lacked many basic services.[159]

OPPORTUNITY TO CORRECT DEFICIENCIES. Some state statutes and regulations require licensing agencies to give the licensed entity an opportunity to correct deficiencies before imposing sanctions. Although this opportunity is not constitutionally required, it must be provided when guaranteed by state law, or any sanctions will be invalid unless immediate action is justified by deficiencies that threaten life or health.

DEGREE OF VIOLATION AND LESSER PENALTIES. Some licensing statutes recognize that it might not be in the public interest to revoke a health care institution's license for minor violations. These statutes provide a range of lesser penalties, such as monetary penalties, and reserve license suspension or revocation for

---

157 Hummel-Jones v. Strope, 25 F.3d 647 (8th Cir. 1994).
158 *E.g.*, Stone v. North Carolina Dep't of Labor, 347 N.C. 473, 495 S.E.2d 711 (1998) [under *public duty doctrine,* workers injured in fire could not sue state agency for failure to inspect plant].
159 Woodiwiss v. Jacobs, 125 Misc. 584, 211 N.Y.S.2d 217 (Sup. Ct. 1961). For a similar result concerning a nursing home, *see* Bethune Plaza, Inc. v. Lumpkin, 863 F.2d 525 (7th Cir. 1988) [issuing conditional license without prior hearing violates due process when no emergency].

"substantial" violations. Definitions of substantial violation vary from state to state. However, in every state sufficiently serious violations lead to license revocation.[160]

AGENCY DISCRETION IN ENFORCEMENT. Generally, agencies have discretion whether to invoke the penalties authorized by law. Private individuals cannot compel licensing agencies to take action.[161] However, agencies cannot exercise this discretion on discriminatory grounds, such as religion. A federal appellate court permitted the orthodox Jewish operators of a nursing home to sue state officials for allegedly citing their facility for reasons the nursing home viewed as discrimination against their religion.[162]

SCOPE OF JUDICIAL REVIEW. When a licensing agency makes an adverse decision, the institution can generally seek judicial review. In most states, courts will review only the administrative hearing record and will not accept additional evidence. Courts will overrule the agency only if the decision was beyond the agency's authority, the agency did not follow proper procedures, or the evidence was insufficient to justify the decision.

CRIMINAL PENALTIES. In addition to fines and license suspension or revocation, some licensing statutes provide criminal penalties for violations. For example, the operation of a hospital without a license can lead to criminal prosecution.

PROTECTION OF THOSE WHO REPORT VIOLATIONS. The law protects persons who report violations to appropriate government agencies. For example, after visiting a nursing home in which they were planning to place a relative, family members reported what they believed to be violations to federal and state officials. The home lost its Medicare and Medicaid eligibility and was not allowed to admit new patients during a state investigation. The nursing home sued the family members, claiming that they had conspired and tortuously interfered with its business relationships. A federal appellate court upheld a summary judgment in the family members' favor because any interference was justified by the greater public interest in the proper operation of such facilities.[163]

---

[160] Harrison Clinic Hosp. v. Texas State Bd. of Health, 400 S.W.2d 840 (Tex. Civ. App.), aff'd, 410 S.W.2d 181 (Tex. 1966) [multiple violations of fire, safety rules, multiple citations for poor sanitation justified license revocation].

[161] E.g., Mullen v. Axelrod, 74 N.Y.2d 580, 549 N.Y.S.2d 953, 549 N.E.2d 144 (1989).

[162] Sherwin Manor Nursing Ctr., Inc. v. McAuliffe, 37 F.3d 1216 (7th Cir. 1994); Illinois settles with nursing home, WIS. ST. J., Oct. 18, 1997, 8A [$250,000 settlement with state.]

[163] Brownsville Golden Age Nursing Home, Inc. v. Wells, 839 F.2d 155 (3d Cir. 1988).

USES OF LICENSING VIOLATIONS IN OTHER CONTEXTS. Private individuals sometimes use licensing requirements in disputes with hospitals and other health care entities. A hospital avoided honoring a contract with a nurse staffing agency because the agency did not have the license that was required by state law.[164] Employee groups and others sometimes use regulatory violations to try to apply pressure.[165] Violations of regulations can sometimes be used to help establish liability in malpractice suits.

2-4.5 Accreditation

Accreditation is a private function that is not legally mandated. Private accrediting bodies assess whether participating institutions and programs meet their standards and issue accreditation to those that do meet the standards. The primary focus of most of the accreditation standards is the quality and safety of services, but many also include additional documentation and other requirements.

Some states accept accreditation by some organizations, such as the Joint Commission on Accreditation of Healthcare Organizations (JCAHO or Joint Commission) [formerly called the Joint Commission on Accreditation of Hospitals (JCAH)], as the basis for full or partial licensing of some providers without further state inspection. Other states coordinate accreditation and state compliance surveys to reduce the burden of multiple inspections. In most states, there is no link between accreditation and institutional licensure.

Accreditation can be helpful with federal compliance. Hospitals that are accredited by JCAHO and some other entities are "deemed" to meet the Medicare Conditions of Participation (COPs). Thus, they can continue to participate in Medicare, unless a Medicare validation survey finds noncompliance with the COPs. On the other hand, Medicare will sometimes approve hospitals that have lost accreditation.[166]

Another incentive for accreditation is that some health care payers will only contract with providers that are accredited.

The Joint Commission includes representatives from the American College of Physicians; American College of Surgeons; American

---

[164] U.S. Nursing Corp. v. Saint Joseph Med. Ctr., 39 F.3d 790 (7th Cir. 1994).

[165] *E.g., Unions search for regulatory violations to pressure firms and win new members,* WALL ST. J., Feb. 28, 1992, B1.

[166] *E.g., King/Drew gets reprieve,* AM. MED. NEWS, Mar. 7, 2005, 14.

Dental Association; American Hospital Association; American Medical Association; and American Nurses Association; plus representatives of the public. Health care organizations seeking accreditation apply to JCAHO, pay a fee, and submit to a survey to determine whether they satisfy the standards established by JCAHO. JCAHO publishes accreditation manuals, such as the *Comprehensive Accreditation Manual for Hospitals.*[167] JCAHO also accredits long-term care facilities; mental health, chemical dependency, and mental retardation/developmental disabilities services; home care; and pathology and clinical laboratory services. When an organization ceases to meet the standards, it can lose its accreditation.[168]

The Joint Commission continues to experiment with new approaches to assess and improve quality of services from the patient's perspective. For example, surveys now use a "tracer methodology" that tracks many aspects of the care of individual patients through their entire stay in the facility.[169]

The American Osteopathic Association (AOA) accredits osteopathic hospitals and functions similarly to JCAHO.

There are accrediting bodies for other health care entities. For example, the National Committee for Quality Assurance (NCQA) and JCAHO accredit managed care entities.

2-5 What Are the Issues When an Organization Is Converted from One Type into Another?

Health care organizations sometimes change in their legal basis and operations. This section discusses some of the legal issues related to conversions between organizational structures. There have been conversions between private nonprofit and for-profit (2-5.1); public and private (2-5.2); types of public organizations (2-5.3); and secular and religious organizations (2-5.4). Many of these conversions have been controversial and have lead to judicial, legislative, and political challenges.

---

[167] Joint Commission on Accreditation of Healthcare Organizations, COMPREHENSIVE ACCREDITATION MANUAL FOR HOSPITALS (2005 ed.) [hereinafter 2005 JCAHO CAMH].

[168] *E.g., Troubled Los Angeles hospital loses accreditation from national commission,* AP, Feb. 2, 2005.

[169] See http://www.jcaho.org/accredited+organizations/svnp/svnp+qa_tracer+methodology.htm [accessed June 9, 2005].

2-5.1 Conversion Between Private Nonprofit and For-Profit

Generally, it is not possible to convert a nonprofit legal entity into a for-profit legal entity. Conversions to for-profit status are accomplished by sale of the business or sale of the assets of the nonprofit entity to a for-profit entity. Likewise, a for-profit entity can sell its business or assets to a nonprofit entity. In the alternative, a for-profit entity can generally be converted into a nonprofit entity if its owners all agree or the contrary minority owners are bought out; in essence, the assets are donated to the charity.

Most of the controversy arises when a for-profit entity takes over a nonprofit facility. The public has contributed to the facility over the years directly though donations and indirectly through tax exemptions. In most cases, the focus is on whether the price is fair and the public interest will continue to be served. Legal battles have been fought over whether technical legal requirements had been met. Many states have enacted laws that require review and approval of such transactions by state officials, usually the attorney general; so more frequently the focus is expressly on fairness of price and ongoing public interest in services.[170]

Frequently, after such transactions the nonprofit entity continues and makes grants or supports services with the proceeds from the sale.[171] These arrangements have generally been upheld.[172] In 1998, the Kansas Supreme Court upheld such an arrangement.[173] A church organization that had founded a hospital, but had later made the hospital independent to avoid church liability for hospital operations, sought to dissolve the hospital corporation after the hospital had sold its assets to a for-profit entity. The church sought to have a portion of the assets distributed to the church rather than using

---

[170] See *Status of state legislation regulating acquisition of nonprofit hospitals by nonprofit companies*, 6 H.L.R. 1166 (1997); *California attorney general approves first nonprofit to for-profit conversion under new conversion law*, 25 HEALTH L. DIG. (June 1997), at 93 [Riverside Comm. Hosp.]; *Hospital conversions spur states to examine community benefit issues*, 7 H.L.R. 653 (1998); *State Attorney General disapproves R.I.-Massachusetts hospital group merger*, 7 H.L.R. 1436 (1998).

[171] *Conversion foundation assets grow, prompt controversy over use of funds*, 7 H.L.R. 235 (1998).

[172] *E.g.*, Attorney General v. Hahnemann Hosp., 397 Mass. 820, 494 N.E.2d 1011 (1986) [conversion to grant-making organization permitted where articles of incorporation permitted this activity].

[173] Kansas East Conf. of United Methodist Church v. Bethany Med. Ctr., 266 Kan. 366, 969 P.2d 859 (1998) [corporate law governs the transaction, trust law not applicable]; *but see* Greil Mem. Hosp. v. First Ala. Bank of Montgomery, 387 So.2d 778 (Ala. 1980) [charitable bequest lapsed when corporation created to treat tuberculosis converted to grant-making foundation].

them for other local health care purposes. The court rejected the challenge.

Nonprofit Blue Cross and Blue Shield plans in many states have been sold to for-profit entities. In some states, this has been controversial. Several states have ultimately permitted the sales to occur.[174] Some states have barred the proposed sales. For example, in 2003, the Kansas Supreme Court blocked a proposed sale, and it was dropped.[175]

2-5.2 Conversion Between Public and Private

The legality of the sale, lease, or other transactions that place public health care organizations under the control of private entities generally is determined by the scope of the laws that create the public entities, although occasionally state constitutional principles are invoked to challenge these transactions. For example, a North Carolina court ruled that a county hospital could not be leased to a for-profit management company because (1) there was no statutory authority for the lease and (2) the lease violated a restriction in the deed to the property that would have caused the loss of the property.[176] A Michigan appellate court upheld the leasing of a county hospital because the patient care management system in the contract fulfilled the county's duties.[177] The Kansas Supreme Court upheld the transfer of assets of a county hospital to a nonprofit corporation because the transfer was authorized by statute.[178] In 1997, the Oklahoma Supreme Court approved a fifty-year lease of the university hospital to a for-profit entity.[179]

Sometimes the legal analysis focuses on public interest more than on technical statutory issues. For example, the Georgia Supreme Court upheld the restructuring of a county hospital in

---

[174] *E.g.,* ABC for Health, Inc. v. Commissioner of Ins., 250 Wis. 2d 56, 640 N.W.2d 510 (App. 2001).

[175] Blue Cross & Blue Shield v. Praeger, 276 Kan. 232, 75 P.3d 226 (2003); J. Hanna, *Blue Cross won't seek new deal after court ruling*, AP, Aug. 7, 2003; *see also* T. Stuckey, *Insurance commissioner rejects CareFirst sale*, AP, Mar. 6, 2003 [Md.]; G. Johnson, *Premera appeals insurance commissioner's decision*, AP, Aug. 14, 2004 [disapproval by Wash. insurance commissioner].

[176] National Med. Enters., Inc. v. Sandrock, 72 N.C. App. 245, 324 S.E.2d 268 (1985).

[177] University Med. Affiliates, P.C. v. Wayne County Executive, 142 Mich. App. 135, 369 N.W.2d 277 (1985). Leases have also been upheld in Kromko v. Arizona Bd. of Regents, 149 Ariz. 319, 718 P.2d 478 (1986) and Local Union No. 2490 v. Waukesha County, 143 Wis. 2d 438, 422 N.W.2d 117 (Ct. App. 1988).

[178] Ullrich v. Board of County Comm'rs, 234 Kan. 782, 676 P.2d 127 (1984).

[179] Petition of University Hospitals Authority, 953 P.2d 314 (Okla. 1997); *Okla. teaching hospitals transferred to Columbia/HCA,* AM. MED. NEWS, Mar. 2, 1998, 10.

which the hospital was leased to a nonprofit corporation governed by a board controlled by members of the county hospital authority.[180] The court found that public hospitals needed to be more competitive and that the lease would enable the hospital to better serve the public health needs of the community.

EMINENT DOMAIN. Federal and state governments have the power to take property for public uses. This is called the power of *eminent domain*. States can authorize local governmental entities to exercise eminent domain. This power can be used in some circumstances to involuntarily convert a private health care facility into a public facility. The Fifth Amendment to the Constitution requires the payment of just compensation in exchange for the property. When there is no agreement on compensation, generally courts set the compensation. Eminent domain can be used to take ongoing businesses as well as land.[181]

Hospitals are usually confronted with eminent domain only when highway authorities take a strip of land to widen a bordering road or when a public hospital authority takes neighboring land for expansion. There have been a few cases where the taking of whole hospitals has been proposed and even completed. In 1981, the Michigan Supreme Court approved the taking of a neighborhood to build an automobile manufacturing plant. A hospital was taken as part of the project and was demolished.[182] In 1985, the city and county of St. Louis, Missouri decided that they needed to replace their inner-city public hospitals. Instead of building a new hospital, they proposed to use eminent domain to take a hospital from a for-profit chain and convert it to a public hospital. Faced with the takeover, the chain sold the hospital to a new nonprofit corporation organized by the city and the county to operate the hospital.[183] In

---

[180] Richmond County Hosp. Auth. v. Richmond County, 255 Ga. 183, 336 S.E.2d 562 (1985).

[181] *E.g.*, Kelo v. City of New London, 125 S. Ct. 2655 (U.S. 2005) [integrated development plan is permitted public use]; Long Island Lighting Co. v. Cuomo, 666 F. Supp. 370 (N.D.N.Y. 1987) [upholding state law authorizing eminent domain to take over power company], *vacated*, 888 F.2d 230 (2d Cir. 1989) [moot due to settlement]. Mandating hospital governing board composition is not considered a taking of the hospital. *See* American Hosp. Ass'n v. Hansbarger, 600 F. Supp. 465 (N.D. W.Va. 1984), *aff'd*, 783 F.2d 1184 (4th Cir. 1986), *cert. denied*, 479 U.S. 820 (1986).

[182] Poletown Neighborhood Council v. City of Detroit, 410 Mich. 616, 304 N.W.2d 455 (1981); *City to settle lawsuit for $68 million*, UPI, Apr. 13, 1993 [settlement with hospital owners twelve years later].

[183] Punch, *Faced with takeover, Charter officials will sell St. Louis hospital for $15 million*, MOD. HEALTHCARE, July 19, 1985, 24; *New corporation purchases Charter hospital in St. Louis*, MOD. HEALTHCARE, Nov. 8, 1985, 11.

1991, there was a proposal in Miami, Florida to use eminent domain to take a hospital for public use, but the proposal was abandoned.[184] In 2002, in California, the newly formed North Sonoma County Hospital District acquired the Healdsburg General Hospital through eminent domain.[185]

In 1998, a Missouri appellate court ruled that a city could not use eminent domain to take over a nonprofit private hospital after it reduced services and entered a lease to another operator. The court found the property already committed to a public use and ruled that eminent domain could not be used to convert such property to another public use without specific statutory authority.[186]

2-5.3 Conversion Between Types of Public Organizations

Some states have converted hospitals that were state agencies into separate public entities, frequently called hospital authorities.[187] The hospitals remain public, but they are governed by a separate public board rather than by the state administrative structure. These reorganizations are usually done to give the institutions more flexibility to deal with market forces than is generally permitted for state agencies.

2-5.4 Conversion Between Secular and Religious Organizations

Conversions from secular to religious and from religious to secular organizations have led to controversies. Some controversies have arisen over control and distribution of proceeds from the transaction.[188] The controversy has often arisen from the desire of religious organizations to prohibit the use of their facilities for certain proce-

---

[184] *Dade may force hospital to sell to ease crowding at Jackson*, MIAMI HERALD [FL], Mar. 4, 1991, 1B [proposal to take Cedars Medical Center]; *Cedars to fight bid to take over hospital*, MIAMI HERALD [FL], Mar. 23, 1991, 4B.

[185] G.V. Moser & T.L. Driscoll, *Going public*, THE RECORDER [San Francisco, CA], Jan. 1, 2003, 4.

[186] City of Smithville v. St. Luke's Northland Hosp. Corp., 972 S.W.2d 416 (Mo. Ct. App. 1998).

[187] *E.g.*, COLO. REV. STAT. 23-21-501 et seq.; WIS. STAT. ch. 233.

[188] *E.g.*, *Methodist ministers reviewing proposed sale of Wesley to HCA*, MOD. HEALTHCARE, Jan. 18, 1985, 9; *Wesley trustees, church approve sale*, MOD. HEALTHCARE, Feb. 15, 1985, 35 [358 to 252 vote by United Methodist Church; church to get payments from part of interest income on proceeds and get some control over foundation]; J. Moore, *Church, hospital clash*, MOD. HEALTHCARE, Oct. 6, 1997, 1 [Bethany Med. Ctr.]; Kansas East Conf. of United Methodist Church v. Bethany Med. Ctr., No. 97-C-308 (Kan. Dist. Ct. Sept. 26, 1997), *as discussed in* 6 H.L.R. 1517 (1997) [hospital allowed to sell assets].

dures that violate their beliefs.[189] Religious organizations have had difficulty entering into transactions that result in the loss of that control.[190] However, some sales of religious hospitals have occurred with loss of control.[191] Mergers present more difficulties because religious organizations generally will not participate in the ongoing operations of facilities that violate their beliefs. This has led to community concerns about the loss of the availability of services, especially when there are no alternate providers nearby.[192] In some cases, it has been possible to facilitate alternate providers.

2-6 What Are the Issues When an Organization Is Merged, Consolidated, Sold, or Dissolved?

MERGER OR CONSOLIDATION. *Merger* occurs when two or more organizations combine and one organization is the survivor. *Consolidation* (sometimes also called a merger in nonlegal contexts) occurs when two or more organizations combine and the result is an entirely new organization.[193] In a merger or consolidation, the resulting organization assumes the assets and liabilities of the former organizations.

SALE. Without any merger or consolidation, an organization or facility can be sold so that it has a new owner. Sometimes the new owner is a large organization.[194] and sometimes it is another local organization. Usually, the organization or facility is sold as an ongoing

---

189 M.C. Jaklevic, *Market forces hospital to lose Catholic status*, MOD. HEALTHCARE, Mar. 6, 1995, 40 [abandoning religious status so it can be sold to non-Catholic system].

190 *As health mergers rise, standards of Catholics face a new challenge*, N.Y. TIMES, Mar. 8, 1995, A11.

191 *E.g.*, *Catholic hospital finalizes sale to for-profit chain*, AM. MED. NEWS, Apr. 13, 1998, 34 [St. Louis Univ. Hosp.]; M. Moran, *Catholic leaders protest teaching hospital's sale to for-profit*, AM. MED. NEWS, Jan. 26, 1998, 4 [St. Louis Univ. Hospital]; V. Foubister, *L.A. hospital deal OK'd after endowment fund established*, AM. MED. NEWS, June 8, 1998, 14 [Queen of Angels Hosp.]; *Attorney General approves Queen of Angels sale to Tenet*, 7 H.L.R. 823 (1998); *Queen of Angels board amends bylaws to eliminate need for bishop's approval*, 7 H.L.R. 493 (1998); *Queen of Angels dispute centers around religious law*, 7 H.L.R. 367 (1998); *Los Angeles Archbishop formally opposes sale of hospital to Tenet*, 7 H.L.R. 322 (1998) [Queen of Angels].

192 E. Fein, *Catholic hospitals in nonsectarian merger deals set off abortion concerns*, N.Y. TIMES, Oct. 14, 1997, A17; L. Kertesz, *Community voices concern over hospital's Catholic affiliation*, MOD. HEALTHCARE, Feb. 13, 1995, 40; *ACLU may sue over dropped services*, MOD. HEALTHCARE, Feb. 13, 1995, 41 [elimination of contraceptive services after merger with Catholic hospital].

193 *E.g.*, Larkin, *Financial woes force L.A. hospitals to merge*, 63 HOSPS. (July 5, 1989), 28.

194 *E.g.*, *Hospital corp. completes sale of 104 hospitals*, WALL ST. J., Sept. 18, 1987, 20 [sale of 104 hospitals by Hospital Corporation of America to Heathtrust, Inc.].

entity with the buyer assuming the assets and liabilities. Sometimes only the assets are sold, and the liabilities are not assumed.[195] This is often not feasible, if the intention is to continue to operate the facility, due to requirements for new licenses, other regulatory approvals, and Medicaid and other payer contracts.

When the owner of a facility has been excluded from Medicare and Medicaid participation, one way for the facility to restore Medicare and Medicaid participation is to change the ownership of the facility to an owner that is not excluded. Sometimes the Center for Medicare and Medicaid Services (CMS) will permit a facility to participate during a transition period while the sale is arranged, provided the facility is operated by independent management that is acceptable to CMS.[196]

PROCEDURES. Proper procedures must be followed in a merger, consolidation, or sale, including procedures required by statutes applicable to constituent organizations, by their articles of incorporation, and by their bylaws. Some governmental organizations have special requirements that can include a vote of the residents of the governmental unit, such as a county. When one or more of the organizations is dissolved in the process, the applicable procedures for dissolution must also be followed.

The selection of the proper approach requires a careful analysis that is beyond the scope of this book.[197] Combination or sale of organizations is often difficult in practice[198] due to (1) philosophical differences, especially religious orientations; (2) reduction in the number of leadership positions; (3) necessary changes in established relationships with physicians, employees, suppliers, the community, and others; and (4) the technical complexity of developing an acceptable approach and obtaining necessary approvals.

Some of the legal considerations in developing the proper approach are restrictions in state statutes, articles of incorporation, bylaws, deeds, grants, gifts, loans, collective bargaining agreements,[199] and other legal documents. For example, if certain

---

[195] *But see* United States v. Vernon Home Health, Inc., 21 F.3d 693 (5th Cir.), *cert. denied*, 513 U.S. 1015 (1994) [asset purchaser liable to U.S. for Medicare overpayments to prior owner, state law preempted].

[196] *E.g.*, *Golden Valley hospital has Medicare reinstated*, AP, May 22, 2002.

[197] *See* Greene, *Administrators, attorneys have different approaches to mergers*, MOD. HEALTHCARE, July 21, 1989, 38.

[198] *E.g.*, D. Burda, *Iowa merger off as boards disagree*, MOD. HEALTHCARE, Feb. 20, 1995, 8.

[199] *E.g.*, Asseo v. Hospital San Francisco, Inc., 1988 U.S. Dist. LEXIS 11873 (D. P.R.) [acquiring hospital found to be successor corporation and obligated to bargain with nurses' union].

changes are made, Hill-Burton hospital construction grants must be repaid to the government,[200] some loans can require accelerated repayment,[201] and some depreciation can be recaptured by governmental payers.[202] There are also complex tax and reimbursement implications. One hospital had to take its case to the California Supreme Court to establish that it did not have to pay sales tax on the sale of its furnishings and equipment as part of the sale of all the assets of the hospital.[203] Proper notification must be given to licensure, certificate-of-need, and other regulatory authorities, and in some cases licenses, certificates, or permits must be obtained. Some types of changes may even involve federal securities law.

In 1950, the Attorney General of Missouri challenged a proposed affiliation of Barnard Free Skin and Cancer Hospital with Washington University Medical Center that involved relocation of Barnard Hospital.[204] The Attorney General asserted that the proposal violated several provisions of the gifts and will of Mr. Barnard that established and supported Barnard Hospital. The Missouri Supreme Court found the affiliation contract to be a reasonable exercise of board powers that did not violate any conditions imposed by gifts and bequests of Mr. Barnard.

In any merger, consolidation, or sale, consideration must be given to antitrust implications. (See Chapter 13.)

DISSOLUTION. An organization can *dissolve* as part of a closure or a reorganization, merger, or consolidation. The facility might continue to operate under another organization, or the services of the facility might be relocated or discontinued. Proper procedures must be followed in any dissolution, including the procedures in applicable statutes, articles of incorporation, and bylaws. The procedures usually include (1) an approval mechanism, which can involve a

---

[200] *E.g.*, 15 U.S.C. § 291i; United States v. St. John's Gen. Hosp., 875 F.2d 1064 (3d Cir. 1989); United States v. Coweta County Hosp. Auth., 603 F. Supp. 111 (N.D. Ga. 1984), *aff'd*, 777 F.2d 667 (11th Cir. 1985); *see also* National Med. Enters., Inc. v. United States, 28 Fed. Cl. 540 (1993), *appeal dismissed*, 14 F.3d 612 (Fed. Cir. 1993) [20-year lease is a transfer of hospital triggering Hill-Burton recovery].

[201] *E.g.*, IRS PLR No. 9427025 (Apr. 11, 1994); *Hospital sale to for-profit firm requires bond redemption in 90 days*, 3 H.L.R. 971 (1994).

[202] *E.g.*, Sandpoint Convalescent Servs., Inc. v. Idaho Dep't of Health & Welfare, 114 Idaho 281, 756 P.2d 398 (1988) [recapture of Medicaid depreciation payments not unconstitutional].

[203] *E.g.*, Creighton Omaha Reg. Health Care Corp. v. Sullivan, 950 F.2d 563 (8th Cir. 1991) [recapture of Medicare depreciation]; Bethesda Found. v. Nebraska Dep't of Social Servs., 498 N.W.2d 86 (Neb. 1993) [state recapture of Medicaid depreciation on sale to for-profit organization].

[204] Taylor v. Baldwin, 362 Mo. 1224, 247 S.W.2d 741 (1952).

state administrative official, a court, or a vote of a specified percentage of the stockholders, members of the corporation, or others; (2) a notification of creditors and others; and (3) clearance by governmental tax departments. Some governmental hospitals have special requirements, including a vote of the residents of the district, city, or county that supports the organization.

Usually, authority to dissolve a corporation is clear, but it is sometimes questioned. When a Missouri nonprofit hospital association chartered to provide hospital services to employees of a railroad company sold its hospital and was distributing the assets to members, several members challenged the dissolution of the association.[205] The court found the dissolution to be beyond the authority of the board under Missouri law because it was not expressly authorized by the articles of incorporation; not approved by a sufficient percentage of the membership; and not of imperative necessity because there was a reasonable prospect of successfully continuing the business.

Dissolution can be voluntarily initiated by the organization. In appropriate circumstances, dissolution of a corporation can be involuntarily initiated by outside parties, such as the state attorney general, shareholders, directors, and creditors.[206] A person called a *receiver* can be appointed to operate the organization during the process of involuntary dissolution. Appointment of a receiver is not limited to dissolutions. For example, as mentioned earlier in this chapter, receivers can be appointed on a temporary basis while a court sorts out who should control the organization.

The corporation continues for a period of time after it ceases to operate the facility so that the affairs of the organization can be concluded. After satisfying any debts and liabilities that have not been assumed by other organizations, the assets of the corporation must be distributed. Some assets might have to be returned to those who gave them to the organization or to others designated by the giver because of restrictions imposed on the grants or gifts. All other assets are distributed under a plan of distribution that might have to be approved by an administrative agency or court. Assets of for-profit corporations are distributed to their shareholders. Assets designated for charitable purposes must usually be distributed to a

---

[205] McDaniel v. Frisco Employees' Hosp. Ass'n, 510 S.W.2d 752 (Mo. Ct. App. 1974).
[206] *E.g.*, WIS. STAT. § 180.1430.

corporation or organization engaged in activities that are substantially similar to those of the dissolving corporation.

Some nonprofit corporations choose not to dissolve after selling their assets. They continue as independent foundations and use the proceeds of the sale of the business for other charitable purposes, such as paying for indigent patient care.[207]

2-7 What Are the Issues When an Organization Closes or Relocates a Hospital or Other Delivery Location?

A hospital building or other health care facility can close (1) as part of relocation of functions or (2) without transfer or replacement of the functions because they are viewed as excess capacity or are otherwise not viable. Some communities have challenged planned closures, causing costly delays. Although courts have seldom found the plans illegal, some of the challenges have resulted in modifications of the plans. It is important to determine community concerns when planning relocations and closures and to consider reasonable accommodations to avoid protracted challenges.[208]

One example that illustrates the extent to which opponents can go in challenging closure is the Wilmington Medical Center cases. Two private hospitals in Wilmington, Delaware planned to replace a large portion of their inner-city facilities with one suburban hospital. Various opponents conducted an extensive legal challenge. The plaintiffs claimed that the Medicare law had been violated,[209] that the relocation discriminated against minorities in violation of Title VI of the Civil Rights Act[210] and against the handicapped in violation

---

[207] *E.g.*, J. Greene, *Are foundations bearing fruit?* MOD. HEALTHCARE, Mar. 20, 1995, 53; Coady, *Not-for-profits, beware - Foundation formed by sale could be short-lived*, MOD. HEALTHCARE, Mar. 29, 1985, 138; Carland, *Computer model used to evaluate foundation had flawed assumptions*, MOD. HEALTHCARE, June 7, 1985), 177; D.W. Coyne & K.R. Kas, *The not-for-profit hospital as a charitable trust: To whom does its value belong?* 24 J. HEALTH & HOSP. L. 48 (1991); *see also Big charities born of nonprofit-to-profit shifts*, WALL ST. J., Apr. 4, 1995, B1 [conversions of Blue Cross and other nonprofit health plans].

[208] *E.g.*, Mussington v. St. Luke's-Roosevelt Hosp. Ctr., 18 F.3d 1033 (2d Cir. 1994), *aff'g*, 824 F. Supp. 427 (S.D.N.Y. 1993) [individuals, three churches sued to stop transfer of hospital services from minority low income neighborhood, but all claims barred by laches or statute of limitations]; Greenpoint Hosp. Comm. Bd. v. New York City Health & Hosps. Corp., 114 A.D.2d 1028, 495 N.Y.S.2d 467 (2d Dept. 1985) [hospital found in contempt of court for violating order on consultations with community board].

[209] 42 U.S.C. § 1320a-1, which was announced not to be enforced, 53 FED. REG. 10,431 (Mar. 31, 1988).

[210] 42 U.S.C. §§ 2000d-2000d-6.

of section 504 of the Rehabilitation Act of 1973,[211] and that an environmental impact statement was required under the National Environmental Policy Act of 1969.[212] A court required the Secretary of the Department of Health, Education, and Welfare (HEW) to determine whether there had been any violation and report to the court.[213] The court ruled that an environmental impact statement was not required because no major federal action was involved[214] and ruled that it was constitutional to provide different administrative appeal procedures for recipients and complainants under Title VI and section 504.[215] The court ruled that the approval of the project by HEW was not subject to judicial review and that it was constitutional not to provide an appeal mechanism for opponents.[216] In the fifth reported decision, the court ruled that there was a private right of action to challenge discrimination that violated Title VI or section 504 and ordered a trial.[217] After the trial, the court ruled that the evidence was adequate to justify the reorganization and relocation plans; so they did not violate Title VI or section 504.[218]

In 1998, a federal appellate court rejected a challenge to a municipal hospital's relocation of services for disabled children, finding that neither the Rehabilitation Act of 1973 nor the Americans with Disabilities Act guaranteed a level of medical care for the disabled.[219]

In June 2001, the inpatient services at D.C. General Hospital were closed. The closure was challenged in court by two city counsel members and a union representing medical residents. In 2001, a federal court rejected the challenge finding that the union did not have standing and the city counsel members did not state a legal claim because the closure was properly authorized.[220]

---

[211] 29 U.S.C. § 794.

[212] 42 U.S.C. § 4332.

[213] NAACP v. Wilmington Med. Ctr., Inc., 426 F. Supp. 919 (D. Del. 1977).

[214] NAACP v. Wilmington Med. Ctr., Inc., 436 F. Supp. 1194 (D. Del. 1977), aff'd, 584 F.2d 619 (3d Cir. 1978).

[215] NAACP v. Wilmington Med. Ctr., Inc., 453 F. Supp. 330 (D. Del. 1978).

[216] Wilmington United Neighborhoods v. United States, Dep't of HEW, 458 F. Supp. 628 (D. Del. 1978), aff'd, 615 F.2d 112 (3d Cir.), cert. denied, 449 U.S. 827 (1980).

[217] NAACP v. Medical Ctr., Inc., 599 F.2d 1247 (3d Cir. 1979), rev'g, 453 F. Supp. 289 (D. Del. 1978).

[218] NAACP v. Wilmington Med. Ctr., Inc., 491 F. Supp. 290 (D. Del. 1980), aff'd, 657 F.2d 1322 (3d Cir. 1981).

[219] Lincoln CERCPAC v. Health & Hosps. Corp., 147 F.3d 165 (2d Cir. 1998).

[220] Chavous v. District of Columbia Fin. Responsibility & Mgmt. Assistance Auth., 154 F. Supp. 2d 40 (D. D.C. 2001).

Some courts find that neither patients nor citizens have a right to challenge decisions to close public hospitals.[221] However, when a court ordered consultation with a community board, failure to do so was contempt of court.[222]

In the 1960s, a New Jersey city sought to enjoin a hospital from relocating outside city limits.[223] The court denied the injunction because the hospital had legally amended its articles of incorporation to give the board authority to relocate and the board had found relocation to be in the hospital's best interests.

Sometimes a hospital is forced to close. In 2001, Edgewater Medical Center in Chicago closed. Medicare had stopped making payments after a grand jury indicted three doctors, an administrator, and a hospital management firm for an alleged kickback scheme. When a federal judge refused to order reinstatement of Medicare payments, all patients were discharged or transferred and the hospital closed.[224]

Public hospitals frequently must obtain voter approval before closing. Some consumer groups have attempted to use these requirements to preclude the hospital from changing its services. For example, a group in Texas sought to bar the closure of an emergency room of a public hospital. The group asserted that closing the emergency room was equivalent to closing the hospital; so the requirement of a vote before the hospital could be closed should apply. In 1984, a Texas appellate court ruled that they were not equivalent; so no vote was required.[225]

Some states impose a duty on local government to provide certain health care services. In 2004, a federal appellate court affirmed a preliminary injunction stopping Los Angeles County from closing a county rehabilitation center or reducing the number of beds at the USC Medical Center. The court said that the proposed closures

---

[221] *E.g.*, Citizens for State Hosp. v. Commonwealth, 123 Pa. Commw. 150, 553 A.2d 496 (1989), *cert. denied*, 494 U.S. 1017 (1990) [citizens]; Punikaia v. Clark, 720 F.2d 564 (9th Cir. 1983), *cert. denied*, 469 U.S. 816 (1984) [patient residents of leprosarium had no property interest in continued operation of facility, so not entitled to hearing before closure].

[222] Greenpoint Hosp. Comm. Bd. v. N.Y.C. Health and Hosps. Corp., 114 A.D.2d 1028, 495 N.Y.S.2d 467 (2d Dept. 1985).

[223] City of Paterson v. Paterson Gen. Hosp., 97 N.J. Super. 514, 235 A.2d 487 (Ch. Div. 1967).

[224] *Edgewater hospital closes*, AP, Dec. 7, 2001.

[225] Jackson County Hosp. Dist. v. Jackson County Citizens for Continued Hosp. Care, 669 S.W.2d 147 (Tex. Ct. App. 1984).

could violate the state law duty of California counties to provide health care services.[226]

Contractual barriers to closure can also arise. An Arkansas court ordered a corporation to continue to operate a nursing home on a certain property because it had promised to do so in the lease to the property.[227] In many circumstances, federal law requires that employees be given sixty days notice of closings or large layoffs.[228] Employee challenges to closure have generally been unsuccessful.[229] However, a federal appellate court ruled that a union was entitled to obtain copies of some transactional documents from a hospital that was closing so that the union could determine worker rights and union responsibilities.[230]

Care must be taken in carrying out the closure. In 1994, all the patients were discharged from a small Florida hospital, but the hospital did not relinquish its license or its Certificate of Need while it pursued sale or consolidation. The city sued to stop the closure. After the hospital refused to treat an emergency patient, the state initiated proceedings to revoke the hospital license. The owner settled with the state, agreeing to transfer ownership by a specified date or lose the license.[231]

2-8 What Is the Impact of Bankruptcy Law?

When health care entities and those with whom they do business become insolvent, it is important to understand the impact of bankruptcy law. Even large hospital systems can become insolvent and enter the bankruptcy process. In 1998, a multihospital system, the

---

[226] Rodde v. Bonta, 357 F.3d 988 (9th Cir. 2004); Harris v. Board of Supervisors, 366 F.3d 754 (9th Cir. 2004).

[227] Lonoke Nursing Home, Inc. v. Wayne & Neil Bennett Family P'ship, 12 Ark. App. 282, 676 S.W.2d 461, *adhered to* (en banc), 12 Ark. App. 286, 679 S.W.2d 823 (1984).

[228] 29 U.S.C. §§ 2101-2109; *but see* Jurcev v. Central Comm. Hosp., 7 F.3d 618 (7th Cir. 1993), *cert. denied*, 511 U.S. 1081 (1994) [hospital closure with two weeks notice did not violate WARN because closure due to unforeseeable business circumstance of foundation decision to stop payments to hospital].

[229] *E.g.*, Brindle v. West Allegheny Hosp., 406 Pa. Super. 572, 594 A.2d 766 (1991) [dismissed claim by six nurses of fraud in closure of hospital].

[230] Mary Thompson Hosp. v. NLRB, 943 F.2d 741 (7th Cir. 1991).

[231] City of Destin v. Columbia/HCA Healthcare Corp., No. 94-17015-CA (Fla. Cir. Ct. Okaloosa County filed June 15, 1994) [city suit]; Agency for Health Care Admin. v. Fort Walton Beach Med. Ctr., HQA No. 01-094-005-HOSP (complaint filed Aug. 22, 1994 & settled Aug. 30, 1994) [license revocation proceeding], *as discussed in* 3 H.L.R 877, 1207 & 1280 (1994).

Allegheny Health, Education & Research Foundation, entered bankruptcy.[232]

For bankruptcy purposes, the Federal Bankruptcy Reform Act of 1978 (called the *Bankruptcy Code*) defines an entity as being "insolvent"

> ...when the sum of such entity's debts is greater than all of such entity's property, at fair evaluation, exclusive of (i) property transferred, concealed, or removed with intent to hinder, delay or defraud such entity's creditors, and (ii) property that may be exempted....[233]

When a health care organization discovers that it is insolvent and cannot work out other arrangements with creditors, it might need to consider bankruptcy to settle its accounts and obligations on an equitable and final basis.Because bankruptcy proceedings are entirely a matter of federal law, they are conducted in the federal district courts under the provisions of the Bankruptcy Code. A petition for bankruptcy can be voluntary (by the debtor) or involuntary (by creditors).

Nonprofit corporations, including charitable hospitals, are not subject to involuntary bankruptcy; so they cannot be forced into bankruptcy by creditors. Domestic insurance companies are not subject to bankruptcy. This restriction has led to numerous cases addressing whether health maintenance organizations and life care facilities are insurance companies and, thus, not subject to federal bankruptcy. The answer depends on how they are treated under state law.[234] The only remedy available to creditors of a nonprofit organization or insurance company is through applicable state law proceedings.[235] Nonprofit corporations, but not insurance companies, can voluntarily petition to be adjudicated bankrupt. Petitions can be filed with the federal court even after state insolvency proceedings have been instituted.

---

[232] *E.g.*, *Hospital bankruptcy crisis examined*, 7 H.L.R. 905 (1998) [American Hosp. Ass'n analysis being examined by congressional committee]. For an example of multihospital system in bankruptcy, *see In re* Allegheny Health, Education & Research Found., No. 98-25773 to 98-25777 (Bankr. W.D. Pa. filed July 21, 1998).

[233] 11 U.S.C. § 101(31).

[234] 11 U.S.C. § 109; *e.g.*, *In re* Estate of Medcare HMO, 998 F.2d 436 (7th Cir. 1993) [HMO not subject to bankruptcy]; *In re* Mich. Master Health Plan, Inc., 90 Bankr. 274 (E.D. Mich.1985) [HMO subject to bankruptcy because not insurance company under state law]; *In re* Florida Brethren Homes, 88 Bankr. 445 (Bankr. S.D. Fla. 1988) [life care facility subject to bankruptcy because not insurance company under state law].

[235] *E.g.*, V. Foubister, *State declares HIP of New Jersey insolvent*, AM. MED. NEWS, Nov. 23/30, 1998, 11.

Bankruptcy does not necessarily require the corporation to dissolve. While bankruptcy under Chapter 7 of the Bankruptcy Code does include dissolution, bankruptcy under Chapter 11 permits the corporation to continue to operate through modification of its operations and debt structure.

Most lawsuits and other actions against a debtor must stop when the petition for bankruptcy is filed. This is called the *automatic stay*.[236] There are some exceptions,[237] and there are procedures creditors can follow to seek permission from the bankruptcy court to pursue their suits, which is generally called "relief from stay."[238] There are also restrictions on others changing their relationships with the debtor. For example, a federal appellate court ruled that a malpractice insurance company could not cancel insurance without notice to the court and creditors.[239] Clauses in contracts that purport to permit termination of the contract if a party becomes bankrupt are not enforceable in most situations.

When the health care organization is a creditor, it is important to file in the bankruptcy court most claims against the debtor, or the claims might be lost.

In bankruptcy proceedings, the debtor or bankruptcy trustee has an opportunity to either assume or reject most ongoing contracts.[240] This has been most controversial when debtors have sought to reject collective bargaining agreements; so the Bankruptcy Code was amended to permit rejections of collective bargaining agreements only after a court finds that certain conditions exist and approves the rejection or modification.[241] Limits have also been placed on the modification of insurance benefits to retired employees.[242]

---

[236] 11 U.S.C. § 362.

[237] *E.g.*, *In re* Grau, 172 Bankr. 686 (Bkrtcy. S.D. Fla. 1994) [not violation of automatic stay for malpractice creditor to have communication with state licensing board concerning failure of debtor doctor to pay judgment where first report filed prepetition].

[238] 11 U.S.C. § 362(c), (d); *e.g.*, *In re* Corporacion de Servicos, 60 Bankr. 920 (D. P.R. 1986), *aff'd*, 805 F.2d 440 (1st Cir. 1986) [exemption from automatic stay for state regulatory actions does not apply when effort to revoke hospital license is subterfuge to force termination of management contract]; *In re* Bel Air Chateau Hosp., Inc., 611 F.2d 1248 (9th Cir. 1979) [NLRB proceedings not subject to automatic stay, but can be stayed if assets threatened].

[239] *In re* Lavigne, 114 F.3d 379 (2d Cir. 1997).

[240] 11 U.S.C. § 365; *e.g.*, *In re* Corporacion de Servicios Medicos Hospitalarios de Fajardo, 60 Bankr. 920 (D. P.R. 1986), *aff'd*, 805 F.2d 440 (1st Cir. 1986) [assumption of hospital management contract]; *In re* Reph Acquisition Co., 134 Bankr. 194 (N.D. Tex. 1991) [debtor's interest in hospital lease deemed rejected when failed to assume lease within allotted time].

[241] 11 U.S.C. § 1113; *e.g.*, *In re* Sierra Steel Corp., 88 Bankr. 337 (Bankr. D. Colo. 1988) [approval of modifications in collective bargaining agreement].

[242] 11 U.S.C. § 1114.

The bankruptcy court has broad powers to undo many transactions that occurred before the filing if they are considered to be preferences that favor one creditor improperly or fraudulent transfers that tried to place assets improperly beyond the reach of creditors.[243]

When a provider continues to operate after filing for bankruptcy, the state Medicaid agency can recoup prior overpayments by reducing current payments. Even though this would be forbidden if done by a private payer,[244] in 1989, the United States Supreme Court ruled that a state agency can do it because the Eleventh Amendment to the Constitution grants states immunity from money judgments, even those handed down by bankruptcy courts. The bankruptcy court cannot order the state to make full payment unless the state waives its immunity by filing a claim against the provider.[245] The United States Department of Health and Human Services (HHS) is also permitted to recoup Medicare overpayments.[246] While bankruptcy courts have broad powers to extend contractual deadlines in some circumstances, they generally cannot extend Medicare deadlines.[247]

While a debtor is in the bankruptcy process, it must obtain court approval for some major business transactions.[248] In some cases, the bankruptcy court appoints a trustee to operate the business.[249]

For the debtor to successfully leave Chapter 11 bankruptcy, the bankruptcy court must approve a plan for its reorganization.[250] The debtor has the first opportunity to propose a plan. If the plan is not approved, the creditors can develop a plan.

---

[243] *E.g.*, 11 U.S.C. §§ 544, 547, 548, 553; *In re* Sheppard's Dental Centers, Inc., 65 Bankr. 274 (Bankr. S.D. Fla. 1986) [transfer of management agreement can be voidable transfer].

[244] *E.g.*, St. Francis Physician Network, Inc. v. Rush Prudential HMO Inc., 213 Bankr. 710 (N.D. Ill. Bankr. 1997) [bankruptcy law limits HMO's right to deduct from capitation payments to physician networks for sums owed network].

[245] 11 U.S.C. § 106, *as amended by* Pub. L. No. 103-394, § 113, 108 Stat. 4117 (1994); Hoffman v. Connecticut Dep't of Income Maint., 492 U.S. 96 (1989). For an example of waiver by filing a claim, *see* St. Joseph Hosp. v. Dep't. of Pub. Welfare, 103 Bankr. 643 (Bankr. E.D. Pa. 1989).

[246] United States v. Consumer Health Servs., 323 U.S. App. D.C. 336, 108 F.3d 390 (1997).

[247] *E.g.*, *In re* Ludlow Hosp. Soc'y, 124 F.3d 22 (1st Cir. 1997) [bankruptcy court cannot extend time to sell capital assets subject to depreciation credits after terminating Medicare participation].

[248] *E.g.*, *AMH seeks court approval for sale of Calif. facility*, MOD. HEALTHCARE, Oct. 14, 1988, 8.

[249] *E.g.*, *Care creditors ask court to remove chain's owners*, MOD. HEALTHCARE, June 2, 1989, 7.

[250] *E.g.*, *Bankruptcy judge OKs hospital reorganization plan*, AP, Aug. 5, 2003 [Crouse Hosp., Syracuse, N.Y.]; *In re* Community Hosp. of the Valleys, 51 Bankr. 231 (Bankr. 9th Cir. 1985), *aff'd*, 820 F.2d 1097 (9th Cir. 1987) [confirmation of reorganization plan]; *In re* Medical Equities, Inc., 39 Bankr. 795 (Bankr. S.D. Ohio 1984) [denial of confirmation]; *Judge says plan to reopen hospital is unworkable*, MOD. HEALTHCARE, Sept. 2, 1988, 14 [bankruptcy court rejected community group reorganization plan].

In a Chapter 7 bankruptcy, the assets of the debtor are sold, and the proceeds are distributed to the creditors in a priority order specified by the Bankruptcy Code.

An important aspect of either Chapter 7 or Chapter 11 is that the court can discharge some debts so that the debtor is protected from personal liability on those debts.[251] Liability for willful and malicious injuries is not discharged in bankruptcy. But in 1998, the United States Supreme Court ruled that medical malpractice judgments generally do not fit in this exception; so they are discharged in bankruptcy.[252] In 2005, the bankruptcy law was extensively amended to reduce the opportunity for the discharge of debts and to make other changes.[253]

Another extraordinary power of the bankruptcy court is that it can authorize the sale of property free and clear of prior interests in the property. Thus, it can extinguish liens, mortgages, judgment, writs of garnishment, and the like. The applicability of bias claims and settlements obligations to the property can also be extinguished. In 2003, a federal appellate court upheld a bankruptcy court ruling that the purchaser of the assets of a bankrupt airline company would be free and clear of twenty-nine bias claims against the bankrupt company pending before the Equal Employment Opportunity Commission and for ongoing obligations arising out of settlement of prior claims.[254]

The bankruptcy court has broad latitude in the sales arrangements that can be approved. In 2003, a federal bankruptcy court authorized an auction to sell a hospital in the District of Columbia.[255]

Health care organizations facing insolvency need to evaluate their options in order to avoid personal liability for directors and to use the available bankruptcy proceedings to optimize the outcome. Directors can be personally liable for voting to authorize improper distribution of corporate assets when the corporation is insolvent.[256] Bankruptcy proceedings can often be used to implement changes that permit the institution to survive.

---

[251] *E.g.*, 11 U.S.C. §§ 523, 524, 727, 1141(d).

[252] Kawaauhau v. Geiger, 523 U.S. 57 (1998).

[253] Bankruptcy Abuse Prevention and Consumer Protection Act of 2005, Pub. L. No. 109-8 [most changes are effective in October 2005]; S. Block, *Filing Chapter 7 bankruptcy will get tougher soon*, USA TODAY, Apr. 21, 2005, 4B.

[254] *In re* Transworld Airlines, Inc., 18 F.3d 208 (3d Cir. 2003).

[255] A. Goldstein, *Judge to allow auction of hospital in SE*, WASHINGTON POST, Nov. 23, 2003, B6; B. Brubaker, *Tuft's group wins auction for hospitals*, WASHINGTON POST, Dec. 18, 2003, E1.

[256] Renger Mem. Hosp. v. State, 674 S.W.2d 828 (Tex. Ct. App. 1984).

Discussion Points

1. What are six types of organizations, and what are their major differences?
2. How do government organizations differ from other organizations?
3. How does government control nonprofit corporations?
4. What rights do shareholders have in for-profit corporations?
5. Discuss the impact of Sarbanes-Oxley on for-profit corporations and nonprofit corporations.
6. What is the source of corporate authority, and what happens when a corporation acts outside that authority?
7. What are the duties of board members? Discuss the "business judgment" rule. When can board members be held personally liable?
8. What are some of the potential self-dealing and conflicts of interest of board members, and how should they be addressed?
9. What are the duties of CEOs, and what is the source of their authority? When can CEOs be held personally liable?
10. What is the difference between licensure and accreditation? What is the role of the Medicare Conditions of Participation?
11. When can licensing rules be successfully challenged?
12. What are the consequences for violating licensing rules?
13. Discuss the issues involved in converting an organization from one type to another. What approvals are usually required?
14. Discuss the issues involved when an organization ceases to exist due to merger, consolidation, sale, or closure. What approvals are usually required?
15. Discuss the issues involved when a service delivery site is closed or relocated. What are the grounds for challenging such changes?
16. What is the effect on the provider and others when a health care provider seeks protection under the bankruptcy law?

CHAPTER THREE

Creation and Maintenance of Physical Resources

Objectives

The objective of this chapter is to provide an overview of the legal aspects of the creation and maintenance of the physical resources necessary to deliver health care services, including land and buildings, equipment, other devices, drugs, supplies, blood, biologicals, and tissues. The reader should learn many of the ways that government regulates these physical resources.

Health care services delivery requires physical resources. Hospitals, skilled nursing facilities, physician offices, and many other providers require land and buildings. Some services, such as home services, might not require land and buildings. Virtually all health care services require equipment, other devices, drugs, and supplies. Some health care services require blood, biologicals, and tissues.

This chapter surveys the types of regulations concerning the creation and maintenance of these physical resources.

Related topics are addressed in other chapters. Relocation and closure of facilities is addressed in Chapter 2. The decision to create or maintain a specific physical resource is often determined by the availability of financing or coverage by third-party reimbursement. These issues are discussed in Chapters 9 and 10. Taxability of property can also be a factor and is discussed in Chapter 9.

This section addresses:

3-1. What land use, construction, and other permitting regulations are applicable to health care facilities?

3-2. What are the licensure requirements for health care facilities?

3-3. What are the regulations concerning the manufacture and use of drugs, medical devices, tissues, and other items used in health care?

3-1 What Land Use, Construction, and Other Permitting Regulations Are Applicable to Health Care Facilities?

There are several types of regulations with which most health care facilities must comply. First, zoning requirements (3-1.1) specify where facilities can be built. Second, building codes (3-1.2) specify how most health care facilities must be designed. Third, when new facilities are built or major modifications are made to existing facilities, usually a building permit (3-1.3) must be obtained. Fourth, in some states, a certificate-of-need (3-1.4) must be obtained from the state before some facilities can be built.

The stated basis for zoning requirements and building permits is usually public health and safety, and in most cases, this is the purpose for which they are used. However, sometimes local governments withhold their approval until the health care entity agrees to financial or operational demands.

3-1.1 Zoning Requirements

Zoning ordinances are laws adopted by local governments that specify where certain types of land use are permitted. Zoning laws are an important part of governmental efforts to assure orderly land development and compatibility of uses that encourages investment in homes, businesses, and other uses. Zoning ordinances can also limit the height, size, and design of buildings. Zoning is what protects hospitals from new incompatible uses of nearby land, but zoning can also be a barrier to opening a new health care building or making substantial changes in some existing services. Frequently, the required approvals are granted without difficulty.[1] Sometimes these

---

[1] *E.g., Commission OKs rezoning for hospital parking lot*, Tampa Tribune, Aug. 19, 2000, 2.

limitations can restrict expansion or require time-consuming efforts to obtain waivers, variances, or amendments to zoning ordinances.

When zoning authorities impose too many restrictions, health care facilities must look for other locations. For example, in 2002, a Wisconsin hospital had to look for a different clinic site when zoning authorities placed severe size and operating hour restrictions on any clinic on the hospital's land.[2]

Local ordinances usually are not permitted to exclude hospitals or other health care uses, but they can require hospitals to be located in specified areas. Local governments can be required to permit certain exceptions to their zoning requirements when necessary to avoid discrimination against the disabled. In 2004, a federal court in Wisconsin ordered the City of Milwaukee to issue a special use permit to a community service program that provided services to persons with mental impairments. The court found that the Americans with Disabilities Act required the city to permit this use as a reasonable and necessary accommodation.[3]

Zoning rulings can also create problems after projects are commenced. In 1988, a Florida hospital obtained a building permit for a staff tower and diagnostic clinic. The tower was designed to provide offices for the medical staff. After construction was commenced, the city attorney issued an opinion that the term "staff offices" in the zoning ordinance permitted offices only for physicians employed full-time by the hospital. Because most of the medical staff members were not full-time employees, this ruling made it impossible to obtain permanent construction funding or to lease the office space. In 1989, a federal court issued a preliminary injunction preventing enforcement of the interpretation because it was likely the hospital could show due process violations.[4] The hospital and city settled, with the city dropping its interpretation, the hospital agreeing to pay property taxes on the building, and the physicians with offices in the building being subject to an annual city occupational license fee.[5]

---

[2] *Council decision prompts hospital to look for new site*, MILWAUKEE JOURNAL SENTINEL, July 19, 2002, 5B.

[3] Wisconsin Cmty. Serv. v. City of Milwaukee, 309 F. Supp. 2d 1096 (E.D. Wis. 2004).

[4] Mount Sinai Med. Ctr. v. City of Miami Beach, 706 F. Supp. 1525 (S.D. Fla. 1989).

[5] *Miami Beach settles with Mount Sinai*, FLA. MED. BUS. (S. Fla. ed.), Feb. 28, 1989, 16. For another zoning settlement, *see* MOD. HEALTHCARE, May 5, 1997, 52 [settlement between Alta Bates hospital, city over whether construction was contrary to zoning, permitting laws].

When zoning laws are changed, usually existing uses are permitted to continue as nonconforming uses either indefinitely or for a specified period of time. Generally, there are limits on the improvements that can be made to nonconforming uses. For example, a Pennsylvania court found that a hospital had sufficiently used its helipad to establish it as a nonconforming use; so the hospital did not have to obtain the special exception required for new helipads. The court also ruled that the adding of paving and lighting to the pad did not exceed permitted improvements.[6]

3-1.2 Building Codes

Health care facilities must comply with applicable building and fire safety codes. The most widely applicable code is the Life Safety Code®[7] that protects from fires. Other building codes address other issues ranging from elevators[8] to earthquakes.[9] These codes can provide for inspections of the hospital and other facilities by building inspectors and fire marshals who can either have authority to initiate action through their own agencies or refer the matter to the licensing agency to initiate action. Building and fire safety codes are often enforced through institutional licensing laws.

Compliance with the Life Safety Code® is also required for institutional Medicare participation and for accreditation by bodies like the JCAHO.[10] There are several levels of Life Safety Code® standards. The most expensive standards apply to space that is used for care of inpatients. There is an intermediate standard that applies to ambulatory care facilities, such as surgical centers, that take care of multiple patients who are unable to look out for their own safety due to their underlying condition or the treatment they are receiving. There is a third standard that applies to general business uses where the users are able to look out for their own safety.

---

6   Appeal of Suburban Gen. Hosp., 48 Pa. Commw. 273, 410 A.2d 85 (1980).
7   Life Safety Code® is a registered trademark of the National Fire Protection Association, Quincy, MA.
8   *Board grants four variances*, CAL-OSHA RPTR., Mar. 5, 2004 [variance granted for oversize platform for wheelchair lift].
9   *E.g.*, CAL. HEALTH & SAFETY CODE § 130000 et seq.; T. Pristin, *Decade after big quake, a hospital building boom*, N.Y. TIMES, Nov. 24, 2004, C6.
10 Joint Commission on Accreditation of Healthcare Organizations, 2005 COMPREHENSIVE ACCREDITATION MANUAL FOR HOSPITALS, EC.5.20 [hereinafter the manual is referred to as 2005 JCAHO CAMH].

The Life Safety Code® is changed from time to time. Facilities are usually required to meet the code applicable at the time the facility is approved for construction. Areas that are subject to major renovation usually must meet the standards applicable at the time the renovation is approved.

Generally, local government authorities must issue a permit, often called a certificate of occupancy (CO), before a new building can be used. Usually, the local authorities require a hospital building to pass an inspection by the hospital licensing agency before granting a CO.[11]

3-1.3 Building Permits

In most situations, health care entities, like others, must obtain a building permit in order to construct new facilities or make major changes in existing facilities. Some governmental hospitals are exempt from building permit requirements.

One of the strangest zoning battles concerning a building permit occurred in New York. A hospital obtained a building permit and built a new emergency department, which opened in 2001. Neighbors challenged the permit; so in 2002, a trial court ruled that the permit was not valid because the state environmental impact assessment requirement had not been satisfied. The court ordered the closure of the emergency department until the permit process was repeated with the required assessment. The court postponed the effect of the closure order until appeals were completed. An appellate court upheld the closure order in 2003, and the highest court refused to review the decision in 2004. The trial court then extended the postponement while the hospital and city sought to fulfill the requirements.[12]

---

[11] *E.g.*, Miami Heart Inst. v. Heery Architects & Eng'rs, Inc., 765 F. Supp. 1083 (S.D. Fla. 1991), *aff'd without op.*, 44 F.3d 1007 (11th Cir. 1994) [alleged breach of contract from failure to draw plans, specifications for hospital in accordance with relevant codes; hospital failed inspections by state hospital licensing agency, City of Miami Beach delaying certificate of occupancy for nearly a year].

[12] Coppola v. Good Samaritan Hosp. Med. Ctr., N.Y.L.J., Nov. 2, 2002, 25 [text of trial court order]; E. Holm, *Planning board turns back the clock; Court-ordered review of already-built wing at hospital begins*, NEWSDAY (New York), Apr. 20, 2003, G23; Coppola v. Good Samaritan Hosp. Med. Ctr., 309 A.D.2d 862, 765 N.Y.S.2d 888 (2d Dept. 2003), *app. denied*, 1 N.Y.3d 506 (2004); A. Guardino, *Zoning and land use; Proceeding with caution after negative declaration*, N.Y.L.J., Feb. 17, 2004, 16; L. Jones, *Legal limbo; four-year battle over emergency room reaches new stage*, N.Y.L.J., Mar. 2, 2004, 16; *Court stays enforcement of injunction against emergency room's continued operation*, N.Y.L.J., Mar. 3, 2004, 21.

In some areas, hospital-related facilities are entitled to building permits in situations where other uses could not get permits. For example, in 2004, a New York court upheld a building permit for a cancer research laboratory issued to a cancer hospital in New York City, finding that the laboratory was hospital-related.[13]

3-1.4 Certificate-of-Need Laws

Some states require some health care providers to obtain a certificate of need (CON) from a state agency before expenditures can be made on certain new buildings, equipment, or services.

In the 1970s, all states had CON laws. The National Health Planning and Resources Development Act of 1974[14] required states to have a CON law to qualify for certain federal health funds. The state CON programs were tied into a national health planning system. When the federal requirement was repealed,[15] many states repealed their CON laws, while others changed the scope of projects subject to the requirement.[16]

In states that still have CON laws, health care organizations that plan capital expenditures or program changes must comply with applicable state CON requirements. These requirements define (1) which expenditures are subject to review, (2) the criteria for evaluating need, and (3) the review procedures. Organizations, other than the applicant, will often participate in the review.

States vary in the extent to which they permit organizations providing the same service to challenge the determination of the need for additional competitors. For example, in 1998, the Mississippi Supreme Court permitted competing hospitals to challenge successfully a primary care center.[17] In 2004, a New York court ruled that a competitor did not have standing to challenge approval of a

---

[13] Abady v. Board of Standards & Appeals, N.Y.L.J., Apr. 14, 2004, 18.

[14] Pub. L. No. 93-641, 88 Stat. 2225, § 1523(a)(1)(4) (1975) (*codified at* 42 U.S.C. § 300m-2(a)(1)(4)). For a short history of the law of health planning, *see* R. Miller, PROBLEMS IN HOSPITAL LAW, 95-108 (5th ed.).

[15] Pub. L. No. 99-660, 100 Stat. 3799 (1986).

[16] J. Preston, *States ease restrictions on hospitals*, N.Y. TIMES, July 27, 1998, C18 [end of requirement of certificate of need for many services]; *Lapse of law could mean increase in nursing homes*, AP, Jan. 1, 2003 [Missouri]; *see also Hospitals lobby to keep planning and review board*, AP, Mar. 18, 2003 [N.H.].

[17] St. Dominic-Jackson Mem. Hosp. v. Mississippi State Dep't of Health, 728 So.2d 81 (Miss. 1998) [successful challenge to primary care center by competing hospitals]; *see also* Methodist Healthcare-Jackson Hosp. v. Jackson-Madison County Gen. Hosp. Dist., 2003 Tenn. App. LEXIS 369.

new dialysis center.[18] When a state permits such involvement, opposition by a competitor is generally not considered illegal antitrust activity. For example, in 1999, a federal appellate court held that it was not a violation of the antitrust law for a hospital to oppose a CON for a competing ambulatory surgery center even when knowingly false statements were made in the process.[19]

Some of the categories of capital expenditures for which review can be required include those that (1) exceed a specified threshold, (2) are for starting a new institution, (3) change bed capacity more than a specified amount, or (4) are for starting new services that will involve ongoing annual operational costs that exceed a defined threshold. Some states also require a CON to close certain services.[20]

The review criteria now vary among the states, but they generally focus on the relationship to the existing health care system and to applicable health plans. Some criteria are numerical, such as bed need formulas based on population, while others are more subjective.

Some states favor institutions that treat Medicaid and indigent patients,[21] but at least one state favored a private nursing home over a facility that projected 65 percent Medicaid utilization because the state had insufficient Medicaid funds.[22]

Procedures also vary, but they generally involve an application, public notice, a hearing with the right to present evidence, a timely decision, and an opportunity to appeal. Most states require technical compliance with the application requirements before an application can be processed.[23] In some states, if the agency does not act on the application within a specified time, the CON is automatically approved.[24]

CONs generally specify the timetable for completing the approved project and the maximum amount of authorized capital

---

[18] Matter of MGNH, Inc. & HCA Genesis, N.Y.L.J., May 24, 2004, 22.

[19] Armstrong Surgical Ctr., Inc. v. Armstrong County Mem. Hosp., 185 F.3d 154 (3rd Cir. 1999), *cert. denied,* 530 U.S. 1261 (2000).

[20] FLA. STAT. § 395.0146 [CON required to close emergency room].

[21] *E.g., In re* Hazlet Manor Ass'n, No. A-1431095T3F (N.J. Super. Ct. App. Div. Jan. 17, 1997), *as discussed in* 25 HEALTH L. DIG. (Feb. 1997), at 35 [affirming rejection of CON for long-term care facility that refused to commit to 55% Medicaid occupancy].

[22] National Health Corp. v. South Carolina Dep't of Health & Environ. Control, 298 S.C. 373, 380 S.E.2d 841 (Ct. App. 1989).

[23] *E.g., In re* Nashua Brookside Hosp., 636 A.2d 57 (N.H. 1993) [error of law to review application to convert substance abuse beds to psychiatric beds without required letters from state mental health agency].

[24] *E.g., In re* VHA Diagnostic Servs., Inc., 65 Ohio St. 3d 210, 602 N.E.2d 647 (1992).

expenditures. If a good faith effort is not made to meet the timetable, the CON can be withdrawn. If the actual expenditures are expected to exceed the maximum, the project can be subject to further review. The withdrawal of a CON after a project is commenced could have a serious adverse effect on a hospital; so a realistic timetable and budget are essential elements of a prudent CON application.

Some states have imposed limits on the total capital expenditures in the state for health care. Other states have imposed moratoria on approvals of all capital expenditures of certain types, such as expenditures for hospitals[25] or nursing homes.[26] These moratoria and limits have been successfully challenged only when they were not authorized by state statute.[27] When there is a moratorium on new CONs, changes can occur only through transfers of existing CONs.[28]

Hospitals that are granted CONs generally can be ordered to comply with them. After an Alabama hospital obtained a CON to operate a long-term facility but operated it with an average length of stay of 6.6 days, a court ordered that the hospital be limited to an average length of stay of thirty days or more.[29] Hospitals that make promises in the course of obtaining a CON are generally required to honor their commitments. To settle a CON challenge, a Florida hospital agreed to provide a certain amount of indigent care or to pay a local governmental hospital any shortfall. When the care was not provided, the hospital was ordered to make the payment.[30]

Failure to have a CON for a service is generally not a defense to a collection action for that service. A federal appellate court ruled in favor of the hospital in its suit to collect for a transplant procedure, even though the hospital did not have a CON for the service.[31]

---

[25] *E.g.,* J. Piazza, *Officials: moratorium on Maine's hospitals will cause drop in issuance,* BOND BUYER, July 9, 2003, 3.

[26] *E.g.,* Sheffield Towers Rehab. & Health Care Ctr. v. Novello, 293 A.D.2d 182, 741 N.Y.S.2d 103 (2d Dept. 2002) [moratorium on nursing homes affirmed].

[27] *E.g.,* Balsam v. Dep't of Health & Rehabilitative Servs., 452 So.2d 976 (Fla. 1st DCA 1984); Arkansas Dep't of Human Servs. v. Greene Acres Nursing Homes, Inc., 296 Ark. 475, 757 S.W.2d 563 (1988).

[28] For an example of the complications involved in transfers, *see* Paragon Health Network, Inc. v. Thompson, 251 F.3d 1141 (7th Cir. 2001).

[29] Hospital Corp. of Am. v. Springhill Hosps., Inc., 472 So.2d 1059 (Ala. Civ. App. 1985).

[30] South Broward Hosp. Dist. v. Nu-Med Penbroke, 603 So.2d 11 (Fla. 4th DCA 1992).

[31] Rush-Presbyterian-St. Luke's Med. Ctr. v. Hellenic Republic, 980 F.2d 449 (7th Cir. 1992).

3-2 What Are the Licensure Requirements for Health Care Facilities?

Some regulatory or accrediting agencies focus on entire institutions. These are discussed in section 2-4. Other agencies focus on individual services or activities, such as pharmacies, laboratories, radiology, or elevators. Some agencies can focus on the institution or on individual activities depending on the circumstances. For example, in a few states, a certificate-of-need agency must give its permission before some new facilities or new services can be started. Numerous other regulations apply to other aspects of health care organizations, such as financing, taxation, waste disposal, communications, transportation, and labor relations.

This section reviews a few of the regulations applying to individual services. Pharmacy regulation is discussed in section 3-3.

CLINICAL LABORATORIES IMPROVEMENT ACT (CLIA). Hospitals and other providers, including physician offices, must meet federal standards for most clinical laboratory services and obtain a federal CLIA certificate to operate those services.[32] The Department of Health and Human Services has broad powers to revoke certificates for noncompliance.[33]

MAMMOGRAPHY QUALITY STANDARDS ACT. Hospitals and other providers, including physician offices, must meet federal standards for mammography and obtain a federal certificate to provide mammography services.[34]

RADIOACTIVE MATERIAL. Hospitals and other providers must obtain a permit to possess use and radioactive material. The Nuclear Regulatory Commission administers this requirement at the federal level. Administrative responsibility has been delegated

---

[32] 42 U.S.C. § 263a; 42 C.F.R. pt. 493; Consumer Federation of Am. v. U.S. Dep't of H.H.S., 317 U.S. App. D.C. 449, 83 F.3d 1497 (1996) [in challenge to CLIA rules, agency ordered to provide rationale or pursue further changes].

[33] *See* Elsenety v. H.C.F.A., 85 Fed. Appx. 405 (6th Cir. 2003) [affirming revocation of CLIA certificates]; Oakland Med. Group, P.C. v. Sec'y of Health & Human Servs., 298 F.3d 507 (6th Cir. 2002) [no right to pretermination hearing].

[34] 42 U.S.C. § 263b; 21 C.F.R. pt. 900; *Newark hospital cited for violation in mammogram unit*, AP, Dec. 28, 2001 [federal citation]; *Chicago mammography facility fined $30,000, suspended for five years*, BREAST IMPLANT LITIGATION RPTR., Aug. 25, 1998, 13; J. Peres, *Panel says medical facilities that hold breast cancer screenings must do better*, CHICAGO TRIB., May 24, 2005 [Institute of Medicine report].

to the state level in states that meet certain standards. The delegated states are called Agreement States.[35]

ELEVATORS. Most states require permits for and periodic inspections of elevators.[36]

3-3 What Are the Regulations Concerning the Manufacture and Use of Drugs, Medical Devices, Tissues, and Other Items Used in Health Care?

The use of drugs and medical devices is heavily regulated. State laws regulate pharmacies. Federal laws regulate the production, distribution, and use of drugs and medical devices, especially drugs and medical devices involved in interstate commerce. State laws usually regulate intrastate commerce involving drugs that is not regulated by federal laws.[37] JCAHO standards and the Medicare conditions of participation also address hospital pharmacies. For example, the Medicare conditions of participation require that hospital pharmaceutical services be under the direction of a qualified pharmacist.[38]

This focus is understandable in light of the estimated 40 percent of Americans who take at least one prescription drug and 17 percent who take more than two.[39]

This section discusses state regulation of pharmacies (3-3.1); formulary systems (3-3.2); the Controlled Substances Act (3-3.3); regulation of drugs and devices by the U.S. Food and Drug Administration (FDA) (3-3.4); and laws related to marketing drugs and devices (3-3.5). Regulation of the use of cells and tissues is discussed in section 15-4.3.

---

[35] *See* http://www.nrc.gov/materials/medical.html [accessed Sept. 11, 2004]; *NRC imposes fine against hospital*, AP, June 18, 2002 [fine for dose of radioactive pharmaceutical to student not approved by a physician]; for other examples of enforcement efforts, *see* http://www.nrc.gov/what-we-do/regulatory/enforcement/current.html#materials [accessed Sept. 11, 2004].

[36] E.g., Cal. Lab. Code §§ 7300.1 et seq.; *Board grants four variances*, CAL-OSHA RPTR., Mar. 5, 2004 [CA hospital granted variance to permit platform size wheelchair lift].

[37] *E.g., Florida allows 2 firms to market interferon under law on cancer*, WALL ST. J., Nov. 4, 1983, 46.

[38] 2005 JCAHO CAMH, MM.1.10 - 8.10; 42 C.F.R. § 482.25.

[39] R. Pear, *Americans relying more on prescription drugs, report says*, N.Y. TIMES, Dec. 3, 2004, A16 [based on National Center for Health Statistics report].

3-3.1 State Regulation of Pharmacies

All states regulate pharmacies. Retail pharmacies are required to have pharmacy licenses. Some states require hospitals to obtain a separate pharmacy license for the hospital pharmacy. Some states regulate hospital pharmacies through the hospital licensing system, exempting hospital pharmacies from the pharmacy licensing system.[40] Some exemptions apply only to dispensing inpatient drugs and take-home drugs in conjunction with a hospital visit, but not to refills, so that a pharmacy license is required for nonexempt dispensing. Some states that license hospital pharmacies require a separate community pharmacy license before the pharmacy can fill prescriptions for staff or others for use outside the hospital. Pharmacies in nonprofit hospitals that fill such prescriptions also need to comply with the limitations on the use of drugs that are acquired at special prices for the hospital's own use. These limitations are discussed in Chapter 13.

Regulations usually include staffing requirements. The scope of permitted uses of unlicensed technical staff varies.

3-3.2 Formulary Systems

Hospitals generally promote rational and cost-effective drug use through a hospital formulary system that selects the drugs to be available for use. When a medical staff committee determines that two or more drugs are equivalent, only one is primarily stocked. It is selected by negotiation with or bidding from competing suppliers. When a physician prescribes a drug for which an equivalent is stocked, the equivalent drug is dispensed unless the physician specifies on the prescription form or orders that no substitutions are permitted. Hospital or medical staff rules determine when such a specification will result in obtaining the specified drug and when it will result in an educational effort or other response. Formulary systems are required by Medicare conditions of participation.[41] The JCAHO requires a procedure for selecting medications available in the hospital.[42]

Formulary systems have been legally challenged on the basis of state antisubstitution or generic substitution laws, federal or state drug laws, and trademark laws. These challenges have not been

---

[40] *E.g.,* Missouri Hosp. Ass'n v. Missouri Dep't of Consumer Affairs, 731 S.W.2d 262 (Mo. Ct. App. 1987).
[41] 42 C.F.R. § 482.25(b)(9).
[42] 2005 JCAHO CAMH, MM.2.10.

successful when there is an agreement between the prescriber and dispenser that an equivalent drug can be dispensed. The equivalent drug is what is actually being prescribed by the symbols on the prescription. Usually, the agreement is in the medical staff bylaws or rules, which each medical staff member accepts to obtain and retain medical staff membership.

Managed care organizations frequently have formularies of the drugs for which they will pay.[43] Some states have sought to limit the use of managed care formularies.[44]

State Medicaid programs also use formularies to control drug utilization and cost.[45] These formularies have been challenged in court and have generally been upheld.[46] There are sometimes intense efforts to influence administrative decisions concerning these lists.[47]

In the absence of an express or implied agreement, substitution is generally unlawful.[48]

3-3.3 Controlled Substances Act

The Comprehensive Drug Abuse Prevention and Control Act of 1970,[49] commonly known as the Controlled Substances Act, regulates distribution systems and also deals with rehabilitation programs, research in and treatment of drug abuse, and importation and exportation of controlled substances. The Act should be reviewed when hospitals create or revise procedures for handling and administering controlled substances.

---

[43] M. Freudenheim, *Not quite what doctor ordered*, N.Y. TIMES, Oct. 8, 1996, C1.

[44] *E.g., Governor signs bill to allow patient access to drugs not listed on plan formularies*, 7 H.L.R. 1058 (1998) [Cal. Senate Bill 625].

[45] 42 U.S.C. § 1396r-8(d)(4) [outpatient formularies]; G Aston, *Medicaid short list*, AM. MED. NEWS, May 3, 2004, 5 [some physicians see preferred-drug lists as barriers to care].

[46] *E.g.,* Karen L. v. Health Net, 78 Fed. Appx. 772 (2d Cir. 2003) [unpub] [affirm denial of injunction of deletions from Conn. Medicaid formulary]; *see also* Pharmaceutical Research & Mfrs. of Am. v. Walsh, 538 U.S. 644 (2003) [affirming denial of preliminary injunction of Maine program requiring prior authorization for drugs from manufacturers that did agree to rebates]; Pharmaceutical Research & Mfrs. of Am. v. Thompson, 360 U.S. App. D.C. 375, 362 F.3d 817 (2004) [approving Michigan program requiring prior authorization for drugs of manufacturers who do not sign rebate agreements].

[47] *See* G. Harris, *States try to limit drugs in Medicaid, but makers resist*, N.Y. TIMES, Dec. 18, 2003, A1 [describing lobbying against removal of drugs from Medicaid lists].

[48] *See Pharmacy closed as 'danger' to public health*, AP, Aug. 27, 2004 [Vir. pharmacy closed for unauthorized substitutions]; L.A. Johnson, *Medco settles accusations by 20 states*, AP, Apr. 26, 2004 [alleged pressure on physicians to substitute medications that were more profitable to the prescription benefits manager; agreed to payment, practice changes without admitting wrongdoing].

[49] Pub. L. No. 90-513, 84 Stat. 1236 (codified as amended in scattered sections of 18, 21, 26, 31, 42, 46, and 49 U.S.C.).

Hospitals are defined as "institutional practitioners"[50] and must register under the Act.[51] Each registrant must take a physical inventory every two years.[52] A separate inventory is required for each registered location and for each independent activity registered. Each registrant must also maintain records of all controlled substances received and disposed of.[53]

Controlled substances are classified into lists, called schedules, by the degree to which they are controlled.[54] The Drug Enforcement Administration (DEA) of the Department of Justice has discretion in determining in which schedule to classify a substance.[55] Schedule I has the tightest controls. Controlled substances in Schedules I through IV can be dispensed only upon the lawful order of a practitioner. For outpatients, the order must be a prescription that complies with legal requirements.[56] For inpatients, a chart order satisfies the requirement.[57] The practitioner who signs the order must be registered with the DEA or exempt from registration.[58] State law determines which professionals can be practitioners.[59] Persons who are registered with the DEA are issued a DEA number. There has been a problematic trend for private entities to use the DEA number for other purposes.[60]

All institutions and individual registrants must provide controls and procedures to guard against theft and diversion of controlled substances. Only authorized personnel should have access to the central storage area and to other areas where drugs are kept in the hospital. Controlled substances stored at nursing units should be securely locked.

Substantial federal criminal penalties, including fines and imprisonment, are imposed for violating the Act.[61] In addition, violators can lose the authority to possess, prescribe, and dispense controlled

---

[50] 21 C.F.R. § 1306.02(c).
[51] 21 U.S.C. § 822.
[52] 21 U.S.C. § 827.
[53] *Id.*; *Harvard settles suit over pharmacy's laxness*, N.Y. TIMES, Oct. 1, 1996, A10 [$775,000 payment for lax security, faulty record-keeping at University pharmacy].
[54] 21 U.S.C. § 812.
[55] *E.g.,* Alliance for Cannabis Therapeutics v. D.E.A., 15 F.3d 1131 (D.C. Cir. 1994) [upholding DEA order refusing to change classification of marijuana to Schedule II].
[56] 21 C.F.R. pt. 1306.
[57] 21 C.F.R. §§ 1306.02(f), 1306.11(c), 1306.21(c), 1306.31(c).
[58] 21 C.F.R. § 1301.24 [exempting medical residents, some agents].
[59] 21 C.F.R. § 1306.2(b).
[60] V. Foubister, *Demands for DEA numbers become hassle*, AM. MED. NEWS, July 13, 1998, 7.
[61] *E.g.,* United States v. Steele, 147 F.3d 1316 (11th Cir. 1998) (en banc) [conviction of pharmacist for unlawful dispensing].

substances. Most states have controlled substances acts that parallel the federal law; so state sanctions are also possible.[62]

One area of tension concerning this federal law has been the federal prohibition of the medicinal use of marijuana for pain control. Some local areas have sought to make this substance available for medicinal use, while other states have supported the federal position.[63] In 1998, the voters in five states passed referenda legalizing medicinal marijuana, but these actions remain preempted by federal law.[64] Congress prohibited the voters of the District of Columbia from voting on the issue; so when a vote was held, the ballots were not counted.[65] Courts have generally ruled that neither the federal nor state constitution grant a right even to the terminally ill to use any substance banned by the government.[66] In 1999, a patient with multiple sclerosis was prosecuted in the District of Columbia for medicinal use of marijuana.[67] In 2001, the United States Supreme Court ruled that there was no medical necessity defense to federal prosecution for marijuana possession.[68] In 2002, the California Supreme Court interpreted the state law that provided a defense to state prosecution for marijuana use and possession.[69] In 2005, the United States Supreme Court ruled that state law provided no protection from federal prosecution for medicinal use of marijuana.[70]

At one time there was concern that even discussing marijuana with a patient could subject a physician to federal penalties, but in 2002, a federal appellate court affirmed a permanent injunction keeping the federal government from revoking a physician's license

---

[62] *E.g.,* Schmidt v. Iowa State Bd. of Dental Examiners, 423 N.W.2d 19 (Iowa 1988) [dental license suspended for 30 days for diversions of drugs due to ineffective office controls]; Schmidt v. Iowa State Bd. of Dental Examiners, 872 F.2d 243 (8th Cir. 1989) [suspension not a denial of due process].

[63] *E.g., Florida cabinet opposes legalizing medical marijuana,* AM. MED. NEWS, Apr. 13, 1998, 35.

[64] L. Page, *Five states approve medical marijuana,* AM. MED. NEWS, Nov. 23/30, 1998, 5.

[65] *D.C. can't count marijuana initiative votes due to provision in omnibus spending law,* 7 H.L.R. 1752 (1998); *Judge refuses to order immediate release of medical marijuana initiative vote results,* 7 H.L.R. 1843 (1998).

[66] *E.g.,* Seeley v. Washington State, 132 Wash. 2d 776, 940 P.2d 604 (Wash. 1997) [terminally ill bone cancer patient has no state constitutional right to medicinal marijuana].

[67] C. Strong, *MS patient goes on trial for smoking joint,* WIS. ST. J., Feb. 10, 1999, 5A.

[68] United States v. Oakland Cannabis Buyers' Coop., 532 U.S. 483 (2001).

[69] People v. Mower, 28 Cal. 4th 457, 49 P.3d 1067, 122 Cal. Rptr. 2d 326 (2002) [state law does not confer complete immunity for cultivation, use of marijuana; confers limited immunity that permits defense at trial, but defendant need only raise a reasonable doubt].

[70] Gonzales v. Raich, 125 S. Ct. 2195 (U.S. 2005).

based solely on the physician's professional recommendation of the use of medical marijuana.[71]

3-3.4 Regulation of Drugs and Devices by the U.S. Food and Drug Administration

The Food and Drug Administration enforces a complex system of federal controls over the testing, manufacturing, labeling, and distributing of drugs, cosmetics, and devices.[72] These controls appear in the Federal Food, Drug, and Cosmetic Act, which includes the Medical Device Amendments of 1976, and in FDA regulations.[73]

DEFINITION OF DRUGS AND DEVICES. The definitions of drugs and devices are broad. For example, human blood is considered a drug. Virtually all equipment and supplies used in patient care are regulated as devices. In addition to such obvious devices as hip prostheses, pacemakers, and artificial hearts, the term includes common equipment and supplies such as catheters, hospital beds, specimen containers,[74] support stockings, scissors, adhesive tape, elastic bandages, tongue depressors, and sutures. In 1992, a federal appellate court upheld a FDA rule defining replacement heart valve allographs as medical devices.[75] A heart valve allograph is a human heart valve that has been processed and preserved so that it can be stored until needed for implantation.

FDA ENFORCEMENT DISCRETION. The FDA has broad discretion to decide whether to use its powers to investigate or penalize specific activities. When the FDA declined to investigate drugs used to execute condemned criminals, the United States Supreme Court was asked to order a FDA investigation. The Court ruled that the FDA and other federal agencies have prosecutorial discretion to decide whether to exercise their discretionary powers in individual cases; so courts cannot review such decisions in most situations.[76]

---

[71] Conant v. Walters, 309 F.3d 629 (9th Cir. 2002), *cert. denied*, 540 U.S. 946 (2003).

[72] *See, e.g.*, D.A. Kessler, S.M. Pape & D. Sudwall, *The Federal regulation of medical devices*, 317 NEW ENG. J. MED. 357 (1987).

[73] Title 21 of the United States Code and Title 21 of the Code of Federal Regulations; *see also* T.K. Gilman & B.R. McCormick, *Federal Food and Drug Act violations*, 38 AM. CRIM. L. REV. 819 (2001) [reviewing criminal penalties for violations].

[74] *E.g.*, United States v. Undetermined Number of Unlabeled Cases, 21 F.3d 1026 (10th Cir. 1994) [specimen containers for testing for HIV are devices].

[75] Alabama Tissue Ctr. v. Sullivan, 975 F.2d 373 (7th Cir. 1992); Annotation, *What is a "drug," a "device," and a "new drug" within the definitions of these terms in sec.201(g)(1), (h), and (p) of the Federal Food, Drug, and Cosmetic Act as amended*, 3 A.L.R. FED. 843; *but see* Northwest Tissue Ctr. v. Shalala, 1 F.3d 522 (7th Cir. 1993) [permitting challenge to the applying of regulations].

[76] Heckler v. Chaney, 470 U.S. 821 (1985).

TIMELINESS OF FDA APPROVAL. The FDA has been attacked for the time it takes to approve new drugs and devices and for the cost of compliance with its requirements, among other factors.[77] It has been defended for its contribution to protecting public safety. In the mid-1990s, the FDA implemented some reforms to speed review, including exempting many low risk devices from review.[78] In 1997, the FDA law was amended to further expedite review and make other changes.[79] The FDA has subsequently been criticized when approved drugs were later demonstrated to have harmful and even lethal side effects.[80] It is clear that there are competing public interests that cannot all be satisfied. The balance between cost, safety, access, and other factors will undoubtedly periodically shift.

Thalidomide is an example of a drug that illustrates the difficulty in striking the appropriate balance. In the 1950s, thalidomide was used in Europe to treat pregnant women and resulted in the birth of children with missing limbs and other birth defects. The FDA had not approved thalidomide for use in the United States, but a few handicapped children were born to American women after they obtained the drug from Europe. In reaction to thalidomide, the FDA law was amended to significantly increase the powers of the FDA to control the introduction of new drugs. It was later discovered that thalidomide was an effective drug to treat leprosy. Understandably in light of the risks associated with use of thalidomide and its high profile role in the history of FDA control of new drugs, there was reluctance to lift the ban on use. In 1997, a FDA panel recommended that use be permitted.[81] In 1998, the FDA approved use

---

[77] *E.g.,* P. Huber, *FDA caution can be deadly, too,* WALL. ST. J., July 24, 1998, A14 [Thalidomide]; *F.D.A. becomes target of empowered groups,* N.Y. TIMES, Feb. 12, 1995, 12; *FDA moves too slowly in approving medical devices, industry critics say,* 3 H.L.R. 884 (1994).

[78] *Administration announces more reforms to speed drug, medical device reviews,* 4 H.L.R. 562 (1995); P. Hilts, *With record speed, F.D.A. approves a new AIDS drug.* N.Y. TIMES, Mar. 15, 1996, A9; *FDA cleared 139 products in 1996, a record increase,* WALL ST. J., Jan. 16, 1997, B10.

[79] FDA Modernization and Accountability Act of 1997, Pub. L. No. 105-115 (1997).

[80] C.L. Bennett, et al., *The research on adverse drug events and reports (RADAR) project,* J.A.M.A., May 4, 2005, 2131 [proposals regarding postmarketing surveillance]; G. Harris, *F.D.A. to create advisory board on drug safety,* N.Y. TIMES, Feb. 16, 2005, A1; S. Stapleton, *Drug recalls raise questions about FDA drug approvals,* AM. MED. NEWS, Aug. 17, 1998, 28; D. Grady, *F.D.A. accused of hasty drug approval,* N.Y. TIMES, Dec. 3, 1998, A24.

[81] S. Stolberg, *Thalidomide, long banned, wins support,* N.Y. TIMES, Sept. 6, 1997, 11; A. Womack, *Panel recommends thalidomide's use in leprosy cases,* WALL ST. J., Sept. 8, 1997, B10.

within strict rules that required registry of patients and special training of prescribing physicians and dispensing pharmacists.[82]

OTHER FDA FUNCTIONS. The FDA performs other important health functions. For example, it has mandated that foods be fortified with various substances that are essential to good health. In 1924, iodizing of salt was required. In 1943, the addition of vitamins and iron to certain foods was required. In 1996, folic acid was ordered to be added to grain foods to cut down on birth defects.[83]

INVESTIGATIONAL DRUGS AND DEVICES. Before new drugs and devices can enter general use, an elaborate procedure must be followed to establish their safety and effectiveness. The investigational new drug (IND) and investigational device exemption (IDE) requirements must be met to use investigational drugs and devices lawfully. With few exceptions, these drugs and devices can be used only in research projects approved by an institutional review board, conducted by a qualified investigator, and sponsored by an appropriate company or institution.[84] Sale or use of unlicensed drugs and devices outside the permitted processes can result in substantial penalties.[85] There is no constitutional right to use unapproved drugs; they can be used only as permitted by law.[86]

Record-keeping. Investigators need to maintain complete and accurate records, and the manufacturer must make full disclosure of the results to the FDA. The FDA can use criminal sanctions to enforce its record-keeping and reporting requirements. A Minnesota investigator was convicted of mail fraud and making false statements to the government for submitting false information concerning a study.[87] Officials of manufacturers have been convicted for submitting false information or failing to submit information that should have been submitted.[88]

---

[82] S. Stolberg, *Thalidomide gets U.S. approval to aid lepers and maybe others*, N.Y. TIMES, July 17, 1998, A1.

[83] G. Kolata, *Vitamin to protect fetuses will be required in foods*, N.Y. TIMES, Mar. 1, 1996, A8.

[84] 21 C.F.R. pts. 50, 56, 312, 812, 813. For a summary of FDA actions for scientific misconduct from 1975 through 1983, *see* M.F. Shapiro & R.P. Charrow, *Scientific misconduct in investigational drug trials*, 312 NEW ENG. J. MED. 731 (1985).

[85] *E.g.*, United States *ex rel.* Zissler v. Regents of Univ. of Minn., No. 3-95-168 (D. Minn. settlement Nov. 17, 1998), *as discussed in* 7 H.L.R. 1897 (1998) [sale of unlicensed drugs].

[86] *E.g.*, Cowan v. United States, 5 F. Supp. 2d 1235 (D. Okla. 1998) [denial of injunction of FDA to permit AIDS patient to use unapproved drug].

[87] United States v. Garfinkel, 29 F.3d 1253 (8th Cir. 1994).

[88] *E.g.*, United States v. Chatterji, 46 F.3d 1336 (4th Cir. 1995) [founder, part owner convicted of fraud for falsifying batches of drug].

Testing phases. New drugs generally have three testing phases.[89] Phase 1 focuses on determining the pharmacologic action of the drug, side effects, and maximum tolerated dose. Phase 1 studies can involve normal volunteers. Phase 2 consists of small controlled clinical studies on patients to evaluate effectiveness for particular indications and side effects. Phase 3 consists of expanded controlled and uncontrolled studies to gather additional information on effectiveness and safety, evaluate the risk-benefit relationship, and provide an adequate basis for labeling. Some drugs that appeared promising in earlier phases have failed in Phase 3.[90] In some circumstances, there are Phase 4 postmarketing studies.[91]

Research on special populations. After years of discouraging research involving children in an effort to protect them from the risks, it was recognized that children were not able to gain access to important drugs because there was insufficient data on their effects on children. In 1998, the FDA mandated pediatric studies on drugs.[92] In 2002, a federal court struck down the pediatric study mandate as being beyond the authority of the FDA.[93] Congress amended the law to give HHS authority concerning pediatric studies and to reward drug companies with a patent extension for some of the pediatric studies.[94]

In 1998, the FDA also mandated that studies include other important demographic subgroups, including groups based on gender and race.[95]

Treatment uses prior to full approval. The FDA can approve treatment with an investigational new drug outside of clinical trials when the drug is for a serious or immediately life threatening disease and there is no satisfactory alternative therapy available. This approval is often called a *treatment IND*.[96] There is also a procedure for approval of emergency shipments prior to IND approval.[97]

---

[89] 21 C.F.R. § 312.21.

[90] *E.g., The tale of a dream, a drug and data dredging*, WALL ST. J., Feb. 7, 1995, B1 [drug designed to heal wounds did well in all tests until it failed to outperform a placebo in its Phase 3 clinical trial].

[91] 21 C.F.R. § 312.85.

[92] 63 FED. REG. 66,631 (Dec. 2, 1998).

[93] Ass'n of Am. Physicians & Surgeons, Inc. v. U.S. F.D.A., 226 F. Supp. 2d 204 (D. D.C. 2002).

[94] 21 U.S.C. §§ 355a, 355c.

[95] 63 FED. REG. 6854 (Feb. 11, 1998).

[96] 21 C.F.R. § 312.34.

[97] 21 C.F.R. § 312.36.

There are rules permitting humanitarian uses of investigational devices.[98]

Subjects in clinical studies generally do not have a legal right to continued access to investigational drugs after they cease to be subjects.[99] However, consent documents can create a contract to continue to supply the drug.[100]

Payment for use. One controversial aspect of use of investigational drugs and devices is that some third-party payers refuse to pay for their use. This has led to suits as discussed in Chapter 10.

In 1994, the Office of Inspector General of the Department of Health and Human Services issued a subpoena seeking the records of all uses of investigational devices at many hospitals.[101] The scope of the subpoena was eventually focused on certain cardiac devices. There was a concern that HHS was taking the position that when a investigational device was used during a hospitalization that the entire hospitalization was not eligible for Medicare or Medicaid payment, even making the submission of a bill for that hospital stay a false claim. This led some hospitals to either stop enrolling Medicare and Medicaid patients in clinical device trials or halting all uses of investigational devices until their status was clarified.[102] Hospitals sued to challenge the federal enforcement effort. In 1996, a federal court invalidated a 1986 HCFA instruction denying payment for services using medical devices under an IDE, on the grounds that it was a new rule and had not been properly promulgated with notice and a comment period.[103] HCFA adopted rules in 1995 that specified the process that would be used to determine coverage for investigational devices and related services.[104] In 1997,

---

[98] 63 FED. REG. 19,185 (Apr. 17, 1998).

[99] *E.g.*, Kraemer-Katz v. United States Public Health Service, 872 F. Supp. 1235 (S.D.N.Y. 1994); A. Pollack, *Judge rejects patients' suit to get test drug*, N.Y. TIMES, June. 8, 2005, C8; *but see* Wagner v. Janssen, N.Y. Sup. Ct., N.Y.L.J., Jan. 2, 2001, 25 [manufacturer ordered to distribute withdrawn drug to individual].

[100] *E.g.*, Dahl v. HEM Pharmaceuticals Corp., 7 F.3d 1399 (9th Cir. 1993).

[101] *IG nationwide hospital investigation seeks data on non-FDA approved devices*, 3 H.L.R. 836 (1994).

[102] *E.g.*, L. Scott, *Hospitals try to devise solutions in device debate*, MOD. HEALTHCARE, Feb. 20, 1995, 34.

[103] Cedars-Sinai Med. Ctr. v. Shalala, 939 F. Supp. 1457 (C.D. Cal. 1996); on appeal, it was ruled that (1) the district court should consider the HHS motion to dismiss on statute of limitations grounds and (2) a person who brought a qui tam action concerning the same issue could not intervene, Cedars-Sinai Med. Ctr. v. Shalala, 125 F.3d 765 (9th Cir. 1997).

[104] 60 FED. REG. 48,417 (Sept. 19, 1995); *see also* FDA, Office of Device Evaluation, *Implementation of FDA/HCFA interagency agreement regarding reimbursement categorization of investigational devices* (Sept. 15, 1995).

the FDA adopted rules concerning treatment uses of investigational devices.[105] In 2000, Medicare issued a national coverage decision to pay for routine costs of patients during clinic trials.[106]

Some states have mandated that private insurers pay for participation in some clinical trials of investigational drugs and devices.[107]

APPROVED DRUGS AND DEVICES. When the FDA is convinced that a new drug or device is safe and effective for certain uses, it approves the drug for general sale. The approval can permit either over-the-counter sales or sales by order of a practitioner. Approval of drugs or devices can include additional restrictions on use.[108]

There are often disputes over whether prescriptions should be required. Granting over-the-counter status makes the items more accessible, removes the protection of practitioner oversight, and usually removes health care insurance coverage for the item.[109]

Labeling. The FDA approval specifies which uses of the drug or device should be included in labeling. In the past, only uses that had been fully proven in controlled studies could be on labels. Special studies on children were required before any uses for children could be on the label; so there was limited label information about uses for children. In 1995, the FDA began permitting more label information about uses for children.[110] In 1998, the FDA amended its regulations concerning disclosure of information concerning uses of approved drugs and devices that vary from the approved uses.[111] However, a few months later, a federal court ruled that the FDA could not enforce its restrictions on dissemination of this information, finding the restrictions violated the First Amendment rights applicable to commercial speech.[112] Note that the First Amendment protects only truthful commercial speech; so the FDA still has the authority to address labeling that is not considered to be accurate.

---

[105] 62 FED. REG. 48,940 (Sept. 18, 1997).

[106] Sec. 30-1, Medicare Coverage Issues Manual (Sept. 19, 2000).

[107] *E.g., Governor signs off on grievance rules, clinical trial coverage, other bills*, 7 H.L.R. 743 (1998) [Md.].

[108] *E.g.*, S. Stolberg, *Thalidomide gets U.S. approval to aid lepers and maybe others*, N.Y. TIMES, July 17, 1998, A1.

[109] *See* R. Cohen, *The ethicist: Drug providers*, N.Y. TIMES MAG., Dec. 7, 2003, 32 [responding to patient requests to shift to prescription drugs covered by insurance]; G. Kolata, *There's a blurry line between Rx and O.T.C.*, N.Y. TIMES, Dec. 21, 2003, 3WK.

[110] 21 C.F.R. § 201.57(9).

[111] 63 FED. REG. 31,143 (June 8, 1998).

[112] Washington Legal Found. v. Friedman, 13 F. Supp. 2d 51 (D. D.C. 1998); *FDA motion seeks clarification of order in decision voiding "off-label" policies*, 7 H.L.R. 1356 (1998); Washington Legal Found. v. Friedman, No. 94-1306(RCL) (D. D.C. Feb. 16, 1999) [upholding 1998 ruling finding some FDA restrictions on off-label information unconstitutional].

In 2004, the California Supreme Court ruled that FDA warning label requirements for nicotine patches preempt stricter state-mandated labeling.[113]

Off-label uses. Usually medical practice changes more rapidly than FDA approval; so drug or device use is often different from the approved uses listed on labels.[114] Such uses are often referred to as *off-label* uses. Drugs are often given for other conditions or in different dosages. It is not a violation of federal law for physicians to order such unapproved uses or for pharmacists to dispense drugs pursuant to such orders. However, unapproved uses that result in injuries to patients can result in liability. Some courts consider FDA-approved labeling to be sufficient evidence of proper use so that no further expert testimony is required.[115] However, when defendants introduce evidence that FDA-approved uses lag behind current medical practice, deviations from FDA-approved uses alone do not conclusively prove negligence. Juries are permitted to consider the FDA position along with other testimony concerning accepted practice in deciding whether the use was negligent.[116] Although there is no requirement to obtain informed consent for off-label drug use, when a particular use is not widely adopted, the prudent practice is for the physician to explain the unapproved use and the reasons for the use to the patient and to obtain the patient's informed consent.

Some payers have refused to pay for some or all off-label uses of approved drugs,[117] even though such uses are part of standard practice. In 1998, a federal circuit court ruled that a health plan limiting drug coverage to FDA approved uses did not unambiguously preclude coverage for prescribed off-label uses; so payment was required.[118] Some states have begun to require plans to cover some off-label uses of approved drugs.[119]

---

[113] Dowhal v. SmithKline Beecham Consumer Healthcare, 32 Cal. 4th 910, 12 Cal. Rptr. 3d 262 (2004).

[114] *E.g.,* T.A. Ratko, *Recommendations for off-label use of intravenously administered immunoglobulin preparations,* 273 J.A.M.A. 1865 (1995).

[115] *E.g.,* DePaolo v. State, 99 A.D.2d 762, 472 N.Y.S.2d 10 (2d Dept. 1984).

[116] *E.g.,* Morlino v. Medical Ctr. of Ocean City, 152 N.J. 563, 706 A.2d 721 (1998) [*Physicians' Desk Reference* drug warnings do not constitute standard of care; physician failure to follow drug use warnings is not by itself negligence]; Young v. Cerniak, 126 Ill. App. 3d 952, 467 N.E.2d 1045 (1st Dist. 1984).

[117] *See 'Off-label' drug use raises a cost flag for managed-care companies,* WALL ST. J., Mar. 12, 1998, A1.

[118] I.V. Servs. of Am., Inc. v. Trustees of Am. Consulting Eng'rs Council of Ins. Trust Fund, 136 F.3d 114 (2d Cir. 1998).

[119] *E.g., New law requires health plans to pay for 'off-label' cancer drugs,* 7 H.L.R. 596 (1998) [Minn.].

FDA immunity. The FDA is generally immune from liability for its decisions to approve drugs and devices.[120]

PRESCRIPTIONS. When prescriptions are required, they must be properly documented. Written prescriptions or orders in the medical record satisfy the documentation requirement. The Act requires oral prescriptions to dispense drugs to be "reduced promptly to writing and filed by the pharmacist."[121] This is generally interpreted not to preclude registered nurses and other appropriate personnel to transcribe oral orders to administer drugs in institutional settings. Hospitals should review these requirements and other state requirements, such as hospital licensing regulations, to assure that telephone orders are accepted by proper personnel.

Electronic prescriptions. In 1998, a Wisconsin court ruled that a community pharmacy could accept an e-mail prescription in the same circumstances that it could accept a telephone order, overruling the pharmacy licensing board ruling that an e-mail order violated the requirement of a written signature.[122] Physicians who prescribe electronically should apply the same standards that apply to telephone prescriptions. They generally need to be personally familiar with the patient. A Wisconsin physician prescribed Viagra, an impotence drug, from a Web site to persons he had never seen. He was investigated in 1998 by the state medical licensing board and was permitted to keep his license when he agreed to stop the practice.[123]

National standards for electronic prescription are being developed. The 2003 amendments to the Medicare program require HHS to develop an electronic prescription program.[124] Proposed rules were published in 2005.[125]

Scope of pharmacist duties. While a pharmacist has a duty to question a prescription that is suspicious on its face, a pharmacist generally does not have a duty to question every prescription. This issue was analyzed in detail by the Utah Supreme Court in a case in

---

[120] *E.g., In re* Orthopedic Bone Screw Products Liab. Litig., MCL Docket No. 1014 (E.D. Pa. Nov. 12, 1998), *as discussed in* 7 H.L.R. 2025 (1998).

[121] 21 U.S.C. § 353(b).

[122] Walgreen Co. v. Wisconsin Pharmacy Examining Board, 217 Wis. 2d 290, 577 N.W.2d 387 (1998) Wisc. App. LEXIS 201 (unpub).

[123] *Doctor who sold Viagra from Web site keeps license,* AM. MED. NEWS, May 25, 1998, 6; *see also* G. Baldwin, *Web Rx,* AM. MED. NEWS, Aug. 3, 1998, 22.

[124] 42 U.S.C. § 1395w-104(e).

[125] 70 FED. REG. 6256 (Feb. 4, 2005).

which a pharmacist attempted to defend his customer relations problems on the grounds that he had a duty to challenge prescriptions.[126]

DEVICE TRACKING. Manufacturers have a duty to put in place a method for tracking certain devices, including permanently implantable devices, life-support devices for use outside of a hospital, and other devices designated by rule.[127] Hospitals and other distributors are required to provide the necessary information to the manufacturer, unless an exemption is obtained.[128]

MANUFACTURING. Every person who owns or operates any establishment engaged in interstate or intrastate "manufacture, preparation, propagation, compounding or processing" of drugs must register each such establishment.[129] The terms *manufacture, preparation, propagation, compounding,* and *processing* include prepackaging or otherwise changing the container, wrapper, or labeling of drugs for distribution to others who will make the final sale or distribution to the ultimate consumer. The Act also requires manufacturers to maintain certain records; file specified reports; be periodically inspected; and satisfy other requirements.[130] Manufacturers must file a list of all drugs they manufacture. The FDA exempts most hospitals from these requirements if the hospitals are "in conformance with any applicable local laws."[131] However, if the hospital pharmacy supplies compounded or repackaged drugs to other institutions or pharmacies under circumstances other than emergencies, it can be considered a manufacturer.

The Prescription Drug Marketing Act of 1988[132] places additional restrictions on transfers of drugs to persons other than patients. Drugs can be resold or even returned to manufacturers and distributors only if the proper procedures are followed.[133]

In 2000, the FDA announced that one year later it would begin treating hospitals that reprocessed single-use devices as manufacturers so that they would need to register as manufacturers with

---

[126] Ryan v. Dan's Food Stores, 972 P.2d 395 (Utah 1999).

[127] 21 U.S.C. § 360i(e); 21 C.F.R. pt. 821.

[128] 21 C.F.R. § 821.30; FDA, *Guidance on medical device tracking*, 7 H.L.R. 400 (1998); the FDA reporting rule was revised, 63 FED. REG. 26,069 (May 12, 1998).

[129] 21 U.S.C. § 360.

[130] *See* M. Petersen, *Drug maker to pay $500 million fine for factory lapses*, N.Y. TIMES, May 18, 2002, A1; *F.D.A. approves Schering-Plough plan on factories*, N.Y. TIMES, June 4, 2003, C4.

[131] 21 C.F.R. § 207.10(b).

[132] Pub. L. No. 100-293, 102 Stat. 95 (*codified at* 21 U.S.C. §§ 331(t), 333(b), 353(c)(3), 353(d), 353(e)).

[133] D. Holthaus, *Network of laws governs resale of products*, 62 HOSPS. (Sept. 20, 1988), at 54.

the FDA and satisfy its manufacturing standards.[134] Many hospitals abandoned such reprocessing and began relying on other registered processors.

Hospital blood banks must register and comply with regulations concerning good manufacturing practices for blood and blood components.[135]

BAR CODING. In 2004, the FDA adopted a rule that required the bar coding of drugs and biologic products. Newly approved drugs must comply within sixty days of their approval. Drugs approved prior to April 26, 2004, must comply by April 26, 2006.[136]

IMPORTS. Canada has negotiated much lower drug prices than are generally available in the United States. There has been substantial political pressure to permit the reimportation from Canada of drugs purchased at Canadian prices. In 2000, Congress authorized HHS to promulgate rules to permit this practice.[137] As of mid-2005, HHS had not yet promulgated such rules, maintaining that it had not yet been able to develop a program to assure the safety of such imports.[138] Instead HHS continued to pursue active enforcement of laws against such importation.[139]

Several states and local governments adopted governmental programs to facilitate such purchases. In 2003, Illinois applied for permission for its program, but as of mid-2005, permission had not been granted.[140] In 2004, Vermont filed suit against HHS seeking the latitude to pursue its program.[141] By mid-2005, HHS had not taken any reported enforcement action against any government program.

POISON PREVENTION PACKAGING ACT. The Poison Prevention Packaging Act[142] requires most drugs to be dispensed in con-

---

[134] 65 FED. REG. 49,583 (Aug. 14, 2000); J.J. Smith & J.A. Agraz, *Federal regulation of single-use medical devices: a revised FDA policy*, 56 FOOD & DRUG L.J. 317 (2001).

[135] 21 C.F.R. pt. 607 [registration]; 21 C.F.R. pt. 606 [manufacturing practices].

[136] 69 FED. REG. 9199 (Feb. 26, 2004); M. Kaufman, *Bar codes favored to cut hospitals' drug errors; health chief maps rules to encourage their use*, WASH. POST, Feb. 26, 2004, A3.

[137] 21 U.S.C. § 384.

[138] *See* D. Henderson, *FDA frets over unsafe drug imports*, AP, Aug. 23, 2004; T. Jones, *Bush rejects imports of prescription drugs*, CHICAGO TRIB., Dec. 22, 2004, § 1, 11.

[139] *E.g.*, T. Albert, *FDA sues Rx sellers to stop importation of drugs from Canada*, AM. MED. NEWS, Oct. 13, 2003, 9; *U.S. grabs 81-year-old's Lipitor pills*, CAPITAL TIMES (Madison, WI), Feb. 7, 2005, 3A [mailed from Canadian pharmacy].

[140] M. Davey, *Illinois to help residents buy drugs from Canada, and afar*, N.Y. TIMES, Aug. 17, 2004, A5; M. Davey, *Illinois seeks permission to buy drugs in Canada*, N.Y. TIMES, Oct. 27, 2003, A11; A.W. Mathews, *As states fight drug imports, Illinois rebels*, WALL ST. J., Oct. 27, 2003, B1.

[141] C. Rowland, *Vermont sues over importing prescription drug*, BOSTON GLOBE, Aug. 20, 2004.

[142] Pub. L. No. 91-601, 84 Stat. 1670 (codified as amended in scattered sections of 7,15, 21 U.S.C.).

tainers designed to be difficult for children to open. Exceptions are permitted when authorized by the prescribing physician.

3-3.5 Laws Related to Marketing Drugs and Devices

There are three main sources of regulation of the marketing of drugs and devices — the FDA, Federal Trade Commission (FTC), and Centers for Medicare and Medicaid Services (CMS). Other regulatory agencies and state and private suits also constrain marketing activities.

FDA. The FDA regulates the labeling of drugs and devices and seeks to regulate advertising of drugs and devices.

The First Amendment restricts the ability to regulate advertising. In 2002, the United States Supreme Court struck down a FDA prohibition of advertising compound drugs, finding it an unconstitutional restriction on commercial speech.[143] Complete prohibition of truthful advertising is generally not permitted. Regulation to prohibit false or misleading advertising is permissible. Labeling requirements of the FDA are generally upheld. The FDA frequently directs changes in labeling, both as to content and format.[144] The FDA also challenges advertising or promotions that it considers to be misleading.[145]

There has been controversy over the extent to which the FDA can regulate the promotion of off-label uses. In 1999, a federal district court found that the FDA's regulatory efforts under the Food and Drug Administration Modernization Act of 1997 (FDAMA) violated the First Amendment and issued an injunction against the FDA. The FDA appealed and stated during the appeal that FDAMA did not provide it with independent authority to proscribe speech. Based on this concession, the appellate court vacated the district court injunction. The FDA maintained that it still could prosecute any promotion of off-label uses outside the scope authorized by

---

[143] Thompson v. Western States Med. Ctrs., 535 U.S. 357 (2002).

[144] *E.g.*, S. Elliott, *The F.D.A. may ask drug advertisers to make information on side effects more prominent*, N.Y. TIMES, Feb. 5, 2004, C5 [proposed rules].

[145] *E.g.*, G. Harris, *Federal drug agency calls ads for the cholesterol pill Crestor 'false and misleading,'* N.Y. TIMES, Dec. 23, 2004, A16; *Genetech warned by F.D.A.*, N.Y. TIMES, Aug. 28, 2003, C11 [warned to stop misleading promotions of growth hormone]; E. Douglass, *Gilead ordered to stop misstatements*, L.A. TIMES, Aug. 8, 2003, pt. 3, 2; J. Bennett, *FDA tells Allergan that Botox ads violate federal law*, AP, June 24, 2003.

FDAMA. Nonetheless, the challengers decided that they did not want to pursue the case any further; so it was dropped as moot.[146]

FEDERAL TRADE COMMISSION. The FTC actively regulates advertising, pursuing claims that are false, misleading, or unproven.[147] The Federal Trade Commission Act provides that "unfair or deceptive acts or practices in or affecting commerce are declared unlawful."[148]

> "Unfair" practices are defined to mean those that "cause[] or [are] likely to cause substantial injury to consumers which is not reason- ably avoidable by consumers themselves and not outweighed by countervailing benefits to consumers or to competition."[149]

For example, in 2000, a drug company was accused of making unproven claims in its advertising. In a settlement with the FTC, the company entered a consent decree that included a national con- sumer education campaign.[150]

Private suits can be brought under some of the laws adminis- tered by the FTC. Companies sometimes use these laws to chal- lenge claims made by their competitors.[151]

CENTERS FOR MEDICARE & MEDICAID SERVICES (CMS). Medicare and Medicaid law prohibits inducements to providers to purchase products and services. This antikickback law is discussed in Chapter 12. This prohibition has a substantial impact on market- ing activities. In 2003, the Inspector General of the Department of Health and Human Services issued marketing guidance for pharma- ceutical manufacturers.[152]

In 2001, a federal district court ruled that a False Claims Act suit could be brought against a drug manufacturer for promoting off-

---

[146] Washington Legal Found. v. Henney, 56 F. Supp. 2d 81, 87 (D. D.C. 1999) [injunction], *vacated*, 340 U.S. App. D.C. 108, 202 F.3d 331, 335 (D.C. Cir. 2000), *on remand*, 128 F. Supp. 2d 11 (D. D.C. 2000); D. Mack, *Appeal dismissed in off-label use case; A constitu- tional question disappears*, CORP. LEGAL TIMES, May 2000, 80.

[147] http://www.ftc.gov/ [accessed Sept. 18, 2004].

[148] 15 U.S.C. § 45(a)(1).

[149] 15 U.S.C. § 45(n).

[150] *Bayer settles FTC charges of unproven claims in aspirin ads*, PHARMACEUTICAL LITIGATION RPTR., Feb. 2000, 6 [United States v. Bayer Corp., No. 00-132 (D NJ, consent decree submit- ted for court approval Jan. 11, 2000)]; http://www.ftc.gov/os/2000/01/sterlingdecree.htm [accessed Sept. 18, 2004].

[151] *See* H.P. Weinberger & J.M. Wagner, *On the false advertising battlefront; fiercest Lanham Act conflicts waged by large pharmaceutical companies over reps' oral claims*, N.Y.L.J., July 24, 2000, S3.

[152] 68 FED. REG. 23,731 (May 5, 2003).

label use.[153] In 2004, the drug manufacturer pled guilty to paying physicians to prescribe the drug for off-label uses and agreed to pay $430 million to settle all criminal and civil charges.[154]

In 2003, another drug company agreed to pay $622 million to settle claims regarding marketing of feeding liquids. The company had given free tubes and pumps to providers who were suspected to have billed Medicare and Medicaid for the tubes and pumps.[155]

STATE LAWS ON PRICE ADVERTISING. In the past, many states had laws limiting prescription price advertising. In 1976, the Supreme Court declared unconstitutional all laws that prohibit or unnecessarily restrict advertising of prescription price information. The Court left room for states to control some aspects of advertising, including restrictions on time, place, manner, and false or deceptive practices.[156] Some states now require the posting of prices in pharmacies.

OTHER STATE LAWS. Some states require a report on the number of gifts made to individual physicians from drug companies.[157]

Discussion Points

1. Discuss the legal constraints on construction of health care facilities. How do zoning requirements, building codes, building permit requirements, and certificate of need laws regulate the creation of health care buildings?
2. What are the limits on government use of these regulations to bar health care buildings?
3. What are some of the health care services that are not authorized by a general institutional license and require special additional licenses?
4. Discuss the legal issues involved in implementing formulary systems.
5. Discuss how the federal Controlled Substances Act regulates the use of controlled substances in health care.

---

153 United States *ex rel.* Franklin v. Parke-Davis, 147 F. Supp. 2d 39 (D. Mass. 2001).
154 G. Harris, *Pfizer to pay $430 million over promoting drug to doctors*, N.Y. TIMES, May 14, 2004, C1 [Pfizer acquired Warner-Lambert, the parent of Parke Davis, in 2000].
155 G. Harris, *Abbott to pay $622 million to end inquiry into marketing*, N.Y. TIMES, June 27, 2003, C1.
156 Virginia State Bd. of Pharmacy v. Virginia Citizens Consumer Council, 425 U.S. 748 (1976).
157 A Robeznieks, *States ask drug firms to report gifts to individual physicians*, AM. MED. NEWS, Mar. 1, 2004, 1 [required reporting in Nevada, New Mexico, Vermont, and Maine].

6. Discuss federal Food and Drug Administration (FDA) regulation of new drugs.
7. Discuss off-label uses of drugs.
8. Discuss FDA regulation of new devices.
9. Discuss what constitutes a valid prescription for a drug.
10. Discuss FDA regulation of the importation of low cost drugs from other countries.
11. Discuss the scope of governmental authority to regulate labeling and advertising of drugs and devices.

CHAPTER FOUR

Individual Providers and Caregivers

Objectives

The objective of this chapter and Chapter 5 is to provide an overview of the legal aspects of the relationship of individual health care providers and caregivers with the health care delivery system. Medical staff members are discussed in the next chapter. The reader should learn the relationship to government through licensure, the relationship to other professionals through private certification, and the relationship to the health care delivery system through employment, independent contract, or volunteer or student status.

Health care is ultimately provided by individuals. There are few situations where an individual can provide health care beyond first aid without the support of others. To provide health care, individual providers must work in interrelated teams within an organization, which provides the infrastructure that is necessary to finance and deliver the complex clinical aspects of medicine and to maintain compliance with regulatory and billing requirements and the standard of care.

Many individual health care providers are licensed by the government and must meet governmental standards. Section 4-1 of this chapter addresses individual licensing. Private organizations certify individuals. In some cases, this private certification is required by government to qualify for certain positions, status, or payment.

Section 4-2 addresses private certification of individuals. Individual providers generally have one of four relationships with health care organizations. Most individuals are employees, independent contractors, owners (e.g., partners or shareholders), or have privileges to practice. Some individuals can have more than one status with the same health care entity. For example, some physicians who have hospital privileges are also employees or independent contractors of the hospital. Many individuals can have different relationships with different entities. For example, some physicians are partners in their medical practice, and their only relationship with a hospital is privileges.

Section 4-3 discusses the employment relationship. Section 4-4 discusses independent contactors. The relationship of partners and shareholders is discussed in Chapter 2. Section 4-5 discusses others who provide services in health care organizations, such as volunteers and students. The organized medical staff and practice privileges are discussed in Chapter 5.

4-1 Individual Licensing

Licensing of individual health care providers is usually intended to assure that only qualified people are engaged in health care practice. The primary purpose is to protect the public health by helping the public identify qualified providers and by prohibiting unqualified persons from providing services that require expertise.

These concerns about quality are also addressed through several other approaches, including the private certification and review of individuals by accrediting bodies (4-2); by employers (4-3); by institutional providers and provider networks through medical staff processes (5); by managed care plans (10-2); by malpractice claims (11); and by criminal prosecutions (12-4.2). In general, it is the role of licensing to maintain basic quality standards. The other approaches are used to strive for higher standards in various settings. Some licensing requirements are criticized as barriers to those who want to enter practice; thus the requirements can constitute a restriction on competition.

This section addresses the following questions:

4-1.1. When is a license required?
4-1.2. What are the requirements for licenses?
4-1.3. What is the scope of practice permitted by a license?

4-1.4. What is the scope of rule-making authority by licensing boards?

4-1.5. What is the scope of the disciplinary power of licensing boards?

4-1.6. What is the impact of licensing on competition and availability of services?

4-1.1 When Is a License Required?

MANDATORY VERSUS PERMISSIVE LICENSING. Public licensing can be either mandatory or permissive. A mandatory licensing law requires that individuals obtain licenses before practicing within the scope of practice reserved for those with licenses, unless the individual is exempted. A permissive licensing law usually regulates use of titles; an individual cannot use the title without a license but can perform the functions. In the past, some licensing laws, both mandatory and permissive, provided for registration with no required special qualifications. Today registration laws are rare. Nearly all licensing laws include educational and examination requirements.

SELECTION OF PROFESSIONS TO LICENSE. States have discretion to determine which professions to license. In 1889, the United States Supreme Court upheld mandatory licensing of physicians.[1] The scope of discretion is illustrated by a 1966 Supreme Court decision permitting states not to recognize naturopathy as a discipline distinct from orthodox medical practice.[2] Thus, naturopaths may be required to qualify for a full medical license; states are not required to offer them a separate license but may do so.[3]

Attempts have been made to use other rights as a basis for requiring separate licensing, but these have been unsuccessful. In 1997, a federal appellate court upheld New York's midwife licensing law; the right of privacy does not include the right to use a midwife.[4] States are not required to provide a religious exemption to licensing laws. In 1996, a Pennsylvania court upheld fining a member of a religious

---

1   Dent v. West Virginia, 129 U.S. 114 (1889); St. George's School of Med. v. Dep't of Registration and Educ., 640 F. Supp. 208 (N.D. Ill. 1986) [authority to license physicians belongs to state].

2   Beck v. McLeod, 240 F. Supp. 708 (D. S.C. 1965), *aff'd*, 382 U.S. 454 (1966); *see also* Peckmann v. Thompson, 745 F. Supp. 1388 (C.D. Ill. 1990) [state has broad police power to regulate healing arts; no constitutional right to have midwives recognized or licensed].

3   *E.g., Judge: Natural health practitioner can keep doors open*, AP, Mar. 30, 2002 [natural health practice may continue but practitioner cannot advertise as doctor of naturopathy in S. Dak.].

4   Lange-Kessler v. Dep't of Educ., 1997 U.S. App. LEXIS 15275.

community who performed dentistry on other members of the community without a license.[5]

Physicians, dentists, registered nurses, and pharmacists are subject to mandatory licensing in all states. Many other professionals, including physical therapists, psychologists, speech pathologists, audiologists, occupational therapists, and podiatrists, are licensed in most states. Some states license technical personnel such as emergency medical technicians and radiology technologists. Further, some localities have licensing requirements.[6]

The federal government also licenses some individual health care providers. For example, professionals who manufacture, prescribe, distribute, or dispense controlled substances must be registered with the Drug Enforcement Administration.[7]

On rare occasions, states suspend specific licensing requirements, especially when they become a threat to patient care. For example, in 2001, Colorado suspended the requirement for licenses for nursing aides because the exam backlog created a shortage that was threatening the well-being of nursing home residents.[8]

LICENSE RENEWAL. Failure to renew licenses in a timely manner not only violates the licensing law, but also can increase liability exposure. The Virginia Supreme Court ruled that the state statutory cap on malpractice damages does not apply to services provided while a physician has an expired license.[9] Billing for services while unlicensed can constitute fraud, leading to prosecution and/or required refunds. A Pennsylvania pharmacist was required to reimburse the state for all prescriptions billed to the state during the period his license had lapsed.[10]

INSTITUTIONAL REVIEW. Health care providers need a system to determine whether or not staff members have the required qualifications and licenses. In some states if a patient is harmed by a staff member who is practicing illegally, the hospital can be liable in situ-

---

[5] Zook v. State Board of Dentistry, 683 A.2d 713 (Pa. Commw. Ct. 1996).

[6] *E.g.*, P. Sutin, *Council is unswayed by patient's opposition to requirement for stretcher van technicians*, ST. LOUIS POST-DISPATCH, Dec. 3, 2001, 1 [county license].

[7] 21 U.S.C. § 823; Pearce v. United States Dep't of Justice, DEA, 867 F.2d 253 (6th Cir. 1988) [example of revocation of DEA license].

[8] A. Imse, *Licensing rule suspended for nurse's aides*, ROCKY MOUNTAIN NEWS [Denver, Colo.], June 28, 2001, 16A.

[9] Taylor v. Mobil Oil Corp., 248 Va. 101, 444 S.E.2d 705 (1994).

[10] Calabro v. Dep't of Aging, 689 A.2d 347 (Pa. Commw. Ct. 1997) [PA pharmacist required to refund for prescriptions billed while unlicensed]; *Optometrist operating without a license indicted for Medicare fraud, reports U.S. attorney*, PR NEWSWIRE, Apr. 23, 2002.

ations where it would not be liable if the staff member was practicing legally.[11] However, in liability cases involving unlicensed staff, most states focus on whether the employee was competent, rather than on lack of a license.[12] Hospitals can be subject to administrative and criminal penalties for using unlicensed staff. For example, a New Jersey hospital was ordered to pay an administrative fine for aiding and abetting the illegal practice of medicine because it employed an unlicensed physician in its emergency room.[13]

In some states, hospitals and other health care organizations have the responsibility to determine whether or not certain professional and technical personnel meet government-imposed qualifications,[14] instead of having a governmental agency evaluate the qualifications and issue a license.

Courts generally understand that hospitals must take action against employees who fail to maintain necessary licenses and other requirements. For example, a Pennsylvania court ruled that a nurse who was terminated for failure to renew her license was not entitled to unemployment compensation.[15] The failure was considered "willful misconduct."

Some hospital staff members are exempt from some licensing requirements. Exemption gives hospitals more flexibility in determining qualifications of those staff.

OUT-OF-STATE ACTIVITIES. Since each state has its own licensing law, professionals generally must obtain a license in each state in which they practice. Some states have exceptions that permit persons licensed in another state to provide some services in consultation with a professional licensed in the state or some emergency services, but the scope of the exceptions vary. Professionals who provide services outside their state of primary licensing need to limit their services to

---

[11] *E.g.*, Central Anesthesia Assocs., P.C. v. Worthy, 173 Ga. App. 150, 325 S.E.2d 819 (1984), *aff'd*, 254 Ga. 728, 333 S.E.2d 829 (1985) [hospital liable for injuries caused by student nurse anesthetist under supervision of physician's assistant when law required physician supervision].

[12] *E.g.*, Turek v. St. Elizabeth Comm. Health Ctr., 241 Neb. 467, 488 N.W.2d 567 (1992); Leahy v. Kenosha Mem. Hosp., 118 Wis. 2d 441, 348 N.W.2d 607 (Ct. App. 1984); *see also* Lingle v. Dion, 776 So. 2d 1073 (Fla. 4th DCA 2001) [failure to comply with office surgery rule not negligence per se].

[13] State Bd. of Med. Exam'rs v. Warren Hosp., 102 N.J. Super. 407, 246 A.2d 78 (Dist. Ct. 1968), *aff'd*, 104 N.J. Super. 409, 250 A.2d 158 (App. Div. 1969).

[14] *E.g.*, Roach v. Kelly Health Care, Inc., 87 Or. App. 495, 742 P.2d 1190 (1987) [home health agency violated regulations by using certified nursing assistant who had not received required additional 60 hours of training on home care].

[15] Adams v. Commonwealth, Unemployment Comp. Bd. of Review, 86 Pa. Commw. 238, 484 A.2d 232 (1984).

those that do not require a license or obtain a license. This is an issue not only when the professional crosses the border but can also apply when services are provided by Internet to an out-of-state patient.[16]

4-1.2 What Are the Requirements for Licenses?

States have discretion in determining the requirements for licensing. Most licensing laws require specified training and tests. Some states impose requirements in addition to education and testing.[17] For example, some states require physicians to participate in Medicare and accept its payment as payment in full.[18] In 1998, a federal appellate court upheld the right of states to require physicians to contribute to a malpractice liability fund in order to be licensed.[19] The Illinois Supreme Court ruled that the state can require good moral character and place the burden on the applicant to prove it.[20] Unless the licensing statute authorizes waiver of requirements, generally the licensing agency does not have the discretion to waive requirements that are set by statute.[21]

The Americans with Disabilities Act (ADA) limits inquiries into physical and mental health and requires some accommodations of disabilities.[22] ADA regulations call for extra time accommodations

---

[16] *E.g., California fines six out-of-state doctors*, AP, Feb. 11, 2003.

[17] *E.g.,* Dittman v. State, 191 F.3d 1020 (9th Cir. 1999) [state may require disclosure of social security number in license application].

[18] *E.g.*, Massachusetts Med. Soc'y v. Dukakis, 637 F. Supp. 684 (D. Mass. 1986), *aff'd*, 815 F.2d 790 (1st Cir.), *cert. denied*, 484 U.S. 896 (1987); McGinn, *R.I. mandates Medicare assignment for all claims*, Am. MED. NEWS, Sept. 22/29, 1989, 3; *but see* Hennessey v. Berger, 403 Mass. 648, 531 N.E.2d 1268 (1988) [nonparticipating physician may refuse to treat Medicaid recipient].

[19] Hayes v. Ridge, 168 F.3d 478, 1998 U.S. App. LEXIS 29684 (3d Cir. Oct. 27, 1998) (unpub.), *earlier decision*, 946 F. Supp. 354 (D. Pa. 1996) [denying injunction]; *see also* Ubel v. State, 547 N.W.2d 366 (Minn. 1996), *cert. denied*, 519 U.S. 1057 (1997) [upholding medical license surcharge].

[20] Abrahamson v. Illinois Dep't of Prof. Reg., 153 Ill. 2d 76, 606 N.E.2d 1111 (1992).

[21] *E.g.*, Dep't of Prof. Reg. v. Florida Dental Hygienist Ass'n, Inc., 612 So. 2d 646 (Fla. 1st DCA 1993) [agency exceeded delegated authority by permitting hygienists graduated from programs with lower standards than legislative requirement]; *but see* Abramson v. Florida Psychological Ass'n, 634 So. 2d 610 (Fla. 1994) [state must honor settlement with psychology applicants that granted license to person not meeting statutory requirements].

[22] *E.g.*, Hason v. Medical Bd., 279 F.3d 1167 (9th Cir. 2002), *cert. dismissed*, 538 U.S. 958 (2003) [MD may challenge license denial based on mental illness]; Medical Soc'y of N.J. v. Jacobs, 1994 U.S. Dist. LEXIS 15261 (D. N.J.) [settlement of ADA challenge to license questions on mental illness, substance abuse, agreed to drop questions, pay legal fees]; *but see* Kotz v. State, 33 F. Supp. 2d 1019 (M.D. Fla. 1998) [federal court will not intervene to stop state licensing board from collecting information about alleged disabilities]; Colorado State Bd. of Med. Exam'rs v. Davis, 893 P.2d 1365 (Colo. Ct. App. 1995) [ADA does not bar medical license revocation for recent history of illegal prescription drug use]; Ramachandar v. Sobol, 838 F. Supp. 100 (S.D. N.Y. 1993) [Rehabilitation Act does not preclude medical license revocation for mental illness]; *see also* Medical Soc'y of N.J. v. Doe, 191 F. Supp. 2d 574 (D. N.J. 2002) [dismiss challenge to policy of making agreements concerning past substance abuse pubic records].

on timed examinations in some circumstances.[23] In 1999, a federal appellate court ruled that it was not discrimination to disclose which tests results involved accommodations.[24]

4-1.3 What Is the Scope of Practice Permitted by a License?

Mandatory licensing laws reserve a scope of practice for those who obtain licenses. The definition and evolution of the scope of practice for some professionals have been controversial. The controversy has focused on two issues. Who is allowed to make the judgment that certain procedures will be performed? Who is allowed to perform the procedures?

Although courts will uphold almost all restrictions on scope of practice adopted under the state police power, occasionally courts will find that some laws have gone too far. In 1992, the Georgia Supreme Court declared a statute unconstitutional that permitted only physicians, dentists, podiatrists, and veterinarians to perform any surgery, operation, or invasive procedure in which human or animal tissue was cut, pierced, or altered.[25] The court concluded that there was no rational basis for this statute, which did not permit nurses to give injections or diabetics to inject themselves with insulin.

In general, medical diagnosing and ordering some diagnostic and therapeutic procedures are reserved for physicians. Podiatrists and dentists usually are permitted to diagnose and treat the parts of the body related to their practice; there continue to be disputes over the boundaries.[26] Other professionals are increasingly being permitted to make some diagnoses and order some treatments.[27] By 2004, two states allowed psychologists to prescribe some drugs, and six states allowed pharmacists to dispense some drugs without

---

[23] 29 C.F.R. § 1630.2(j)(3)(i); *compare* Rush v. National Bd. Med. Exam'rs, 268 F. Supp. 2d 673 (N.D. Tex. 2003) [ADA testing accommodation ordered] *with* Powell v. National Bd. of Med. Exam'rs, 364 F.3d 79 (2d Cir. 2004) [affirming denial of ADA testing accommodation].

[24] Doe v. National Bd. of Med. Exam'rs, 199 F.3d 146 (3d Cir. 1999).

[25] Miller v. Medical Ass'n of Ga., 262 Ga. 605, 423 S.E.2d 664 (1992).

[26] *E.g.*, J. Spencer, *Decision lets Texas podiatrists continue treating the ankle*, COX NEW SERVICE, July 1, 2002 [county judge refused to throw out settlement between state, podiatrists]; *Camarillo men fined in cosmetic surgeries*, L.A. TIMES, Feb. 5, 2004, B3 [Calif. dentists performed cosmetic surgery].

[27] M. Croasdale, *Empowered by insurers and states, nonphysicians push practice limits*, AM. MED. NEWS, Feb. 9, 2004, 1; M. Croasdale, *Nonphysicians eager to pick up prescription pad*, AM. MED. NEWS, Feb. 7, 2005, 1.

a prescription.[28] States vary concerning which procedures may be ordered by physicians' assistants and nurse practitioners and under what circumstances.[29]

Nursing diagnosis is generally recognized as different from physician diagnosis. Generally, nurses determine what nursing care is needed and when nursing care is insufficient so that medical attention or instructions must be sought. In some states, nurses are permitted to make some judgments traditionally reserved for physicians when acting pursuant to standing orders or established protocols.[30] Many states license nurse practitioners to independently make some judgments traditionally reserved to physicians, including prescribing many drugs.[31]

There has been considerable controversy over the degree of supervision required for nurse anesthetists. Medicare requires physician supervision unless the state has elected to opt out of the physician supervision requirement, which some states have elected to do.[32]

Most medical procedures are restricted to physicians when they are first introduced. As experience with them grows and they become better defined, nurses tend to be permitted to perform the procedures, and in some situations, other professional and technical personnel are permitted to perform them. This evolution has varied from state to state and has been recognized in several ways — licensing statute amendments, state attorney general opinions, medical and/or nursing licensing board rules or statements,[33] joint statements of private professional organizations, and judicial decisions. Sometimes established practices are overturned by subsequent rulings. For example, the Iowa Supreme Court affirmed an injunction prohibiting a chiropractor from performing acupuncture,

---

[28] J. Spencer, *Getting drugs without the doctor*, WIS. ST. J., June 1, 2004, D1 [extension of prescription-writing powers to others; six states allow pharmacists to give out morning-after pill; two states allow psychologists to prescribe some drugs - La. & N. Mex.].

[29] *E.g.,* Rockefeller v. Kaiser Found. Health Plan of Ga., 554 S.E.2d 623 (Ga. App. 2001) [violation for PA to provide treatment without supervision by approved physician].

[30] *E.g.,* Sermchief v. Gonzales, 600 S.W.2d 683 (Mo. 1983).

[31] *E.g.,* WIS. STAT., § 441.16.

[32] 66 FED. REG. 56762 (Nov. 13, 2001) [CMS rule granting option]; *State Board of Medicine and Surgery supports removing physician supervision for Nebraska's nurse anesthetists*, U.S. NEWSWIRE, Feb. 25, 2002 [2d state to opt out of MD supervision]; *see also Hospital says nurses gave anesthetic without doctor's order*, AP, Oct. 4, 2003 [14 nurses fired, 9 disciplined].

[33] *E.g.,* State *ex rel.* Lakeland Anesthesia Group, Inc. v. Ohio State Med. Bd., 74 Ohio App. 3d 643, 600 N.E.2d 270 (1991).

drawing blood specimens, and giving advice on diet and nutrition even though the Board of Chiropractic Examiners had issued a declaratory ruling that these practices were permitted.[34] In 1996, an Arizona appellate court upheld rules of the chiropractic board permitting chiropractic assistants to administer physical therapy.[35] Many sources may need to be examined to determine the scope of practice in a particular state.

DELEGATION. Some states have given physicians broad authority to delegate functions to nurses and sometimes others.[36] For example, Michigan permits physicians to delegate functions to others under proper supervision if permitted by standards of acceptable and prevailing practice.[37] The Michigan attorney general has interpreted this to permit physicians to delegate to nurses the prescribing of any drugs except controlled substances if the prescription identifies the supervising physician.[38] Other states have given licensing boards the broad authority to expand nursing functions. For example, Iowa gives the Board of Nursing authority to expand nursing roles by rule when the expanded roles are recognized by the medical and nursing professions.[39] Oregon has gone one step farther and permitted nurse practitioners to be selected as the "attending physician" of an injured worker under the workers' compensation law.[40]

Delegation should be limited to the permitted scope. A physician's assistant was convicted for prescribing a controlled substance without statutory authority when he authorized refilling a prescription for Tylenol with codeine in accordance with written instructions from the supervising physician. The physician and the physician's assistant were excluded from participation in Medicare for five years as a result of the conviction.[41] In 1999, an Illinois physician's license was suspended for permitting a pharmacist assistant to diagnosis and treat patients, including writing prescriptions, giving injections,

34 State *ex rel.* Iowa Dep't of Health v. Van Wyk, 320 N.W.2d 599 (Iowa 1982).
35 State Farm Mutual Auto. Ins. Co. v. Arizona Bd. of Chiropractic Exam'rs, 931 P.2d 426 (Ariz. App. Ct. 1996).
36 *E.g.,* Wis. Stat. § 448.03(2)(e).
37 MICH. COMP. LAWS § 333.16215(1).
38 Opinion No. 5630 (Jan. 22, 1980).
39 IOWA CODE ANN. § 152.1(6)(d).
40 Cook v. Workers' Compensation Dep't, 306 Or. 134, 758 P.2d 854 (1988).
41 Mullen v. Inspector General, HHS D.A.B., Civil remedies Div. No. C-94-299, Dec. No. CR227 (Oct. 5, 1994), *as reprinted in* MEDICARE & MEDICAID GUIDE (CCH) ¶43,008.

and removing stitches.[42] In 2002, an Iowa physician was fined for permitting an unlicensed EMT student to treat a patient.[43]

When acts can be delegated, there usually are supervision requirements. In 2002, a California physician lost his license in part for permitting medical assistants to perform tests without supervision.[44]

4-1.4 What Is the Scope of Rule-making Authority by Licensing Boards?

Some rules promulgated by licensing boards have been challenged on the basis that they are believed to be beyond the boards' authority. Licensing boards generally have broad authority.

A New Jersey appellate court upheld a rule requiring licensed radiologists who provide diagnostic services for other physicians to provide them for licensed chiropractors.[45] Although this service was inconsistent with the practice of many radiologists, the court ruled that it was reasonable, within the board's authority, and promulgated using proper procedures. The Ohio Supreme Court upheld a rule prohibiting the prescription of anabolic steroids for the enhancement of athletic ability.[46] In 1990, the New Jersey Supreme Court upheld a Board of Physical Therapy rule that reduced physician supervision and permitted therapists to modify the prescribed treatment.[47] In 2000, a Florida appellate court upheld an emergency moratorium on all complex physician office surgery.[48] In 2004, a federal appellate court ruled that it was not a violation of the First Amendment to limit advertising of medical specialty certification to recognized certifying boards.[49]

[42] Siddiqui v. Illinois Dep't of Prof. Reg., 307 Ill. App. 3d 753, 718 N.E.2d 217 (4th Dist. 1999).

[43] *Doctor fined for allowing unlicensed student to treat woman*, AP, Oct. 2, 2002.

[44] *Medical board accusation leads to surrender of Burbank physician's medical license*, BUSINESS WIRE, June 27, 2002 [pulmonary function tests, ultrasound tests]; *see also* M. Lasalandra, *State warns heart doctors; Too many complex tasks performed by assistants*, BOSTON HERALD, July 17, 2000, 1 [alleged PAs performing invasive heart procedures]; M. Crane, *Board revokes doctor's license*, COLUMBUS [Ohio] DISPATCH, July 13, 2000, 1C [left patients in care of unsupervised assistant].

[45] Brodie v. State Bd. of Med. Exam'rs, 177 N.J. Super. 523, 427 A.2d 104 (App. Div. 1981).

[46] State Med. Bd. v. Murray, 66 Ohio St. 3d 527, 613 N.E.2d 636 (1993).

[47] Medical Soc'y of N.J. v. New Jersey Dep't of Law & Pub. Safety, 120 N.J. 18, 575 A.2d 1348 (1990).

[48] Florida Med. Ass'n v. State, 766 So. 2d 406 (Fla. 1st DCA 2000); *see also Board places 90-day ban on in-office cosmetic procedure*, AP, Feb. 7, 2004 [Fla. 90-day moratorium on office combined tummy tuck, liposuction procedures in MD offices after several deaths].

[49] American Academy of Pain Management v. Joseph, 353 F.3d 1099 (9th Cir. 2004).

Occasionally, specific controversial rules have been found to exceed the board's authority. A Florida appellate court ruled that the licensing board did not have authority to prohibit chelation therapy for arteriosclerosis unless the board found the therapy was harmful or hazardous to patients.[50] The prohibition was not justified by the lack of proof of effectiveness or the limited number of physicians who used it. An Illinois appellate court invalidated a rule that excluded from the dental licensing examination all persons who were not graduates of schools approved by the American Dental Association or schools with a curriculum equivalent to that of the University of Illinois College of Dentistry.[51] The statute limited the examination to graduates of "reputable" schools. The board could not arbitrarily determine that a school was not reputable; it had to evaluate the school. A Florida appellate court ruled that a Board of Optometry rule authorizing optometrists to use certain drugs was beyond the authority of the board.[52] A Pennsylvania court invalidated a rule requiring physicians to obtain permission from the board on a patient-by-patient basis before prescribing amphetamines.[53] In 2004, a Florida appellate court invalidated a rule that required anesthesia for outpatient surgery to be supervised by an anesthesiologist; a statute specifically limited the board's authority on this issue.[54]

Decisions in one state are of limited help in addressing these issues in other states, but these examples show that it is possible to challenge some rulings of licensing boards.

4-1.5 What Is the Scope of the Disciplinary Power of Licensing Boards?

Licensing boards have broad authority to discipline licensed professionals when they violate professional standards specified in licensing laws or board rules. The discipline can be a reprimand,

---

[50] Rogers v. State Bd. of Med. Exam'rs, 371 So. 2d 1037 (Fla. 1st DCA 1979), *aff'd*, 387 So. 2d 937 (Fla. 1980); *see also* P. Simms, *Board allows chelation therapy*, WIS. ST. J., Nov. 25, 2003, C1.

[51] Garces v. Dep't of Registration & Educ., 118 Ill. App. 2d 206, 254 N.E.2d 622 (1st Dist. 1969).

[52] Board of Optometry v. Florida Med. Ass'n, Inc., 463 So. 2d 1213 (Fla. 1st DCA 1985).

[53] Pennsylvania Med. Soc'y v. Commonwealth, State Bd. of Med., 118 Pa. Commw. 635, 546 A.2d 720 (1988).

[54] Ortiz v. Dep't of Health, 882 So. 2d 402 (Fla. 4th DCA 2004).

revocation,[55] suspension, fine,[56] or probationary period during which conditions must be met.[57] Most licensing boards have authority to impose various conditions, including prohibiting types of practice[58] or requiring substance abuse rehabilitation efforts; practice monitoring; record review; consultation or supervision of specified procedures; completion of education programs; and increased malpractice insurance.[59] Before imposing disciplinary sanctions, licensing boards must provide due process to licensed professionals, including notice of the wrongful conduct and an opportunity to present information.[60]

Many states impose stricter requirements that must be followed for the board's action to be valid. For example, the Colorado Supreme Court ordered a nurse's license to be reinstated, in part because the statute required the full licensing board to attend the revocation hearing and the full board had not done so.[61] Most licensing laws do not require the presence of the full board, but if this is required, the law must be followed. In some states, the licensing board cannot attend the evidentiary hearing.[62]

---

[55] *E.g., Doctor's license revoked for wrong-finger surgery*, AP, June 25, 2002 [NY].

[56] *E.g., Boca doctor fined for surgery mistake*, PALM BEACH [FL] POST, Feb. 14, 1995, 1B [neurosurgeon fined $5,000 for operating on wrong side of skull].

[57] *E.g.*, Kite v. DeBuono, 233 A.D.2d 783, 650 N.Y.S.2d 384 (3d Dept. 1996) [medical license revoked for violating probation by disregarding supervisor]; Birchard v. Louisiana State Bd. of Med. Exam'rs, 609 So. 2d 980 (La. Ct. App. 1992) [physician on probation with condition he obtain board approval for changes of employment not entitled to hearing on denial of approval].

[58] *E.g.*, Sternberg v. Administrative Rev. Bd. for Prof. Med. Conduct, 235 A.D.2d 945, 652 N.Y.S.2d 855 (3d Dep't 1997) [barring private practice, limiting to institutional practice]; *Doctor disciplined for death of patient after surgery*, AP, Apr. 8, 2004 [emergency order restricted Fla. physician license after death during office breast augmentation, cannot perform procedures with general anesthesia].

[59] *E.g.*, Caselnova v. New York State Dep't of Health, 91 N.Y.2d 441, 672 N.Y.S.2d 79, 694 N.E.2d 1320 (1998) [medical licensing board may condition probation on monitoring, record review, increased malpractice insurance].

[60] Annotation, *Rights as to notice and hearing in proceeding to revoke or suspend license to practice medicine*, 10 A.L.R. 5TH 1; Fleury v. Clayton, 847 F.2d 1229 (7th Cir. 1988) [right to notice, hearing applies when only sanction is censure]; Jensen v. California Bd. of Psychology No. B091019 (Calif. Ct. App. 2d Dist. May 14, 1996), *cert. denied*, 519 U.S. 1058 (1997), *as discussed in* 6 HEALTH LAW RPTR. [BNA] 72 (1997) [notice sent by certified mail to last address provided to board was sufficient] [hereinafter HEALTH LAW RPTR. will be cited as H.L.R.].

[61] Colorado State Bd. of Nursing v. Hohu, 129 Colo. 195, 268 P.2d 401 (1954); *see also In re* Grimm, 138 N.H. 42, 635 A.2d 456 (1993) [violation of due process for some members of hearing panel, acting in fact-finding capacity, to fail to attend all testimony, especially cross-examination of respondent]; Pet v. Dep't of Health Servs., 228 Conn. 651, 638 A.2d 6 (1994) [remand where no board member attended all hearings, record did not indicate whether voting members had read entire record].

[62] *E.g.*, Virginia Bd. of Med. v. Fetta, 244 Va. 276, 421 S.E.2d 410 (1992) [proceedings against chiropractor dismissed because board violated law when four of sixteen members sat with hearing officer at evidentiary hearing].

NOTICE. To provide due process, licensed professionals must have two types of notice. They must have individualized notice of the specific questioned acts and omissions which form the basis for discipline.[63] In addition, the statute and regulations must provide generalized advance notice that conduct of that type will lead to discipline. Courts usually rule that prohibition of "unprofessional conduct" gives adequate notice that a wide range of inappropriate behavior is prohibited. "Unprofessional conduct" is not considered too vague when it is applied to conduct widely recognized as unprofessional. In 1997, the Montana Supreme Court held that conviction for Medicare false claims was unprofessional conduct justifying license revocation.[64] In 1996, a Missouri appellate court held that pushing a nurse in the operating room was unprofessional conduct, justifying suspension of the surgeon's license for one day.[65] The Oregon Supreme Court upheld the revocation of a nurse's license for "conduct derogatory to the standards of professional nursing."[66] She had instructed, recommended, and permitted her daughter to serve as a registered nurse, knowing that her daughter had no nursing license. However, "unprofessional conduct" is not adequate notice for all possible violations. The Idaho Supreme Court ordered reinstatement of a nursing license that had been suspended for six months for unprofessional conduct.[67] The Board of Nursing had found that the nurse had discussed laetrile treatment with a hospitalized leukemia patient without physician approval, interfering with the physician-patient relationship. The board considered this to be unprofessional conduct. The court ruled that the board could have prohibited this conduct by rule but that a prohibition of unprofessional conduct did not give nurses adequate warning that this conduct was prohibited.

GROUNDS FOR DISCIPLINE. Some licensing boards specify by rule more detailed grounds for discipline, but some courts have

---

[63] *E.g.*, Devous v. Wyoming State Bd. of Med. Exam'rs, 845 P.2d 408 (Wyo. 1993) [violation of due process not to notify physician of facts, nature of charges against him].

[64] Erickson v. State *ex rel.* Bd. of Med. Exam'rs, 282 Mont. 367, 938 P.2d 625 (1997); *accord*, Teruel v. DeBuono, 244 A.D. 2d 710, 664 N.Y.S.2d 381 (3d Dept. 1997) [Medicaid fraud conviction justified revocation of medical license].

[65] Hoffman v. State Board of Registration for the Healing Arts, 936 S.W.2d 182 (Mo. App. Ct. 1996).

[66] Ward v. Oregon State Bd. of Nursing, 226 Or. 128, 510 P.2d 554 (1973).

[67] Tuma v. Board of Nursing, 100 Idaho 74, 593 P.2d 711 (1979).

considered the statutory criteria to be sufficiently clear so that no rules are needed.[68]

With or without rules, licensing boards have sought to impose discipline in several areas.

States have adopted different positions on whether medical directors of managed care organizations can be disciplined for their coverage decisions. For example, in 2001, the Missouri Supreme Court approved review of such coverage decisions.[69] On the other hand, in 1997, a District of Columbia court reached a decision that apparently precludes licensing board review of such decisions in that jurisdiction. The court ruled that a health plan medical director was not practicing medicine; so no license was required.[70]

Boards in some jurisdictions have explored applying discipline for actions taken during litigation. In 1998, a Pennsylvania court upheld the authority of the medical licensing board to discipline a physician for disclosing confidential patient records in the course of business litigation that did not involve the patient.[71] The court ruled that judicial immunity did not provide protection from licensing board discipline. In 1997, the Washington Supreme Court agreed, finding that there could be professional discipline for testimony as an expert witness in a child custody case.[72] In 2000, an Ohio appellate court upheld revocation of a podiatrist's license for perjury during a deposition.[73] In 2003, North Carolina suspended the license of a physician for the content of expert testimony.[74] Absolute immunity for witnesses protects from civil liability but not from discipline.

Some commentators evaluate the licensing process by the number of disciplinary actions that are taken, criticizing jurisdictions that take fewer actions. In reaction, more physicians are being disciplined.[75]

---

[68] *E.g.*, Kibler v. State, 718 P.2d 531 (Colo. 1986).

[69] State Bd. of Reg. for the Healing Arts v. Fallon, 41 S.W.3d 474 (Mo. 2001), *accord*, Murphy v. Arizona Bd. of Med. Examiner, 190 Ariz. 441, 949 P.2d 530 (Ct. App. 1997); *see also* D. Gianelli, *HMO directors must stand behind their decisions*, AM. MED. NEWS, June 21, 1999, 9 [AMA ethics council report].

[70] Morris v. District of Columbia Bd. of Med., 701 A.2d 364 (D.C. 1997).

[71] Huhta v. Pennsylvania Bd. of Med., 706 A.2d 364 (Pa. Commw. Ct. 1998).

[72] Deatherage v. State Examining Bd. of Psychology, 134 Wash. 2d 131, 948 P.2d 828 (1997).

[73] Hayes v. State Med. Bd. of Ohio, 138 Ohio App. 3d 762, 742 N.E.2d 238 (2000).

[74] *N.C. board suspends license for neurosurgeon's expert testimony*, AP, Nov. 22, 2003.

[75] A. Goldstein, *D.C. is ranked last on punishment of doctor misconduct; nonprofit also faults process in Md., Va.*, WASH. POST, Sept. 5, 2002, B5; D. Adams, *Medical board discipline up; lawmakers demand even more*, AM. MED. NEWS, May 9, 2005.

Another interesting development in licensing is the effort by some patients to pressure licensing boards to discipline individual providers.[76]

APPEALS. When licensed professionals prevail in challenges to board actions, they usually cannot get payment from the state or the board members.[77] They are limited to reversal of improper discipline and invalidation of improper rules. In most states, board members have broad immunity from monetary liability.[78]

4-1.6 What Is the Impact of Licensing on Competition and Availability of Services?

States have broad authority to determine which professions to license.[79] The state is confronted with a difficult analysis whenever it is requested to license a health discipline.

Many professional and technical disciplines seek to be licensed. They claim that licensing is necessary to protect the public from unqualified practitioners. Licensing is also sought because it provides status and often is accompanied by expansion of the scope of practice into areas previously reserved for other licensed professionals. Licensing can be an economic benefit to those licensed because licensure reduces the number of people permitted to perform specific tasks. The educational and testing requirements designed to protect the public increase the time and expense of becoming qualified and thus reduce the number of people available to provide the service. This can have a detrimental effect on the public if the subsequent increase in costs charged by the licensed

---

[76] *See Fremont woman wants licenses revoked for two nurses in Javed clinic*, AP, Nov. 25, 2003 [NE]; S. Allen, *House approves patients' rights bill: 'Taylor's law' allows testimony before disciplinary board*, BOSTON GLOBE, Feb. 26, 2004, B3 [Mass.].

[77] *But see* Burns v. Board of Psychologist Examiners, 116 Or. App. 422, 841 P.2d 680 (1992) [licensing board not liable for tort damages for testing irregularities, but authorized ancillary relief could include repayment for direct losses]; *Medical board must pay Raleigh doctor*, AP, Dec. 22, 2001 [federal court ordered W. Va. medical bd. to pay $277K in fees, costs].

[78] *E.g.*, Berthiaume v. Caron, 142 F.3d 12 (1st Cir. 1998) [qualified immunity for nursing board in challenge to making sexual arousal test a condition of license renewal]; Watts v. Burkhart, 978 F.2d 269 (6th Cir. 1992) [quasi-judicial immunity for licensing board members in suspension of physician's license]; Horowitz v. State Bd. of Med. Examiners, 822 F.2d 1508 (10th Cir.), *cert. denied*, 484 U.S. 964 (1987) [absolute immunity from civil rights liability]; Duncan v. Mississippi Bd. of Nursing, 982 F. Supp. 425 (D. Miss. 1997); *but see* Rindley v. Gallagher, 890 F. Supp. 1540 (D. Fla. 1995) [immunity lost due to allegations of public boasting of illegal input into adjudicative process].

[79] *E.g.*, Sutker v. Illinois State Dental Soc'y, 808 F.2d 632 (7th Cir. 1986) [state need not offer separate license to denturists].

professionals is too great. It can have a catastrophic effect if too few people meet the requirements for licensure because some members of the public will then receive no service. Licensing can be a barrier to innovation because of the difficulty in changing statutes and rules that define what licensees may do.

The barriers to entry imposed by licensing are widely accepted for some health professions, especially for professionals who often function independently, such as physicians, dentists, and nurses. The appropriateness of state licensing of dependent practitioners who function under the supervision of other licensed practitioners has been questioned. Some commentators believe that the public health could be adequately protected by placing responsibility on the institution and supervising independent health professionals instead of the system of state licensure. In addition, they say the public interest in innovative, cost-effective health services could be advanced by more flexibility in the use of dependent health personnel. However, the trend appears to continue toward licensing of more health disciplines.

In many cases, the focus is not on the barriers to enter a particular profession, such as the educational requirements to become a physician or a nurse. Instead, sometimes a profession seeks to perform functions that are restricted to another profession. Chiropractors have sought to be permitted to perform functions restricted to physicians. Nurse practitioners, especially nurse anesthetists and nurse midwives, have sought to practice without a supervising or collaborating physician. Lay midwives have sought to practice without nursing or medical training.

Usually, these questions are decided by the legislature or by regulators. As discussed in 4-1.1, courts will generally defer to legislative judgments about licensure and to regulatory actions taken within the scope of those laws. In one unusual case in 1996, the Kansas Supreme Court addressed permissibility of unlicensed lay midwifery by a creative interpretation of the state licensing laws. The court concluded that lay midwifery was not a healing art and did not fall within the definition of medical or nursing practice; so no license was required.[80]

---

[80] State Board v. Reubke, 259 Kan. 599, 913 P.2d 142 (1996); *contra,* People v. Odam, 69 Cal. App. 4th 1192, 82 Cal. Rptr. 2d 184 (4th Dist. 1999) (unpub), *app. dismissed,* 33 P.3d 450, 113 Cal. Rptr. 2d 26 (2001) [conviction of midwife for practicing medicine without a license].

In summary, licensure rules have been challenged as barriers to competition and to consumer access. The rules have been defended on the basis that they maintain quality by requiring additional training for those who perform specific functions. Evaluating the quality of health delivery and determining the appropriate levels of cost and availability are difficult public policy decisions.

4-2 Private Certification of Individuals

In addition to the individual licensing by government agencies, there are many private methods of credentialing, including accreditation of educational programs, certification of individuals, and credentialing by institutions. Credentialing by institutions is addressed in 4-3 and 4-4.

ACCREDITATION OF EDUCATIONAL PROGRAMS. Private professional organizations have established criteria to evaluate educational programs. Periodically an individual or a team investigates programs that desire to be accredited. Programs that meet the criteria are accredited. Although accreditation is voluntary, most educational programs strive to obtain and retain accreditation from established accrediting bodies because students tend to choose accredited programs. Graduates of accredited programs often find it easier to obtain permission to take licensing examinations or to be admitted for advanced study because their degrees are generally accepted without additional proof of their education. Graduates of accredited programs often find it easier to convince employers that they are prepared for employment in the discipline. Others will usually have to provide more information concerning their training programs to demonstrate the adequacy of their training.

Not all accrediting bodies have earned the wide acceptance given to the longer-standing bodies that accredit medicine and nursing programs. Health care organizations should not automatically assume that accreditation assures high standards. If the health care organization is not familiar with the accrediting body, it should make inquiries before relying on its accreditation.

There have been legal challenges to denial of accreditation. Most courts defer to the accrediting bodies. A Pennsylvania hospital that lost accreditation of a general surgery residency program challenged the action in state and federal court. The challenge started with a petition to the state medical licensing board to review the accrediting body's action. The board denied review. A lower state court ordered the board to review the action, but the Pennsylvania Supreme Court reversed, finding the board did not have authority to review individual residency accreditation decisions.[81] A lower federal court granted an injunction of withdrawal of accreditation of a residency program, which the federal appellate court vacated, finding that the accreditation decision was not state action.[82] When a Maryland Roman Catholic hospital lost accreditation of its obstetrics-gynecology residency program because it failed to prove training in family planning, a federal court found that the loss of accreditation did not violate any constitutional or statutory rights of the hospital.[83]

CERTIFICATION OF INDIVIDUALS. Private professional organizations sponsor programs to certify that individuals meet certain criteria and are considered prepared to practice in the discipline. Individual certification is generally related to performance, usually including passing a test. Some certifications, especially certifications by medical specialty boards, have become so widely accepted that it can be difficult to practice without them. However, Medicare-participating hospitals cannot adopt an absolute requirement of board certification for specialty clinical privileges.[84] Instead, hospitals can avail themselves of the value of certification, while avoiding the absolute requirement, by requiring "board certification or equivalent training and experience."

Some managed care plans will pay physicians only when they have board certification.[85]

Certifying bodies have proliferated, resulting in a certifying body for virtually every professional and technical health care discipline.[86] Not all of these bodies have earned the same acceptance as the longer-standing certification bodies. There is also variation in the acceptance of medical specialties. In 2005, the American Board of Medical Specialties recognized 24 medical specialty boards, while over 180 others existed that have not

---

[81] McKeesport Hosp. v. Pennsylvania State Bd. of Med., 539 Pa. 384, 652 A.2d 827 (1995), *rev'g*, 156 Pa. Commw. 480, 628 A.2d 476 (1993).

[82] McKeesport Hosp. v. A.C.G.M.E., 24 F.3d 519 (3d Cir. 1994).

[83] St. Agnes Hosp. v. Ruddick, 748 F. Supp. 319 (D. Md. 1990).

[84] 42 C.F.R. § 482.12(a)(7).

[85] H. Larkin, *All aboard?* AM. MED. NEWS, Mar. 13, 1995, 11 [options for those without board certification to deal with managed care, since 35 to 40 percent of physicians are not board certified].

[86] *E.g.*, J.L. Fickeissen, *56 ways to get certified*, AM. J. NURSING, Mar. 1990, 50.

been recognized.[87] Health care organizations should be familiar with a certifying body before giving it substantial weight in evaluating applications. One advantage of the private certification system is that the organization generally has the discretion to use its own evaluation system.

States can require private certification as a condition of state licensing.[88]

Individuals who challenge denial of certification are generally unsuccessful.[89] Courts will generally enforce the releases that boards require as part of the application process, except as to antitrust claims.[90] Unsuccessful applicants have generally been unable to state antitrust claims.[91]

In 2004, a federal appellate court upheld a California requirement that physicians could advertise board certification only when the state recognized the board. It was found not to be a violation of the First Amendment to bar advertising certification by an unrecognized board.[92]

4-3 Employment Relationship

Health care organizations provide patient care through their employees. The quality and performance of the employed staff and the relationship between the organization and its employees determine whether satisfactory, compassionate care can be provided to patients. Health care organizations should carefully select, train, supervise, and discipline employees. Many aspects of employee relations are now subject to detailed state and federal regulation,

---

[87] *See* www.abms.org (accessed Sept. 3, 2005); R. Abelson, *New board for surgeons denied again*, N.Y. TIMES, Mar. 18, 2005, C4 [vascular surgeons].

[88] Gilliam v. National Com'n for Certification of Physician's Assistants, 727 F. Supp. 1512 (E.D. Pa. 1989), *aff'd*, 898 F.2d 140 (3d Cir.), *cert. denied*, 495 U.S. 920 (1990).

[89] *E.g.*, Poindexter v. American Bd. of Surgery, 911 F. Supp. 1510 (D. Ga. 1994); Patel v. American Bd. of Psychiatry & Neurology, Inc., 975 F.2d 1312 (7th Cir. 1992); Goussis v. Kimball, 813 F. Supp. 352 (E.D. Pa. 1993); Sammons v. National Com'n on Certif. of Physician's Assistants, 104 F. Supp. 2d 1379 (N.D. Ga. 2000); Gilliam v. National Com'n for Certification of Physician's Assistants, Inc., 727 F. Supp. 1512 (E.D. Pa. 1989), *aff'd*, 898 F.2d 140 (3rd Cir.), *cert. denied*, 495 U.S. 920 (1990) [not a state actor so not subject to constitutional or § 1983 claims].

[90] *E.g.*, Sanjuan v. American Bd. of Psychiatry and Neurology, Inc., 40 F.3d 247 (7th Cir. 1994), *amended, reh'g denied* (en banc), 1995 U.S. App. LEXIS 565 (7th Cir.).

[91] *E.g.*, *id.*; Marrese v. American Acad. of Orthopaedic Surgeons, 977 F.2d 585 (*without op.*), 1992 U.S. App. LEXIS 25530 (7th Cir.).

[92] American Academy of Pain Management v. Joseph, 353 F.3d 1099 (9th Cir. 2004).

including equal employment opportunities, compensation and benefits, occupational safety, labor-management relations, and other matters.

This section discusses some general concerns regarding employee relations and then reviews the pertinent federal laws. Some state laws are mentioned, but a detailed state-by-state analysis is not attempted.

This section is divided into general employee relations issues (4-3.1); equal opportunity employment laws (4-3.2); compensation and benefits (4-3.3); occupational safety and health (4-3.4); labor-management relations (4-3.5); and selected state laws (4-3.6).

4-3.1 General Employee Relations Issues

SELECTION. Health care organizations must exercise care in selecting their employees. The organization should verify any required licenses and should check references and other information provided by the applicant to confirm that it is reasonable to believe the applicant is qualified.[93] The Immigration Reform and Control Act of 1986 requires all employers to verify the identity and work authorization of each employee.[94] Selection should comply with applicable equal employment opportunity laws that are discussed later in this chapter.

In 1990, a federal appellate court ruled that an employer does not have a duty to the prospective employee to determine whether he is qualified before planning to hire him; so the hospital employer was not liable to a prospective physician when he was not permitted to start the job because he did not have the qualifications.[95] Employers should be truthful in their promises during recruitment. Some courts will impose liability for breaches of such promises.[96]

One controversial area is the extent to which an employer should or may make inquiries concerning the criminal record of applicants and use the information in employment decisions.[97] Some states do

---

[93] *As value of diplomas grows, more people buy bogus credentials*, WALL ST. J., Apr. 2, 1987, 1.

[94] 8 U.S.C. § 1324a; *see Calif. hospital assessed largest immigration fine*, MOD. HEALTHCARE, June 23, 1989, 12 [$183,200 fine for 259 violations].

[95] Carlson v. Arnot-Ogden Mem. Hosp., 918 F.2d 411 (3d Cir. 1990).

[96] *Employers face new liability: Truth in hiring*, WALL. ST. J., July 9, 1993, B1.

[97] *See* G. Fields, *Security vetting of employees is highly prized*, WALL ST. J., Feb. 24, 2004, B1 [twelve-month backlog for swamped government background checking staff].

not permit collection or use of such information. In 2003, the Pennsylvania Supreme Court ruled that a criminal background check requirement was an infringement on the individual's rights under the state constitution to pursue an occupation.[98] Some states require collection and use of criminal background information for some health care workers.[99] In states where it is permitted, employers have been held liable for crimes by employees when no background check has been made,[100] and employees have been discharged for failing to disclose their criminal record on the employment application form.[101] In 2002, the Iowa Supreme Court ruled that an arbitrator could not order the reinstatement of an employee who was discovered to have a criminal background through such checks.[102]

HEALTH SCREENING. Employers should screen employees to identify conditions, such as contagious diseases, that can constitute a risk to patients and take appropriate steps to assure that persons who constitute risks do not have contact with patients or objects that could transmit their condition. However, employers should be prepared to defend their policies, especially when national guidelines have been adopted, such as the guidelines for AIDS.[103]

The Americans with Disabilities Act requires health screening of applicants to be postponed until after a contingent offer of employment has been made and requires that any screening be for all applicants for covered positions.[104]

Consent of the applicant or employee should be obtained for testing. In 1998, a federal appellate court found that an employer violated employee rights by testing for genetic disorders, venereal disease, or pregnancy without consent.[105]

---

[98] Nixon v. Commonwealth, 576 Pa. 385, 839 A.2d 277 (2003).

[99] *E.g.,* WIS. STAT. §§ 48.685, 50.065; WIS. ADMIN. CODE HFS 12; Miller v. DeBuono, 90 N.Y.2d 783, 666 N.Y.S.2d 548, 689 N.E.2d 518 (1997) [state may bar future nursing home employment by aide on abuse registry].

[100] Tallahassee Furniture v. Harrison, 583 So. 2d 744 (Fla. 1st DCA 1991).

[101] *E.g.,* Curry v. Almance Health Servs., No. 2:92CV00351 (M.D. Ga. April 1, 1994), *as discussed in* 3 HEALTH L. RPTR. [BNA] 519 (1994).

[102] State v. AFSCME Iowa Council 61, 648 N.W.2d 119 (Iowa 2002).

[103] *E.g,* Leckelt v. Board of Comm'rs, 909 F.2d 820 (5th Cir. 1990), *aff'g,* 714 F. Supp. 1377 (E.D. La. 1989) [not violation of Rehabilitation Act to discharge LPN who refused to disclose her HIV test results]; Bradley v. University of Tex. M.D. Anderson Cancer Ctr., 3 F.3d 922 (5th Cir. 1993), *cert. denied,* 510 U.S. 1119 (1994) [hospital properly reassigned surgical technician with HIV to purchasing department]; *see also* Fedro v. Reno, 21 F.3d 1391 (7th Cir. 1994) [need not create new position for employee with hepatitis B].

[104] 42 U.S.C. §§ 12101-12117; 29 C.F.R. pt. 1630.

[105] Norman-Bloodsaw v. Lawrence Berkeley Laboratory, 135 F.3d 1260 (9th Cir. 1998); *Blood tests of workers restricted by court,* N.Y. TIMES, Feb. 5, 1998, A19.

TRAINING AND SUPERVISION. Employers can be liable for injuries caused by negligent or intentional acts of their employees in the course of employment. To optimize patient care and minimize liability exposure, health care providers arrange for their employees to have the necessary training and supervision and to participate in continuing education so they maintain and improve their skills.

Regular performance appraisals are important. The Joint Commission on the Accreditation of Healthcare Organizations requires performance evaluations for hospital employees at least every three years.[106] When human resources personnel learn of employee problems that pose a risk to patients, they need to initiate appropriate action. In 1998, the Idaho Supreme Court ruled that a hospital could be sued for the sexual relationship a fired respiratory therapist developed with a minor former patient that he had met while a patient. The therapist had told an Employee Assistance Program counselor that he been terminated from a prior job for sexually molesting a patient.[107]

STAFFING. As health care organizations respond to pressures to reduce costs and to shortages of nurses and other professional and technical staff, new ways of structuring care are being developed, and staffing patterns are changing.[108] In most areas, there is some latitude to make changes, but appropriate levels must be maintained.[109] Legally mandated staffing ratios have been proposed, but these efforts have generally been unsuccessful, except for the California experiment described in the following paragraph. In 2005, New Jersey mandated public disclosure of staffing levels.[110] Some courts have protected individual employees who objected to staffing decisions.[111]

In 1999, California adopted a statute that mandated nurse-to-patient staffing ratios that began to be phased in January 1, 2004.

---

[106] Joint Commission on Accreditation of Healthcare Organizations, COMPREHENSIVE ACCREDITA-TION MANUAL FOR HOSPITALS (2005 ed.), Elements of Performance #1 for HR.3.20.

[107] Doe v. Garcia, 131 Idaho 578, 961 P.2d 1181 (1998).

[108] *E.g.*, L. Tarkan, *Nursing shortage forces hospitals to cope creatively*, N.Y. TIMES, Jan. 6, 2004, D5.

[109] *E.g.*, *Health department cites hospital for violations of patient care laws*, 7 H.L.R. 1219 (1998) [nurse staffing].

[110] N.J. STAT. § 26:2H-5g (eff. July 23, 2005); *Hospitals, nursing homes in New Jersey must post data on nurse staffing levels*, H.L.R., Jan. 27, 2005, 131.

[111] *E.g.*, Dabbs v. Cardiopulmonary Management Servs., 188 Cal. App. 3d 1437, 234 Cal. Rptr. 129 (4th Dist. 1987) [respiratory therapist could not be discharged for refusing to work night shift as only experienced therapist].

On July 1, 2003, the ratios were published. It was estimated that the ratios would cost California hospitals over \$400 million in 2004, escalating to nearly one billion dollars in 2008. The state interpreted the rule to apply even during short breaks. The hospital association sued to challenge this interpretation. In 2004, a California trial court upheld the interpretation. Surveys indicated that in early 2004 many hospitals were not in compliance. Los Angeles County Hospital sought relief in early 2004. One hospital that closed in early 2004 announced that one reason was the staffing requirements. The governor attempted to postpone the effective date of the rule. In 2005, a trial court declared the postponement invalid, and an appellate court refused to intervene. The state announced its intent to appeal. The ultimate impact on cost, availability, and quality of services remains to be seen.[112]

Some nurses and their organizations have sought to reduce or eliminate mandatory overtime. Many health care organizations through policies or collective bargaining agreements have sought to minimize mandatory overtime, but the unpredictability of the workload in many hospitals and the unpredictability of staff time off for illness, family medical leave, and other purposes makes it virtually impossible to eliminate all of the situations where patient safety demands some mandatory overtime. Several states have considered such laws. By mid-2004, at least seven states had passed laws restricting mandatory overtime.[113] These laws differ in when they apply and the permitted exceptions.

SEARCHING THE WORKPLACE. Public employers need to limit searches of employee workplaces to appropriate purposes and means. In 1987, the United States Supreme Court ruled that public employees have a reasonable expectation of privacy in their desks and file cabinets that is protected by the Fourth Amendment prohibition against unreasonable searches and seizures, but that a search

---

[112] J. Coleman, *Health regulators unveil nurse-to-patient ratios*, AP, July 1, 2003; S. Fox, *Hospitals may fail to meet nurse-staffing standard*, L.A. TIMES, Nov. 14, 2003, pt. 2, 4; California Healthcare Assn. v. California Dep't of Health Servs., No. 03-CS-01814 (Cal. Super. Ct. May 26, 2004); D. Vrana, *Hospital staffing law is upheld*, L.A. TIMES, May 27, 2004, C2; *L.A. hospital closes acute care operations, claims new staffing requirements to blame*, H.L.R., Jan. 15, 2004, 90; *Staffing has improved, but many hospitals not complying with ratios, surveys say*, H.L.R., Feb. 12, 2004, 230; D. Thompson, *Schwarzenegger to appeal final ruling on nurse-patient ratio*, AP, June 7, 2005.

[113] 26 MAINE R. S. § 603; MD. LABOR & EMP. CODE ANN. § 3-421; MINN. STAT. §181.275; N.J. STAT. §§ 34:11-56a33 - 34:11-56a37; Ore. R.S. § 441.160 - § 441.170; REV. CODE WASH. §§ 49.28.130 - 49.28.140; W. VA. CODE §§ 21-5F-1 - 21-5F-5.

warrant is not required for noninvestigatory, work-related purposes or for work-related misconduct, provided the search is reasonable under all the circumstances in both its inception and scope.[114] The case arose out of a state hospital's search of the office of a psychiatrist, who was chief of professional education. There were concerns about the management of the psychiatry residency program. While the employee was on administrative leave, the hospital inventoried the property in his office and seized personal items. The court remanded the case for a determination of the reasonableness of the search. The first trial resulted in a verdict for the hospital employees that had directed and conducted the search. This verdict was overturned on evidentiary grounds.[115] The second trial generated a verdict for the searched employee that was upheld on appeal.[116]

Lower federal court decisions have indicated that this reasonable expectation of privacy generally does not apply to open, accessible areas but only to enclosed areas given over to the employee's exclusive use.[117] Where there would otherwise be a reasonable expectation of privacy, the expectation can also be overcome by promulgated regulations expressly authorizing random searches in some circumstances.[118]

DISCIPLINE AND DISMISSAL. Health care providers should take appropriate steps to enforce institutional policies to maintain appropriate patient care and institutional integrity. Proper procedures should be followed, and actions should be based on legally permissible grounds.

Generally, employees are considered to be employees *at will* unless they have contracts for a specified time period. Employers may terminate employees at will at any time without cause,[119]

---

[114] O'Connor v. Ortega, 480 U.S. 1492 (1987).

[115] Ortega v. O'Connor, 50 F.3d 778 (9th Cir. 1995).

[116] Ortega v. O'Connor, 146 F.3d 1149 (9th Cir. 1998).

[117] *E.g.*, Vega-Rodriguez v. Puerto Rican Telephone Co., 110 F.3d 174 (1st Cir. 1997) [no reasonable expectation of privacy against video surveillance to monitor open work area]; Shepard v. Beerman, 18 F.3d 147 (2d Cir. 1994) [no reasonable expectation of privacy in open work areas]; United States v. Taketa, 923 F.2d 665 (9th Cir. 1991) [reasonable expectation of privacy against video surveillance of office reserved for exclusive use]; Gossmeyer v. McDonald, 128 F.3d 481 (7th Cir. 1997) [state worker had no reasonable expectation of privacy in her locked desk, part of "workplace," not part of "personal domain"].

[118] *E.g.*, American Postal Workers Union v. United States Postal Serv., 871 F.2d 556 (9th Cir. 1989); DeMaine v. Samuels, 2000 U.S. Dist. LEXIS 16277 (D. Conn.); United States v. Thorn, 2004 U.S. App. LEXIS 14295 (8th Cir.) [no reasonable expectation of privacy in office computer contents, employer policy on computer use].

[119] *E.g.*, Burrell v. Carraway Methodist Hosp., 607 So. 2d 193 (Ala. 1993); Lampe v. Presbyterian Med. Ctr., 590 P.2d 513 (Colo. Ct. App. 1978).

unless (1) the employer is bound by contract or statute to follow certain procedures or standards in terminations or (2) the termination violates public policy.

Many courts view some personnel policy manuals and other procedures for discipline or dismissal to be contracts with the employees that the employer must follow.[120] However, courts have disagreed on what constitutes an enforceable policy or procedure.[121] The Delaware Supreme Court ruled that statements in employee handbooks do not change an employee's at-will status unless they specify a definite term of employment.[122] Some courts have found a health care organization's employee manual to be a contract without this specificity.[123] Several courts have ruled that handbooks or manuals are not contracts when they contain disclaimers or other clear indications they are not intended to be contracts.[124]

Some public health care employees are covered by civil service laws that require certain procedures. Absent statutory or contractual requirements, public employees are generally not entitled to a formal hearing prior to termination. For example, in 1985, the United States Supreme Court ruled that public employees must be given oral or written notice of the charges, an explanation of the employer's evidence, and a pretermination opportunity to present their side of the story, but a formal hearing was not required.[125] Employees do not have a constitutional right to due process concerning termination by private employers.[126]

---

[120] *E.g.*, Jones v. Central Peninsula Gen. Hosp., 779 P.2d 783 (Alaska 1989); Duldulao v. St. Mary of Nazareth Hosp. Ctr., 115 Ill. 2d 482, 505 N.E.2d 314 (1987); Annotation, *Right to discharge allegedly "at-will" employee as affected by employer's promulgation of employment policies as to discharge*, 33 A.L.R. 4TH 120.

[121] *E.g.*, Hunsucker v. Josephine Sunset Home, 89 Wash. App. 1041 (1998) [employee manual specifying termination procedures not implied employment contract].

[122] Heideck v. Kent Gen. Hosp., 446 A.2d 1095 (Del. 1982); *see also* Mursch v. Van Dorn Co., 851 F.2d 990 (7th Cir. 1988) [guidelines in employee handbook not a contract].

[123] *E.g.*, Carlson v. Lake Chelan Comm. Hosp., 66 P.2d 1080 (Wash. App. 2003); Watson v. Idaho Falls Cons. Hosps., 111 Idaho 44, 720 P.2d 632 (1986); Jewell v. North Big Horn Hosp. Dist., 935 P.2d 135 (1998).

[124] *E.g.*, Bowe v. Charleston Area Med. Ctr., 428 S.E.2d 773 (W. Va. 1993); Lee v. Sperry Corp., 678 F. Supp. 1415 (D. Minn. 1987); *See* Annotation, *Effectiveness of employer's disclaimer of representations in personnel manual or employee handbook altering at-will employment relationship*, 17 A.L.R. 5TH 1; *but see* Doyle v. Holy Cross Hosp., 186 Ill. 2d 104; 708 N.E.2d 1140 (1999) [old handbook may create contract despite disclaimer in current handbook]; *accord*, Robinson v. Ada S. McKinley Community Servs., Inc., 19 F.3d 359 (7th Cir. 1994).

[125] Cleveland Bd. of Educ. v. Loudermill, 470 U.S. 532 (1985); *see also cases finding adequate due process*, Bradley v. Colonial Mental Health & Retardation Servs. Bd., 856 F.2d 703 (4th Cir. 1988); Phares v. Gustafsson, 856 F.2d 1003 (7th Cir. 1988).

[126] *E.g.*, Simpkins v. Sandwich Comm. Hosp., 854 F.2d 215 (7th Cir. 1988).

When staff members are covered by individual employment contracts or collective bargaining agreements, procedures specified in the contract or agreement should be followed.[127] Usually, employees will be required to exhaust contractual remedies before being allowed to sue.[128] Such contracts do not have to be in writing to be enforceable. A Louisiana court found a hospital liable for breaching an oral promise to five certified registered nurse anesthetists that they would be given a six-month notice of termination.[129] However, if the oral contract is for a specified period of more than one year, instead of at will, it will not be enforceable in most states because the Statute of Frauds requires that such contracts be in writing to be enforceable.[130]

As the Louisiana case illustrates, courts generally will not order employees reinstated unless authorized by statute; instead, former employees who are wrongfully discharged are awarded payment of lost wages and other damages. However, some statutes do authorize reinstatement.[131]

Employees have protection from retaliatory discharge in some situations. In 1998, the United States Supreme Court ruled that at-will employees have a constitutionally protected interest in continued employment so that an at-will former employee of a home health agency could use the federal civil rights statutes to challenge firing in retaliation for participation in criminal prosecution of the employer for Medicare fraud.[132] Some statutes forbid retaliatory discharge for making certain reports to governmental agencies,[133] and some courts have extended such protection to employees who make other reports,[134] who refuse to testify untruthfully in malprac-

---

[127] *E.g.*, Musgrave v. HCA Mideast, Inc., 856 F.2d 690 (4th Cir. 1988); Jackam v. Hospital Corp. of Am. Mideast, Inc., 800 F.2d 1577 (11th Cir. 1986).

[128] *E.g.*, Dearden v. Liberty Med. Ctr., 75 Md. App. 528, 542 A.2d 383 (1988).

[129] Hebert v. Woman's Hosp. Found., 377 So. 2d 1340 (La. Ct. App. 1979).

[130] 72 Am. Jur. 2d *Statute of frauds* (1974); *e.g.*, Santa Monica Hosp. v. Superior Court, 173 Cal. App. 3d 239, 218 Cal. Rptr. 543 (1985).

[131] *E.g.*, 29 U.S.C. § 626(b) [age discrimination].

[132] Haddle v. Garrison, 525 U.S. 121 (1998).

[133] *E.g.*, Fla. Stat. § 440.205 [no retaliation for workers' compensation claims]; *but see* Allan v. SWF Gulf Coast, Inc., 535 So. 2d 638 (Fla. 1st DCA 1988) [employee may be terminated for other reasons even after claim].

[134] *E.g.*, Shores v. Senior Manor Nursing Ctr., 164 Ill. App. 3d 503, 518 N.E.2d 471 (5th Dist. 1988) [patient abuse]; Palmer v. Brown, 242 Kan. 893, 752 P.2d 685 (1988) [fraudulent Medicaid billing]; Kelsay v. Motorola, Inc., 74 Ill. 2d 172, 384 N.E.2d 353 (1979) [workers' compensation claim]; *contra* Washington v. Union Carbide Corp., 870 F.2d 957 (4th Cir. 1989) [no recovery in West Virginia for discharge for reporting safety violations].

tice cases,[135] who refuse to handle radioactive materials in violation of federal regulations,[136] who refuse to prepare or file false claims with the government,[137] who participate in abuse investigations,[138] or who refuse to work with inadequate staffing.[139] Not all statements are protected.[140] Moreover, courts generally scrutinize claims that discipline is for legally required behavior.[141] In 1998, the Utah Supreme Court rejected a pharmacist's challenge to termination for rudeness to clients that he claimed was due to fulfilling his legal duty to question the validity of prescriptions. The court gave a detailed analysis of the scope of the pharmacist's legal duties and found that the objectionable behavior was not legally mandated.[142]

Employees of public institutions who are discharged for exercising their rights of free speech have some protection under the First Amendment.[143] Employee grievances that are not matters of public concern are not protected.[144] Employees engaging in protected speech are not protected from being discharged for reasons independent of their speech.[145] The First Amendment does not apply to employment actions by private employers.[146] For example, an Illinois appellate court ruled that even if a nurse had been terminated

---

[135] *E.g.*, Sides v. Duke Hosp., 72 N.C. App. 331, 328 S.E.2d 818 (1985).

[136] *E.g.,* Wheeler v. Caterpillar Tractor Co., 108 Ill. 2d 502, 485 N.E.2d 372 (1985).

[137] *E.g.*, Jones v. Lake Park Care Center Inc., 569 N.W.2d 369 (Iowa 1997); Webb v. HCA Health Services of Midwest, 300 Ark. 613, 780 S.W.2d 571 (1989).

[138] *E.g.*, Fisher v. Lexington Health Care, 301 Ill. App. 3d 547, 703 N.E.2d 988 (2d Dist. 1998).

[139] *See supra* note 111; *but see* Fineman v. New Jersey Dep't of Human Servs., 272 N.J. Super. 606, 640 A.2d 1161 (App. Div. 1994) [physician may be terminated for refusing to provide temporary medical care to 300 nursing home patients].

[140] *E.g.*, Goodman v. Wesley Med. Ctr., 2003 Kan. LEXIS 591.

[141] *E.g.*, Parent v. Mount Clemens Gen. Hosp., 2003 Mich. App. LEXIS 1862 [affirmed at-will lab tech firing for insubordination, refused to use "tray method," not within public policy exception].

[142] Ryan v. Dan's Food Stores, 972 P.2d 395 (Utah 1999).

[143] *E.g.*, Waters v. Churchill, 511 U.S. 661 (1994); Rodgers v. Banks, 344 F.3d 587 (6th Cir. 2003); Paradis v. Montrose Mem. Hosp., 157 F.3d 815 (10th Cir. 1998); Annotation, *First Amendment protection for public hospital or health employees subjected to discharge, transfer, or discipline because of speech*, 107 A.L.R. FED. 21.67.

[144] *E.g.*, Rahn v. Drake Ctr., 31 F.3d 407 (6th Cir. 1994), *cert. denied*, 515 U.S. 1142 (1995); Havekost v. United States Dep't of Navy, 925 F.2d 316 (9th Cir. 1991) [mere workplace grievance about dress code, staffing policies not protected]; Ganthier v. North Shore-Long Island Jewish Health Sys., 298 F. Supp. 2d 342 (E.D. N.Y. 2004).

[145] *E.g.*, Pilarowski v. Macomb County Health Dep't, 841 F.2d 1281 (6th Cir.), *cert. denied*, 488 U.S. 850 (1988) [layoffs for budget cuts were permitted]; Black v. City of Wentzville, 686 F. Supp. 241 (E.D. Mo. 1988) [documented poor work performance].

[146] *E.g.*, Wright v. Shriners Hosp. for Crippled Children, 412 Mass. 469, 598 N.E.2d 1241 (1992) [reversing award to nurse for dismissal after critical remarks to internal survey team, termination did not violate public policy]; Willis v. University Health Servs., 993 F.2d 837 (11th Cir.), *cert. denied,* 510 U.S. 976 (1993) [private entity managing county hospital that fired nurse allegedly for free speech was not a public employer].

solely in retaliation for reporting incidents to a newspaper, she would not be entitled to any more protection than other at-will employees of private employers.[147]

An employer generally does not have a legal duty to inform an employee that it is conducting an investigation of the employee's conduct.[148] However, when an employer conducts an investigatory interview of an employee that the employee reasonably believes might result in discipline and the employee is part of a unit represented by a union, the employee has a right to have a representative present during the interview if the employee so requests.[149] The employer does not have to advise the employee of that right, and the employer may decide not to conduct the interview if the right is invoked. In a collective bargaining agreement, a union can waive the right to representation in such interviews.[150] Nonunion employees generally do not have a right to representatives.[151]

Some provisions of the National Labor Relations Act also apply when employees are not represented by a union. The equal employment opportunity laws apply to all aspects of employment, including discipline and dismissal; so the provisions of these laws also must be considered. Employers should also be aware of what grounds for dismissal will be considered "just cause" by the unemployment compensation agency in their state so that they know whether they will be required to pay unemployment compensation to a dismissed staff member.

Supervision and discipline must be handled in a civilized manner. The Alabama Supreme Court upheld an award to a nurse from a physician who struck her and yelled at her to turn on a suction machine.[152]

Some employee terminations and other discipline must be reported to state agencies.

---

[147] Rozier v. St. Mary's Hosp., 88 Ill. App. 3d 994, 411 N.E.2d 50 (5th Dist. 1980); *see also* Maus v. National Living Ctrs., 633 S.W.2d 674 (Tex. Ct. App. 1982) [nurse's aide discharged for complaints to superiors concerning patient care].

[148] *E.g.*, Dobinsky v. Rand, 248 A.D.2d 903, 670 N.Y.S.2d 606 (3d Dept. 1998) [not intentional infliction of emotional distress for hospital to investigate death allegedly implicating plaintiffs, not keeping them abreast of investigation].

[149] NLRB v. J. Weingarten, Inc., 420 U.S. 251 (1975).

[150] Prudential Ins. Co., 275 NLRB 30 (1985).

[151] *E.g.*, IBM Corp., 341 NLRB No. 148 (2004) [no right], *rev'g*, Epilepsy Found. of Northeastern Ohio, 331 NLRB 676 (2000) [right], *rev'g*, E.I. DuPont, 289 NLRB 627 (1988) [no right]; Slaughter v. NLRB, 876 F.2d 11 (3d Cir. 1989) [upholding NLRB position of no right]; Epilepsy Found. of Northeastern Ohio v. NLRB, 268 F.3d 1095 (D.C. Cir. 2001), *cert. denied*, 536 U.S. 904 (2002) [upholding NLRB position of right].

[152] Peete v. Blackwell, 504 So. 2d 222 (Ala. 1986).

DRUG TESTING. In a 1989 United States Supreme Court case, Customs Service workers challenged a requirement that employees applying for promotion to positions involving interdicting drugs or carrying firearms submit to drug analysis of urine specimens. Because the employer was the government, the Fourth Amendment protected the employees from unreasonable searches.[153] The Court concluded that the urine-testing requirement was a reasonable search, even without suspicion of wrongful conduct by the individual, for persons in these sensitive positions, especially because the procedures for collection and analysis minimized intrusion on privacy interests. The government interest in the integrity and capacity of persons in these positions outweighed the employees' privacy rights. In a companion case, the Court ruled that the Fourth Amendment protections also applied to a private employer's testing that was mandated or authorized by governmental regulations.[154] The regulations required tests of railway employees after certain train accidents and incidents and authorized tests after violations of certain safety rules. The Court concluded that the tests were reasonable without individualized suspicion of impairment because of the government's interest in the safety of the traveling public. The Court did not address whether the government could require testing of health care employees, but the factors the Court viewed as important to justify testing (such as the need for unimpaired employees to assure public safety and the highly regulated nature of the industry) appear to apply in the health care context.[155]

When an employer wants to begin a drug-testing program in a situation where there is no governmental mandate for the program, the employer in general can do so if there is no collective bargaining agreement and no law forbidding the program. In 1989, the National Labor Relations Board (NLRB) ruled that drug tests of union workers are a mandatory subject of bargaining; so employers without a governmental mandate cannot, without union concurrence or a legal mandate, start testing union workers.[156] On the same day, the Supreme Court ruled that when the existing collective bargaining

---

[153] National Treasury Employees Union v. Von Raab, 489 U.S. 656 (1989).
[154] Skinner v. Railway Labor Executives' Ass'n, 489 U.S. 602 (1989).
[155] *See* Kemp v. Caliborne County Hosp., 763 F. Supp. 1362 (S.D. Miss. 1991) [applying *Von Raab* and *Skinner* to uphold a hospital screening program].
[156] Johnson-Bateman Co., 295 NLRB No. 26 (June 19, 1989); *see also, e.g.*, Utility Workers v. Southern Cal. Edison Co., 852 F.2d 1083 (9th Cir. 1988), *cert. denied*, 489 U.S. 1078 (1989).

agreement can be construed to permit drug testing that the employer is not obligated in some situations to bargain with the union before starting the program, but the union can challenge the contract interpretation through the arbitration provisions of the contract after the program is initiated.[157] Also, on the same day the NLRB ruled that a program to test job applicants is not a mandatory subject of bargaining, but unions are entitled to information concerning the program to monitor employer practices.[158] If there is no collective bargaining agreement, a private employer can start a program within any limitations imposed by state and local laws.[159] A governmental employer must also consider the limits of the Fourth Amendment discussed in the previous paragraph, which can restrict the ability to extend the program beyond those employees with patient contact or in other safety sensitive positions.

State and local laws vary.[160] For example, in 1997, the California Supreme Court upheld drug testing of all applicants, but not of all current employees.[161]

OTHER BEHAVIORAL SCREENING. Some employers screen applicants and/or employees for unhealthy behaviors. For example, some employers have excluded smokers from their work force, even when the smoking only occurs off the employer's premises.[162] Although this is a controversial practice, courts have generally upheld these policies.[163] Some states have passed laws barring employment decisions based on the use of legal products off the employer's premises during nonworking hours.[164]

---

[157] Conrail v. Railway Labor Executives' Ass'n, 491 U.S. 299 (1989); *see also, e.g.*, Laws v. Calmat, 852 F.2d 430 (9th Cir. 1988); Utility Workers v. Southern Cal. Edison Co., 852 F.2d 1083 (9th Cir. 1988), *cert. denied*, 489 U.S. 1078 (1989).

[158] Cowles Media Co., Star Tribune Div., 295 NLRB No. 63 (1989).

[159] *E.g.*, Greco v. Halliburton Co., 674 F. Supp. 1447 (D. Wyo. 1987); Stevenson v. Panhandle E. Pipe Line Co., 680 F. Supp. 859 (S.D. Tex. 1987); *but see* CONN. GEN. STAT. ANN. § 31-51x [prohibition of employee drug testing without showing good cause for suspected drug use].

[160] *E.g.*, Wilcher v. City of Wilmington, 139 F.3d 366 (3d Cir. 1998) [required direct observation of urine collection does not violate federal rights, remand to reconsider state law invasion of privacy claim].

[161] Loder v. City of Glendale, 14 Cal. 4th 846, 59 Cal. Rptr. 2d 696, 927 P.2d 1200 (1997).

[162] *See* B. Wysocki, *Companies get tough with smokers, obese to trim costs*, WALL ST. J, Oct. 12, 2004, B1; K. Maher, *Companies are closing doors on job applicants who smoke*, WALL ST. J, Dec. 21, 2004, B6.

[163] *E.g.*, Grusendorf v. City of Oklahoma City, 816 F.2d 539 (10th Cir. 1987); City of North Miami v. Kurtz, 653 So. 2d 1025, 1028 (Fla. 1995), *cert denied*, 516 U.S. 1043 (1996).

[164] *E.g.*, Wis. Stat., § 111.321; Colo. Rev. Stat. § 24-34-402.5.

POLYGRAPH TESTS. The Employee Polygraph Protection Act of 1988[165] prohibits most uses of polygraph tests on employees. There are some limited exemptions where such tests can still be used, but most employers avoid using the exemptions because (1) the situations that justify a polygraph test generally will justify adverse action against the employee and (2) tested employees can bring federal lawsuits in which the employer must prove the exemption applied.

COMMUNICATIONS ABOUT FORMER STAFF. Employers have been sued for libel or slander by former staff members based on unfavorable evaluations, termination notices, and responses to inquiries from prospective employers.[166] Some supervisory personnel have been reluctant to communicate deficiencies accurately because of liability concerns.

In general, communicating the truth cannot result in liability for libel or slander.[167] However, because absolute truth is often difficult to prove, certain communications have a *qualified privilege*. This means there is liability only if the communication was made with malice. The qualified privilege applies to communications to persons who have a legitimate interest in the information given, but such communications must be limited in scope commensurate with that interest and must be made in a proper manner so that others do not also learn of them inappropriately. Courts have recognized that an employer or prospective employer has a legitimate interest in employment-related information.[168] The best way to avoid exceeding the qualified privilege is to limit the communication to factual statements and avoid statements concerning personality or personal spite. Usually, neutral factual statements can communicate the deficiencies that need to be communicated without creating the

---

[165] 29 U.S.C. §§ 2001-2009; *but see* Hossaini v. Western Mo. Med. Ctr., 140 F.3d 1140 (8th Cir. 1998) [county hospital is political subdivision, not subject to Act]; Theisen v. Covenant Medical Center Inc., 636 N.W.2d 74 (Iowa 2001) [required voice print analysis not violation of lie detector prohibition].

[166] K.B. Stickler & M.D. Nelson, *Defamation in the workplace: Employer rights, risks, and responsibilities*, 21 J.HEALTH & HOSP.L. 97 (1988).

[167] *E.g.*, McCullough v. Visiting Nurse Serv., 691 A.2d 1201 (Me. 1997) [statement that nurse had been terminated for "several" incidents when she had been terminated for two incidents was substantially true, so not defamatory]; Mayer v. Morgan Stanley & Co., 703 F. Supp. 249 (S.D. N.Y. 1988).

[168] *E.g.*, Gengler v. Phelps, 92 N.M. 465, 589 P.2d 1056 (Ct. App. 1978), *cert. denied,* 92 N.M. 353, 588 P.2d 554 (1979) [communication concerning nurse anesthetist].

appearance of malice. Knowing communication of false information can be construed to indicate malice and can lead to liability.[169]

Most former employers require a written authorization from the former employee before releasing information. This authorization provides some additional protection,[170] but care must still be taken in the wording of any information released.[171]

If a former employee has filed a discrimination complaint, some negative job references can be viewed as retaliation for the complaint, permitting a federal civil rights suit. In 1997, the United States Supreme Court decided that a former employee could also sue under Title VII for posttermination retaliation, such as negative job references.[172]

EMPLOYEE LIABILITY. Employees can be liable criminally and civilly for their conduct. For example, a 1988 federal appellate court decision addressed an employee who had arranged for his employer to purchase laser paper at $14.25 per thousand sheets and for the vendor to pay him a kickback of $2.00 per thousand sheets. The court upheld the conviction of the employee for engaging in a conspiracy to defraud.[173] Civil liability is discussed in Chapter 11, and criminal liability is discussed in Chapter 12.

4-3.2 Equal Opportunity Employment Laws

The federal government has enacted several laws to expand equal employment opportunities by prohibiting discrimination on various grounds. These laws include Title VII of the Civil Rights Act of 1964; the Equal Pay Act of 1963; the Age Discrimination in Employment Act; sections 503 and 504 of the Rehabilitation Act of 1973; and the Americans with Disabilities Act. In addition, numerous state laws address equal employment opportunities.

The older Civil Rights Acts from the 1860s and 1870s provide remedies for a broad range of discrimination, which includes

---

169 *E.g.*, Burger v. McGilley Mem. Chapels, Inc., 856 F.2d 1046 (8th Cir. 1988); *see also* Annotation, *Defamation: loss of employer's qualified privilege to publish employee's work record or qualification*, 24 A.L.R. 4TH 144.

170 *E.g.*, Eitler v. St. Joseph Reg. Med. Ctr., 789 N.E.2d 497 (Ind. App. 2003) [release form barred defamation claim].

171 *E.g.*, Kellums v. Freight Sales Ctrs., 467 So. 2d 816 (Fla. 5th DCA 1985) [release form did not preclude liability for deliberate falsehood].

172 Robinson v. Shell Oil Co., 519 U.S. 337 (1997) [former employee can sue under Title VII for posttermination retaliation, including negative job references].

173 United States v. Kibby, 848 F.2d 920 (8th Cir. 1988).

employment discrimination. These older acts are applied in several other contexts involving health care organizations, including some medical staff cases.

42 U.S.C. § 1981. Section 16 of the Civil Rights Act of 1870[174] guaranties individuals equal rights under the law, including the right to make and enforce contracts. Because employment is based on contract, this law provides a remedy for some kinds of employment discrimination. This act is codified as 42 U.S.C. § 1981, as amended; so it is usually referred to as *§ 1981.*

Section 1981 has generally been interpreted to apply only to discrimination that is based on race, although some courts have also applied it to alienage (citizenship or immigration status).[175] In 1988, a federal appellate court upheld a judgment under § 1981 against a hospital for discharging an African-American employee due substantially to racial motivation, even though there were nondiscriminatory reasons for the discharge. The employee had been a security guard. He failed three polygraph tests concerning thefts. However, Caucasian guards who had also failed had not been fired.[176]

Due to the impossibility of developing a satisfactory definition of race, the United States Supreme Court in 1987 decided that § 1981 protects against discrimination based on being a member of an ethnically or physiognomically distinctive subgroup of a population but that distinctive physiognomy is not essential.[177] Section 1981 does not apply to discrimination based on such factors as age, gender, and religion.

In 1989, the Court narrowly interpreted making and enforcing contracts so that § 1981 did not apply, for example, to discriminatory conditions of continuing employment.[178] In the same year, the Court also decided another case limiting the reach of § 1981.[179] In an effort to reverse these decisions and to make certain other traditional interpretations expressly part of the statute, the Civil Rights

---

[174] Act of May 31, 1879, c.114, § 16, 16 Stat. 144.

[175] *E.g.*, Anderson v. Conboy, 156 F.3d 167 (2d Cir. 1998).

[176] Edwards v. Jewish Hosp., 855 F.2d 1345 (8th Cir. 1988); *see also* Roberts v. Gadsden Mem. Hosp., 835 F.2d 793 (11th Cir. 1988), *amended on reh'g*, 850 F.2d 1549 (11th Cir. 1988) [violation not to give promoted African-American employees same raise as whites who were promoted]; *but see* Armstrong v. Turnage, 690 F. Supp. 839 (E.D. Mo. 1988), *aff'd without op.*, 873 F.2d 1448 (8th Cir. 1989) [disparate treatment of African-American, Caucasian hospital pharmacists after errors insufficient to prove motive where rules consistently applied].

[177] St. Francis College v. Al-Khazraji, 481 U.S. 604 (1987).

[178] Patterson v. McClean Credit Union, 491 U.S. 164 (1989).

[179] Wards Cove Packing Co. v. Atonio, 490 U.S. 642 (1989).

Act of 1991 was passed.[180] It amended § 1981 to (a) expand the definition of "make and enforce contracts" to include the enjoyment of the benefits of the contractual relationship and (b) extend express protection from nongovernmental discrimination.

42 U.S.C. § 1983. Section 1 of the Civil Rights Act of 1871[181] addresses deprivation under *color of state law* of rights, privileges, or immunities secured by the Constitution or laws. Thus, a plaintiff must show (a) the existence of some right secured by the Constitution or law, (b) deprivation of that right, and (c) that the deprivation is under color of state law. Purely private action cannot be remedied under this Act.[182] This Act is codified as 42 U.S.C. § 1983, as amended; so it is usually referred to as *§ 1983.*

Actions of public health care entities are generally under color of state law. For example, a discharged quality assurance director was able to sue a county hospital under § 1983 due to the alleged (a) lack of pretermination notice of charges and opportunity to respond and (b) arbitrary, capricious, and improperly motivated basis for her discharge.[183]

Private health care providers are generally considered not to act under color of state law; receiving Medicare and Medicaid funds is not sufficient.[184] Being designated by the state as the emergency receiving facility for the mentally ill was held not to be sufficient in one 1994 case.[185] When a nurse sued to challenge her termination, a federal appellate court ruled that the lease of a public hospital to a private corporation did not make the actions of that corporation under color of state law.[186]

Private individuals and entities can act under color of state law when they act in concert with governmental officials. Thus, private

---

[180] Pub. L. No. 102-166, 105 Stat. 1071 (1991); Andrews v. Lakeshore Rehabilitation Hosp., 140 F.3d 1405 (11th Cir. May 15, 1998) [former hospital employee claiming retaliatory discharge for filing race discrimination claim with EEOC permitted to sue under 1991 amendments].

[181] Act Apr. 20, 1871, c. 22, § 1, 17 Stat. 13.

[182] *E.g.*, Hamm v. Lakeview Commun. Hosp., 950 F. Supp. 330 (D. Ala. 1996) [dismissal of former emergency room nurse, claim under § 1983 against physician for alleged harassment when physician not employed by state or not acting under color of state law; physician was employed by private company under contract with community hospital].

[183] Anglemyer v. Hamilton County Hosp., 848 F. Supp. 938 (D. Kan. 1994), *aff'd*, 58 F.3d 533 (10th Cir. 1995).

[184] *E.g.*, Wheat v. Mass, 994 F.2d 273 (5th Cir. 1993).

[185] Trimble v. Androscoggin Valley Hosp., 847 F. Supp. 226 (D. N.H. 1994); *but see* Snyder v. Albany Med. Ctr. Hosp., 206 A.D.2d 816, 615 N.Y.S.2d 139 (3d Dep't 1994) [holding involuntarily committed patient at private hospital was under color of state law].

[186] Willis v. University Health Servs., 993 F.2d 837 (11th Cir.), *cert. denied*, 510 U.S. 976 (1993).

hospital paramedics were found to be acting under color of state law when they acted in concert with police to detain a person under the emergency detention state statute.[187]

42 U.S.C. § 1985. The Civil Rights Act of 1861[188] forbids conspiracies to interfere with civil rights, including deprivation of equal protection of the laws or equal privileges and immunities under the laws. This Act is codified as 42 U.S.C. § 1985, as amended; so it is usually referred to as *§ 1985.*

A conspiracy needs to be shown, which means that two or more entities must be acting together. Some courts recognize an intracorporate conspiracy exception so that all of the employees and agents of a corporation generally are treated as one entity,[189] similar to the exception recognized for antitrust (see Chapter 13).

The conspiracy does not have to involve state action or be under color of state law to violate § 1985.[190] However, when the conspiracy is aimed at interfering with a right that protects only against state interference, the conspiracy must involve state action in order to state a claim under § 1985. For example, the Fourteenth Amendment creates the right to be free from state action that interferes with equal protection or due process; so a purely private conspiracy would not interfere with Fourteenth Amendment rights. State action would have to be shown to state a claim under § 1985 for a conspiracy to interfere with Fourteenth Amendment rights. A federal appellate court applied this rule to conclude that a physician had failed to state a claim under § 1985 for the termination of his clinical privileges by a private hospital. There was no state involvement, and he based his claim on the Fourteenth Amendment.[191] On the other hand, some federal laws create rights to be free from private action; so no state action would need to be shown.

There generally must be a racial or other class-based invidiously discriminatory animus behind the conspiracy.[192]

---

[187] Moore v. Wyoming Med. Ctr., 825 F. Supp. 1531 (D. Wyo. 1993).

[188] Acts July 31, 1861, ch. 33, 12 Stat. 284; Acts Apr. 20, 1871, ch. 22, § 2, 17 Stat. 13.

[189] *E.g.*, Travis v. Gary Community Mental Health Ctr., 921 F.2d 108 (7th Cir, 1990), *cert. denied*, 502 U.S. 812 (1991); *but see* Fobbs v. Holy Cross Health Sys. Corp., 29 F.3d 1439 (9th Cir. 1994), *cert. denied*, 513 U.S. 1127 (1995) [claim stated against hospital, 27 individual staff physicians]; Saville v. Houston County Healthcare Auth., 852 F. Supp. 1512 (M.D. Ala. 1994) [intracorporate conspiracy exception not available in Eleventh Circuit in § 1985(3) suit].

[190] Griffin v. Breckenridge, 403 U.S. 88 (1971).

[191] Wong v. Stripling, 881 F.2d 200 (5th Cir. 1989).

[192] *E.g.*, United Brotherhood v. Scott, 463 U.S. 825 (1983).

TITLE VII OF THE CIVIL RIGHTS ACT OF 1964. Title VII[193] prohibits disparate employment treatment based on race, color, religion, sex, national origin, or pregnancy. It applies to hiring, dismissal, promotion, discipline, terms and conditions of employment,[194] and job advertising. It applies to nearly all employers; governmental agencies were included by the 1972 amendments.

The primary enforcement agency is the Equal Employment Opportunity Commission (EEOC). In some situations, the EEOC can defer to enforcement by local or state agencies or through individual suits. Generally, employees must exhaust the administrative remedies from the EEOC before they can sue under Title VII. False claims can result in criminal penalties.[195]

Three legal theories are used as the basis for finding employment discrimination. First, violations can be found on the basis of *disparate treatment* when work rules or employment practices are not applied in a consistent fashion due to a discriminatory motive. Consistent treatment avoids liability for disparate treatment.[196] Second, violations can be found on the basis of *disparate impact* when an employment practice, such as a written employment test, has an adverse impact on minorities and cannot be justified as job related. In 1988, the United States Supreme Court ruled that an employee had to present more than statistics to establish a disparate impact case.[197] The employee must prove specific employment practices that caused the disparate impact. If such practices are proved, then the employer has the burden of presenting legitimate nondiscriminatory reasons for the practices but need not present formal studies validating the practices. The burden then returns to the employee to prove that the reasons are just a pretext for discrimination. Third, *carryover* from past discrimination can constitute a violation when minorities are in a disadvantageous position because of prior discriminatory practices.

---

[193] 42 U.S.C. §§ 2000e–2000e-17.

[194] *E.g.*, Judie v. Hamilton, 872 F.2d 919 (9th Cir. 1989) [restrictions on supervisory responsibilities of African-American hospital food manager could be violation].

[195] *E.g., False EEO claims earn former DOE worker heavy sentence*, FEDERAL EEO ADVISOR, June 6, 2003.

[196] *E.g.*, Fitten v. Chattanooga-Hamilton County Hosp., 75 Fed. Appx. 384, 2003 U.S. App. LEXIS 18818 (6th Cir.) [affirming dismissal of racial discrimination employment claim, failure to identify comparable nonprotected person who was treated better]; Beene v. St. Vincent Mercy Med. Ctr., 111 F. Supp. 2d 931 (D. Ohio 2000) [terminated African-American registered nurse did not show white nurses treated more favorably for mixing up telemetry strips].

[197] Watson v. Ft. Worth Bank & Trust, 487 U.S. 977 (1988).

Prior to 1991, there was no liability under Title VII in *mixed motive* cases where both prohibited (e.g., race) and nonprohibited factors (e.g., job performance) motivated the employer's action. Title VII was amended by the Civil Rights Act of 1991, so that other factors, if proven, do not eliminate liability but restrict the available remedies.[198]

Employees can waive Title VII rights in private settlements, but the release must be knowingly and voluntarily entered.[199]

Employees can agree to arbitration of Title VII claims.[200] In 2001, the United States Supreme Court ruled that the Federal Arbitration Act applies to employment claims; so state barriers to arbitration do not apply to contracts that are in interstate commerce.[201] In 1995, a federal court ruled that an employer could not retaliate against employees who refused to agree to arbitration of discrimination complaints.[202] However, other courts have disagreed on whether to enforce arbitration requirements in employment manuals.[203]

Some provisions in arbitration agreements can render them unenforceable. Agreements that give the employer discretion whether to insist on arbitration are generally viewed as one-sided and unenforceable.[204] Agreements that do not provide for

---

[198] 42 U.S.C. §§ 2000e-2(m), 2000e-5(g)(2)(B); Desert Palace, Inc. v. Costa, 539 U.S. 90 (2003) [direct evidence of discrimination not required to submit mixed motive issue to jury].

[199] *E.g.*, Vital v. Interfaith Med. Ctr., 168 F.3d 615 (2d Cir. 1999) [error to dismiss employee claim; employer must show knowing, voluntary release of right to bring Title VII action]; Beadle v. City of Tampa, 42 F.3d 633 (11th Cir.), *cert. denied,* 515 U.S. 1152 (1994).

[200] *E.g*, Metz v. Merrill Lynch Pierce Fenner & Smith, 39 F.3d 1482 (10th Cir. 1994); *see also* Norton v. AMISUB St. Joseph Hosp., 155 F.3d 1040 (8th Cir. 1998) [participation in arbitration of Title VII claim without objection or timely motion to vacate award waived right to object to arbitration].

[201] 9 U.S.C. §§ 1 et seq.; Circuit City Stores, Inc. v. Adams, 532 U.S. 105 (2001) [FAA exemption for some employment contracts applies only to transportation workers], *on remand,* 279 F.3d 889 (9th Cir. 2002) [arbitration agreement not enforceable because contract unconscionable since not equally binding on both sides].

[202] EEOC v. River Oaks Imaging & Diagnostic, 1995 U.S. Dist. LEXIS 6140 (S.D. Tex.) [preliminary injunction of employer's alternative dispute resolution policy, retaliation against employees who refused to sign agreement].

[203] *E.g.*, Patterson v. Tenet Healthcare Inc., 113 F.3d 832 (8th Cir. 1997) [arbitration procedure in employee handbook binding for Title VII claim, even when handbook not contract under state law]; Gibson v. Neighborhood Health Clinics, Inc., 121 F.3d 1126 (7th Cir. 1997) [refusal to enforce agreement to arbitrate job bias claims for lack of consideration]; *Ex parte* Beasley, 712 So. 2d 338 (Ala. 1998) [employee handbook that is not binding on employer cannot be basis for mandatory arbitration].

[204] Circuit City Stores, Inc. v. Adams, 279 F.3d 889 (9th Cir. 2002), *on remand* from, 532 U.S. 105 (2001).

neutral arbitrators are generally unenforceable; the employer cannot insist that the arbitrator be picked from a list that it generates.[205] Agreements that are viewed as placing too much of the costs of the arbitration on the employee may not be enforceable.[206]

Title VII overlaps with the older civil rights acts. Thus, for example, most claims of ethnic-based discrimination in employment can be made under either § 1981 or Title VII. Frequently, claims are made under both statutes. Some courts have considered the elements of the claims to be identical. There are procedural differences; a plaintiff does not have to pursue the EEOC administrative procedure before filing a § 1981 suit. There are some differences in the remedies granted. Some claims can only be brought under Title VII. For example, a religion discrimination claim against a private hospital that could be brought under Title VII probably could not be brought under the older civil rights acts.

Who Is an Employee? Courts apply several different tests to determine whether a person is an *employee* and, thus, entitled to the protection of these employment nondiscrimination laws. Clearly if the employer withholds employment taxes from the person's income, the person is an employee. In less clear cases, the courts apply one or both of the common law control test and the economic realities test. Under the *control test*, persons are employees if the employer controls the details and means by which the work is performed. Under the *economic realities test*, persons are employees if they are dependent on the business to which they render service.[207] Some courts use a *hybrid test* that combines elements of the other two tests.[208] In 1998, one federal court ruled that remuneration was required to make a person an employee; so

---

[205] *E.g.*, Murray v. United Food & Commercial Workers Internat'l Union, 289 F.3d 297 (4th Cir. 2002).

[206] *E.g.*, McGaskill v. SCI Mgmt. Corp., 285 F.3d 623 (7th Cir. 2002) [limits on prevailing employee recovery of attorney fees rendered arbitration unenforceable under Title VII]; *see also* Bond v. Twin Cities Carpenters' Pension Fund, 307 F.3d 704 (8th Cir. 2002) [required split of arbitration cost violated ERISA].

[207] *E.g.*, Diggs v. Harris Hosp.-Methodist, Inc., 847 F.2d 270 (5th Cir.), *cert. denied*, 488 U.S. 956 (1988); Amiable v. Long & Scott Farms, 20 F.3d 434 (11th Cir.), *cert. denied*, 513 U.S. 943 (U.S. 1994).

[208] *E.g.*, Deal v. State Farm County Mut. Ins. Co., 5 F.3d 117 (5th Cir. 1993).

it rejected the claim by an unpaid volunteer without looking at the other tests.[209]

Generally, nonemployee physicians have been unable to use Title VII to challenge medical staff decision because they are not employees.[210] However, Title VII also applies to interference with employment opportunities. Thus, in some circumstances, physicians who have been denied or lost medical staff membership have been able to use Title VII to sue hospitals even when they are clearly not employees of the hospital.[211]

Who Is an Employer? In most cases, the answer to this question is clear. Small employers of less then fifteen employees are exempt. In 1997, the United States Supreme Court ruled on how employees would be counted to determine the fifteen employee threshold.[212]

Coworkers are not employers; they are not liable under Title VII.[213] Generally, a parent company of the employer is not liable as an employer under Title VII.[214]

Race and National Origin. While most racial discrimination suits are brought by persons of African descent, the courts have

---

[209] O'Connor v. Davis, 126 F.3d 112 (2d Cir. 1997), *cert. denied*, 522 U.S 1114 (1998) [unpaid hospital volunteer (student intern) could not bring sexual harassment claim against hospital for acts of staff physician because volunteer was not paid and, thus, not an employee].

[210] *E.g.*, Cilecek v. Inova Health Sys. Servs., Inc., 115 F.3d 256 (4th Cir. 1997), *cert. denied*, 522 U.S. 1049 (1998) [independent contractor ER physician could not make Title VII employment discrimination charges].

[211] *E.g.*, Pardazi v. Cullman Med. Ctr., 838 F.2d 1155 (11th Cir. 1988) [Title VII claim stated when denial of medical staff membership led to loss of employment opportunity with medical group]; Doe on behalf of Doe v. St. Joseph's Hosp., 788 F.2d 411 (7th Cir. 1986), *on remand*, 113 F.R.D. 677 (N.D. Ind. 1987) [physicians terminated from medical staff may sue under Title VII if they show interference with employment by others]; Gomez v. Alexian Bros. Hosp., 698 F.2d 1019 (9th Cir. 1983) [rejection of contract proposal by emergency medical professional corporation can violate Title VII as to Hispanic physician employee of corporation]; Sibley Mem. Hosp. v. Wilson, 160 U.S. App. D.C. 14, 488 F.2d 1338 (1973) [hospital can violate Title VII by interfering with private duty nurse's employment opportunities]; Annotation, *Who is "employee" as defined in sec. 701(f) of the Civil Rights Act of* 1964, 72 A.L.R. Fed. 522; *but see* Diggs v. Harris Hosp.-Methodist, Inc., 847 F.2d 270 (5th Cir. 1988) [physician's "employment" relationship with patients not sufficient to permit Title VII action against hospital]; Mitchel v. Frank R. Howard Mem. Hosp., 853 F.2d 762 (9th Cir. 1988) [relationship with patients and with wholly-owned professional corporation insufficient]; Shrock v. Altru Nurses Registry, 810 F.2d 658 (7th Cir. 1987) [nurse referral agency not employer, not liable under Title VII].

[212] Walters v. Metropolitan Educ. Enters. Inc., 519 U.S. 202 (1997) [payroll method adopted for determining 15-employee threshold].

[213] *E.g.*, Smith v. St. Bernards Reg. Med. Ctr., 19 F.3d 1254 (8th Cir. 1994).

[214] *E.g.*, Garcia v. Elf Atochem N. Am., 28 F.3d 446 (5th Cir. 1994).

recognized that other races are protected, including Arabs and Asians.[215] In addition, reverse discrimination suits have been brought by Caucasians.[216]

When mistakes are promptly corrected, liability can often be avoided. In 1996, a federal appellate court found no violation because mistaken payment of higher wages to later hired Caucasian unit secretaries had been promptly reduced, with retroactive payment to African-American unit secretaries of the differential for the period of higher wages. The court found that there was no evidence of racial bias by those involved in the salary decision and bias by others was not relevant.[217]

Employers can require experience as a qualification when it is needed,[218] but a neutral requirement of experience for promotion can become discriminatory when the employer discriminates in the opportunities to gain the experience.[219] The Immigration Reform and Control Act[220] also bars some employment discrimination based on national origin or citizenship status, but citizens can be preferred over equally qualified aliens.

Request of the patient for discrimination is no excuse. Employers cannot accede to patient racial preferences concerning their providers. In 2003, a Pennsylvania hospital complied with a man's demand that no African-American staff members assist in the deliv-

---

[215] *E.g.*, St. Francis College v. Al-Knazraji, 481 U.S. 604 (1987) [Arabs are a race for purposes of 42 U.S.C. § 1981 suits; "distinctive physiognomy is not essential"]; Jatoi v. Hurst-Euless Bedford Hosp. Auth., 807 F.2d 1213 (5th Cir.), *as modified*, 819 F.2d 545 (5th Cir. 1987) [East Indians]; Doe on behalf of Doe v. St. Joseph's Hosp., 788 F.2d 411 (7th Cir. 1986), *on remand*, 113 F.R.D. 677 (N.D. Ind. 1987) [Asians]; MacDissi v. Valmont Indust., Inc., 856 F.2d 1054 (8th Cir. 1988) [Lebanese]; Janko v. Illinois State Toll Highway Auth., 704 F. Supp. 1531 (N.D. Ill. 1989) [Gypsies].

[216] *E.g.*, Adarand Constructors, Inc. v. Pena, 515 U.S. 200 (1995); Lawrence v. University of Tex. Med. Branch, 163 F.3d 309 (5th Cir. 1999) [Caucasian nurse challenged selection of African-American nurse as nursing supervisor as reverse discrimination; defendants prevailed because reason for selection — best qualified candidate — was not pretext]; Harding v. Gray, 9 F.3d 150 (D.C. Cir. 1993) [hospital shop foreman; allegations of superior qualifications, if supported by facts, can constitute sufficient background circumstances to establish prima facie case]; McNabola v. Chicago Transit Auth., 10 F.3d 501 (7th Cir. 1993) [affirming reverse discrimination judgment for Caucasian physician terminated as per diem medical examiner].

[217] Trotter v. Board of Trustees of Univ. of Ala., 91 F.3d 1449 (11th Cir. 1996).

[218] *E.g.*, Mosley v. Clarksville Mem. Hosp., 574 F. Supp. 224 (M.D. Tenn. 1983); Dotson v. Blood Ctr., 988 F. Supp. 1216 (E.D. Wis. 1998). [African-American medical technologist who had applied for five openings, but had not been hired, failed to state racial discrimination claim where he did not allege he was qualified or that positions remained open after he was not selected].

[219] *E.g.*, Walker v. Jefferson County Home, 726 F.2d 1554 (11th Cir. 1984).

[220] 8 U.S.C. § 1324b.

ery of his child. No reported suit resulted. The action was widely criticized in the media, and the hospital publicly apologized.[221]

Religion. Employers must make reasonable accommodations for employee religious observances, short of incurring undue hardship.[222] This includes accommodating religious practices that preclude working on certain days. The offering of a reasonable accommodation satisfies the requirement even if it is not the accommodation the employee prefers.[223] Not everything that is claimed to be a religious observance is given this protection.[224] A federal district court rejected a woman's claim that her belief in adultery was religious; so it ruled that her discharge was not religious discrimination.[225]

Not all religious practices have to be accommodated. A federal appellate court upheld the termination of a Veterans Administration psychiatric hospital chaplain.[226] The court accepted the hospital's explanation that the chaplain's evangelical approach was not appropriate in the hospital and antithetical to its philosophy of care. In 1999, a federal appellate court ruled that a person could be refused employment based on a religious refusal to provide a Social Security number.[227]

---

[221] *Hospital apologizes for keeping black workers from patient's room*, AP, Oct. 3, 2003; *see also* R. Cohen, *The ethicist: Dying wish*, N.Y. Times Mag., May 11, 2003, 22 [family of African-American patient requested African-American nursing assistant rather than planned Latino]; E. Kane, *Hospital case shows danger of power, bias*, Milwaukee J. Sentinel, Dec. 14, 2000, 1B [Tenn. surgeon asked black staff to leave room at patient request].

[222] Trans World Airlines, Inc. v. Hardison, 432 U.S. 63 (1977); Shelton v. University of Med. & Dentistry, 223 F.3d 220 (3d Cir. 2000) [offer of lateral transfer accommodated nurses religious belief against abortions]; Bruff v. North Mississippi Health Services, Inc., 244 F.3d 495 (5th Cir. 2001) [EAP counselor may be terminated for religious refusal to counsel on homosexual and extramarital relationship issues, would be undue burden to accommodate].

[223] *E.g.*, Brener v. Diagnostic Ctr. Hosp., 671 F.2d 141 (5th Cir. 1982); Mathewson v. Florida Game & Fresh Water Fish Comm'n, 693 F. Supp. 1044 (M.D. Fla. 1988), *aff'd without op.*, 871 F.2d 123 (11th Cir. 1989); Murphy v. Edge Mem. Hosp., 550 F. Supp. 1185 (M.D. Ala. 1982).

[224] *E.g*, Tribulak v. Minirth-Meier-Rice Clinic, 113 F.3d 135 (*without op.*), 1997 U.S. App. LEXIS 6932 (8th Cir.) [religious counseling clinic employee resigned after being told to include more prayer; failed to establish bona fide belief his religion would be violated by compliance with employer requirements].

[225] McCrory v. Rapides Reg. Med. Ctr., 635 F. Supp. 975 (W.D. La.), *aff'd without op.*, 801 F.2d 396 (5th Cir. 1986).

[226] Baz v. Walters, 782 F.2d 701 (7th Cir. 1986); *accord,* Grant v. Fairview Hosp, 2004 U.S. Dist. LEXIS 2653 (D. Minn.) [prohibiting antiabortion proselytizing on the job not religious discrimination, adequate accommodation to permit employee to leave room].

[227] Sutton v. Providence St. Joseph Medical Center, 192 F.3d 826 (9th Cir.1999); *see also* EEOC v. Allendale Nursing Ctr., 996 F. Supp. 712 (W.D. Mich. 1998) [may terminate for religious refusal to obtain Social Security number].

Religious employers are exempt from the federal religious discrimination laws.[228] In 1987, the United States Supreme Court ruled that this exemption was constitutional, including its application to secular nonprofit activities, such as hospitals.[229] In 1988, a federal court ruled that a religious hospital does not forfeit its exemption from the religious discrimination statutes by accepting Medicare payments.[230]

Discrimination in favor of a religion can also violate Title VII. A supervisor's preferential promotion of persons of the same religion can be a violation without showing that a specific religion was the target of the discrimination.[231]

Sex. In addition to the unjustified preference of one sex for certain jobs, sex discrimination can also take the form of sexual harassment. The two forms of sexual harassment are (1) *quid pro quo* sexual harassment when job conditions are altered due to refusal to submit to sexual demands and (2) *hostile environment* sexual harassment when the employer's conduct unreasonably interferes with performance or creates an intimidating or offensive environment. Employers are generally liable for any quid pro quo sexual harassment by supervisors.[232] In some situations, employers may be liable for harassment of employees by third parties such as patients and suppliers.[233] In some circumstances, harassment by medical staff members can lead to hospital liability.[234]

---

[228] 42 U.S.C. § 2000e-1; *see also* McKeon v. Mercy Healthcare Sacramento, 19 Cal. 4th 321, 965 P.2d 1189, 79 Cal. Rptr. 2d 319 (1998) [Catholic hospital exempt from nurse's state claims of race, gender bias]; Tacoma v. Franciscan Found., 94 Wash. App. 663, 972 P.2d 566 (1999) [state law exempting religious nonprofit organizations from job bias suits preempts application of city discrimination ordinance to religious hospital].

[229] Corporation of Presiding Bishop v. Amos, 483 U.S. 327 (1987).

[230] Young v. Shawnee Mission Med. Ctr., No. 88-2321-S (D. Kan. Oct. 21, 1988), *as discussed in* 22 J. HEALTH & HOSP. L. 160 (1989).

[231] *E.g.*, Mandell v. County of Suffolk, 316 F.3d 368 (2d Cir. 2003).

[232] *E.g.*, Steele v. Offshore Shipbuilding, Inc., 867 F.2d 1311 (11th Cir.), *reh'g denied* (en banc), 874 F.2d 821 (11th Cir. 1989); Sparks v. Pilot Freight Carriers, Inc., 830 F.2d 1554 (11th Cir. 1987).

[233] *E.g.*, Turnbull v. Topeka State Hosp., 255 F.3d 1238 (10th Cir. 2001) [employer may be liable for sexual harassment of psychologist by patient]; Cal. Gov. Code § 12940(j)(1); Salazar v. Diversified Paratransit, Inc., 117 Cal. App. 4th 318, 11 Cal. Rptr. 3d 630 (2d Dist. 2004) [employers may be sued by employees under state law for some harassment by clients].

[234] *E.g.*, Kopp v. Samaritan Health Sys., Inc., 13 F.3d 264 (8th Cir. 1993) [hospital could be liable for hostile environment sexual harassment based on conduct of cardiologist, hospital's response]; *but see* Sparks v. Regional Med. Ctr. Bd., 792 F. Supp. 735 (N.D. Ala. 1992 [hospital's prompt response to sexual harassment by pathologist prevented hospital liability for physician conduct].

In 1986, the United States Supreme Court held that sexual harassment that created a hostile or offensive working environment could violate Title VII.[235] It is not necessary to show that the sexual harassment is tied to the granting or denial of an economic benefit. Employers are not strictly liable for hostile environment sexual harassment by their supervisors, but employers are not always shielded from suit by lack of knowledge of the behavior. If the employer has a policy against sexual harassment and has implemented a reasonable procedure to resolve harassment claims, the employer will usually be shielded from liability absent actual knowledge of misconduct. The procedure should not require that the first step be a complaint to the supervisor who is the source of the harassment.

In 1993, the United States Supreme Court made it easier to prove sexual harassment by determining that it was not necessary to prove injury or a serious effect on the employee's psychological well-being.[236]

Federal appellate courts have generally ruled behavior that is merely offensive or boorish is generally not a violation of Title VII.[237] The behavior must be so severe or pervasive as to alter the conditions of employment. However, in some cases, a single egregious incident can be sufficient.[238]

Although most claims are by females, males may also bring sexual discrimination and sexual harassment claims.[239]

---

[235] Meritor Sav. Bank v. Vinson, 477 U.S. 57 (1986), *on remand*, 25 U.S. App. D.C. 397, 801 F.2d 1436 (1986). For EEOC regulations, *see* 29 C.F.R. § 1604.11. For examples, *see* Ross v. Twenty Four Collection, Inc., 681 F. Supp. 1547 (S.D. Fla. 1988), *aff'd without op.*, 875 F.2d 873 (11th Cir. 1989) [liability for sexual harassment]; Dockter v. Rudolf Wolff Futures, Inc., 684 F. Supp. 532 (N.D. Ill. 1988), *aff'd*, 913 F.2d 456 (7th Cir. 1990) [hostile working environment not shown]; *see also* Scott v. Western State Hosp., 658 F. Supp. 593 (W.D. Va. 1987) [duty to investigate racial harassment charges, take steps].

[236] Harris v. Forklift Sys., Inc., 510 U.S. 17 (1993).

[237] *E.g.*, Patt v. Family Health Systems, Inc., 280 F.3d 749 (7th Cir. 2002); Duncan v. General Motors Corp., 300 F.3d 928 (8th Cir. 2002); Ocheltree v. Scollon Productions, 308 F.3d 351 (4th Cir. 2002).

[238] *E.g.*, Little v. Windermere Relocation, Inc., 301 F.3d 958 (9th Cir. 2002).

[239] *E.g.*, Carey v. Mt. Desert Island Hosp., 156 F.3d 31 (1st Cir. 1998) [affirming award to male executive claiming discharge due to sex discrimination]; Lynn v. Deaconess Med. Ctr., 160 F.3d 484 (8th Cir. 1998) [terminated male nurse may bring sex discrimination claim]; *see also* Rene v. MGM Grand Hotel, Inc., 305 F.3d 1061 (9th Cir. 2002) [same sex harassment included].

Most courts have held that preferential treatment of an employee on the basis of a consensual romantic relationship between a supervisor and employee is not sexual discrimination.[240]

Some groups have sought to convince courts that Title VII requires adoption of a *comparable worth doctrine*. This doctrine would require employers to revise wage scales so that pay is based on a comparison of the work done by persons in different job classifications without regard to the labor market. This doctrine goes beyond the Equal Pay Act (discussed in the following section) that requires equal pay for essentially identical work. Courts generally have ruled that Title VII does not require wage scales based on comparable worth.[241]

Pregnancy. In 1978, Title VII was amended to prohibit discriminatory treatment of pregnant women for all employment-related purposes. Employers are not required to provide special considerations.[242] However, for example, if leaves are offered for disability, similar leaves must be offered for disabling maternity. Mandatory maternity leaves not based on inability to work violate Title VII.[243] Pregnancy itself is not considered a disability, but if a pregnant worker becomes unable to work, then disability benefits must be offered the pregnant worker. Some states require employers to offer a leave of absence for pregnancy.

One federal court found that job absence for infertility treatments was protected.[244]

---

[240] *E.g.*, DeCintio v. Westchester County Med. Ctr., 807 F.2d 304 (2d Cir. 1986), *cert. denied*, 484 U.S. 965 (1987) [writing job description to favor girlfriend not sex discrimination]; Autry v. North Carolina Dep't of Human Resources, 820 F.2d 1384 (4th Cir. 1987); *contra* King v. Palmer, 598 F. Supp. 65 (D. D.C. 1984), *rev'd on other grounds*, 250 U.S. App. D.C. 257, 778 F.2d 878 (1985).

[241] *E.g.*, Lemons v. City of Denver, 620 F.2d 228 (10th Cir.), *cert. denied*, 449 U.S. 888 (1980); Briggs v. City of Madison, 536 F. Supp. 435 (W.D. Wis. 1982); American Nurses Ass'n v. Illinois, 783 F.2d 716 (7th Cir. 1986) [case settled in 1989, MOD. HEALTHCARE, Mar. 10, 1989, 14]; AFSCME v. Washington, 770 F.2d 1401 (9th Cir. 1985), *reh'g denied* (en banc), 813 F.2d 1034 (9th Cir. 1987) [case settled in 1985, N.Y. TIMES, Jan. 2, 1986, 7].

[242] *E.g.*, Garcia v. Woman's Hosp. of Tex., 143 F.3d 227 (5th Cir. 1998) [not pregnancy discrimination to require all employees to be able to lift 150 pounds]; Spivey v. Beverly Enterprises, Inc., 196 F.3d 1309 (11th Cir. 1999) [pregnant employee has no right to light duty work]; Stout v. Baxter Healthcare Corp., 282 F.3d 856 (5th Cir. 2002) [pregnant employees may be discharged for absenteeism unless absences of nonpregnant employees overlooked].

[243] *E.g.*, Floca v. Homecare Health Servs., 845 F.2d 108 (5th Cir. 1988) [violation to terminate pregnant director of nursing]; Carney v. Martin Luther Home, Inc., 824 F.2d 643 (8th Cir. 1987) [violation to force unpaid medical leave while still able to work]; *but see* McKnight v. North Charles Gen. Hosp., 652 F. Supp. 880 (D. Md. 1986) [hospital hired replacement head nurse for CCU when return from pregnancy delayed; not discrimination to place returning nurse in staff position in same unit].

[244] Pacourek v. Inland Steel Co., 858 F. Supp. 1393 (N.D. Ill. 1994); *but see*, Tyndall v. National Educ. Ctrs., 31 F.3d 209 (4th Cir. 1994) [discharge for health-related absences not protected by ADA]; Zatarain v. WDSU-Television, Inc., 881 F. Supp. 240 (E.D. La. 1995) [employer not required by ADA to accommodate employee's infertility treatment].

In 1991, the United States Supreme Court ruled that Title VII was violated by fetal protection programs that prohibit female employees capable of childbearing from some jobs, such as those with exposure to toxic chemicals or high blood lead levels.[245] In 1994, a federal appellate court ruled that a pregnant home health nurse could be terminated for refusal to treat an AIDS patient.[246]

Employer health plans that cover employee's spouses must cover pregnancy-related disabilities of spouses.[247]

In 1997, a federal appellate court ruled that the pregnancy discrimination law does not apply after birth; so it does not apply to a woman's decisions concerning care for the child after birth.[248]

Bona Fide Occupational Qualifications. In some circumstances, sex or features related to religion or national origin can be bona fide occupational qualifications (BFOQ) reasonably necessary to the normal operation of a particular business. When employers can demonstrate this necessity, the use of the qualification is not a violation of the law. For example, a federal district court ruled that it was not illegal sex discrimination for a hospital to employ only female nurses in its obstetrics-gynecology department.[249] The court noted that the policy was based on the privacy rights of the patients, not just patient preference. An appellate court vacated the decision because the case became moot when the male nurse voluntarily quit his job.[250]

A federal appellate court ruled that it was not illegal discrimination based on national origin for a hospital to require all employees

---

245 International Union United Auto Workers v. Johnson Controls, Inc., 499 U.S. 187 (1991).

246 Armstrong v. Flowers Hosp., 33 F.3d 1308 (11th Cir. 1994).

247 Newport News Shipbuilding & Dry Dock Co. v. EEOC, 462 U.S. 669 (1983).

248 *E.g.*, Piantanida v. Wyman Ctr., Inc., 116 F.3d 340 (8th Cir. 1997).

249 Backus v. Baptist Med. Ctr., 510 F. Supp. 1191 (E.D. Ark. 1981); *accord* Jones v. Hinds Gen. Hosp., 666 F. Supp. 933 (S.D. Miss. 1987); *Hospitals can ban male nurses from delivery room*, AM. MED. NEWS, Oct. 3, 1994, 19 [Cal. Fair Employment and Housing Comm'n]; *see also* Jennings v. N.Y. State Office of Mental Health, 977 F.2d 731 (2d Cir. 1992) [state mental health facility could require at least one security treatment assistant assigned to each ward to be of same gender as patients]; *see also* EEOC v. Columbia Lakeland Med. Ctr., 1999 U.S. Dist. LEXIS 663 (E.D. La.) [deny hospital its attorney fees against EEOC for defense of suit seeking to force hiring male nurse for maternity ward]; *but see* Little Forest Med. Ctr. v. Ohio Civil Rights Comm'n, 61 Ohio St. 3d 607, 575 N.E.2d 1164 (1991), *cert. denied*, 503 U.S. 906 (1992) [gender not BFOQ for nurse's aide]; Slivka v. Camden-Clark Mem. Hosp., 594 S.E.2d 616 (W.Va. 2004) [under state law, insufficient evidence presented to dismiss male nurse challenge to denial of obstetrics job, sent back to trial court for further review].

250 Backus v. Baptist Med. Ctr., 671 F.2d 1100 (8th Cir. 1982).

to have some facility in communication in the English language.[251] The court recognized that ability to communicate in English was a bona fide occupational qualification for virtually every position in a sophisticated medical center. However, requiring employees to speak only English on the job can be national origin discrimination unless the employer can demonstrate business necessity.[252]

Retaliation. Employers are prohibited from retaliating against employees who oppose discrimination by engaging in reasonable activities.[253] A federal appellate court found that a hospital had violated this provision when it fired an African-American registered nurse who had complained about African-American patient care.[254] However, filing a discrimination complaint does not shield an employee from all adverse actions. Employees can be disciplined or discharged, even after a complaint has been filed, if there are sufficient nonpretextual reasons for the action.[255] In 1997, the United

---

[251] Garcia v. Rush-Presbyterian-St. Luke's Med. Ctr., 660 F.2d 1217 (7th Cir. 1981); *see also* Velasquez v. Goldwater Mem. Hosp., 88 F. Supp. 2d 257 (S.D. N.Y. 2000) [dismiss challenge to firing for violating hospital English-only policy]; Tran v. Standard Motor Products, Inc., 1998 WL 293244 (D. Kan. 1998) [English-only policy during work and meeting did not create a hostile environment in violation of § 1981 or Title VII]; E. Fein, *Lack of a common language can hinder care at hospitals*, N.Y. TIMES, Nov. 23, 1997, 1; *English-only, a touchy work issue, touches more legal nerves*, WALL ST. J., Mar. 10, 1998, A1.

[252] 29 C.F.R. § 1606.7; Dimaranan v. Pomona Valley Hosp. Med. Ctr., 775 F. Supp. 338 (C.D. Cal. 1991) [hospital rule restricting use of Tagalog language by Filipino nurses was not prohibited English-only rule in violation of Title VII where shift-specific directive addressed conflicts among identified nurses]; McNeil v. Aguilos, 831 F. Supp. 1079 (S.D. N.Y. 1993) [non-Filipino nurse did not state claim for hospital policy of allowing nurses to communicate in workplace in Tagalog]; Reed v. Driftwood Convalescent Hosp., EEOC Charge No. 377-93-0509 (July 13, 1994) [Calif. Dep't of Health Services policy; employees may speak other languages away from patients, but not to patients]; EEOC v. Premier Operator Servs., 113 F. Supp. 2d 1066 (N.D. Tex. 2000) [business necessity for English-only rule not shown in non-health care case]; *see also* Yniguez v. Arizonans for Official English, 69 F.3d 920 (9th Cir. 1995) (en banc) [amendment to state constitution making English the official language of state violates U.S. constitution].

[253] 42 U.S.C. § 2000e-3; *but see* Lewis v. Holsum of Fort Wayne, Inc., 278 F.3d 706 (7th Cir. 2002) [no inference of retaliation solely from timing of firing three months after EEOC charge filed].

[254] Wrighten v. Metropolitan Hosp., 726 F.2d 1346 (9th Cir. 1984); *see also* Sparrow v. Piedmont Health Sys. Agency, 593 F. Supp. 1107 (M.D. N.C. 1984) [refusal to give reference letter was prohibited retaliation].

[255] *E.g.*, Whittlington v. Dep't of Veterans Affairs, 132 F.3d 54 (*without op.*), 1997 U.S. App. LEXIS 34353 (Fed. Cir.) [upheld discharge of nurse for patient abuse, rejecting claim of retaliation]; Stevens v. St. Louis Univ. Med. Ctr., 97 F.3d 268 (8th Cir. 1996) [hospital proved nondiscriminatory reason for terminating nurse who had filed sexual discrimination claim, sufficient evidence of misconduct, job performance issues]; Vislisel v. Turanage, 930 F.2d 9 (8th Cir. 1991) [VA did not retaliate for discrimination complaint by requesting physical, mental exam after peculiar behavior]; Davis v. State Univ. of N.Y., 802 F.2d 638 (2d Cir. 1986) [low productivity, inability to accept supervision, angry response to conflict were sufficient nonpretextual reasons]; Klein v. Trustees of Ind. Univ., 766 F.2d 275 (7th Cir. 1985) [refusal to reschedule private practice hours to accommodate student health service hours was nonpretextual reason for discharge].

States Supreme Court decided that a former employee could also sue under Title VII for posttermination retaliation, such as negative job references.[256]

Firing Discriminating Employees. Since employers can sometimes be found liable for discriminatory acts of employees, it is fortunate that most courts recognize such discriminatory acts to be grounds for discipline and even termination of the offending employees.[257] For example, a federal district court ruled that an employer's reasonable belief that an African-American employee was making unwelcome sexual overtures to female employees was a legitimate, nondiscriminatory reason to terminate the offending employee; so there was no racial discrimination in the discharge.[258] However, some courts have ruled that discrimination is not good cause for termination of a physician's contract; so there may be liability for breach of contract.[259] In those jurisdictions, contracts can be written to expressly permit appropriate action to deal with discrimination.

State Law. Title VII does not preempt the entire field of equal employment opportunity. While state law cannot permit something prohibited by Title VII, state law can assure more opportunities. Thus, many state laws that limit the types of work women may perform are superseded, but state laws requiring employers to offer

---

[256] Robinson v. Shell Oil Co., 519 U.S. 337 (1997).

[257] *E.g.,* O'Sullivan v. Cook County Bd. of Comm'rs, 239 Ill. App. 3d 1, 687 N.E.2d 1103 (1st Dist. 1997) [upholding dismissal of chief engineer for violating policy on sexual harassment, abusive behavior; reversing lower court order to demote without back pay, benefits].

[258] Baker v. McDonald's Corp., 686 F. Supp. 1474 (S.D. Fla. 1987), *aff'd without op.,* 865 F.2d 1272 (11th Cir. 1988), *cert. denied,* 493 U.S. 812 (1989); *accord* Stroehmann Bakeries Inc. v. Local 776, 969 F.2d 1436 (3d Cir. 1992), *cert. denied,* 506 U.S. 1022 (1992) [public policy violated by arbitrator order reinstating accused sexual harasser]; Anderson v. Hewlett-Packard Corp., 694 F. Supp. 1294 (N.D. Ohio 1988) [personnel manager's constant sexual remarks, innuendos, suggestions to female subordinates created hostile or offensive work environment justifying termination]; *see also* Davis v. Monsanto Chem. Corp., 858 F.2d 345, 350 (6th Cir. 1988), *cert. denied,* 490 U.S. 1110 ["In essence, while Title VII does not require an employer to fire all 'Archie Bunkers' in its employ, the law does require that an employer take prompt action to prevent such bigots from expressing their opinions in a way that abuses or offends their coworkers."]; Stockley v. AT&T Information Sys., Inc., 687 F. Supp. 764 (E.D. N.Y. 1988) [since employer obligated to investigate sexual harassment claims, report of investigation protected by qualified privilege in defamation action].

[259] Flanagan v. Aaron E. Henry Comm. Health Servs. Ctr., 876 F.2d 1231 (5th Cir. 1987) [termination of Caucasian physician for race discrimination was not good cause under employment contract]; Szczerbaniuk v. Memorial Hosp. of McHenry County, 180 Ill. App. 3d 706, 536 N.E.2d 138 (2d Dist. 1989) [action by radiologist for termination of three-year exclusive contract by CEO after allegations of sexual harassment by hospital employees]; Charter Southland Hosp., Inc. v. Eades, 521 So. 2d 981 (Ala. 1988) [psychologist independent contractor made sexual advances to hospital employees; termination of contract not justified because contract permitted termination for only death, disability, or conviction for felony].

pregnancy leaves are not suspended.[260] Some state and local laws protect from discrimination based on sexual orientation.[261]

EQUAL PAY ACT OF 1963. This Act[262] is designed to prohibit discriminatory compensation policies based on sex. It requires equal pay for equal work. Equal work is defined as work requiring equal skill, equal effort, and equal responsibility that is performed under similar working conditions. A federal district court in Georgia upheld paying physician's assistants more than nurse practitioners because of the greater training and skills required, even though they provided substantially similar services.[263] The payment of higher wages to male orderlies than to female aides has been challenged in several cases.[264] In general, the courts have required equal pay except when the hospital has been able to prove actual differences in the work performed during a substantial portion of work time.

AGE DISCRIMINATION IN EMPLOYMENT ACT. This Act (ADEA)[265] prohibits discriminatory treatment of persons forty years of age and older for all employment-related purposes.[266] Mandatory retirement is prohibited except for certain exempted executives. The law applies to employers of twenty or more persons. There are exceptions for BFOQs,[267] bona fide seniority systems, and reasonable factors other than age, such as physical fitness. In 1984, a federal appellate court found a hospital guilty of age discrimination because its medical director had fired a 56-year-old secretary and replaced her with a 34-year-old individual.[268] The replacement testi-

---

[260] *E.g.*, California Fed. Sav. & Loan Ass'n v. Guerra, 479 U.S. 272 (1987) [state statute requiring pregnancy leave, reinstatement not preempted by Title VII].

[261] *E.g.*, Walsh v. Carney Hosp. Corp., No. CA-94-2583 (Mass. Super. Ct. jury verdict Dec. 30, 1996), *as discussed in* 6 H.L.R. 107 (1997) [housekeeping manager at Roman Catholic hospital fired because he was believed to be homosexual awarded $1.275 million by jury for violation of state law against discrimination based on sexual orientation].

[262] 29 U.S.C. § 206(d); *see* Lambert v. Genesee Hosp., 10 F.3d 46 (2d Cir. 1993), *cert. denied*, 511 U.S. 1052 (1994) [female employee in duplicating services department failed to establish Equal Pay Act claim]; Jones v. Westside-Urban Health Ctr., 760 F. Supp. 1575 (S.D. Ga. 1991) [employed male physician stated prima facie case under Equal Pay Act].

[263] Beall v. Curtis, 603 F. Supp. 1563 (M.D. Ga. 1985).

[264] *E.g.*, Marshall v. St. John Valley Security Home, 560 F.2d 12 (1st Cir. 1977) [no violation]; Brennan v. Prince Williams Hosp., 501 F.2d 282 (4th Cir. 1974), *cert. denied*, 420 U.S. 972 (1975) [violation]; EEOC v. Harper Grace Hosps., 689 F. Supp. 708 (E.D. Mich. 1988) [violation].

[265] 29 U.S.C. §§ 621-634, 663(a).

[266] *E.g.*, Stamey v. Southern Bell Tel. & Tel. Co., 859 F.2d 855 (11th Cir.), *reh'g denied* (en banc), 867 F.2d 1431 (11th Cir.), *cert. denied*, 490 U.S. 1116 (1989).

[267] *E.g.*, Trans World Airlines, Inc. v. Thurston, 469 U.S. 111 (1985) [age of less than 60 years not a bona fide occupational qualification for flying engineers].

[268] O'Donnell v. Georgia Osteopathic Hosp., Inc., 748 F.2d 1543 (11th Cir. 1984).

fied that the medical director told her she was selected for her appearance. Violations can also be found for discriminating in favor of those who are older. An Oregon appellate court found a retirement home guilty of age discrimination under a state nondiscrimination law because it had refused to hire a beautician, saying she was too young for its residents.[269]

The employer is not liable for termination of a protected person if the employer presents valid reasons, such as reduction in force or inability to do the job, that are not pretexts.[270]

Employers must be careful not to give the impression of age discrimination. After a 62-year-old day-shift nurse supervisor resigned, she sued the hospital for age discrimination;[271] a federal appellate court ruled in 1985 that a jury should decide whether the CEO's statements concerning the need for "new blood" and her "advanced age" created intolerable working conditions in violation of the Act that forced her to resign.

In 1996, a federal appellate court upheld a jury award in favor of a fired director of a hospital radiology department. The court concluded that the hospital personnel manager had adversely altered the evaluation notes of the employee by his supervisor; so the jury was entitled to conclude that the reasons the employer gave for the firing were a pretext.[272]

Some employers have tried to settle age discrimination suits and have obtained from the employee a signed waiver of the right to sue for damages. These unsupervised waivers may not be effective. Waivers must satisfy statutory standards.[273] Thus, prior approval

---

269 Ogden v. Bureau of Labor, 680 Or. App. 235, 682 P.2d 802 (1984), *aff'd in part/rev'd in part*, 299 Or. 98, 699 P.2d 189 (1985).

270 *E.g.*, Stafford v. Radford Comm. Hosp., 120 F.3d 262 (*without op.*), 1997 U.S. App. LEXIS 19741 (4th Cir.) [50-year-old nurse could not show she was performing job at employer's legitimate expectations]; Vaughan v. MetraHealth Cos., 145 F.3d 197 (4th Cir. 1998) [57-year-old woman fired during downsizing; no ADEA claim stated, no age motivation shown]; Lesch v. Crown Cork & Seal Co., 282 F.3d 467 (7th Cir. 2002) [overqualification for position is nonpretextual reason for selecting another person for retention in reduction in force]; Gehring v. Case Corp., 43 F.3d 340 (7th Cir. 1994), *cert. denied*, 515 U.S. 1159 (1995) [theory of disparate impact of reduction in force not an ADEA theory.]; Rhodes v. Guiberson Oil Tools, 39 F.3d 537 (5th Cir. 1994) [reduction in force nonpretexual; to show pretext must show reason false, discrimination was real reason]; Anderson v. Baxter Healthcare Corp., 13 F.3d 1120 (7th Cir. 1994) [goal of reducing salary costs is not age discrimination]; Grohs v. Gold Bond Bldg. Prods., 859 F.2d 1283 (7th Cir. 1988), *cert. denied*, 490 U.S. 1036 (1989) [difficulty getting along with peers was nonpretextual].

271 Buckley v. Hospital Corp. of Am., 758 F.2d 1525 (11th Cir. 1985).

272 Shaw v. HCA Health Servs., 79 F.3d 99 (8th Cir. 1996).

273 29 U.S.C. § 626(f), as amended by Pub. L. No. 101-433, § 201, 104 Stat. 983 (1990).

from the enforcement agency or a court may be necessary to make such waivers binding.

In 2004, the Supreme Court ruled that younger workers cannot use the ADEA to challenge better benefit packages that are given to older workers.[274]

AMERICANS WITH DISABILITIES ACT. This Act (ADA)[275] prohibits discrimination on the basis of disabilities in employment, transportation, and public accommodations. Title I provides that employers of fifteen or more employees may not "discriminate against a qualified individual with a disability because of the disability in regard to job application procedures, the hiring, job assignment, advancement, or discharge of employees, employee compensation or fringe benefits, job training, and other terms conditions, and privileges of employment."[276] The ADA applies to public employers, but in 2001, the United States Supreme Court decided that remedies against some public employers are limited.[277]

Disability/Qualified Person. Employees and applicants who are *qualified* individuals with *disabilities* are protected. A *disability* is (a) having a physical or mental impairment that substantially limits one or more major life activities, (b) having a record of such an impairment, or (c) being regarded as having a substantially limited impairment.[278] *Major life activities* include self-care, performing manual tasks, walking, seeing, hearing, speaking, breathing, sitting, standing, lifting, reaching, learning, and working. A *qualified person with a disability* means "an individual with a disability who meets the skill, experience, education, and other job-related requirements of a position held or desired, and who, with or without reasonable accommodation, can perform the essential functions of the positions."[279]

There has been a large volume of litigation about all of these terms. In 1999, the United States Supreme Court ruled that cor-

---

[274] General Dynamics Land Sys. v. Cline, 124 S. Ct. 1236 (U.S. 2004).

[275] 42 U.S.C. §§ 12101-12117; 29 C.F.R. pt. 1630; *see* M.A. Dowell, *The Americans with Disabilities Act: The responsibilities of health care providers, insurers and managed care organizations*, 25 J. HEALTH & HOSP. L. 289 (1992).

[276] 42 U.S.C. § 12112(a).

[277] Board of Trustees of the Univ. of Ala. v. Garrett, 531 U.S. 356 (2001) [Eleventh Amendment protects state from suits for money damages under Title I].

[278] 42 U.S.C. § 12102(2); Summers v. A. Teichert & Sons, Inc., 127 F.3d 1150 (9th Cir. 1997) [ADA claimant must prove only one of three prongs of disability definition].

[279] 42 U.S.C. § 12111(8); 29 C.F.R. § 1630.2(m).

rectable conditions are not disabilities under the ADA.[280] In 1997, a federal court ruled that a person who required treatment that was disabling could be disabled even if the underlying condition was not itself disabling.[281]

The scope of major life activities has been the focus of many cases, as employees have sought to expand the scope of protection of the Act.[282] In 1998, the United States Supreme Court ruled that reproduction is a major life activity that is substantially limited by HIV; so a symptomatic HIV-positive person can be covered as disabled.[283] In 1999, a federal appellate court decided that the inability to work more than forty hours per week did not substantially limit a major life activity; so the director of human resources who could no longer work more than forty hours was not disabled.[284] Also in 1999, another federal appellate court ruled that the employer's cancellation of a promotional video that included the employee allegedly because the employee was too obese did not substantially limit a major life activity.[285] In 1997, another federal appellate court decided that the ability to lift more than 25 lbs. was not a major life activity; so a nurse with a lifting limitation was not disabled.[286]

A person currently engaged in the illegal use of drugs is not qualified.[287] An employer may prohibit the use of alcohol and illegal drugs in the workplace; may prohibit employees from being under

---

[280] Sutton et al. v. United Air Lines Inc., 527 U.S. 471 (1999) [correctable myopia not a disability]; Albertson's v. Kirkingburg, 527 U.S. 555 (1999) [correctable condition not protected by ADA]; *see also* Krocka v. City of Chicago, 203 F.3d 507 (7th Cir. 2000) [police officer taking Prozac that controls symptoms of depression is not disabled for ADA]; Tangires v. Johns Hopkins Hosp., 79 F. Supp. 2d 587 (D. Md. 2000) [asthmatic employee who refuses to take medication not disabled under ADA].

[281] Christian v. St. Anthony Med. Ctr., 117 F.3d 1051 (7th Cir. 1997), *cert. denied,* 523 U.S. 1022 (1998).

[282] *E.g.,* Watson v. Hughston Sports Med. Hosp., 231 F. Supp. 2d 1344 (M.D. Ga. 2002) [latex allergy not disability, not substantially limited in major life activity or regarded as disabled].

[283] Bragdon v. Abbott, 524 U.S. 624 (1998).

[284] Tardie v. Rehabilitation Hosp. of R.I., 168 F.3d 538 (1st Cir. 1999).

[285] Walton v. Mental Health Ass'n, 168 F.3d 661 (3d Cir. 1999).

[286] Thompson v. Holy Family Hosp., 121 F.3d 537 (9th Cir. 1997); *but see* Deane v. Pocono Med. Ctr., 142 F.3d 138 (3d Cir. 1998) (en banc) [nurse with wrist injury that restricted heavy lifting could pursue ADA claim; employee regarded as disabled need only show she could perform essential functions of the job].

[287] 42 U.S.C. §§ 12110(a), 12114(a); Shafer v. Preston Mem. Hosp. Corp., 107 F.3d 274 (4th Cir. 1997) [illegal drug use prior to being placed on leave for rehabilitation was "current" illegal use permitting termination on completion of rehabilitation]; *see also* Johnson v. New York Hosp., 1998 U.S. Dist. LEXIS 19099 (S.D. N.Y.) [refusal to rehire recovering alcoholic nurse not ADA violation, where pursuant to policy against reinstating employees with unsatisfactory work record].

the influence of illegal drugs in the workplace; and may require compliance with the Drug Free Workplace Act of 1988.[288]

Essential Functions. A key part of the analysis of whether an individual is qualified is the determination of the essential functions of the position.[289] This determination is also a key part of assessing whether any proposed accommodation is sufficient to enable the person to perform the essential functions and actually is proposing to change the essential functions. This issue is discussed in the section on Reasonable Accommodations.

Safety Issues/Direct Threat. An individual who poses a *direct threat* to the health or safety of others is not *qualified.*[290] The employer generally has the burden of proof on this issue because it is viewed as a defense against an ADA claim. However, in 1997, a federal appellate court recognized that safety issues are not limited to this direct threat defense context. The court ruled that when the essential functions of the job necessarily implicate the safety of others that safety issues are included in the plaintiff's burden to prove ability to perform the essential functions of the job in order to be qualified. Thus, it was proper to require a former behavior therapist who had previously attempted suicide with drugs to prove that she was qualified to safely perform a job that required the handling of medications for patients.[291] There are other conditions that have been found to raise direct threat or other safety issues.[292] For example, courts have found that there are some positions in hospitals where HIV-positive persons are a direct threat to the health and safety of others or are otherwise not qualified.[293]

---

[288] 42 U.S.C. § 12114(c); 29 C.F.R. § 1630.16(b).

[289] *E.g.*, Stafne v. Unicare Homes, 266 F.3d 771 (8th Cir. 2001) [RN had no ADA claim where rheumatoid arthritis made it impossible for her to perform essential functions of job with accommodation].

[290] 42 U.S.C. §§ 12111(3), 12113.

[291] EEOC v. Amego Inc., 110 F.3d 135 (1st Cir. 1997).

[292] *E.g.*, Hutton v. Elf Atochem North America, Inc., 273 F.3d 884 (9th Cir. 2001) [diabetic worker posed direct threat].

[293] *E.g.*, Estate of Mauro v. Burgess Med. Ctr., 137 F.3d 398 (6th Cir. 1998), *cert. denied*, 525 U.S. 815 (1998) [HIV-positive surgical technician posed a direct threat to health and safety of others]; Bradley v. University of Tex. M.D. Anderson Cancer Ctr., 3 F.3d 922 (5th Cir. 1993), *cert. denied*, 510 U.S. 1119 (1994) [reassignment of an HIV-positive surgical technician to be a procurement technician did not violate the ADA]; Waddell v. Valley Forge Dental Assocs., 276 F.3d 1275 (11th Cir. 2001) [dental hygienist posed direct threat].

In 2002, the United States Supreme Court upheld an EEOC regulation permitting employers to refuse to hire a person when the job poses a direct threat to the person's health.[294]

Hiring Process/Other Inquiries. The law imposes numerous restrictions on the hiring process. While inquiries can be made about the ability to perform job-related functions, no inquiry can be made about whether the applicant has a disability or has any history of workers' compensation. Job criteria and employment tests are scrutinized to determine that they are job related and consistent with business necessity; in addition, tests that screen out disabled people are not permitted when alternate tests are available that disabled people can pass. The use of medical examinations is limited. They cannot be used until after a job offer is made and then only if they are required for all entering employees for the job regardless of disability, and access to and use of the resulting information is limited.

The law has been interpreted to put other restrictions on employer inquiries of employees. In 1997, a federal appellate court ruled that an employer cannot require disclosure or restrict use of prescription drugs by employees.[295] In 1998, another federal appellate court ruled that in some limited circumstances a medical examination can be required of an existing employee.[296]

Job applicants may volunteer information.[297] Employers must be careful in how they use volunteered information.

Reasonable Accommodations. As part of nondiscrimination, covered employers must provide *reasonable accommodations* that do not involve undue hardship on the employer. In 1999, the EEOC published enforcement guidelines concerning reasonable accommodations.[298] The employee must request the accommodation. In 1999, a federal appellate court ruled that the ADA does not

---

[294] Chevron U.S.A. v. Echazabal, 536 U.S. 73 (2002) [upholding EEOC regulation permitting refusal to hire person when job poses direct threat to person's health].

[295] Roe v. Cheyenne Mountain Conference Resort, Inc., 124 F.3d 1221 (10th Cir. 1997); *but see* Doe v. Southeastern Pa. Transp. Auth., 72 F.3d 1133 (3d Cir. 1995) [use of prescription benefit may be monitored].

[296] *E.g.*, EEOC v. Prevo's Family Market, Inc., 135 F.3d 1089 (6th Cir. 1998).

[297] *See* J.S. Lublin, *Should job hunters reveal chronic illnesses? The pros and cons,* WALL ST. J., Jan. 13, 2004, B1.

[298] Equal Employment Opportunity Comm'n, *Enforcement guidance: Reasonable accommodation and undue hardship under the Americans with Disabilities Act* (Mar. 2, 1999) [http://www.access.gpo.gov/eeoc/docs/accommodation.html] [hereinafter cited as *EEOC 1999 Guidance*].

apply to an employee who effectively resigns before requesting an accommodation.[299] The employer need not provide the requested accommodation; the employer is required only to provide a reasonable accommodation. An employer is not required to exempt the employee from the essential functions of the job.

Employers can generally implement temporary accommodations without compromising their position that the accommodation is not required under the ADA. Most courts encourage such temporary accommodations while the employer investigates the circumstances by not allowing the temporary accommodation to be used as proof that such an accommodation can be continued indefinitely. Courts recognize that temporary accommodations would be discouraged if they had to be continued indefinitely. In 1999, a federal appellate court found that an employer who had granted unpaid leave was not required to continue the leave.[300] In 1998, another federal court ruled that the temporary assignment of a nurse to a days-only schedule did not compromise the hospital's position that rotating shifts were an essential function of the job.[301]

Here are some examples where accommodations were not required. Employees have sought to change their work schedules. While in some positions this can be done without undue hardship, there are many positions in health care settings where the schedule is an essential part of the job. In 1998, a federal appellate court ruled that a nurse with fatigue-related seizures was not entitled to an accommodation of a days-only shift schedule because rotating shifts were an essential function for her maternity unit job.[302] In 1999, a federal appellate court ruled that working more than forty hours per week was an essential function of the job of director of human resources; so the employee was not entitled to have the job restructured to a forty-hour per week job.[303]

Employees have sought exemption from physical aspects of their jobs. In 1998, a federal appellate court found that a practical nurse with joint disease and arthritis could not perform the essential functions of the job; so no accommodation was required.[304] In

---

[299] Hammon v. DHL Airways, Inc., 165 F.3d 441 (6th Cir. 1999); *accord* Taylor v. Prenapal Financial Group. Inc., 93 F.3d 155 (5th Cir. 1996) [employee must request reasonable accommodations].

[300] Walton v. Mental Health Ass'n, 168 F.3d 661 (3d Cir. 1999).

[301] Laurin v. Providence Hosp., 150 F.3d 52 (1st Cir. 1998).

[302] *Id.*

[303] Tardie v. Rehabilitation Hosp. of R.I., 168 F.3d 538 (1st Cir. 1999).

[304] Jones v. Kerrville State Hosp., 142 F.3d 263 (5th Cir. 1998).

1993, a federal appellate court ruled that requiring firefighters to be clean shaven did not violate ADA rights of persons with a skin condition that precluded shaving. There was a business necessity in order to safely use respirators and no showing that a reasonable accommodation was available.[305] Employers are not required to exempt employees from the physically demanding parts of essential training for their positions.[306] Employers are not required to hire assistants to perform part of the essential functions of the job.[307]

Some employees have sought to use the ADA to change their supervisors. Courts have generally rejected that this is a reasonable accommodation.[308]

Reasonable accommodations may include reassignment to open existing positions for which the employee is qualified.[309] Reassignments sometimes trigger seniority rights. In 2002, the United States Supreme Court decided that when a requested accommodation conflicts with a seniority rule that it ordinarily, but not necessarily, is not a reasonable accommodation.[310] Thus, in most circumstances, the ADA does not require violation of seniority rules.

Generally, when the condition of the employee results in frequent absences without warning, most courts recognize that no reasonable accommodation can be made without undue hardship.[311] However, in some circumstances, paid or unpaid leave can be a reasonable accommodation.[312] The EEOC recognizes that some positions cannot be

---

[305] Fitzpatrick v. City of Atlanta, 2 F.3d 1112 (11th Cir. 1993).

[306] *E.g.*, Jones v. Kerrville State Hosp., 142 F.3d 263 (5th Cir. 1998) [licensed vocational nurse not otherwise qualified under ADA, not reasonable accommodation to exempt from physical portion of training in managing aggressive behavior of mental patients].

[307] *E.g.*, Reigel v. Kaiser Found. Health Plan, 859 F. Supp. 963 (E.D. N.C. 1994) [HMO did not violate ADA by firing internist with shoulder injury precluding performance of duties; not required to create position with just supervision, administration, or to hire assistant to perform physical tasks of job].

[308] *E.g.*, Mancini v. General Electric Co., 820 F. Supp. 141 (D. Conn. 1993) [employer fired employee with emotional impairment after fight with supervisor; ability to follow orders an essential function of job so not qualified; transfer away from supervisor not a reasonable accommodation]; Ceazan v. Saint John's Hosp. & Health Ctr., 2004 Cal. App. Unpub. LEXIS 3601 (2d Dist.) [not required to give depressed employee a new supervisor].

[309] Aka v. Washington Hosp. Ctr., 332 U.S. App. D.C. 256, 156 F.3d 1284 (D.C. Cir. 1998) (en banc); *accord*, Gale v. United Airlines, 95 F.3d 492 (7th Cir. 1996); Community Hosp. v. Fall, 969 P.2d 667 (Colo. 1998) [if no positions available at existing pay rate, may be position at reduced pay]; *see also* Webster v. Methodist Occupational Health Ctrs., Inc., 141 F.3d 1236 (7th Cir. 1998) [not violation to terminate nurse who could not work independently after stroke and refused nonnursing job].

[310] US Airways, Inc. v. Barnett, 535 U.S. 391 (2002).

[311] *E.g.*, Carr v. Reno, 306 U.S. App. D.C. 217, 23 F.3d 525 (1994); Tyndall v. National Educ. Ctrs., 31 F.3d 209 (4th Cir. 1994); *see also* Earl v. Mervyns, Inc., 207 F.3d 1361 (11th Cir. 2000 [not required to permit tardiness as accommodation for obsessive-compulsive disorder].

[312] *E.g.*, Chers v. Northeast Ohio Alzheimer's Research Ctr., 155 F.3d 775 (6th Cir. 1998).

held open without undue hardship. The EEOC takes the position that if the employer has another equivalent or lower level vacant position for which the employee is qualified that the employee should be reassigned to that position for the remainder of the leave, but if no such position exists, the leave may be terminated when the position can no longer be left open.[313] It is generally recognized that an indefinite leave is not a reasonable accommodation.[314]

Insurance Benefits. In 1999, a federal appellate court ruled that caps on the employee health benefits coverage for HIV did not violate the ADA.[315]

Former employees have sought to use the ADA to challenge disability coverage. Federal courts have disagreed whether a totally disabled former employee is still an employee covered by Title I employment provisions of the ADA.[316] Those courts that do not apply Title I have examined whether the Title III public accommodations provisions apply. Courts have generally limited public accommodations to places; so Title III does not apply to the terms of insurance policies.[317]

REHABILITATION ACT OF 1973. This Act[318] prohibits discrimination on the basis of handicap. Section 503 prohibits discrimination by government contractors, while Section 504 prohibits discrimination by entities that receive federal financial assistance.[319] This law overlaps with the ADA but remains an independent requirement. Because of the overlap in terminology, court decisions under this law are often considered in deciding ADA cases, but the detailed requirements are different. Hospitals are generally subject to both laws and need to comply with both.

In 1984, the United States Supreme Court ruled that any entity receiving federal financial assistance cannot discriminate in either services or employment.[320] In 1990, the law was amended to prohibit the entire health care facility from discriminating, not just the pro-

---

[313] *EEOC 1999 Guidance*, question 18.

[314] *E.g.,* Walsh v. United Parcel Service, 201 F.3d 718 (6th Cir. 2000).

[315] Doe v. Mutual of Omaha, 179 F.3d 557 (7th Cir. 1999), *cert. denied*, 528 U.S. 1106 (2000).

[316] *E.g.*, EEOC v. CNA Ins. Co., 96 F.3d 1039 (7th Cir. 1996) [not covered]; *contra*, Castellano v. New York, 142 F.3d 58 (2d Cir.), *cert. denied*, 525 U.S. 820 (1998) [covered].

[317] *E.g.*, Parker v. Metropolitan Life Ins. Co., 121 F.3d 1006 (6th Cir. 1997) (en banc); Ford v. Schering-Plough Corp., 145 F.3d 601 (3d Cir. 1998); Weyer v. Twentieth Century Fox Film Corp., 198 F.3d 1104 (9th Cir. 2000).

[318] 29 U.S.C. §§ 701-794.

[319] 29 U.S.C. § 793 [section 503]; 29 U.S.C. § 794 [section 504].

[320] Conrail v. Darrone, 465 U.S. 624 (1984).

gram receiving federal financial assistance.[321] Medicare and Medicaid reimbursement have been interpreted to be federal financial assistance.[322]

When the Rehabilitation Act applies, the institution is prohibited from discriminating against any qualified handicapped person who, with reasonable accommodation, can perform the essential functions on the job in question.[323] Preemployment inquiries about handicaps are prohibited except that applicants can be asked if they are able to perform the job. Preemployment physical examinations may be required only if all applicants for similar positions undergo the same examination.

In 1994, a federal appellate court ruled against a blood bank administrator who was terminated after stating she was unable to work because the ventilation system made her asthma worse. She was not handicapped because she was not substantially limited in any major life activity and because her condition was exacerbated only in this one setting.[324]

In 1987, the United States Supreme Court ruled that a discharged teacher with a history of tuberculosis was otherwise qualified to teach and therefore must be reasonably accommodated.[325] Persons with HIV infections have been determined to be handicapped and protected.[326] In 1995, a federal appellate court decided that the FBI violated the Act when it asked a physician under contract to examine a FBI agent to determine whether the agent had AIDS and then terminated his contract based on reports he had AIDS. The court ruled that the contract could not be terminated for his evasiveness about AIDS. In 1996, the United States Supreme Court vacated the decision and directed the appellate court to review the case. The appellate court then ruled in favor of the defendants based on sovereign immunity.[327]

---

[321] Pub. L. No. 100-259, § 4, 102 Stat. 29 (1988).

[322] United States v. Baylor Univ. Med. Ctr., 736 F.2d 1039 (5th Cir. 1984), *cert. denied*, 469 U.S. 1189 (1985).

[323] *E.g.*, Tuck v. HCA Health Servs., 7 F.3d 465 (6th Cir. 1993) [hospital violated Act by terminating nurse].

[324] Heilweil v. Mount Sinai Hosp., 32 F.3d 718 (2d Cir. 1994), *cert. denied*, 513 U.S. 1147 (1995).

[325] *E.g.*, School Bd. of Nassau County v. Arline, 480 U.S. 273 (1987), *after remand*, 692 F. Supp. 1286 (M.D. Fla. 1988) [discharged teacher with history of tuberculosis otherwise qualified, entitled to reinstatement, back pay].

[326] Bragdon v. Abbott, 524 U.S. 624 (1998).

[327] Doe v. Attorney General, 95 F.3d 29 (9th Cir. 1996), *after remand,* Reno v. Doe, 518 U.S. 1014 (1996), *vacating*, Doe by Laverty v. Attorney General, 1995 U.S. App. LEXIS 16264 (9th Cir.).

Numerous other conditions have been ruled to be protected handicaps.[328]

When a handicap precludes a function, the courts look closely to determine whether that function is needed for the job. Thus, a federal appellate court questioned whether heavy lifting was really necessary for a postal job for a person with a back injury.[329] However, generally standards do not have to be lowered, and the nature of the job does not have to be changed. The *Federal Register* was not required to lower its accuracy standards to accommodate an editor with cerebral palsy.[330] The FBI was not required to change the role of special agents to accommodate an insulin-dependent diabetic.[331]

An employer may refuse to hire or retain a person on the basis of behavioral manifestations of the handicap, such as sleeping on the job by a diabetic[332] or excessive absenteeism.[333] Employers may also refuse to hire or retain persons whose current use of alcohol or drugs

---

[328] *E.g.*, Carter v. Casa Cent., 849 F.2d 1048 (7th Cir. 1988) [director of nursing at nursing home with multiple sclerosis handicapped, otherwise qualified]; Chalk v. United States Dist. Court, 840 F.2d 701 (9th Cir. 1988) [teacher with AIDS was handicapped, otherwise qualified to teach; discrimination to assign to administrative job]; Harrison v. Marsh, 691 F. Supp. 1223 (W.D. Mo. 1988) [surgical removal of part of muscle of arm made typist handicapped; inadequate efforts to accommodate handicap]; Hall v. Veterans Admin., 693 F. Supp. 546 (E.D. Mich. 1988), *aff'd*, 1991 U.S. App. LEXIS 26,046 (6th Cir.) [denial of dismissal of suit seeking a smoke-free environment as accommodation of obstructive lung disease]; Wallace v. Veterans Admin., 683 F. Supp. 758 (D. Kan. 1988) [recovering addict could not be denied nursing position because authority to administer narcotics had been restricted; otherwise qualified].

[329] *E.g.*, Hall v. U.S. Postal Serv., 857 F.2d 1073 (6th Cir. 1988) [on-the-job back injury precluded heavy lifting; lower court should decide whether lifting requirement essential, whether employee could perform function, if essential, whether reasonable accommodation possible, if not essential].

[330] Bruegging v. Burke, 696 F. Supp. 674 (D. D.C. 1987) [FEDERAL REGISTER not required to lower standards of accuracy to accommodate editor with cerebral palsy], *aff'd without op.*, 298 U.S. App. D.C. 97, 976 F.2d 95 (1988), *cert. denied*, 488 U.S. 1009 (1989).

[331] Davis v. Meese, 692 F. Supp. 505 (E.D. Pa. 1988), *aff'd*, 865 F.2d 592 (3d Cir. 1989) [insulin-dependent diabetic applicant for FBI special agent position not otherwise qualified; employer not required to make fundamental alteration in nature of job as accommodation]; *accord* Serrapica v. City of New York, 708 F. Supp. 64 (S.D. N.Y.), *aff'd without op.*, 888 F.2d 126 (2d Cir. 1989) [diabetic not otherwise qualified for sanitation worker job because of heavy vehicles]; *see also* Matzo v. Postmaster Gen., 685 F. Supp. 260 (D. D.C. 1987), *aff'd without op.*, 274 U.S. App. D.C. 95, 861 F.2d 1290 (1988) [discharged postal service legal secretary manic-depressive, not otherwise qualified because disruptive and had poor attendance, good faith efforts had been made to accommodate her handicap]; Bailey v. Tisch, 683 F. Supp. 652 (S.D. Ohio 1988) [postal service applicant not otherwise qualified where heart condition never diagnosed as stable, exercise-related extra heartbeats made him unsuitable].

[332] *E.g.*, Reese v. U.S. Gypsum Co., 705 F. Supp. 1387 (D. Minn. 1989) [state Human Rights Act not violated by discharge of diabetic who slept on job].

[333] *E.g.*, Jackson v. Veterans Admin., 22 F.3d 277 (11th Cir.), *reh'g denied* (en banc), 30 F.3d 1500 (11th Cir. 1994) [housekeeping aide not otherwise qualified because did not satisfy presence requirement for job, no duty to accommodate unpredictable absences]; Lemere v. Burnley, 683 F. Supp. 275 (D. D.C. 1988) [alcoholic employee lost status as qualified handicapped employee by pattern of unscheduled absences].

prevents them from performing job duties or constitutes a direct threat to property or the safety of others. Employers may strictly enforce rules prohibiting possession or use of alcohol or drugs in the workplace.

In 1985, the United States Supreme Court ruled that state agencies could not be sued for violating Section 504 because of their Eleventh Amendment sovereign immunity from being sued.[334] However, the law was amended and subsequently federal appellate courts have permitted suits against state agencies.[335]

4-3.3 Compensation and Benefits

Compensation and benefits of employees are regulated by several federal laws, including the Fair Labor Standards Act, Federal Wage Garnishment Law, Employee Retirement Income Security Act of 1974, Health Insurance Portability and Accountability Act of 1996, Family and Medical Leave Act of 1993, and Internal Revenue Code. In addition, numerous state laws address these issues.

Courts have generally upheld reasonable efforts by employers to monitor benefits use. In 1995, a federal appellate court held that a self-insured employer may monitor employee pharmaceutical use under its health insurance plan, provided the information is used only for monitoring the plan by those with a need to know.[336] The employer had discovered that employee had AIDS from the drugs he was using, but there was not evidence of any discrimination against the employee.

FAIR LABOR STANDARDS ACT. This Act (FLSA)[337] establishes minimum wages, overtime pay requirements, and maximum hours of employment. Employees of all nonprofit and for-profit hospitals are covered by this Act. Bona fide executive, administrative, and professional employees are exempt from the wage and hour provisions when they are salaried.[338] While physicians and administrators

---

[334] Atascadero State Hosp. v. Scanlon, 473 U.S. 234 (1985).

[335] 42 U.S.C. § 2000d-7(a)(1); *e.g.*, Stanley v. Litscher, 213 F.3d 340 (7th Cir. 2000).

[336] Doe v. Southeastern Pa. Transp. Auth., 72 F.3d 1133 (3d Cir. 1995); *but see* Roe v. Cheyenne Mountain Conf. Resort, Inc., 124 F.3d 1221 (10th Cir. 1997) [ADA bars employer requirement of disclosure of employee prescription drug use, unless business necessity].

[337] 29 U.S.C. §§ 201-219.

[338] *See* Auer v. Robbins, 519 U.S. 452 (1997) [upholding Department of Labor interpretation that a "salary basis" requires that "compensation . . . not [be] subject to reduction because of variations in the quality or quantity of the work performed."]; de Jesus-Rentas v. Baxter Pharmacy Servs. Corp., 400 F.3d 72 (1st Cir. 2005) [pharmacists are professionals]; Graziano v. Society of N.Y. Hosp., 1997 U.S. Dist. LEXIS 15926 (S.D. N.Y.) [salaried professional nurses not eligible for overtime compensation despite employee accrual of leave to cover partial day absences].

are clearly exempt, Department of Labor regulations must be consulted to determine the status of other employee classifications.[339] In 2003, the rules defining the scope of the exempt categories were significantly changed, by modifying the income tests and the analysis of duties.[340]

The 1974 amendments to the Fair Labor Standards Act extended minimum wage and overtime coverage to almost all employees of state and local governments. The coverage of governmental employees was declared constitutional by the United States Supreme Court in 1985.[341] However, in 1999, the Supreme Court decided that states retain their Eleventh Amendment immunity from most private suits.[342]

Most employers are required to pay overtime rates for work that exceeds forty hours in seven days. However, hospitals may enter agreements with employees to establish an alternative work period of fourteen consecutive days. If this option is chosen, the hospital pays the overtime rate for hours worked in excess of eighty hours during the fourteen-day period. Even with this option, the hospital must pay overtime rates for hours worked in excess of eight in any one day.

There is still some disagreement among the courts over when persons in on-call status may not have to be paid or may be paid at a different rate. A federal district court ruled that security staff members in one hospital were not entitled to compensation for lunch breaks.[343] The possibility of being called to duty did not make the time compensable. However, another federal district ruled that hospital employees should be paid for their lunch breaks if they were still on call.[344] One federal appellate court ruled that a hospital could pay "on-premises-on-call" operating room technicians and nurses at one and one-half times minimum wage for periods in

---

[339] *E.g.*, Klein v. Rush-Presbyterian-St. Luke's Med. Ctr., 990 F.2d 279 (7th Cir. 1993) [hospital staff nurse not exempt as professional from FLSA, so entitled to overtime]; *but see* Reich v. Newspapers of New England, Inc., 44 F.3d 1060 (1st Cir. 1995) [listing nursing as example of exempt professional].

[340] 69 Fed. Reg. 22122 (Apr. 23, 2004); D.K. Haase, *Final overtime rules*, National L.J., May 24, 2004, 14; D. Rogers, *House defeats bid to overturn rules limiting overtime*, Wall St. J., July 11, 2003, A2.

[341] Garcia v. San Antonio Metro. Transit Auth., 469 U.S. 528 (1985), *rev'g*, National League of Cities v. Usery, 426 U.S. 833 (1976).

[342] Alden v Maine, 527 U.S. 706 (1999).

[343] Kaczmerak v. Mount Sinai Med. Ctr., 1988 U.S. Dist. LEXIS 18680 (E.D. Wis.).

[344] Hoffman v. St. Joseph's Hosp., 1998 U.S. Dist. LEXIS 7911 (N.D. Ga.).

which they did no work, instead of at one and one-half times their regular hourly wage.[345]

The Fair Labor Standards Act also addresses child labor by regulating the hours and conditions of employment of children. The Fair Labor Standards Act does not preempt more protective state or local laws that establish a higher minimum wage,[346] a shorter minimum work week, or more protection for children. There are other federal rules that regulate hours and conditions of employment for specific jobs. For example, the Federal Aviation Administration requires flight crew members, including crews of emergency medical helicopters, to have eight consecutive hours of rest every twenty-four hours.[347]

FEDERAL WAGE GARNISHMENT LAW. One way to enforce a court judgment against another person is to impose garnishment of the debtor's wages. Garnishment is a court order to an employer to pay a portion of the debtor's paycheck to the creditor until the debt is paid. The Federal Wage Garnishment Law[348] and various state laws restrict how much of a paycheck can be garnisheed. When there are multiple garnishments, proper priorities must be observed not to exceed the limit on aggregate garnishments. Federal law prohibits employers from discharging employees because of garnishment for one debt. The limits on garnishment do not apply to certain bankruptcy court orders or debts due for state or federal taxes.

EMPLOYEE RETIREMENT INCOME SECURITY ACT OF 1974. This Act (ERISA)[349] regulates nearly all pension and benefit plans for employees, including pension, profit-sharing, bonus, medical or hospital benefit, disability, death benefit, unemployment, and other plans. ERISA applies to all plans except for governmental plans, some plans of churches, and some § 401(k) retirement plans. The law regulates many features of these plans, including nondiscrimination, benefit accrual, vesting of benefits, coverage, responsibilities of plan managers, termination of plans, descriptions of plans,

---

[345] Townsend v. Mercy Hosp., 862 F.2d 1009 (3d Cir. 1988), *aff'g* 689 F. Supp. 503 (W.D. Pa. 1988).

[346] *See* L. Uchitelle, *Some cities pressuring employers to pay a higher minimum wage*, N.Y. TIMES, Apr. 9, 1996, A1.

[347] *E.g.*, United States v. Rocky Mountain Helicopters, 704 F. Supp. 1046 (D. Utah 1989).

[348] 15 U.S.C. §§ 1671-1677.

[349] Pub. L. No.93-406, 88 Stat. 829 (1974) (codified as amended in scattered sections of 5, 18, 26, 29, 31, and 42 U.S.C.); 29 C.F.R. pts. 2509 - 2677.

and required reports. ERISA requirements should be considered before changing any pension or benefit plan that is not exempt.

Some health benefit plans have attempted to use ERISA to attack state laws that mandate certain benefits. In 1985, the United States Supreme Court ruled that neither ERISA nor the National Labor Relations Act preempts state laws that mandate that insured plans provide certain benefits, such as mental illness coverage.[350] However, states cannot require self-insured or uninsured health plans to provide the specific benefits because such plans are not covered by the savings clause in ERISA that allows state regulation of insurance.[351]

Furnishing false information to a health or welfare fund subject to ERISA is a federal crime. The administrator of a provider of outpatient services was convicted of this crime because he did not report actual costs in a utilization report to a fund, but instead reported the estimated value of the services based on charges.[352]

ERISA forbids retaliation against employees for exercising their rights under a benefit plan. Thus, it is a violation of ERISA to discharge an employee to prevent coverage under a medical benefits plan.[353] A federal appellate court held it a violation to fire an employee who refused to become an independent contractor where more than an incidental reason for the change was to eliminate health coverage.[354] However, it is not a violation of ERISA for the employer to change a welfare benefit plan to the extent permitted by the plan. A discriminatory change that reduces benefits for one disease, such as AIDS, does not violate ERISA[355] but generally violates the ADA.

HEALTH INSURANCE PORTABILITY AND ACCOUNTABILITY ACT OF 1996. One focus of this Act (HIPAA)[356] is on making health insurance coverage "portable" and continuous for workers. Employ-

---

[350] Metropolitan Life Ins. Co. v. Massachusetts, 471 U.S. 724 (1985); *see also* Washington Physicians' Service Ass'n v. Washington, 147 F.3d 1039 (9th Cir. 998), *cert. denied*, 525 U.S. 1141 (1999) [state law requiring HMOs and health care service contractors to offer alternate medical services not preempted by ERISA].

[351] *See also* American Med. Security v. Bartlett, 111 F.3d 358 (4th Cir. 1997), *cert. denied*, 524 U.S. 936 (1998) [ERISA preempts state regulation of stop-loss coverage levels of self-insured employee benefit plans].

[352] United States v. Martorano, 767 F.2d 63 (3d Cir.), *cert. denied*, 474 U.S. 949 (1985).

[353] *E.g.*, Kross v. Western Electric Co., 701 F.2d 1238 (7th Cir. 1983).

[354] Seaman v. Arvida Realty Sales, 985 F.2d 543 (11th Cir.), *reh'g denied* (en banc), 993 F.2d 1556 (11th Cir.), *cert. denied*, 510 U.S. 916 (1993).

[355] McGann v. H.& H. Music Co., 742 F. Supp. 362 (S.D. Tex. 1990), *aff'd*, 946 F.2d 401 (5th Cir. 1991), *cert. denied*, 506 U.S. 981 (1992).

[356] Pub. L. No. 104-191.

ees who change or lose jobs and who meet eligibility conditions have to be accepted into either a group plan or be offered an individual policy.

FAMILY AND MEDICAL LEAVE ACT OF 1993. This Act (FMLA) requires that eligible employees be provided twelve work weeks of leave during any twelve-month period to provide care for a serious health condition of the employee, spouse, child, or parent, or for a birth or adoption. The leave need not be compensated, but health care benefits must be continued during the leave.[357]

The statute defines a *serious medical condition* as "any physical or mental condition that involves inpatient care or continuing treatment by a health care provider."[358] *Continuing treatment* has been further defined by regulations and court decisions.[359] Courts have generally required some degree of incapacity.[360] An employer may require that the requested leave "be supported by a certification issued by the health care provider of the eligible employee." An employer can generally rely on an employee's physician's certification that the employee qualifies for FMLA leave.[361] However, the employer may require a second opinion, and disagreements are resolved by a binding third opinion.[362] An employer can require an employee on leave to obtain subsequent recertifications "on a reasonable basis." Although generally when an employee has a chronic serious health condition, the employer must wait at least thirty days between requests for recertification.[363]

The employee is not required to mention the FMLA to request unpaid leave.[364] The employee need only provide the employer with enough information to put the employer on notice that FMLA-qualifying leave is needed.[365] Advance notice can be required in

---

[357] Pub. L. No. 103-3, 107 Stat. 6 (1993) [codified as amended at 29 U.S.C. §§ 2611-2619 and in scattered sections of 2, 5, and 29 U.S.C.]; 60 Fed. Reg. 2180 (Jan. 6, 1995) [final regulations].

[358] 29 U.S.C. § 2611(11).

[359] 29 C.F.R. § 825.114; Thorson v. Gemini, Inc., 123 F.3d 1140 (8th Cir.1997) [combination of conditions that would not each be sufficient can together meet requirement]; Victorelli v. Shadyside Hosp., 128 F.3d 184 (3d Cir. 1997) [ongoing treatable medical condition (peptic ulcer) requiring occasional sick leave can be sufficient].

[360] *E.g.,* Martyszenko v. Safeway, Inc., 120 F.3d 120 (8th Cir. 1997).

[361] Stoops v. One Call Communications, Inc., 141 F.3d 309 (7th Cir. 1998).

[362] 29 U.S.C. § 2613.

[363] 29 U.S.C. § 2613(e); 29 C.F.R. § 825.308(a).

[364] 29 C.F.R. § 825.303(b).

[365] *E.g.,* Price v. City of Ft. Wayne, 117 F.3d 1022 (7th Cir. 1997).

some circumstances; prompt notice after the fact is permitted in some circumstances.[366]

In 2003, the United States Supreme Court ruled that FMLA applies to state employees and that private suits can be brought against states to enforce the part of FMLA related to the care of close family members.[367] It remains an open issue whether private suits can be used to enforce other parts of FMLA against states. One federal appellate court has ruled that states are immune from private suits concerning other parts of FMLA.[368]

INTERNAL REVENUE CODE. The Internal Revenue Code requires employee benefit plans to meet certain standards to qualify as deductible business expenses.[369]

The Internal Revenue Service (IRS) is more closely scrutinizing the classification of workers as employees or independent contractors in an effort to require employers to pay employment taxes on more workers.

The IRS continues to scrutinize pension plans, deferred compensation, and other benefits.

4-3.4 Occupational Safety and Health

OCCUPATIONAL SAFETY AND HEALTH ACT OF 1970. Congress enacted this Act (OSHA)[370] to establish standards for occupational health and safety and to enforce the standards. Standards developed for various industries are mandatory for all covered employers. When no federal standard has been established, state safety rules remain in effect. OSHA does not apply to employees of states and their political subdivisions, but many states enforce most OSHA standards through state enforcement agencies.[371]

The Act requires each state to enact legislation to implement the standards and procedures promulgated by the Department of

---

[366] 29 C.F.R. § 825.303; Holmes v. Boeing Company, 166 F.3d 1221 (*without op.*), 1999 U.S. App. LEXIS 377 (10th Cir. 1999) [employer may require notice of absences in nonemergency situations; Hopson v. Quitman County Hosp. and Nursing Home, 119 F.3d 363 (5th Cir. 1997) [reduction of thirty day notice for planned surgeries under FMLA not limited to medical emergencies, can be justified by deadline for insurance coverage].

[367] Nevada Dep't of Human Res. v. Hibbs, 538 U.S. 721 (2003).

[368] Brockman v. Wyoming Dep't of Family Services, 342 F.3d 1159 (10th Cir. 2003).

[369] *E.g.*, 26 U.S.C. §§ 401-425.

[370] Pub. L. No. 91-596, 84 Stat. 1590 (1970) (codified as amended at 29 U.S.C. §§ 651-678 and in scattered sections of 5, 15, 29, 42, and 49 U.S.C.).

[371] 29 U.S.C. § 652(4); 29 C.F.R. § 1975.5.

Labor. Litigation has arisen over the issue of inspections used by federal and state officials to enforce OSHA standards. Courts have ruled that an employer can refuse an inspection unless the inspector obtains consent from an authorized agent of the employer or the inspector has a valid search warrant. The United States Supreme Court ruled unconstitutional an OSHA provision that permitted spot checks by OSHA inspectors without a warrant.[372]

OSHA regulations prohibit employers from discriminating against employees who refuse to expose themselves to conditions presenting a real danger of death or serious injury in urgent situations where there is insufficient time to pursue correction through OSHA.[373] This regulation was upheld by the United States Supreme Court in 1980.[374] However, an Indiana appellate court ruled that a lab technician could be terminated for refusing to test vials of bodily fluids with AIDS warnings because the lab had provided appropriate safety manuals and precautions; so there was insufficient danger to justify the refusal.[375]

Where OSHA applies, OSHA preempts all state occupational safety and health regulations. In 1992, the United States Supreme Court decided that states must obtain the approval of the Secretary of Labor for any such state regulations. There is no public safety exception. A nonoccupational impact is not sufficient to defeat preemption.[376]

OSHA adopted rules to protect health care employees from blood-borne diseases.[377] A federal appellate court upheld the blood-borne disease regulations, except as to sites not controlled by the employer or another entity subject to the employer's rules.[378] Thus, the regulations could not be applied to home care by home health workers. In 1998, a federal appellate court ruled that employees who refuse to wear protective clothing required by OSHA can be terminated.[379]

---

[372] Marshall v. Barlow's Inc., 436 U.S. 307 (1978).

[373] 29 C.F.R. § 1977.12(b)(2).

[374] Whirlpool Corp. v. Marshall, 445 U.S. 1 (1980).

[375] Stepp v. Review Bd., 521 N.E.2d 350 (Ind. Ct. App. 1988).

[376] Gade v. National Solid Waste Mgmt. Ass'n, 505 U.S. 88 (1992).

[377] 26 C.F.R. § 1910.1030, as amended 61 FED. REG. 5507 (Feb. 13, 1996).

[378] American Dental Ass'n v. Secretary of Labor, 984 F.2d 823 (7th Cir. 1993) [dissent questioned OSHA's involvement in an area already addressed by CDC and its competence to do so], *cert. denied*, 510 U.S. 859 (1993).

[379] Taylor v. St. Vincent's Med. Ctr., 145 F.3d 1333 (*without op.*), 1998 U.S. App. LEXIS 7991 (6th Cir.).

OSHA has focused on other areas that have special impact on health care areas including latex allergies, needle stick injuries, tuberculosis, and waste anesthetic gasses. Other OSHA initiatives that will impact health care but are not primarily aimed at the health care environment, include workplace violence and ergonomics.[380]

There is a general duty clause in OSHA. Under it, hospitals have been cited for not protecting workers from tuberculosis,[381] not protecting workers from patient violence,[382] and not vaccinating employees.[383]

Employers cannot retaliate against employees who make OSHA complaints.[384]

STATE OCCUPATIONAL SAFETY LAWS. Employers have a statutory duty in some states to furnish employees with a safe place to work.[385] Even in states that do not have such statutes, employers are liable for most injuries suffered by employees as a result of employment unless the employer is protected by governmental immunity. In most situations, employees can pursue compensation only through the workers' compensation system, not through courts.

Other state statutes require that specific facilities be provided to employees. These facilities, such as lavatories, must be provided for the convenience and safety of employees. Local governmental ordinances and laws can also include requirements, such as sanitary and health codes, to promote and safeguard the health and safety of employees and others. In most states, state institutions are exempt from local regulation unless state laws grant local governments the authority to encompass state institutions.

---

[380] For a NIOSH summary of initiatives in the area listed in this paragraph, see pages on each topic at http://www.osha.gov/SLTC/.

[381] *E.g.*, *TB control plans focus of settlements between OSHA, two Wisconsin hospitals*, 2 H.L.R. 1342 (1993) [hospitals cited under general duty clause for not protecting workers from hazard of TB infection through contact with patients at high risk for TB; failure to record on occupational illness and injury logs workers who tested positive for TB; allowed unapproved respirators and allowed facial hair, skull cap with respirators]; *see also* 59 FED. REG. 54242 (Oct. 28, 1994) [CDC guidelines on TB].

[382] *Psychiatric hospital in Chicago cited by OSHA for workplace violence*, 2 H.L.R. 1479 (1993) [cited for failure to protect workers from patient violence; abatement program worked out].

[383] *E.g.*, Secretary of Labor v. Froedtert Mem. Lutheran Hosp., No. 97-1839 (OSHA Rev. Comm. Jan. 16, 2004), *as discussed in* H.L.R., Jan. 29, 2004, 161 [hepatitis B vaccines and bloodborne pathogen training for temporary housekeeping staff].

[384] *E.g.*, Labor Secretary v. Skyline Terrace Inc., No. 95-C-676-K (N.D. Okla. May 22, 1997), *as discussed in* 6 H.L.R. 912 (1997) [punitive damages awarded against nursing home for firing nurse in retaliation for filing OSHA complaint about lack of gloves].

[385] *E.g.*, WIS. STAT. § 101.11.

4-3.5 Labor-Management Relations

Unions are a significant factor in the employee relations of health care providers in some parts of the United States. Various labor organizations have been recognized as collective bargaining representatives for groups of health care employees. There are craft unions that devote their primary organizing efforts to skilled employees, such as carpenters and electricians; industrial unions and governmental employee unions that seek to represent large groups of relatively unskilled or semiskilled employees; and professional and occupational associations and societies, such as state nurses associations, that represent their members and sometimes others.

LABOR-MANAGEMENT RELATIONS ACT. This Act[386] regulates many aspects of the relationship between employers and employees. It prohibits unfair labor practices by employers and employees. It provides hearings for complaints that such practices have occurred. The Act consists of the National Labor Relations Act of 1935 (NLRA),[387] the Taft-Hartley amendments of 1947,[388] and numerous other amendments, including the Labor-Management Reporting and Disclosure Act of 1959.[389] The Act is administered by the National Labor Relations Board (NLRB). The NLRB (1) investigates and adjudicates complaints of unfair labor practices and (2) conducts secret ballot elections among employees to determine whether they wish to be represented by a labor organization and, if so, to determine which organization.

Government hospitals are exempt from the Act. This exemption has been interpreted by the NLRB to apply only to hospitals that are owned and operated by governmental entities.[390] For example, a municipal hospital operated under contract can be considered a private entity subject to the NLRB if a private contractor exercises overall daily control. Exempt governmental hospitals are usually subject to state labor laws.

Nonprofit hospitals were exempt until the amendments of 1974 eliminated the exemption.[391] The 1974 amendments attempted to

---

[386] 29 U.S.C. §§ 141 – 187.
[387] Act of July 5, 1935, ch. 372, 49 Stat. 449.
[388] Act of June 23, 1947, ch. 120, 61 Stat. 136.
[389] Pub. L. No. 86-257, 73 Stat. 519.
[390] *E.g.*, Pikeville United Methodist Hosp. v. United Steelworkers of Am., 109 F.3d 1146 (6th Cir. 1997) [active municipal oversight of private hospital not sufficient to make it governmental].
[391] 29 U.S.C. §§152(2), 158.

deal with some of the unique aspects of health care by providing legislative direction about collective bargaining, mediation, conciliation, and strikes.

Some religious hospitals have challenged these laws. Federal appellate courts have found that it is not a violation of First Amendment religious freedoms to apply these laws to hospitals owned and operated by religious entities.[392]

The law directs the NLRB to give hospitals some special consideration because of their sensitive mission, but individual NLRB rulings will continue to be made on the basis of many factors in addition to the uniqueness of health care.

EXEMPT STAFF. Several groups of staff members are excluded from the NLRB's jurisdiction, including independent contractors, supervisors, managerial employees, confidential employees, and some students. Each of these groups has been defined by numerous NLRB and court decisions; so familiarity with those decisions is necessary to determine whether a particular staff member is exempt.

Supervisors. The NLRA imposes a three-part test for determining which employees are supervisors. Employees are statutory supervisors if (1) they hold the authority to engage in any one of the twelve listed supervisory functions, (2) their "exercise of such authority is not of a merely routine or clerical nature, but requires the use of independent judgment," and (3) their authority is held "in the interest of the employer."[393]

The NLRB interpreted the second test to require that the independent judgment pertains to the other employee's job status or pay. In 1994, the United States Supreme Court rejected this interpretation and decided that nurses who direct other employees' treatment of patients can be supervisors without any involvement in determining job status.[394] The NLRB then interpreted there not to be exercise of independent judgment when the employee only applied "ordinary professional or technical judgment in directing less-skilled employees to deliver services in accordance with employer-specified standards." In 2001, the Court ruled that the NLRB could not exclude this type of judgment from the scope of judgment that could satisfy the second test and found that regis-

[392] St. Elizabeth Comm. Hosp. v. NLRB, 708 F.2d 1436 (9th Cir. 1983); St. Elizabeth Hosp. v. NLRB, 715 F.2d 1193 (7th Cir. 1983).
[393] 29 U.S.C. § 152(11); NLRB v. Health Care & Retirement Corp. of Am., 511 U.S. 571 (1994).
[394] NLRB v. Health Care & Retirement Corp. of Am., 511 U.S. 571 (1994).

tered nurses in a residential mental health center could be supervisors.[395] The Court also ruled that the employer must prove supervisory status. However, the NLRB continues to find registered nurses in nursing homes not to be supervisors in many cases.[396]

The federal appellate courts have split on whether licensed practical nurses who serve as charge nurses in nursing homes can be supervisors.[397] The NLRB generally finds that they are not supervisors.[398]

UNFAIR LABOR PRACTICES. Section 7 of the National Labor Relations Act established four fundamental rights of employees: (1) the right to self-organize, (2) the right to engage in concerted activities for the purpose of collective bargaining or other mutual aid or protection, (3) the right to engage in collective bargaining, and (4) the right to refrain from union activities.

Employer Unfair Labor Practices. An employer commits an unfair labor practice through:

1. interference with any of the four rights recognized in section 7;
2. domination of a labor organization;
3. discouragement or encouragement of union activity;
4. discrimination against employees who file charges or testify in an NLRB proceeding; or
5. violation of the other obligations, including good faith bargaining, specified in section 8(a) of the NLRA.

The NLRA also applies to employers that do not have employees represented by a labor organization. The employee's right to engage in concerted activities for the purposes of mutual aid or protection can apply to isolated incidents; so employers should obtain legal advice before disciplining employees who might be engaged in protected activities. For example, the NLRB ruled that a small group of unorganized staff was protected by the NLRA when members of the group left their workstations to complain to hospital officials concerning

---

[395] NLRB v. Kentucky River Community Care, Inc., 532 U.S. 706 (2001).

[396] *E.g.*, Madison Ctr. Genesis Eldercare, Inc., Case No. 22-RC-11729 (NLRB Reg. Dir. Jan. 31, 2002).

[397] *E.g.*, Beverly Enterprises v. NLRB, 165 F.3d 307 (4th Cir. 1999) (en banc) [supervisors]; *contra*, NLRB v. GranCare, Inc., 170 F.3d 662 (7th Cir. 1998) [not supervisors].

[398] *E.g.*, Beverly Enterprises v. SEIU, 1-RC-21704 (NLRB Reg. Dir. Feb. 4, 2004); Integrated Health Servs., Inc. v. District 1199P, Case No. 6-UC-445 (NLRB Reg. Dir. Dec. 19, 2002).

work conditions.[399] Not all employee actions are protected. The NLRB upheld the dismissal of two hospital employees for continual criticism of the program director.[400] The NLRB found this activity unprotected because it was aimed at influencing administration of the program, rather than at working conditions.

A federal appellate court found that an employer had violated the NLRA by discharging a supervisor in retaliation for refusing to engage in unfair labor practice.[401]

Permanent replacement workers have been a contentious issue. A federal appellate court found that a hospital had committed an unfair labor practice by refusing to reinstate striking nurses to prestrike positions and giving those positions to nonstriking nurses. During the strike, the hospital had closed until it was compelled by community needs to open two units and later to open the whole hospital with supervisory personnel, new hires, and striking nurses who crossed picket lines. The hospital had guaranteed returning nurses they could keep their new positions. The court ruled that those who had actually worked in the new positions could have permanent replacement status but that others were nonpermanent and not entitled to keep positions they were promised.[402] In another case, after finding unfair labor practices by the employer, a nursing home was ordered to reinstate former strikers who had been permanently replaced.[403]

There is frequently litigation regarding to what information the union is entitled. For example, a federal appellate court ruled on the scope of information about nonunit employees that the union could access.[404] The NLRB ruled that a hospital had committed an unfair labor practice by not giving information on its benefit plans.[405] A federal appellate court ruled that the union was not entitled to the home addresses of strike replacement workers.[406]

---

[399] Mercy Hosp. Ass'n, Inc., 235 NLRB 6781 (1978).

[400] Good Samaritan Hosp. & Richey, 265 NLRB 618 (1982); *see also* Bob Evans Farms, Inc. v. NLRB, 163 F.3d 1012 (7th Cir. 1998) [workers who walked out to protest firing of popular supervisor not protected].

[401] Marshall Durbin Poultry Co. v. NLRB, 39 F.3d 1312 (5th Cir. 1994).

[402] Waterbury Hosp. v. NLRB, 950 F.2d 849 (2d Cir. 1991).

[403] Kobell v. Beverly Health & Rehab. Servs., 987 F. Supp. 409 (W.D. Pa. 1997) [order to reinstate former strikers who had been permanently replaced due to ULPs], *aff'd*, 142 F.3d 428 (3d Cir. 1998), *cert. denied*, 525 U.S. 1121 (1999).

[404] East Tenn. Baptist Hosp. v. NLRB, 6 F.3d 1139 (6th Cir. 1993).

[405] Swedish Hosp. Med. Ctr., NLRA Cases 19-CA-22412, 22823 (Oct. 14, 1993), *as discussed in* 2 H.L.R. 1419 (1993).

[406] Chicago Tribune Co. v. NLRB, 79 F.3d 604 (7th Cir. 1996).

A federal appellate court refused to enforce a nationwide NLRB cease and desist order directed at a nursing home chain. The court ruled that the order had to be directed at specific facilities that had engaged in unfair labor practices, since there was no showing of unlawful acts at a substantial number of facilities.[407] Another federal appellate court upheld a nationwide NLRB order based on a finding of a geographically broad history of widespread unfair labor practices.[408]

Employers should also obtain legal advice before working with employee advisory committees. If their role is not appropriately limited, such committees can be considered labor organizations, and many of the employer's interactions with them could be interpreted as unfair labor practices. For example, the NLRB ruled that a hospital had engaged in the unfair labor practice of management domination of a labor organization because the hospital ran the election for an employee committee and wrote its bylaws.[409] A federal appellate court found that an employer-formed forum for nurses to discuss and consider professional nursing practice issues was not a "labor organization" because it did not deal with the employer on matters affecting employment. There was no pattern or practice of making proposals to which the hospital responded, and isolated instances did not constitute "dealing."[410]

A federal appellate court ruled that a hospital had committed an unfair labor practice by unilaterally deciding to stop supplying surgical garbs without bargaining with the union, but that the hospital's decision to reduce the number of teams receiving eighty hours pay for seventy hours work to zero was within its authority under the collective bargaining agreement.[411]

Employees do not have the right to falsely and publicly disparage their employer or its products or services. A federal appellate court decided that it was not an unfair labor practice to fire a nurse who had appeared on a local news broadcast and accused her employer hospital of "jeopardizing the health of mothers and babies" by altering the shift assignments and responsibilities of labor and delivery registered nurse first assistant.[412]

---

[407] Torrington Extend-A-Care Employee Ass'n v. NLRB, 17 F.3d 580 (2d Cir. 1994).
[408] Beverly Health & Rehab. Servs., Inc. v. NLRB, 354 U.S. App. D.C. 414, 317 F.3d 316 (2003).
[409] Rideout Mem. Hosp., 227 NLRB 1338 (1977).
[410] NLRB v. Peninsula Gen. Hosp. Med. Ctr., 36 F.3d 1262 (4th Cir. 1994).
[411] Gratiot Comm. Hosp. v. NLRB, 51 F.3d 1255 (6th Cir. 1995).
[412] St. Luke's Episcopal-Presbyterian Hosps., Inc. v. NLRB, 268 F.3d 575 (8th Cir. 2001).

Labor Organization Unfair Labor Practices. A labor organization commits an unfair labor practice through:

1. restraining or coercing interference with the exercise of the four rights recognized in Section 7 or interfering in management's selection of its representative;
2. attempting to cause the employer to discriminate to encourage or discourage membership in a labor organization;
3. failing to bargain in good faith;
4. engaging in prohibited secondary boycotts;
5. charging excessive union initiation fees;
6. causing employers to pay for services not performed; or
7. picketing solely to compel an employer to recognize a union (recognitional picketing) or to persuade employees to join the union (organizational picketing) without filing a petition for an election within the appropriate time limit.

The United States Supreme Court ruled that a union committed an unfair labor practice by prohibiting members from resigning from the union during a strike or when a strike was imminent.[413]

A federal appellate court affirmed an order that a union not picket a nursing home for one year following its defeat in a decertification election.[414]

A labor organization cannot be liable for the misconduct of its members unless the organization actually participated, gave prior authorization, or ratified such acts after actual knowledge of their perpetration.[415] Applying this rule, an Ohio appellate court ruled that the union could not be liable for the misconduct of its members at a hospital construction site because the required participation, authorization, or ratification had not been shown.[416]

EMPLOYEE REPRESENTATION. A labor organization seeking representation rights for employees may petition the NLRB for a secret ballot election. The petition must make a "showing of interest" supporting the petition. At least 30 percent of the workers who will ultimately make up the bargaining unit must support it and show their interest by signing union authorization cards.

---

[413] Pattern Maker's League v. NLRB, 473 U.S. 95 (1985).
[414] NLRB v. 1115 Nursing Home & Serv. Employees Union, 44 F.3d 136 (2d Cir. 1995).
[415] 29 U.S.C. § 106.
[416] Callen v. Internat'l Brotherhood of Teamsters, 144 Ohio App. 3d 575, 761 N.E.2d 51 (2001).

Bargaining Unit Designation. The employer can take the position that certain persons (supervisors, confidential employees, temporary employees) should be excluded from the unit as inappropriate because of the institutional organization. The NLRB will then conduct a representation hearing to determine the appropriate bargaining unit. The NLRB must implement the congressional intent in the 1974 amendments to avoid "proliferation of bargaining units" in the health care industry.[417] In addition, Section 9 of the NLRA forbids including professional employees in bargaining units with nonprofessionals unless a majority of the included professionals vote in favor of inclusion.[418]

Until 1984, the NLRB determined whether the proposed unit was appropriate by applying a "community of interest" test. That is, a proposed unit was appropriate if its members had a community of interest. This resulted in the recognition of five basic units in health care institutions, as follows:

1. clerical;
2. service and maintenance;
3. technical;
4. professional; and
5. registered nurses.

In 1984, the NLRB abandoned the "community of interest" test, replacing it with a "disparity of interest" test.[419] Under this test, the NLRB began with the broadest possible unit and excluded only those groups that were shown to have disparate interests. No unit was automatically assumed to be appropriate; all were examined on a case-by-case basis.

In 1989, the NLRB abandoned the disparity of interest test and case-by-case determination. The NLRB published rules that the following eight units were presumed to be appropriate in acute care hospitals:

---

[417] S. Rep. No. 93-766, 93d Cong., 2d Sess. 5, *reprinted in* 1974 U.S. CODE CONG. & ADMIN. NEWS 3,946, 3,950.
[418] 29 U.S.C. § 159(b)(1); Leedom v. Kyne, 358 U.S. 184 (1958); Pontiac Osteopathic Hospital, 327 NLRB No. 194 (March 31, 1999).
[419] St. Francis Hosp. & Int'l Brotherhood of Elec. Workers, 271 NLRB 948 (1984); Health-Care Enters., 275 NLRB No. 194 (1985).

1. registered nurses;
2. physicians;
3. professionals, except registered nurses and physicians;
4. technical employees;
5. skilled maintenance employees;
6. business office clerical employees;
7. guards; and
8. other nonprofessional employees.[420]

In 1991, the United States Supreme Court upheld the rules.[421] However, in 1993, the NLRB ruled that it would not upset pre-existing appropriate units based on the new rules.[422]

Geographic scope of units can also be an issue. In some circumstances, the NLRB applies a single facility presumption. However, the NLRB found the presumption to be overcome by a showing of function integration as to services and employees; so it rejected an attempt to create a unit of the employees of one clinic, insisting that the employees in the entire network of clinics be included in one unit.[423] In another case, the union agreed to a multifacility unit of the employees in the main campus, but the NLRB ruled that employees in off-campus facilities and outlying clinics needed to be included.[424] The single facility presumption was ruled not to apply to a multifacility unit.

Solicitation and Distribution. Most health care organizations have rules concerning solicitation of employees and distribution of materials in the facility to avoid interference with patient care. These rules become especially important during campaigns to organize employees; so they should be written to be enforceable under the NLRA. Each policy is examined on a case-by-case basis by the NLRB.[425] Some general guidelines can be derived from past decisions. Nonemployees are generally prohibited access to the facility for solicitation or distribution. Employees can be prohibited from these activities during work time. Work time does not include meal-

---

[420] 29 C.F.R. § 103.30.
[421] American Hosp. Ass'n v. NLRB, 499 U.S. 606 (1991).
[422] Kaiser Found. Hosps., 312 NLRB No. 139 (1993).
[423] St. Luke's Health Sys., Inc., 340 NLRB No. 139 (2003).
[424] Stormont-Vail HealthCare, Inc., 340 NLRB No. 143 (2003).
[425] *E.g.*, Manchester Health Ctr. v. NLRB, 861 F.2d 50 (2d Cir. 1988) [rule upheld]; for an example of the analysis, *see* The Cooper Health System, 327 NLRB No. 189 (1999) [non-solicitation policy too broad].

times or work breaks.[426] Solicitation or distribution can be limited to nonpatient care areas at all times. The United States Supreme Court ruled that solicitation and distribution could be prohibited in areas devoted to patient care.[427] Areas to which visitors have general access, such as cafeterias and lounges, usually cannot be prohibited where a genuine likelihood of patient disturbance cannot be shown.[428] Solicitation at entrances is generally permitted.[429] Another important factor in the exclusion of certain areas is whether reasonable alternative space is designated. A federal appellate court decided that a hospital could enforce its nonsolicitation rule in a cafeteria because no nonemployees had been permitted to solicit there and the presumption of access to the union's message elsewhere had not rebutted.[430]

However, selective enforcement of such rules will generally preclude enforcement against unions.[431]

Election. A labor organization can become the exclusive bargaining agent for a bargaining unit by winning a secret ballot election conducted by the NLRB. After an election, the employer or the labor organization can challenge the outcome by filing an objection.[432] If misconduct is found, the election can be set aside with a new election ordered.[433]

A labor organization can also be decertified as the collective bargaining agent by an election of its members.[434]

Recognition without an Election. An employer can voluntarily recognize a labor organization as the exclusive bargaining agent without an election.[435] Some employer actions, such as checking

---

[426] *E.g.*, Cooper Tire & Rubber Co. v. NLRB, 957 F.2d 1245 (5th Cir. 1992); *see also* One Way, Inc., 268 NLRB 394 (1983) [policy can refer to "work time," but not to "work hours"].

[427] NLRB v. Baptist Hosp., 442 U.S. 773 (1979).

[428] *E.g.*, Stanford Hosp. & Clinics v. NLRB, 325 F.3d 334 (D.C. Cir. 2003).

[429] *E.g.*, Brockton Hosp. v. NLRB, 352 U.S. App. D.C. 302, 294 F.3d 100 (2002).

[430] Oakwood Hosp. v. NLRB, 983 F.2d 698 (6th Cir. 1993).

[431] *E.g.*, Fairfax Hosp. v. NLRB, 14 F.3d 594 (*without op.*), 1993 U.S. App. LEXIS 31,936 (4th Cir. 1993), *cert. denied*, 512 U.S. 1205 (1994); Mt. Clemens Gen. Hosp. v. NLRB, 328 F.3d 837 (6th Cir. 2003).

[432] *E.g.*, Dacas Nursing Support Sys. v. NLRB, 7 F.3d 511 (6th Cir. 1993); Indiana Hosp. v. NLRB, 10 F.3d 151 (3d Cir. 1993).

[433] *E.g.*, Lasalle Ambulance, Inc., d/b/a Rural/Metro Medical Services, 327 NLRB No. 18 (Oct. 30, 1998); Evergreen Healthcare, Inc. v. NLRB, 104 F.3d 867 (6th Cir. 1997); *see also* Beverly Enterprises Inc. v. NLRB, 139 F.3d 135 (2d Cir. 1998).

[434] *E.g.*, Americare Pine Lodge Nursing & Rehab. Ctr. v. NLRB, 164 F.3d 867 (4th Cir. 1999).

[435] *E.g.*, Exxel/Atmos, Inc. v. NLRB, 307 U.S. App. D.C. 376, 28 F.3d 1243 [new president committed unfair labor practice by refusal to bargain with union that predecessor had voluntarily recognized within prior year], *reh'g denied* (en banc), 308 U.S. App. D.C. 411, 37 F.3d 1538 (1994).

union authorization cards or polling employees, can sometimes constitute recognition of a labor organization. Recognition without an election can be challenged as a possible unfair labor practice in some circumstances, especially when other labor organizations are also seeking to represent the employees. Most employers avoid all actions that could be interpreted as voluntary recognition. A second way that a labor organization can be recognized without an election is by NLRB order. When the NLRB finds serious unfair labor practices, it can order the extraordinary remedy of recognition. A third way is accretion.[436] If a labor organization has negotiated a contract with an employer that later acquires a new facility, under some circumstances the new facility is considered to be accreted to the existing one, and new unit employees are automatically covered by the preexisting contract. However, where there is a history of separate bargaining at the two sites, they can sometimes remain separate.[437] A fourth way is that a successor corporation can be required to continue to recognize a union in some circumstances.[438]

COLLECTIVE BARGAINING AND MEDIATION. After a labor organization has been recognized as the exclusive bargaining agent, the employer and labor organization have a duty to negotiate in good faith.[439] They must bargain concerning mandatory subjects, including wages, hours, and other terms and conditions of employment. They may bargain concerning other permissive subjects but are not legally obligated to do so. It is unlawful to bring negotiations to an impasse, strike, or lock out employees over permissive subjects.

Several special notice, mediation, and conciliation safeguards were built into the law to help the health care industry avoid strikes when possible. For example, ninety days notice is required if a party intends to terminate or modify a bargaining agreement, and the Federal Mediation and Conciliation Service (FMCS) must be given sixty days notice.[440] When notified, the FMCS attempts to bring

---

[436] *E.g.*, Local 144 v. NLRB, 9 F.3d 218 (2d Cir. 1993).
[437] *E.g.*, Staten Island Univ. Hosp. v. NLRB, 24 F.3d 450 (2d Cir. 1994).
[438] *E.g.*, NLRB v. Hospital San Rafael, Inc., 42 F.3d 45 (1st Cir. 1994); Midwest Precision Heating & Cooling, Inc., 341 NLRB No. 52 (2004) [successor liability for successor company found to be alter ego of prior employer]; United Steelworkers v. St. Gabriel's Hosp., 871 F. Supp. 335 (D. Minn. 1994) [state law requiring business purchaser to honor existing labor contract until expiration conflicts with federal labor law, so preempted; successor liability under federal law only if continuity of workforce].
[439] *E.g.* Marion Hosp. Corp. v. NLRB, 355 U.S. App. D.C. 233, 321 F.3d 1178 (2003).
[440] 29 U.S.C. § 158(d).

about an agreement, and all parties must participate fully and promptly in meetings called by the FMCS to pursue a settlement. If a strike is threatened, the FMCS can, under certain conditions, establish an impartial board of inquiry to investigate issues and provide a cooling-off period of up to thirty days.[441]

Another special provision for health care institutions is a ten-day advance notice of intention to engage in concerted economic activities, including strikes, picketing, or any other concerted refusal to work.[442] This provision is designed to allow a hospital to make plans for continuity of patient care. Hospitals that use this opportunity to take "extraordinary steps" to stock up on ordinary supplies for an unduly extended period of time may, however, be engaging in an unfair labor practice that would permit the union to strike without notice or during the ten-day period. A Minnesota court ruled that nurses were entitled to unemployment compensation during a layoff where the hospital had laid them off when union gave the ten-day notice of intent to strike.[443] A federal appellate court decided that there was no duty to rehire workers who strike without giving the required notice.[444] In 2005, a federal appellate court upheld an NLRB ruling that when the notice is given that any strike must occur at the designated time or a new notice must be given. The union started the strike four hours after the time stated in its notice pursuant to a prearranged plan that was not disclosed to the clinic employer. Twenty-two striking nurses lost their status as protected employees; so their health care employer did not violate the Act by terminating them.[445]

Some courts have ruled that individual unorganized employees do not have to give a ten-day notice of work stoppage. In 1980, a federal appellate court ruled that two physicians who walked out of the hospital and joined the picket line of a lawful strike by other employees did not have to give the notice.[446] The court noted that

---

[441] 29 U.S.C. § 183; 29 C.F.R. pt. 1420.

[442] 29 U.S.C. § 158(g); *see also* NLRB v. Stationary Eng'rs, 746 F.2d 530 (9th Cir. 1984) [notice must specify date].

[443] Metropolitan Med. Ctr. v. Richardville, 354 N.W. 2d 867 (Minn. Ct. App. 1984).

[444] Beverly Health & Rehab. Servs., Inc. v. NLRB, 354 U.S. App. D.C. 414, 317 F.3d 316 (2003); *see also* Alexandria Clinic, P.A., 339 NLRB No. 162 (2003) [may discharge employees who begin strike after originally set tie without giving new ten-day notice].

[445] Minnesota Licensed Practical Nurses Ass'n v. NLRB, 406 F.3d 1020 (8th Cir. 2005).

[446] Montefiore Hosp. v. NLRB, 621 F.2d 510 (2d Cir. 1980); *see also, e.g.*, East Chicago Rehab. Ctr. v. NLRB, 710 F.2d 397 (7th Cir. 1983), *cert. denied*, 465 U.S. 1065 (1984) [wildcat strike by seventeen nurse's aides].

the action of the physicians was inconsiderate and ethically suspect, but protected.

In some circumstances, the *ally doctrine* allows a union to strike against a secondary employer not involved in the original dispute. The strike is permitted when the secondary employer loses its neutrality by performing work during the course of the labor dispute that would have been performed by striking employees of the primary employer. The legislative history of the 1974 amendments modifies the ally doctrine by permitting a hospital to accept the critically ill patients of a struck hospital without losing its status as a neutral employer. In an advice memorandum issued by the NLRB in September 1977, a union was said to violate the Act when it threatened to picket two neutral hospitals because they received critically ill patients and forty-six pregnant women transferred from the struck hospital.[447]

When a valid impasse is reached in negotiations, the employer may unilaterally implement its final offer.[448]

ADMINISTERING THE CONTRACT. After negotiating a labor agreement, the employer and labor organization should spend no less care on its administration. Managerial rights that have been established at the bargaining table, sometimes at a high price, can be eroded or entirely lost through inattention. The entire managerial team, especially supervisors, should know the aspects of the contract applicable to their responsibilities. Managers should be trained to ensure that discipline is administered for proper reasons and by appropriate procedures under the contract.

Frequently, collective bargaining agreements provide for arbitration of grievances. Courts defer to arbitration decisions unless they violate public policy, but courts seldom find superseding public policies. For example, a federal appellate court upheld an arbitrator decision reinstating an employee caught with marijuana with presumed intent to sell, finding no superseding public policy.[449] Two federal district courts refused to overturn arbitration decisions ordering reinstatement of (1) a nursing attendant who changed an intravenous bag in violation of the state nursing practice act and (2) a nurse who failed to notify a physician of a sudden change in a patient's blood pressure and who committed other violations of

---

[447] Memorandum from Dietz, Associate General Counsel, NLRB, to Siegel, Director, Region 31 (Sept. 2, 1977) [concerning cases No. 31-CC-820, 821, 31-CG-7, 8].

[448] *E.g.*, Pleasantview Nursing Home, Inc. v. NLRB, 351 F.3d 747 (6th Cir. 2003).

[449] Saint Mary Home Inc. v. SEIU, Dist. 1199, 116 F.3d 41 (2d Cir. 1997).

proper nursing practices.[450] The Illinois Supreme Court confirmed an arbitration award reinstating two mental health workers whose patient had died while they were on an unauthorized errand.[451] The United States Supreme Court upheld an arbitrator's reinstatement of an employee who had been found with traces of marijuana in his automobile.[452] This did not violate public policy because there was insufficient connection with use of the drug.

However, sometimes a superseding public policy is found. A New York court reversed an arbitrator's reinstatement of a respiratory therapist who, after being warned, continued to engage in the life-threatening practice of reusing a syringe to draw blood from multiple patients.[453] The Ohio Supreme Court reversed an arbitrator's reinstatement of an aide terminated for abuse of a mentally retarded patient.[454] A federal district court vacated an arbitration decision ordering reinstatement of a nurse discharged for negligent medication administration because reinstatement would violate state "public policy in favor of providing safe and competent nursing care."[455] A Minnesota court ruled that an arbitrator had improperly reinstated a paramedic. Where all of the paramedic's functions were under the medical director's license and he was responsible for quality of care, the decision concerning competence was for the medical director.[456]

There are frequently disputes over the scope of arbitration.[457] At least one court has ruled that the duty to arbitrate can continue beyond the end of the collective bargaining agreement.[458]

---

[450] Flushing Hosp. v. Local 1199, 685 F. Supp. 55 (S.D. N.Y. 1988) [nursing attendant]; Brigham & Women's Hosp. v. Massachusetts Nurses Ass'n, 684 F. Supp. 1120 (D. Mass. 1988) [nurse].

[451] AFSCME v. Illinois, 124 Ill. 2d 246, 529 N.E.2d 534 (1988).

[452] United Paperworkers v. Misco, Inc., 484 U.S. 29 (1987).

[453] State Univ. of N.Y. v. Young, 170 A.D.2d 510, 566 N.Y.S.2d 79 (2d Dept. 1991), *appeal denied*, 80 N.Y.2d 753, 587 N.Y.S.2d 905, 600 N.E.2d 632, *cert. denied*, 506 U.S. 1035 (1992).

[454] Ohio Office of Collective Bargaining v. Ohio Civil Serv. Employees Ass'n, 59 Ohio St. 3d 177, 572 N.E.2d 71 (1991).

[455] Russell Mem. Hosp. Ass'n v. United Steelworkers, 720 F. Supp. 583 (E.D. Mich. 1989); *accord*, Boston Med. Ctr. v. Service Employees Internat'l Union, 113 F. Supp. 2d 169 (D. Mass. 2000) [against public policy to reinstate nurse after substandard practice led to preventable death of infant].

[456] County of Hennepin v. Hennepin County Ass'n of Paramedics & Emergency Med. Technicians, 464 N.W.2d 578 (Minn. Ct. App. 1990).

[457] *E.g.*, Fairview Southdale Hosp. v. Minnesota Nurses Ass'n, 943 F.2d 809 (8th Cir. 1991) [arbitrator did not exceed his authority in determining hospital could not terminate free parking without bargaining about termination despite contract silence on parking]; Trustees of Columbia Univ. v. Local 1199, 805 F. Supp. 216 (S.D. N.Y. 1992) [suit claiming breach of no-strike clause was dismissed, referred to arbitration under broad arbitration clause in contract, despite employer claim arbitration clause intended to apply only to employee grievances]; Clark County Pub. Employees Ass'n v. Pearson, 106 Nev. 587, 798 P.2d 136 (1990) [elimination of nursing clinical ladder program subject to binding arbitration].

[458] Luden's Inc. v. Local Union No. 6, 28 F.3d 347 (3d Cir. 1994).

REPORTING AND DISCLOSURE. The Labor-Management Reporting and Disclosure Act of 1959[459] places some controls on labor unions and their relationship with their members. It also requires employers to report payments and loans made to representatives of labor organizations. Payments to employees for the purpose of persuading them or causing them to persuade other employees to exercise or not to exercise their rights to organize and bargain collectively must also be reported. Many of these payments are illegal, and the reporting requirement does not make them legal. Reports must also be made of (1) expenditures to interfere with employee rights to organize and bargain collectively and (2) certain agreements with labor relations consultants. Reports are made public. Failure to report and false reports can lead to substantial penalties. Governmental hospitals are not subject to these provisions.

4-3.6 State Laws

While federal laws have preempted many state labor laws,[460] state laws still apply in at least two situations. First, when federal law does not cover an activity, states may regulate it. Second, when courts rule that state law does not conflict with federal law, the state law will be enforceable. Despite the broad scope of federal preemption, states may regulate labor relations activity that also falls within the NLRB jurisdiction when the regulated conduct touches interests deeply rooted in local feeling and responsibility. Thus, violence, threats of violence, mass picketing, and obstructing streets may be regulated by states.

In some states, there are no labor relations statutes, but in others, two types directly affect the rights of employees to organize and bargain collectively: (1) anti-injunction acts and (2) laws regulating union security agreements. Other state labor laws deal with equal employment opportunity, child labor, safety, workers' compensation, and unemployment compensation. Many states have laws concerning the relationship between public employees and governmental employers that apply to governmental hospitals.

---

[459] 29 U.S.C. §§ 401-531; *see* International Union v. Dole, 276 U.S. App. D.C. 178, 869 F.2d 616 (1989) [scope of reportable activities defined].

[460] *E.g.,* United Steelworkers v. St. Gabriel's Hosp., 871 F. Supp. 335 (D. Minn. 1994) [state law requiring business purchaser to honor existing labor contract until expiration conflicts with federal labor law, so preempted].

ANTI-INJUNCTION ACTS. The federal government and many states have enacted anti-injunction acts that narrowly define the circumstances in which courts may enjoin strikes, picketing, and related activities in labor disputes. The federal statute is the Norris-LaGuardia Act.[461] Some aspects of state anti-injunction statutes can be preempted. Anti-injunction acts generally apply to health care providers.[462] Occasionally, judges find the standards to have been met and issue injunctions related to labor activities. For example, in 2004, a California judge ordered nurses at a county hospital to end their sickout.[463]

UNION SECURITY CONTRACTS AND RIGHT-TO-WORK LAWS. Some labor organizations seek union security contracts with employers in the form of either (1) the *closed shop contract*, which provides that only members of a particular union can be hired, or (2) the *union shop contract*, which makes continued employment dependent on union membership but does not require the employee to become a member until after being hired. Many states have constitutional provisions or statutes, generally called *right-to-work laws*, making such contracts unlawful.[464] Other states have statutes or decisions that restrict such contracts or specify procedures that must be followed before such agreements may be made. Some states require an employee election. Some states permit a union shop agreement, but not a closed shop. State right-to-work laws are not preempted by the NLRA because Section 14(b) of the NLRA explicitly authorizes them.[465] In states where such agreements are illegal, any request for such a contract must be refused, and the employer can obtain an injunction to stop a strike or picketing designed to induce such agreements. In states that permit such agreements, there is no legal obligation to agree. It is one of the matters on which there can be bargaining. When these provisions are accepted, employers can be forced to fire noncompliant employees.[466]

---

[461] 29 U.S.C. §§ 101-111; *e.g.*, Modeste v. Local 1199, 38 F.3d 626 (2d Cir. 1994) [dismissal of suit against union for alleged intentional torts during strike; Norris-LaGuardia Act does not preempt state law requirement of showing liability of each member of union in order to hold union liable].

[462] *E.g.*, District 1199E v. Johns Hopkins Hosp., 293 Md. 343, 444 A.2d 448 (1982).

[463] M. Landsberg, *Judge tells County-USC nurses to end sickouts*, L.A. TIMES, July 6, 2004, B3.

[464] *E.g.*, FLA. CONST. art. 1, § 6.

[465] 29 U.S.C. § 164(b).

[466] St. John's Mercy Med. Ctr., 344 NLRB No. 44 (Mar. 31, 2005) [hospital ordered to terminate fourteen nurses who did not pay union dues].

WORKERS' COMPENSATION. Every state has workers' compensation legislation to compensate employees for accidental on-the-job injuries. These acts replace the employee's common law remedy of suing the employer for negligence, which was usually an unsuccessful process. Most employers are subject to these acts. Many employers purchase workers' compensation insurance, although self-insurance is usually an option. An employee generally must give written notice of injury to the employer. In cases not routinely paid, the matter will be heard by a state commission to determine liability. State statutes define "employee," "injury," and other terms and have schedules of payment amounts for types of injuries. When the workers' compensation law applies, the employee is barred from suing the employer for the injury.[467] Courts become involved only when there is an appeal concerning a decision of the state commission.

Several issues are frequently litigated. One question is whether the injury arose out of and occurred in the course of employment.[468] A related issue is whether the injury was caused by an accident. Numerous exclusions are usually stated for preexisting or congenital physical conditions and for injuries caused by horseplay or other nonemployment causes.

Workers' compensation laws generally do not bar suits against persons who are not employers. A nurse anesthetist was permitted to sue a psychiatrist for injuries she received while administering electroconvulsive therapy because he was not the employer or a fellow employee.[469] States vary on when fellow employees may be sued.

The California Supreme Court held that a child could sue for in utero injuries that occurred when the mother was injured during her employment. Because there was injury to the child separate from the injury to the mother and the child was not an employee, the court ruled that under California law the workers' compensation law did not bar the suit.[470]

Workers' compensation acts and other benefit programs under which injured workers may seek compensation are often complex.

---

[467] *E.g.,* Chambers v. Hermann Hosp. Estate, 961 S.W.2d 177 (Tex. Ct. App. 1996).
[468] *E.g.,* Herman v. Sherwood Indus., Inc., 244 Conn. 502 701 A.2d 1338 (1998) [workers' compensation covers injury to terminated employee while retrieving personal items].
[469] Salih v. Lane, 244 Va. 436, 423 S.E.2d 192 (1992).
[470] Snyder v. Michael's Stores, Inc., 16 Cal. 4th 991, 68 Cal. Rptr. 2d 476, 945 P.2d 781 (1997).

Familiarity with applicable state law is necessary to appropriately address employee injuries.

The United States Supreme Court ruled that workers are not entitled to notice and an opportunity to be heard before their workers' compensation benefits are suspended during utilization review.[471]

UNEMPLOYMENT COMPENSATION. State law generally provides for payment of unemployment compensation to many unemployed individuals. Generally, persons who have been discharged for misconduct forfeit all or part of the compensation they would have otherwise received. There is considerable litigation concerning what constitutes misconduct. For example, the Pennsylvania Supreme Court found a nursing assistant guilty of misconduct for smoking in a patient's room contrary to hospital rules; so she was denied compensation.[472] The Vermont Supreme Court ruled that a nurse who had been discharged for giving a patient medication by intravenous (IV) push instead of IV drip was entitled to unemployment compensation because her error had been in good faith.[473] The Nebraska Supreme Court ruled that a change of hours from the 3:00 p.m. to 11:00 p.m. shift to the 11:00 p.m. to 7:00 a.m. shift was not good cause for a licensed practical nurse to resign; so she was not entitled to compensation.[474] The Florida unemployment agency ruled that a hospital laboratory technologist who resigned due to fear of AIDS was not entitled to compensation.[475] A Pennsylvania court decided that it was willful misconduct for a phlebotomist to mislabel a blood sample after three prior reprimands for mislabeling; so compensation was denied.[476] A North Carolina court ruled that a hospital employee was disqualified from compensation for violating the hospital policy against fighting with coworkers.[477]

---

[471] American Manufacturers Mutual Ins. Co. v. Sullivan, 526 U.S. 40 (1999).

[472] Selan v. Unemployment Comp. Bd., 495 Pa. 338, 433 A.2d 1337 (1981).

[473] Porter v. Dep't of Employment Sec., 139 Vt. 405, 430 A.2d 450 (1981).

[474] Montclair Nursing Ctr. v. Wills, 220 Neb. 547, 371 N.W.2d 121 (1985); *accord* Baptist Med. Ctr. v. Stolte, 475 So. 2d 959 (Fla. 1st DCA 1985), *rev. denied*, 486 So. 2d 598 (Fla. 1986) [nurse who refuses to accept offered 3-11 position is not "available for work" and, thus, ineligible for unemployment compensation].

[475] Vinokurov v. Mt. Sinai Hosp., No. 88-3158U (Fla. Dep't of Labor & Employment Sec. Apr. 1, 1988); *see also* R.D. Gagliano, *When health care workers refuse to treat AIDS patients*, 21 J. HEALTH & HOSP. L. 255 (1988).

[476] Holly v. Unemployment Compensation Bd. of Review, 151 Pa. Commw. 450, 617 A.2d 80 (1992), *appeal denied*, 534 Pa. 643, 626 A.2d 1160 (1993).

[477] Fair v. St. Joseph's Hosp., 113 N.C. App. 159, 437 S.E.2d 875 (1993).

However, due to the peculiar features of the unemployment compensation process in some states, strange outcomes do occur. The Michigan Supreme Court ruled that under Michigan law a nurse who failed the state licensing exam and, thus, could not legally function as a nurse was entitled to unemployment compensation because the court viewed that she had not lost her job voluntarily.[478] The Nevada Supreme Court ruled that an employee who failed to report to work due to incarceration was entitled to unemployment compensation.[479]

OTHER STATE AND LOCAL LAWS. Some state and local governments regulate the employment relationship in other ways. Here are examples.

Some state and local governments have enacted minimum wage laws that require higher wages than federal law.[480] At least two states have restricted such local laws.[481]

Some states and localities prohibit discrimination based on sexual orientation.[482] Some localities require domestic partner benefits.[483]

Some states extend protection from disability discrimination to conditions that do not qualify as disabilities under federal law.[484]

PUBLIC EMPLOYEES. Because the NLRA does not apply to employees of state and local governmental agencies, the relations

---

[478] Clarke v. North Detroit Gen. Hosp., 437 Mich. 280, 470 N.W.2d 393 (1991).

[479] State Emp. Sec. Dep't v. Evans, 901 P.2d 156 (Nev. 1995); *contra,* Fennel v. Board of Rev., 297 N.J. Super. 319, 688 A.2d 113 (App. Div. 1997) [hospital housekeeper who failed to report to work due to incarceration not entitled to unemployment compensation].

[480] *E.g.,* N.Y. Labor §§ 650 - 665; 19 Del. C. §§ 901 - 914; *Mayor of Baltimore signs groundbreaking 'living wage' bill into law,* U.S. Newswire, Dec.. 14, 1994; *Mayor signs living wage bill,* AP, Nov. 27, 2002 [New York City]; Z. Zhao, *New minimum wage for health care workers,* N.Y. Times, Dec. 1, 2002, 5WC [Westchester County, N.Y.]; *Court upholds Santa Fe wage ordinance; landmark ruling confirms power of cities to raise pay for low-wage residents,* U.S. Newswire, June 24, 2004.

[481] *E.g.,* New Orleans Campaign for a Living Wage v. City of New Orleans, 825 So. 2d 1098 (La. 2002) [state ban on local minimum wage law is constitutional (La. R.S. 23:642); New Orleans ordinance invalid]; Wis. Stat., § 104.001, added by 2005 Wis. Act 12; *see also* D. Lieb, *Supreme Court dismisses appeal in living wage case,* AP, Sept. 5, 2002 [lower court overturned both Missouri state law banning local ordinances and St. Louis ordinance]; *Granholm vetoes bill that would have kept locals from setting minimum wage,* AP, May 7, 2004 [Mich.].

[482] *E.g.,* Wis. Stat. §§ 111.321, 111.36; Hyman v. City of Louisville, 53 Fed. Appx. 740 (6th Cir. 2002) [lacked standing to challenge local ordinance banning employment discrimination based on sexual orientation].

[483] *E.g.,* Catholic Charities of Maine v. City of Portland, 304 F. Supp. 2d 77 (D. Me. 2004) [city may require domestic partnership benefits for all benefits not subject to ERISA preemption; *but see* Phillips v. Wisconsin Personnel Comm'n, 167 Wis. 2d 205, 482 N.W.2d 121 (Ct. App. 1992) [Wis. Stat. § 111.321 does not require family benefits for domestic partners].

[484] *E.g.,* Colmenares v. Braemar Country Club, Inc., 29 Cal. 4th 1019, 63 P.3d 220, 130 Cal. Rptr. 2d 662 (2003).

between these public employees and their governmental employers are controlled by state law. Some states prohibit collective bargaining by public employees; so employee rights are determined by state civil service laws and individual agency policies. Many states authorize representation by a labor organization and collective bargaining. A state agency similar to the NLRB is usually established to administer the law. State laws frequently limit the subjects that can be determined by collective bargaining, and they are different from the NLRA in other ways. Many states prohibit strikes by all or some public employees and require that bargaining impasses be resolved by arbitration.

4-4 Independent Contractors

Health care providers frequently retain independent contractors to provide services. The relationship between an organization and an independent contractor is very different from the relationship with an employee.

The primary distinguishing feature of an independent contractor is that the contractor exercises control over the manner in which the work is completed.[485] This control test is not the only test that is used; other factors are considered in various contexts.[486] In some contexts, withholding taxes or providing some employment benefits is considered determinative, and the control test is not even addressed.

It is important to structure the relationship with independent contractors so that they are consistently treated as independent contractors. When they are treated like employees in one aspect, there is an increased risk that they will considered to be employees for other purposes.

TAXES. Income taxes are not withheld from independent contractors. The contractor is responsible for making estimated tax payments. The employer does not pay employment taxes on independent contractors; only the contractor pays. Independent contractors can deduct business expenses that employees are not permitted to deduct.[487] Retroactive finding of that the incorrect

---

[485] *See* Clackmas Gastroenterology Assocs., P.C. v. Wells, 538 U.S. 440 (2003).

[486] *E.g.*, Nationwide Mutual Ins. Co. v. Darden, 503 U.S. 318 (1992) [ERISA term "employee" incorporates traditional agency-law criteria].

[487] *See* Weber v. C.I.R., 103 T.C. 378 (1994) [since not independent contractor, individual must pay tax deficiencies for deductions].

status was used can lead to tax liability for the business and/or the contractor.

BENEFITS. Employment benefit plans do not apply to independent contractors. Independent contractors must make their own insurance arrangements. Nonemployees sometimes seek retroactive employment status and benefits.[488]

Independent contractors are generally not covered by workers' compensation or unemployment compensation.[489]

DISCRIMINATION. Employment discrimination laws generally apply only to employees; so they generally do not apply to independent contractors.[490] Independent contractor are protected by some discrimination laws that apply to discrimination in contracting.[491]

LABOR LAW. Independent contractors cannot organize for collective bargaining under the NLRA. However, the NLRB has considerable discretion in determining whether particular workers are employees or independent contractors.[492]

WHISTLEBLOWERS. Most of the laws that protect whistleblowers apply only to employees so that independent contractors do not have this protection.[493]

CONFIDENTIALITY OF MEDICAL RECORDS. Independent contractors who need to have access to protected health information can satisfy the requirements of the Health Insurance Portability and

---

[488] *E.g.*, Hensley v. Northwest Permanente P.C. Retirement Plan & Trust, 258 F.3d 986 (9th Cir. 2001) [not arbitrary and capricious for ERISA plan administrator to interpret "employee" to mean only persons for whom taxes were withheld; nurse practitioners, physician's assistants not entitled to pension benefits]; Vizcaino v. Microsoft, 97 F.3d 1187 (9th Cir. 1996) *aff'd on reh'g*, 120 F.3d 1006 (9th Cir. 1997), *cert. denied*, 522 U.S.1098 (1998) [suit seeking inclusion in 401(k) after settlement of employment status of temporary workers with IRS].

[489] *E.g.*, Health Care Associates, Inc. v. Oklahoma Employment Security Comm'n, 26 P.3d 112 (Okla. 2001) [nurses were independent contractors, not eligible for unemployment compensation].

[490] *E.g.*, Alberty-Velez v. Corporacion de Puerto Rico para la Difusion Publica, 361 F.3d 1 (1st Cir. 2004) [not covered by Title VII]; Weary v. Cochran, 2004 U.S. App. LEXIS 15589 (6th Cir) [insurance agent is independent contractor; not covered by ADEA]; Lerohl v. Friends of Minn. Sinfonic, 322 F.3d 486 (8th Cir. 2003) [musicians are independent contractors despite control over rehearsals, performances; not covered by ADA, Title VII].

[491] *E.g.*, 42 U.S.C. § 1981; Gomez v. Alexian Bros. Hosp., 698 F.2d 1019 (9th Cir. 1983) [rejection of contract proposal by emergency medical professional corporation can violate Title VII as to Hispanic physician employee of corporation]; *see also* O'Hare Truck Serv., Inc. v. City of Northlake, 518 U.S. 712 (1996) [independent contractor protected by First Amendment form retaliation by city for political association or expression]; Board of Comm'rs, Wabaunsee Cty. v. Umbehr, 518 U.S. 668 (1996) [local officials may not terminate an independent contractor for criticizing government policy].

[492] *See* NLRB v. United Ins. Co., 390 U.S. 254 (1968); Time Auto Transportation, Inc. v. NLRB, 2004 U.S. App. LEXIS 15270 (6th Cir).

[493] *E.g.*, Bedrossian v. Northwestern Mem. Hosp., 2004 U.S. Dist. LEXIS 5542 (N.D. Ill.) [dismiss whistleblower protection claim under False Claims Act against hospital, hospital not employer].

Accountability Act (HIPAA) privacy regulations in one of two ways. They can be treated as part of the workforce and receive the training that is mandated for the workforce. Alternatively, they can sign a business associate agreement. See Chapter 8 for more details on HIPAA.

LIABILITY. Employers are liable for most of the acts of their employee in the course of employment under the doctrine of *respondiat superior*. Businesses are usually not liable for the acts of independent contractors except in unusual circumstances, such as where the contractor is acting as an agent or apparent agent.[494] Businesses can also be liable when their own negligence contributes to the injury. A New Mexico court found a hospital liable for negligent selection of a contract therapist.[495] These liability issues are discussed in more detail in Chapter 11.

4-5 Others Who Provide Services in Health Care Organizations

In addition to employee and independent contractors, there are several other categories of persons who provide services in health care organizations. Three of these categories are nonemployee medical staff, volunteers, and students. Medical staff members are addressed in Chapter 5.

VOLUNTEERS. Volunteers present some of the same issues as independent contractors. Volunteers are not protected by most of the employment discrimination laws.[496] When health care providers give volunteers employment benefits, there is a risk the volunteers will be considered employees for other purposes. Sometimes former volunteers seek to be retroactively characterized as employees to gain payment or other benefits. These efforts have generally been unsuccessful.[497]

---

[494] *E.g.,* United States v. Thomas, 2004 U.S. App. LEXIS 15542 (2d Cir.) [contractor can be agent for crime].

[495] Eckhardt v. Charter Hosp. of Albuquerque, Inc., 953 P.2d 722 (N.M. Ct. App. 1997).

[496] *E.g.,* York v. Association of Bar of City of N.Y., 2001 U.S. Dist. LEXIS 9457 (S.D. N.Y.) [volunteer not protected by Title VII]; O'Connor v. Davis, 126 F.3d 112 (2d Cir. 1997) [student volunteering at hospital to fulfill degree requirements of college is not an employee or student of the hospital, so neither Title VII nor Title IX applies to harassment by supervising physician].

[497] *E.g.,* Silbar v. Office of Personnel Management, 89 Fed. Appx. 692 (Fed. Cir. 2003) [VA employee not entitled to service credit for time spent volunteering]; Rodriguez v. Township of Holiday Lakes, 866 F. Supp. 1012 (S.D. Tex. 1994) [volunteer police chief found to be employee for FLSA, but exempt from FLSA under another section]; *but see* Lance v. United States, 70 F.3d 1093 (9th Cir. 1995) [volunteers at VA hospitals are employees for purposes of the Federal Employees Compensation Act]; McNichols v. United States, 226 F. Supp. 965 (N.D. Ill. 1964) [VA hospital volunteer is an employee for purposes of the Federal Tort Claims Act].

Issues have also been raised about institutional liability for acts of volunteers. Some states have granted volunteers immunity for liability under some circumstances.[498] When immunity does not apply, courts have reached different results concerning institutional liability and insurance coverage.[499]

States vary on the extent of workers' compensation coverage for volunteers. In some states, volunteers are covered only if institutions elect to include them.[500]

States sometimes regulate the use of volunteers. For example, New York limited the use of volunteers in proprietary nursing homes.[501]

STUDENTS. Some students are employees. Some students are volunteers. Some students are simply in training programs sponsored by the institution or an affiliated institution and are neither employees nor volunteers.

All students are subject to academic supervision, evaluation, and consequences that are different from nonstudents. Courts generally show great deference to bona fide academic judgments concerning academic performance.[502]

Otherwise students who are employees are subject to most of the same rules as other employees discussed in Section 4-3. In some states, students who are employees are subject to somewhat different rules than other employees.[503]

For nonacademic matters, students who are not employees are generally subject to the same principles as volunteers.[504]

There is one significant difference from volunteers. Generally, formal education programs are considered a service program; so some of the discrimination laws concerning programs and services can apply to decisions regarding nonemployee students. Thus, a

---

[498] *E.g.,* WIS. STAT. § 181.0670(2).

[499] *E.g.,* Maynard v. Ferno-Washington, Inc., 22 F. Supp. 2d 1171 (E.D. Wash. 1998) [jury question whether sufficient control exercised to make hospital liable for acts of volunteer EMT].

[500] *E.g.,* WIS. STAT. §§ 102.07(11), (11m).

[501] Greater N.Y. Health Facilities Ass'n v. Axelrod, 770 F. Supp. 183 (S.D. N.Y. 1991) [rejecting challenge to state policy memo limiting activities of volunteers].

[502] *E.g.,* McGuinness v. University of N.M. School of Med., 170 F.3d 974 (10th Cir. 1998), *cert. denied,* 526 U.S. 1051 (1999).

[503] *E.g.,* WIS. STAT. § 40.22(2)(g) [exclusion from state retirement system].

[504] *E.g.,* O'Connor v. Davis, 126 F.3d 112 (2d Cir. 1997) [student volunteering at hospital to fulfill degree requirements of college is not an employee or student of the hospital, so neither Title VII nor Title IX applies to harassment by supervising physician]; *but see* Silbar v. Office of Personnel Management, 89 Fed. Appx. 692 (Fed. Cir. 2003) [approved VA hospital practice of granting service credit to formal students, but not to other volunteers].

federal appellate court concluded that a medical school could be sued for violating the ADA but that the school was not required to accommodate a disability when it would alter the service. Requiring the school to permit continued studies after the National Board exam was failed would alter the school's service of educating physicians.[505] In addition, some training programs are educational programs that are subject to Title IX.[506]

In 2003, some students filed an antitrust challenge to the graduate medical education matching program through which students completing medical school are matched with first-year house staff positions. In early 2004, the federal court dismissed the case as to some defendants but permitted the case to proceed against the remaining defendants. Congress passed a law prohibiting antitrust attacks against the matching program. The federal court then dismissed the suit.[507]

In 1999, the NLRB ruled that house staff in institutions subject to the NLRB could organize into unions.[508] The status of house staff in other institutions varies based on state law.

Most training programs are subject to accreditation standards that regulate aspects of the programs. For example, the accrediting body for medical residency programs has limited the number of hours that house staff in accredited programs may be on duty.[509] It has taken steps to actively enforce this requirement.[510] At least one state, New York, also has laws regulating house staff hours.[511] The restrictions had unintended consequences that interfered with teaching; so a few exceptions were introduced.[512]

---

[505] Powell v. National Board of Medical Ex'ers, 364 F.3d 79 (2d Cir. 2004).

[506] *E.g,* Gossett v. Oklahoma, 243 F.3d 1172 (10th Cir. 2001) [nursing school could be sued under Title XI for alleged discrimination against male students].

[507] Jung v. Association of Am. Med. Colleges, 300 F. Supp. 2d 119 (D. D.C. 2004), 339 F. Supp. 2d 26 (D. D.C. 2004), 226 F.R.D. 7 (D.D.C. 2005); 15 U.S.C. § 37b.

[508] Boston Med. Ctr. Corp., 330 NLRB No. 30 (1999), *overruling* Cedars-Sinai Med. Ctr., 223 NLRB 251 (1976).

[509] L.K. Altman & D. Grady, *Hospital accreditor will strictly limit hours of residents*, N.Y. TIMES, June 13, 2002, A1.

[510] *E.g.,* A. Barnard, *Surgery residents' long hours draw warning for Yale*, BOSTON GLOBE, May 20, 2002, A1; M. Croasdale, *Johns Hopkins penalized for resident hour violations*, Am. Med. News, Sept. 15, 2003, 10.

[511] *See* T. Kelley, *State says many hospitals violate laws on work hours*, N.Y. TIMES, June 27, 2002, B6.

[512] M. Croasdale, *Beat the clock*, AM. MED. NEWS, Mar. 8, 2004, 9 [barrier to learning]; M. Croasdale, *Some work-hour limits could change*, AM. MED. NEWS, Apr. 12, 2004, 13 [ACGME considers longer hours for some specialists]; *Residencies pinpoint work-hour hurdles*, AM. MED. NEWS, Apr. 19, 2004, 12 [AAMC survey – decrease in patient contact, more handoffs, lack of continuity of care, increased faculty hours, and reduced morale].

Discussion Points

1. What are the goals of individual licensing? How well does it accomplish these goals? What other effects does individual licensing have?
2. Discuss the selection of roles to license.
3. What are the consequences for the individual and the institution where he or she works when the individual does not have the required license?
4. What limits are there on the legislatures or regulators who define the scope of licensed practice? What are the abilities of these entities to otherwise limit the actions of licensed persons by regulation?
5. When can licensed persons delegate licensed functions to others who are not licensed?
6. What steps must licensing boards follow in disciplining licensed persons?
7. What is the difference between accrediting educational programs and certifying individuals?
8. What are the responsibilities of employers in hiring new health care employees? What should be checked?
9. Discuss the effect of mandated staffing levels and restrictions on mandatory overtime.
10. What are the restrictions on discipline and dismissal of staff members?
11. Under what circumstances can employees be tested for drugs?
12. What characteristics of a person trigger the protection of equal employment opportunity laws? When may these characteristics be taken into account in employment decisions?
13. What characteristics must a person have to qualify for protection under the Americans with Disabilities Act? What accommodations are considered reasonable and, thus, required for the employer to undertake?
14. What impact does the Fair Labor Standards Act have on employee compensation?
15. What impact does the Employee Retirement Income Security Act have on employee benefits?
16. Under what circumstances must an employee be given a leave of absence according to the requirements of the Family and Medical Leave Act?
17. What major areas of health care employment practice are regulated by the Occupational Safety and Health Act?

18. Describe the framework of federal labor-management relations legislation.
19. Which employees are exempt from National Labor Relations Board (NLRB) jurisdiction?
20. What are unfair labor practices?
21. Discuss the evolution of the bargaining units in health care.
22. How is a labor organization certified as the bargaining agent? How is a labor organization decertified?
23. What is the effect of a union security contract and right-to-work law?
24. What is the function of workers' compensation and unemployment compensation laws?
25. What factors make a person an independent contractor? How does the law treat independent contractors differently from employees?
26. What is the relationship between health care organizations and volunteers or students?

CHAPTER FIVE

Medical Staff

Objectives

The objective of this chapter is to provide an overview of the relationship between health care organizations and their medical staff. The reader will learn about the organization of the medical staff, appointment process, delineation of clinical privileges, review and reappointment, modification and termination of clinical privileges, procedures for adverse actions against members, and liability exposure of participants. Some relationships with medical staff members outside the medical staff organization are also covered.

Physicians and other independent practitioners who practice in hospitals are organized into a medical staff. Only staff members are permitted to admit patients to and practice in the hospital. A physician is appointed to the medical staff and granted clinical privileges by the hospital governing board. A physician is permitted to provide only services for which clinical privileges have been granted. The board has the responsibility to exercise discretion in deciding whether to grant an appointment and what scope of clinical privileges to grant. The board also assures that the physician is periodically reviewed and that clinical privileges are adjusted when needed. The board nearly always relies on the medical staff to conduct reviews and recommend board action.

Other health care organizations, such as skilled nursing facilities, can also have a medical staff so that membership and privileges are required to practice in the organization.[1] These organizations generally do not have as elaborate structures as hospitals.[2]

This section addresses the organization and role of the medical staff (5-1); appointment to the medical staff (5-2); delineation of clinical privileges (5-3); periodic review and reappointment (5-4); modification and termination of clinical privileges (5-5); review procedures for adverse actions (5-6); potential liability of those involved in the process of making medical staff appointment and clinical privilege decisions (5-7); and relationships with physicians outside the medical staff relationship (5-8).

5-1 The Organization and Role of the Medical Staff

Physicians in hospitals are organized into a medical staff in order to comply with Joint Commission on Accreditation of Healthcare Organizations (JCAHO) standards, Medicare conditions of participation, and state hospital licensing rules. The organized medical staff has collective accountability to the governing board for the quality of care delivered by the medical staff.

The board has ultimate authority over the hospital; this authority must be exercised consistent with satisfactory patient care. Through bylaws, the board delegates to the medical staff the authority and duty to carry out medical aspects of patient care. The board retains authority and responsibility to approve appointments to the medical staff, grant or decrease clinical privileges, and assure that there is a procedure for monitoring quality of care. The board normally looks to the medical staff to monitor quality of care and provide expert advice on appointment and clinical privilege decisions. The medical staff organization usually includes officers; an executive committee to act in matters that do not require approval of the entire staff; and other committees to address specific issues, such as infection control, pharmaceutical utilization, and credentials review. In smaller hospitals, these functions can be performed by the entire medical staff. In larger hospitals, several specialty departments with their own organizations are often coordinated by the overall medical staff

---

[1] *E.g.,* Rotwein v. Sunharbor Manor Res. Health Care Facility, 181 Misc. 2d 847, 695 N.Y.S.2d 477 (Sup. Ct. 1999) [podiatrist lost privileges in nursing home].

[2] *E.g.,* WIS. ADMIN. CODE HFS 132.61(1) [organized medical staff optional for nursing home; only medical director required].

organization. Functions of the organized medical staff include (1) facilitating communication among the medical staff members and with the hospital, (2) implementing hospital and medical staff policies and procedures, (3) recommending appointments to the medical staff and scope of clinical privileges, (4) providing continuing medical education, and (5) taking other actions necessary to govern the medical staff and relate to the hospital board.

MEDICAL STAFF BYLAWS. The organization of the medical staff is set forth in medical staff bylaws that are approved by the medical staff and the hospital. In some states, the bylaws are considered a contract between the medical staff and the hospital, which courts will enforce as a contract. In other states, the bylaws are not considered a contract, and there is somewhat more flexibility in changing the document and taking actions that are not specified by the bylaws.[3]

Changes that are not mutually agreeable are generally inadvisable. Since 1985, JCAHO has required that medical staff bylaws be adopted and changed only with the mutual consent of the medical staff and hospital.[4] Some courts had recognized the legal right and even the duty of the hospital board to change the medical staff bylaws unilaterally when necessary.[5] Even when the board has authority to make unilateral changes, hospitals generally seek mutually acceptable changes even when this requires prolonged negotiations. The resulting changes are more likely to be implemented fully when commitment to them is mutual. Unilateral changes are an extraordinary last resort, usually adopted at great cost to deal with impasses.

One of the limits of the contract approach to bylaws is illustrated by a 2003 Illinois appellate court case.[6] According to the court decision, when the hospital found that it had a higher mortality rate for cardiac surgery, it retained an outside peer review group who concluded that some of the problems were due to the practice of the

---

[3] *E.g.,* Miller v. St. Alphonsus Reg. Med. Ctr., Inc., 87 P.3d 934 (Id. 2004); Vakil v. Anesthesiology Assocs. of Taunton, Inc., 51 Mass. App. Ct. 114, 744 N.E.2d 651 (2001).

[4] Joint Commission on Accreditation of Healthcare Organizations, 2005 COMPREHENSIVE ACCREDITATION MANUAL FOR HOSPITALS [hereinafter cited as 2005 JCAHO CAMH], MS.1.30.

[5] *E.g.,* Weary v. Baylor Univ. Hosp., 360 S.W.2d 895 (Tex. Civ. App. 1962); *contra* St. John's Hosp. Med. Staff v. St. John's Reg. Med. Ctr., 90 S.D. 674, 245 N.W.2d 472 (1976).

[6] Lo v. Provena Covenant Med. Ctr., 342 Ill. App. 3d 975, 796 N.E.2d 607 (4th Dist. 2003), *lv. denied,* 207 Ill. 2d 605, 807 N.E.2d 976 (2004); T. Albert, *Doctors fear precedent in privileges case,* AM MED. NEWS, Nov. 17, 2003, 9 [discussion of *Lo* case from the perspective of organized medicine].

head of the Department of Surgery. The head initially agreed to have some surgeries supervised. When he withdrew this agreement and refused supervision, the hospital consulted with medical staff leadership who are alleged to have refused to get involved. Based on imminent danger to patients and the noncooperation of the medical staff leadership, the hospital imposed summary suspension. A trial court issued a temporary restraining order based on its interpretation that the bylaws required all summary suspensions to be initiated by the medical staff. The appellate court reversed the restraining order. The appellate court ruled that under state law the ultimate responsibility rested with the hospital; so the bylaws could not bar action by the hospital. Any bylaw provision that barred hospital action would be unenforceable because it would be against public policy. However, the court interpreted the bylaws to permit the action the hospital had taken. Thus, even in states where bylaws are contracts, there are limits to what can be put in bylaws and be enforceable. Medical staff bylaws are subject to the general contract doctrine that says some contracts are against pubic policy and are unenforceable.

One physician challenged the legality of public hospital bylaws that had been adopted without following the formal rule-making procedures of the state administrative procedure act. The Hawaii Supreme Court ruled that bylaws were internal procedures and, thus, not subject to the act.[7]

COOPERATION AND CONFLICT. Hospital and organized medical staff efforts generally should not be focused on defining ultimate legal rights; they should be focused on minimizing misunderstandings and conflicts, seeking mutually acceptable solutions, and resolving impasses without resort to the judicial process. However, while it is important to be fair to individual medical staff applicants and members, the same effort to reach mutually acceptable solutions to problems with individuals is not required. The hospital and medical staff must take appropriate steps to maintain standards within the hospital.

In some cases, this collegial approach breaks down.[8] There are cases where medical staffs have sought the removal of hospital CEOs and even boards.[9] There are cases where medical staff mem-

---

[7] Rosa v. Oba, 68 Haw. 422, 717 P.2d 1029 (1986).

[8] *E.g.,* D. Adams, *Doctors fight for enforcement of staff bylaws,* AM. MED. NEWS, Jan. 19, 2004, 9; *Study finds power shift,* AM. MED. NEWS, Apr. 26, 2004, 20; T. Albert, *Med staff-hospital fights turn nasty and more litigious,* AM. MED. NEWS, Apr. 19, 2004, 1.

[9] *E.g., Beleaguered hospital exec. resigns,* AM. MED. NEWS, Oct. 27, 2003, 10 [Cal.]; *Medical staff to consider resolution on hospital CEO,* AP, Mar. 31, 2003 [S. Dak.].

bers have become competitors of the hospital and sought to retain their hospital privileges to support their competing businesses. When hospitals have sought to restrict this use of the hospital, it has been called economic credentialing. Bylaws that forbid economic credentialing may be an antitrust violation.[10] Economic credentialing is discussed later in this chapter.

Some medical staff members have even filed complaints with regulatory agencies during battles over governance.[11]

Some medical staffs have sought to be recognized as a separate legal entity. A few states have permitted this. The medical staff then has standing to sue the hospital, and the hospital can sue the medical staff.[12] Other states have rejected this concept, finding the medical staff to be part of the hospital. One benefit of the latter approach is that in most jurisdictions the hospital and medical staff cannot be found to be engaged in a conspiracy for antitrust in other purposes due to the intracorporate conspiracy doctrine that says that an entity cannot conspire with itself.

Unfortunately, some hospital medical staffs or parts of medical staffs have chosen to boycott hospitals.[13] Some hospitals have been reluctant to use the antitrust laws to challenge such boycotts, but some hospitals, other effected entities, and government agencies have initiated action. Most of these enforcement actions have been settled with the boycotting physicians agreeing not to engage boycotts.[14]

---

10 FTC letter to Georgia Hosp. Ass'n, May 28, 1993, *as discussed in* 2 H.L.R. 1161 (1993).

11 *E.g.,* J. Olson, *Doctors want Alegent bosses out: Bergan Mercy's staff declares "no confidence" in the parent company after decisions they say could jeopardize care,* OMAHA WORLD HERALD, Mar. 20, 2003, 1B; N. Aksamit, *Alegent criticizes doctors' complaints,* OMAHA WORLD HERALD, Sept. 17, 2003, 3B [MDs filing complaints against hospital with state and federal agencies].

12 *E.g.,* D. Kelley, *Doctors' lawsuit may go forward; A judge rules that Community Memorial Hospital's medical staff is a legal entity with the right to sue the Ventura facility,* L.A. TIMES, Aug. 8, 2003, pt. 2, 1; D. Kelley, *Doctors, hospital settle rights lawsuit; The accord, subject to ratification, is aimed at stopping the flow of disgruntled physicians and their patients from the Ventura facility,* L.A. TIMES, Aug. 18, 2004, B1.

13 *E.g.,* Duson v. Poage, 318 S.W.2d 89 (Tex. Civ. App. 1958).

14 *E.g,* In re Med. Staff of Good Samaritan Med. Ctr., FTC, File No. 901 0032 (settlement Sept. 7, 1994), *as discussed in* 3 HEALTH L.RPTR. [BNA] 1257 (1994) [agreement of medical staff not to combine to prevent or restrict services of hospital or multispecialty clinic] [hereinafter HEALTH L.RPTR. cited as H.L.R.]; B. McCormick, *Doctors settle FTC boycott case,* AM. MED. NEWS, Oct. 3, 1994, at 10 [Good Samaritan]; S. Lutz, *Antitrust concerns pit Texas hospital against staff doctors in legal fight,* MOD. HEALTHCARE, Mar. 6, 1995, at 18 [hospital accusing eight doctors of conspiring to fix prices, boycott the hospital, pay bribe to CEO]; *see also* P. Guinta, *District sees admissions drop after irking MDs,* FLA. MED. BUSINESS (S.FLA.ED.), Mar. 28, 1989, at 6 [drop in admissions at North Broward Hospital District hospitals after privileges granted to Cleveland Clinic physicians]; D.A. Gilmore, *The antitrust implications of boycotts by health care professionals: Professional standards, professional ethics and the First Amendment,* 14 LAW, MED. & HEALTH CARE 221 (1988).

LIABILITY. The board cannot abdicate its responsibility by relying completely on the medical staff. JCAHO accreditation standards, Medicare conditions of participation, and most hospital licensing rules require board involvement. Hospitals have been found liable for physician actions when they failed to evaluate the physicians properly prior to appointment or to monitor physician performance properly after appointment. The Wisconsin Supreme Court found a hospital liable for injuries to a patient by a physician because the hospital should never have appointed him to the medical staff.[15] The hospital had not checked his professional credentials and references. A check would have uncovered discrepancies and misrepresentations that would have led to denial of appointment. An Arizona court found a hospital liable for failing to curtail the clinical privileges of a physician who had several bad results with a procedure, resulting in suits.[16] The absence of a medical staff recommendation to curtail privileges was not an effective excuse. Most states find liability if a hospital fails to act when it has actual knowledge of or reason to suspect serious problems.

EXTERNAL REVIEW. Sometimes the board employs outside experts to assist in medical care review. Usually, this is done with the advice and concurrence of the medical staff. Outside experts often review specialists when other staff members do not feel able to review them or when those who are able to conduct the review appear to be biased. Some specialty societies have established programs to provide this consultation. One example of such external review is the 2003 Illinois case discussed earlier in this section.

OFFICERS. The organized medical staff has officers, and they are selected in a variety of ways. One area of dispute has been this selection process. Sometimes physicians object when the hospital appoints officers or rejects the officers they prefer. JCAHO does not

---

[15] Johnson v. Misericordia Comm. Hosp., 99 Wis. 2d 708, 301 N.W.2d 156 (1981); *see also* Sheffield v. Zilis, 170 Ga. App. 62, 316 S.E.2d 493 (1984) [hospital not liable because it demonstrated adequate review of physician's credentials]; Annotation, *Hospital's liability for negligence in selection or appointment of staff physician or surgeon*, 51 A.L.R. 3D 981.

[16] Purcell v. Zimbelman, 18 Ariz. App. 75, 500 P.2d 335 (1972); *see also* Pedroza v. Bryant, 101 Wash. 2d 226, 677 P.2d 166 (1984) [hospital can be liable for granting privileges to physician who is not competent, but liability does not extend to treatment provided off hospital premises].

require a particular selection procedure. A California court approved rejection by a hospital board of the medical staff's choice for president because the bylaws reserved this authority, but the board later settled the suit and accepted the elected president.[17] A Florida appellate court refused to order a hospital to hold a medical staff election.[18] The hospital had appointed temporary officers due to disruption of operations. However, the court indicated that if the medical staff held its own election, a court could then decide which set of officers should preside. Hospitals should review individual contracts with physicians as well as bylaws before considering these actions.

In most jurisdictions, if an impasse occurs, the hospital can probably remove medical staff officers.[19] If this results in a breach of contract, the hospital might have to pay damages, but it is unlikely that a court will order the person reinstated to the office. In 1994, a Wisconsin court refused to reinstate a chief of staff who had been removed by a hospital.[20] It is rare for circumstances to arise where such removal is appropriate, but such circumstances can occur. Such hospital actions are often disruptive to the relationship between the hospital and other medical staff members.

DEPARTMENT STRUCTURE. In most hospitals, the medical staff is divided into departments along specialty lines. There is generally discretion to reorganize departments, but disputes can arise from such changes.[21]

Medical departments have heads. JCAHO requires clinical department heads to be certified by the appropriate specialty board or to have "affirmatively established comparable competence through the credentialing process."[22]

The selection and removal of heads sometimes leads to disputes. Generally, courts will not order the reinstatement of removed

---

17 *Eisenhower medical staff to appeal court decision*, MOD. HEALTHCARE, Apr. 14, 1989, 24; Staver, *Hospital board settles, OKs staff president*, AM. MED. NEWS, Nov. 10, 1989, at 6.

18 Lawnwood Med. Ctr., Inc. v. Cassimally, 471 So. 2d 1346 (Fla. 4th DCA 1985).

19 *E.g.*, Triplett v. Camp Wood Convalescent Ctr., 2000 Tex. App. LEXIS 3176 [deny injunction to medical director removed by nursing home]; *See* R.D. Miller, *Removing physicians from medical staff offices*, 1 MEDSTAFF NEWS (Winter 1995), at 1.

20 *E.g.*, Keane v. St. Francis Hosp., 186 Wis. 2d 637, 522 N.W.2d 517 (Ct. App. 1994) [removal of chief of staff].

21 *E.g.*, Ann Arundel Gen. Hosp. v. O'Brien, 49 Md. App. 362, 432 A.2d 483 (1981) [combined radiology and nuclear medicine, entered exclusive contract].

22 2005 JCAHO CAMH, Elements of Performance 8 for MS.1.20.

department heads,[23] but there have been exceptions.[24] When there is a contract between the hospital and the department head, removal can also lead to a claim for damages for breach of contract.[25]

JCAHO standards require each department head to perform a variety of administrative functions.[26] Thus, it is important to have a head who will actually perform the required functions. Most physicians who accept such positions conscientiously perform their duties, but when one fails to do so due to time pressures, conflicting loyalties, or other factors, the medical staff and ultimately the hospital must be able to put someone in the position who will do the job.

JCAHO standards also require department heads to make recommendations concerning all applicants for clinical privileges in the departments.[27] In single specialty departments, this means that the head can be an economic competitor of the applicant, and a negative recommendation can lead to an antitrust claim. If the department head stays out of the later steps of the application process and those steps do not automatically defer to the department head, the risk of a successful antitrust claim will lessen.

Departmental rules have led to litigation. For example, a federal appellate court upheld a departmental rule requiring twenty-four-hour notice of desire to use a particular anesthesiologist.[28] A New York court ruled that the head of a medical department could be sued by a patient injured through treatment by another member of the department based on the head's failure to develop and implement appropriate rules when the responsibility for rule-making had been delegated by the hospital.[29]

---

[23] *E.g., Former CU med chair loses latest try for reinstatement*, AP, May 20, 2003 [denial of reinstatement by U.S. magistrate]; Hrehorovich v. Harbor Hosp. Ctr., 93 Md. App. 772, 614 A.2d 1021 (1992).

[24] Shoemaker v. Los Angeles County, No. BC096101 (Cal. Super. Ct. Jan. 31, 1994), *as discussed in* 3 H.L.R. 186 (1994) [injunction of county hospital from removing chief of emergency medicine, based on due process, civil service requirements despite threatened loss of accreditation of emergency medicine residency because chief was not board certified]; *Agency restores Drew Medical School emergency residency accreditation*, 3 H.L.R. 317 (1994) [on Feb. 23, appellate court granted stay of injunction, so board certified interim chair, program director appointed and accreditation was restored the next day]; Shoemaker v. County of Los Angeles, 37 Cal. App. 4th 618; 43 Cal. Rptr. 2d 774 (2d Dist. 1995).

[25] *E.g.*, Finley v. Giacobbe, 827 F. Supp. 215 (S.D. N.Y. 1993) [bylaws may be contract of employment], *later op.*, 848 F. Supp. 1146 (S.D. N.Y. 1994) [partial summary judgment for defendant on contract claim].

[26] 2005 JCAHO CAMH, Elements of Performance 8 for MS.1.20.

[27] 2005 JCAHO CAMH, Elements of Performance 8 for MS.4.20.

[28] Faucher v. Rodziewicz, 891 F.2d 864 (11th Cir. 1990).

[29] Maxwell v. Cole, 126 Misc. 2d 597, 482 N.Y.S.2d 1000 (1984); *but see* Latiff v. Wyckoff Heights Hosp., 144 A.D.2d 650, 535 N.Y.S.2d 2 (2d Dept. 1988) [no liability where delegation not shown].

COMMITTEE STRUCTURE. In the past, JCAHO and Medicare conditions of participation required an elaborate medical staff committee structure, but now only the medical executive committee is required.[30] The functions that were performed by committees can now be performed in other ways. Many hospitals still have a complex committee structure.

The executive committee is not a separate legal entity; it generally does not have standing to bring suit.[31]

WHAT DISCIPLINES ARE ELIGIBLE FOR MEMBERSHIP? Medical staffs are primarily composed of physicians, that is, medical doctors and doctors of osteopathy. In its early years, the Joint Commission on Accreditation of Hospitals (which later changed its name to JCAHO) and organized medicine sought to keep osteopathic physicians off the medical staff.[32] During the 1960s, most of the barriers were removed.[33] This has not been an issue for many years.

Podiatrists and dentists are generally permitted to be members of the medical staff. Some states require this.[34] Prior to 2004, JCAHO required podiatrists and dentists to have a physician involved in the care of patients they admit to the hospital. In 2004, JCAHO deleted this requirement, leaving the determination of the scope of podiatry and dental privileges to state law and hospital policy.[35]

Some hospitals permit psychologists to be members of the medical staff. Some states require this.[36] When psychologists are permitted to admit patients, they are also generally required to have a physician involved in the care of admitted patients.[37]

---

[30] 2005 JCAHO CAMH, MS.1.40; Medicare conditions of participation require a Utilization Review Committee, but it can be a hospital committee, 42 C.F.R. § 482.30(b).

[31] *E.g.,* Board of Surgeon Directors v. Board of Directors (N.Y. Sup. Ct. June 1999), *as reported in* N.Y.L.J., June 11, 1999, 25 [no standing to challenge sale of hospital assets, but note the sale was later blocked on petition of the state attorney general - *In re* Manhattan Eye, Ear & Throat Hosp, 186 Misc. 2d 126, 715 N.Y.S.2d 575 (Sup. Ct. 1999)].

[32] *E.g.,* Wallington v. Zinn, 146 W.Va. 147, 118 S.E.2d 526 (1961).

[33] *See* F. Helminski, *"That peculiar science:" Osteopathic medicine and the law,* 12 LAW, MED. & HEALTH CARE, Feb. 1984, 32.

[34] *E.g.,* FLA. STAT. § 395.0191; CAL. HEALTH & SAFETY CODE § 1316; *but see* New Hampshire Podiatric Med. Ass'n v. New Hampshire Hosp. Ass'n, 735 F. Supp. 448 (D. N.H. 1990) [not violation of equal protection to deny podiatrists privileges].

[35] 2004 JCAHO CAMH, MS.2.10; 2005 JCAHO CAMH, MS.2.10.

[36] *E.g.,* FLA. STAT. § 395.0191.

[37] *E.g.,* WIS. STAT. § 50.36(3g)(c); *but see* California Ass'n of Psychology Providers v. California Hosp. Ass'n, 51 Cal. 3d 1; 793 P.2d 2 (1990) [state could not require physician involvement].

Hospitals are generally not required to permit other disciplines to be members of the medical staff,[38] but some have permitted chiropractors,[39] midwives,[40] and persons from other disciplines to be members.

JCAHO and other accrediting bodies have increased their attention on nurse practitioners and physician's assistants. Accredited hospitals are required to have a system for reviewing their credentials and determining the scope of what they are permitted to do,[41] but in most states, hospitals are not required to make them members of the medical staff.[42]

CONFIRMATION OF MEMBERSHIP. In some circumstances, hospitals can be liable for not promptly responding to requests for confirmation of present or past membership and privileges.[43]

DIFFERENCE BETWEEN PUBLIC AND PRIVATE HOSPITALS. Lawsuits arising out of board decisions concerning appointments and clinical privileges of physicians usually focus on (1) the right of the board to impose the rules applied or (2) the procedures followed in reaching the decision. In most states, public hospital boards have less discretion than private hospital boards. Many states have also limited the discretion of private hospitals.

---

[38] *E.g.,* Petrocco v. Dover Gen. Hosp., 273 N.J. Super. 501, 642 A.2d 1016 (App. Div. 1994) [exclusion of chiropractors from hospital privileges upheld]; Cohn v. Bond, 953 F.2d 154 (4th Cir. 1991), *cert. denied,* 505 U.S. 1230 (1992) [no conspiracy in denial to chiropractor because intracorporate immunity applied].

[39] *E.g., Easing into the medical mainstream: Chiropractors gain acceptance at hospitals,* THE HERALD (Miami, FL), Feb. 18, 1995, 1C [hospital adding a chiropractic department]; D. Fiely, *Community hospital extends privileges to chiropractors,* COLUMBUS [OHIO] DISPATCH, May 17, 1993, 1E.

[40] *E.g., Midwives allowed to admit, discharge patients at Meriter,* AP, Aug. 29, 2003 [WI]; *but see, Legislator says hospital breaks law in midwife squabble,* AP, Oct. 1, 2003 [IA - midwives permitted to practice under supervision, but not as independent members]; J. Gould, *Midwife strife — city hospital bans birthing assistants,* N.Y. POST, Nov. 28, 2003, 16 [midwives barred from most deliveries]; Nurse Midwifery Assocs. v. Hibbett, 918 F.2d 605 (6th Cir. 1990), *op. modified on reh'g,* 927 F.2d 904 (6th Cir.), *cert. denied,* 502 U.S. 952 (1991) [intracorporate conspiracy doctrine protected pediatricians, but not obstetricians, who recommended against nurse's privileges; could find conspiracy between obstetricians, hospital].

[41] 2005 JCAHO CAMH, LD.3.70, Element of Performance 2.

[42] *But see* Fla. Stat. § 395.0191(2) [application of advanced registered nurse practitioners must be considered].

[43] *E.g.,* Purgess v. Sharrock, 33 F.3d 134 (2d Cir. 1994); *see also* Mishler v. Nevada State Bd. of Med. Examiners, 896 F.2d 408 (9th Cir. 1990) [right to confirmation of license]; *contra* Chuz v. St. Vincent's Hosp., 186 A.D.2d 450, 589 N.Y.S.2d 17 (1st Dep't 1992) [liability only if delay due to malice]; Humana Med. Corp. v. Peyer, 155 Wis. 2d 714, 456 N.W.2d 355 (Wis. 1990) [hospital may refuse to release information until physician repaid money hospital loaned him to establish practice].

Public hospitals are subject to some constitutional constraints or have governmental immunities that do not apply to private hospitals.

Due Process. Public hospitals must satisfy the Fourteenth Amendment to the United States Constitution, which says that no state shall "deprive any person of life, liberty, or property, without due process of law." An action by a public hospital is considered a state action. The interest of a physician in practicing in a hospital can be a liberty or property interest, entitling the physician to "due process of law" when a public hospital makes a decision concerning medical staff appointment or clinical privileges. However, a physician does not have a constitutional right to practice in any public hospital.[44] Physicians must demonstrate that they satisfy valid hospital rules before they may practice in the hospital.

Some federal courts have ruled that an applicant does not have a property or liberty interest in being appointed or being granted privileges.[45] Usually, the property right is in continuation of membership or privileges that have been granted.[46]

To provide physicians with due process, hospital rules must be reasonable and adequately express the intent of the hospital. Rules that are too arbitrary or vague may be unenforceable. Physicians must be offered fair procedures when they are being deprived of a liberty or property interest. In some circumstances, summary action may be taken immediately with the due process provided later.[47]

In some states, it may be possible to structure clinical privileges in a public hospital so that no property interest is created, if there is no understanding not to revoke the privileges without due process.[48]

Equal Protection. The Fourteenth Amendment also says that no state shall "deny to any person within its jurisdiction the equal protection of the laws." Equal protection means that like persons must be dealt with in like fashion. The equal protection clause is concerned with the justifiability of classifications used to distinguish persons for

---

[44] *E.g.,* Hayman v. Galveston, 273 U.S. 414 (1927) [state medical license does not give constitutional right to practice in public hospital].

[45] *E.g.,* Shahawy v. Harrison, 778 F.2d 636 (11th Cir. 1985), *corrected*, 790 F.2d 75 (11th Cir. 1986); *see also*, Randall v. United States, 30 F.3d 518 (4th Cir. 1994), *cert. denied*, 514 U.S. 1107 (1995) [provisional privileges in army hospital created no property interest in request for full privileges].

[46] *E.g.,* Shahawy v. Harrison, 875 F.2d 1529 (11th Cir. 1989) [property interest in continuation of privileges].

[47] *E.g.,* Moore v. Middlebrook, 2004 U.S. App. LEXIS 8558 (10th Cir.) [unpub].

[48] *See* Lowe v. Scott, 959 F.2d 323 (1st Cir. 1992).

various legal purposes. Determining whether a particular difference between persons can justify a particular difference in rules or procedures can be difficult. Courts generally require government agencies to justify differences with a *rational reason*. The major exception to this standard is the *strict scrutiny* courts apply to distinctions based on *suspect classifications*, such as race, and the intermediate level of scrutiny applied to sex-based classifications. Because of comprehensive legislation prohibiting discrimination based on many characteristics, most challenges to alleged discriminatory actions are based on legislation, rather than directly on this constitutional principle. Nondiscrimination legislation is discussed in Chapter 4.

Public Hospital Immunities. Public hospitals have some protections from suits. The Eleventh Amendment to the Constitution forbids many private suits in federal courts against states and entities that are considered arms of the state. This has been applied to bar some suits against hospitals that are considered arms of the state,[49] but not against local governmental hospitals.[50] Moreover, in some circumstances, Congress may abrogate the immunity to permit suits against states and their instrumentalities.[51]

The Local Government Antitrust Act of 1984[52] protects public hospitals from most antitrust damage claims, and the state action doctrine discussed in Chapter 13 protects public hospitals from many other antitrust suits.

Sovereign immunity protects public hospitals in some states from many claims under state common law (see Chapter 11).

State Action. Medical staff actions of most private hospitals are subject to fewer legal constraints than are actions by public hospitals. The Fourteenth Amendment does not apply to private hospitals except in the unusual circumstance when the hospital activity is found to be state action. In some states, private hospitals are required only to follow their own rules in medical staff actions. In other states, legislatures and courts require some procedures in medical staff decisions.

---

[49] *E.g.,* Atascadero State Hosp. v. Scanlon, 473 U.S. 234 (1985); Sullivan v. University of Miss. Med. Ctr., 617 F. Supp. 554 (S.D. Miss. 1985).

[50] *E.g.,* Laje v. R.E. Thomason Gen. Hosp., 665 F.2d 724 (5th Cir. 1982); Howard v. Liberty Mem. Hosp., 752 F. Supp. 1074 (S.D. Ga. 1990); Magula v. Broward Gen. Med. Ctr., 742 F. Supp. 645 (S.D. Fla. 1990).

[51] *E.g.,* Fitzpatrick v. Bitzer, 427 U.S. 445 (1976); Brinkman v. Dep't of Corrections, 21 F.3d 370 (10th Cir. 1994), *cert. denied,* 513 U.S. 927 (1994) [Fair Labor Standards Act]; Davidson v. Board of Governors, 920 F.2d 441 (7th Cir. 1990) [Age Discrimination in Employment Act].

[52] 15 U.S.C. §§ 34-36; Sandcrest Outpatient Servs., P.A. v. Cumberland County Hosp. Sys., Inc., 853 F.2d 1139 (4th Cir. 1988).

Private hospitals are rarely found to be engaged in state action and, thus, subject to the Fourteenth Amendment. In 1974, the United States Supreme Court ruled that state regulation or funding alone did not establish state action. The Court said that there must be a "sufficiently close nexus between the state and the challenged action of the regulated entity so that the action of the latter may be fairly treated as that of the state itself." The Court gave the following examples of such a connection: (1) when the private entity exercises powers traditionally reserved for the state, (2) when the state directly benefits by sharing in the rewards and responsibilities of the private venture, and (3) when the state directs or encourages the particular act.[53]

In rare circumstances, private hospitals can engage in state action. If a majority of the governing board is appointed by a governmental agency, the courts will be likely to find the hospital to be engaged in state action.[54] Appointment of a minority of the governing body is not likely to be sufficient.[55] If the hospital is leased from a governmental entity, it may be found to be engaged in state action,[56] but some courts do not consider this sufficient.[57] However, a public hospital that is managed by a private corporation is generally still public; so the actions of the management corporation are state actions.[58]

State Law Requirements. There is a great range of state law requirements concerning the relationship of public and private hospitals with physicians. Some states have not imposed any requirements, but most states will enforce hospital rules. By statute or court decision, some states have limited the latitude of all hospitals.[59] For example, New York requires hospitals to process all applications for membership or clinical privileges from physicians, podiatrists, and dentists.[60] Membership or clinical privileges may be denied, curtailed, or terminated only after reasons have been stated. The only permissible reasons are "standards of patient care, patient welfare,

---

53 Jackson v. Metropolitan Edison Co., 419 U.S. 345 (1974).
54 *E.g.,* Downs v. Sawtelle, 574 F.2d 1 (1st Cir.), *cert. denied,* 439 U.S. 910 (1978).
55 *E.g.,* Aasum v. Good Samaritan Hosp., 395 F. Supp. 363 (D. Or. 1975), *aff'd,* 542 F.2d 792 (9th Cir. 1976).
56 *E.g.,* Jatoi v. Hurst-Euless-Bedford Hosp. Auth., 807 F.2d 1214 (5th Cir.), *modified & reh'g denied* (en banc), 819 F.2d 545 (5th Cir. 1987), *cert. denied,* 484 U.S. 1010 (1988).
57 *E.g.,* Greco v. Orange Mem. Hosp., 513 F.2d 873 (5th Cir.), *cert. denied,* 423 U.S. 1000 (1975).
58 *E.g.,* Milo v. Cushing Mun. Hosp., 861 F.2d 1194 (10th Cir. 1988).
59 *E.g.,* CAL. BUS. & PROF. CODE § 809.05; Nicholas v. North Colo. Med. Ctr., Inc., 1995-1 Trade Cases ¶ 70.899 (Colo. Ct. App. Feb. 2, 1995) [upholding decision of Board of Medical Examiner's Committee on Anticompetitive Conduct that hospital peer review decision to restrict staff privileges of cardiologist was motivated by personal animosity of opposing cardiologist, those acting in concert with him].
60 N.Y. PUB. HEALTH LAW § 2801-b.

the objectives of the institution or the character or competency of the applicant." The Public Health Council is authorized to investigate complaints alleging violations and to order a hospital to review actions if the council finds "cause exists for the crediting of the allegations." The New York courts require physicians to pursue review by the council before they will permit suits against hospitals.[61]

Some state courts require private hospitals to provide some procedural protections for medical staff members, including notice of alleged shortcomings and an opportunity to be heard.[62] New Jersey requires the right to be represented by a lawyer.[63]

5-2 Appointment to the Medical Staff

An identified, competent practitioner must be responsible for the care of each hospital patient to satisfy most definitions of a hospital and of a medically necessary admission. The practitioners will usually be physicians, but in some situations, they may be dentists and other practitioners. The following discussion concerning physicians also applies to other practitioners who are permitted to admit patients. Hospitals must screen physicians before appointment to the medical staff and allow only medical staff members to admit patients. The admitting physician then assumes continuing responsibility for medical care of that patient until responsibility is transferred to another medical staff member or until the patient is discharged. Because most physicians practice in groups or have other coverage arrangements to permit some time off duty, in practice such transfers of responsibility are common.

A medical license does not give a physician the right to practice in a particular hospital. Each physician must apply for medical staff appointment. Each physician must prove that he or she satisfies the hospital appointment criteria or that the criteria are not permitted. The burden of proof is on the applying physician, especially if the

---

[61] *E.g.,* Guibor v. Manhattan Eye, Ear & Throat Hosp., Inc., 56 A.D.2d 359, 392 N.Y.S.2d 628 (1st Dep't 1977), *aff'd,* 46 N.Y.2d 736, 413 N.Y.S.2d 638, 386 N.E.2d 247 (1978); Johnson v. Nyack Hosp., 964 F.2d 116 (2d Cir. 1992) [applies to claims in federal court, including federal antitrust claims].

[62] Sussman v. Overlook Hosp. Ass'n, 95 N.J. Super. 418, 231 A.2d 389 (App. Div. 1967); Anton v. San Antonio Comm. Hosp., 19 Cal. 3d 802, 140 Cal. Rptr. 442, 567 P.2d 1162 (1977); Silver v. Castle Mem. Hosp., 53 Haw. 475, 563, 497 P.2d 564, *motion denied,* 53 Haw. 675, 501 P.2d 60, *cert. denied,* 409 U.S. 1048 (1972).

[63] Garrow v. Elizabeth Gen. Hosp., 79 N.J. 549, 401 A.2d 533 (1979).

medical staff bylaws so provide. Many court cases have involved such medical staff issues. Procedural issues are discussed later in the chapter. This section reviews some criteria for initial appointment.

PERMITTED CRITERIA. In addition to the obvious criteria of licensure, education, training, and experience, some of the permitted criteria for review of applicants include:

1. complete and accurate application,
2. verification of credentials,
3. references,
4. a demonstrated ability to work with others,
5. board certification or equivalent training and experience,
6. payment of dues and assessments,
7. geographic proximity to the hospital,
8. agreement to provide indigent care,
9. malpractice insurance,
10. the need for additional staff in the specialty,
11. economic credentialing,
12. health status, and
13. background check.

Some of these criteria are subject to limitations and are not permitted in all states. The same standards should apply to all applicants.[64]

Application. Hospitals require a complete and accurate application form, including an agreement to abide by hospital and medical staff rules.[65] Courts have upheld denial of appointment or termination based on incomplete or falsified applications.[66] Physicians should be required, along with providing other information, to

---

[64] *E.g.,* Weiss v. York Hosp., 745 F.2d 786, 821 (3d Cir. 1984), *cert. denied,* 470 U.S. 1060 (1985).

[65] *E.g.,* Evers v. Edward Hosp. Ass'n, 247 Ill. App. 3d 717, 617 N.E.2d 1211 (2d Dist. 1993), *app. denied,* 153 Ill. 2d 559, 624 N.E.2d 806 (1993) [declined to evaluate application because deemed incomplete]; Smith v. Cleburne County Hosp., 870 F.2d 1375 (8th Cir., *cert. denied,* 493 U.S. 847) (1989) [failure to submit papers for reappointment was voluntary withdrawal].

[66] *E.g.,* Johnson v. Galen, 39 S.W.3d 828 (Ky. App. 2001) [misrepresentation on application]; Pariser v. Christian Health Care Sys., Inc., 816 F.2d 1248 (8th Cir. 1987), *after remand,* 859 F.2d 78 (8th Cir. 1988) [falsely denied prior denial of privileges]; Lapidot v. Memorial Med. Ctr., 144 Ill. App. 3d 141, 494 N.E.2d 838 (4th Dist. 1986) [false denial of prior suspension of privileges]; Brooks v. Arlington Hosp. Ass'n. 850 F.2d 191 (4th Cir. 1988) [failure to complete delineation of privileges form]; Untertiner v. Desert Hosp. Dist., 33 Cal. 3d 285, 188 Cal. Rptr. 590, 656 P.2d 554 (1983); Yeargin v. Hamilton Mem. Hosp., 225 Ga. 661, 171 S.E.2d 136 (1969), *cert. denied,* 397 U.S. 963 (1970) [exception to agreement to abide by rules]; Spindle v. Sisters of Providence, 61 P.2d 431 (Alaska 2002) [reasonable to require applicant to provide discharge diagnoses and summaries on prior cases and to consider application incomplete in absence of this information].

(1) present evidence of medical education, training, experience, current competence, current licensure, and health status and (2) disclose professional liability actions and pending and completed governmental, institutional, and professional disciplinary actions against them. In some cases, the health status information may need to be collected later in the process, as discussed later in this section. Some states will suspend or revoke a physician's medical license for false answers on an application for hospital clinical privileges.[67] Refusal to release information concerning discipline at other hospitals may be grounds for denial of an application.[68]

Another important aspect of most applications is a waiver of liability. Waivers are discussed in section 5–7 of this chapter, which deals with liability.

Hospitals generally do not have to process incomplete applications or applications from persons who made previous commitments not to reapply.[69]

A history of malpractice complaints or judgments does not necessarily disqualify a physician from membership of privileges.[70] Malpractice histories should be examined on a case-by-case basis.

Verification. Hospitals need to carefully check information supplied by applicants. JCAHO requires primary source verification of many items.[71] In 2004, JCAHO added a requirement that the identity of the applicant be verified.[72] Hospitals can be liable for injuries to patients by physicians who would have been denied membership if application information had been properly checked.[73] Generally, hospitals are liable for failing to check applications only when a reasonable check would have led to rejection of the applicant.[74]

Hospitals must make an inquiry to the National Practitioner Data Bank concerning each applicant and, at least every two years, con-

---

[67] *E.g.*, Abdelmessih v. Board of Regents, 205 A.D.2d 983, 613 N.Y.S.2d 971 (3d Dep't 1994); Radnay v. Sobol, 175 A.D.2d 432, 572 N.Y.S.2d 489 (3d Dep't 1991); *contra* Elmariah v. Dep't of Prof. Reg., 574 So. 2d 164 (Fla. 1st DCA 1990).

[68] *E.g.*, Scott v. Sisters of St. Francis Health Servs., Inc., 645 F. Supp. 1465 (N.D. Ill. 1986), *aff'd without op.*, 822 F.2d 1090 (7th Cir. 1987).

[69] *E.g.*, Khouw v. Methodist Hosp., 126 Fed. Appx. 657, 2005 U.S. App. LEXIS 4206 (5th Cir. 2005) (unpub) [resignation agreement effectively barred reapplication].

[70] *E.g., Dr. allegedly had three prior medmal complaints: Neff v. Johnson Memorial Hospital*, CONN. L. TRIB., Apr. 26, 2004, 507 [hospital not negligent in credentialing MD with three priors where no expert testimony that it breached standard of care]; *but see* Fletcher v. South Peninsula Hosp., 71 P.3d 833 (Alaska 2003) [hospital should investigate disclosed prior malpractice claims].

[71] 2004 JCAHO CAMH, MS.4.10.

[72] 2004 JCAHO CAMH & 2005 JCAHO CAMH, MS 4.10, Element of Performance 3.

[73] Rule v. Lutheran Hosps. & Homes Soc'y, 835 F.2d 1250 (8th Cir. 1987).

[74] *E.g.*, Ferguson v. Gonyaw, 64 Mich. App. 685, 236 N.W.2d 543 (1975).

cerning each member in order to qualify for the antitrust immunity discussed later in this chapter.[75] Hospitals are presumed to know information they would have obtained by making such inquiries.[76]

References. Satisfactory references may be required,[77] but not from the present medical staff.[78]

Ability to Work with Others. Courts in many states have accepted a requirement that applicants and members demonstrate ability to work harmoniously with other physicians and hospital staff.[79] Most states have not limited the degree of inability to work with others that justifies denial, but a few states have placed limits. A New Jersey court accepted that "prospective disharmony" was a reasonable basis for denial if "valid and constructive criticism of hospital practice" is not equated with disharmony.[80] The court noted that "a person has a right to disagree with the policy or practice, but he does not have a right to be disagreeable in doing so." The California Supreme Court accepted inability to work with others as a basis for denial when it presents "a real and substantial danger that patients treated by him might receive other than a 'high quality of medical care' at the facility."[81]

Board Certification. Many hospitals require that physicians be board eligible or board certified before being granted specialty privileges. Some hospitals require board certification to be obtained within a specified time.

Most courts have upheld hospital requirements of board certification or completion of an approved residency before specialty clinical privileges are granted.[82] A California appellate court upheld a hospital requirement that dilation and curettage privileges be granted only to physicians who had completed a residency in obstetrics and gynecology.[83] A few courts have invalidated board certification requirements of public hospitals.[84]

---

[75] 42 U.S.C. § 1135(a).

[76] 42 U.S.C. § 1135(b).

[77] *E.g.,* Truly v. Madison Gen. Hosp., 673 F.2d 763 (5th Cir.), *cert. denied*, 459 U.S. 909 (1982).

[78] *E.g.,* Ascherman v. St. Francis Mem. Hosp., 45 Cal. App. 3d 507, 119 Cal. Rptr. 507 (1st Dist. 1975).

[79] *E.g.,* Johnson v. Galen, 39 S.W.3d 828 (Ky. App. 2001); Landefeld v. Marion Gen. Hosp, Inc., 994 F.2d 1178 (6th Cir. 1993) [stealing internal mail indicated inability to work with others].

[80] Sussman v. Overlook Hosp. Ass'n, 95 N.J. Super. 418, 231 A.2d 389 (App. Div. 1967).

[81] Miller v. Eisenhower Med. Ctr., 27 Cal. 3d 614, 166 Cal. Rptr. 826, 614 P.2d 258 (1980); *applied in* Pick v. Santa Ana-Tustin Comm. Hosp., 130 Cal. App. 3d 970, 182 Cal. Rptr. 85 (4th Dist. 1982) [sufficient danger shown to justify denial].

[82] *E.g.,* Khan v. Suburban Comm. Hosp., 45 Ohio St. 2d 39, 349 N.E.2d 398 (1976).

[83] Hay v. Scripps Mem. Hosp., 183 Cal. App. 3d 753, 228 Cal. Rptr. 413 (4th Dist. 1986).

[84] *E.g.,* Armstrong v. Board of Directors, 553 S.W.2d 77 (Tenn. Ct. App. 1976).

One way to avoid controversy is to require board certification or equivalent training and experience.[85] This requirement permits the hospital to avail itself of the strengths of the private certification system while leaving open a channel to deal with individual applicants on a case-by-case basis.

A workable exceptions process also avoids facing the threat of disqualification from participation in Medicare. Medicare conditions of participation specifically forbid basing clinical privilege decisions solely on board status.[86] It is not clear whether individual physicians can use this as a basis for judicial relief from such requirements.[87] It is probable that only the federal government can enforce the Medicare rules, and its only sanction is to terminate Medicare participation.

JCAHO states that heads of departments should be board certified in the specialty or prove comparable competence.[88]

Some managed care entities require board certification for participation.[89]

Dues. Physicians may be required to pay dues, fees, and assessments to apply for and retain medical staff membership.[90] For example, a Michigan appellate court upheld the suspension of a physician who refused to pay a $100 assessment levied by the medical staff executive committee to furnish a medical library.[91]

Geographic Proximity. Some courts have upheld geographic criteria that require an applicant to live or practice within a certain distance of the hospital, stated in terms of miles, travel time, or location close enough that the applicant is reasonably able to provide

---

[85] *E.g.,* Sarasota County Pub. Hosp. Bd. v. Shahawy, 408 So. 2d 644 (Fla. 2d DCA 1981) [public hospital may require board certification or unusual qualifications for cardiac catheterization privileges] [partially superseded by statute, Fla. Stat. § 395.0191(3), that requires acceptance of equivalent osteopathic training].

[86] 42 C.F.R. § 482.12(a)(7).

[87] *See, E.g.,* Evelyn V. v. Kings County Hosp. Ctr., 819 F. Supp. 183 (E.D. N.Y. 1993) [Medicaid Act requirement that state plan provide for maintaining health standards of providers did not authorize suit by recipients against city for deficiencies at municipal hospital]; *contra* Fulkerson v. Comm'r, 802 F. Supp. 529 (D. Me. 1992) [Medicaid recipients may enforce equal access to care provision].

[88] 2005 JCAHO CAMH, Elements of Performance 8 for MS.1.20.

[89] H. Larkin, *All aboard?* AM. MED. NEWS, Mar. 13, 1995, 11 [options for those without board certification to deal with managed care, where 35 to 40 percent of physicians are not board certified]; S. McIlrath, *Board-certified only need apply,* AM. MED. NEWS, Dec. 12. 1994, 1 [medical groups seeking to block requirement of board-certification for managed care participation].

[90] Rev. Rul. 65-264, 1965-2 C.B. 159 [nondiscriminatory fees do not jeopardize federal tax exemption]; *see also* Brooks & Morrisey, *Credentialing: Say good-bye to the "rubber stamp,"* 59 HOSPS., June 1, 1985, 50, 52.

[91] Chapman v. Peoples Comm. Hosp. Auth., 139 Mich. App. 696, 362 N.W.2d 755 (1984).

continuity of care.[92] These rules are intended to assure response to patient needs, especially during emergencies. In the past, JCAHO expressly recognized geographic location as an appropriate criterion, but now does not address the issue.[93] Geographic limits based on political boundaries are less likely to be enforceable.[94]

Because the goal of geographic criteria is to assure timely coverage of patient needs, some hospitals accept coverage arrangements as an alternative means of compliance. For example, coverage may include (1) a nearby individual or group that agrees to provide coverage for a more distant applicant or (2) a group of more distant applicants may agree to have one person on duty at the hospital or on call nearby at all times.

Indigent Care. Physicians can be required to provide uncompensated care to those who are unable to pay.[95] Since all hospitals are required to provide some emergency services to those who are unable to pay and many hospitals are required to provide other services to these patients, arrangements must be made for medical coverage. Although some of these services are provided by employed physicians or physicians with special contracts, many of the services are provided by members of the medical staff without a separate contract. Agreement to provide these services can be a requirement for medical staff membership.

Malpractice Insurance. Since 1975, appellate courts have consistently upheld reasonable requirements of malpractice insurance as a condition of medical staff membership.[96] In a malpractice suit,

---

92 *E.g.,* Kennedy v. St. Joseph Mem. Hosp., 482 N.E.2d 268 (Ind. Ct. App. 1985) [moved personal residence too far away], *disapproved on other grounds*, Pepple v. Parkview Mem. Hosp., 536 N.E.2d 274 (Ind. 1989); *but see* Quinn v. Kent Gen. Hosp., Inc., 617 F. Supp. 1226 (D. Del. 1985) [factual issue of whether fifteen-mile rule was reasonable precluded summary judgment in antitrust case].

93 *E.g.,* 1995 JCAHO CAMH, at 488.

94 *E.g.,* Sams v. Ohio Valley Gen. Hosp. Ass'n, 413 F.2d 826 (4th Cir. 1969) [county boundary not valid geographic limit], *disapproved on other grounds*, Modaber v. Culpeper Mem. Hosp., 674 F.2d 1023 (4th Cir. 1982); Berman v. Valley Hosp., 103 N.J. 100, 510 A.2d 673 (1986) [geographic limits to control utilization unenforceable under unique New Jersey review of private hospitals as quasi-public entities].

95 Clair v. Centre Comm. Hosp., 317 Pa. Super. 25, 463 A.2d 1065 (1983); *accord* Coker v. Hunt Mem. Hosp., No. CA-3-86-1200-H (N.D. Tex. July 29, 1986), *as discussed in* 14 HEALTH L. DIG., Sept. 1986, at 4; Rooney v. Medical Ctr. Hosp of Chillicothe, 1994 U.S. Dist. LEXIS 7420 (S.D. Ohio).

96 *E.g.,* Backlund v. Board of Comm'rs, 106 Wash. 2d 632, 724 P.2d 981 (1986), *appeal dismissed*, 481 U.S. 1034 (1987) [religious objections to insurance do not excuse compliance]; Scales v. Memorial Med. Ctr., 690 F. Supp. 1002 (M.D. Fla. 1988) [insurance with risk retention group not approved by state is not compliance]; Pollock v. Methodist Hosp., 392 F. Supp. 393 (E.D. La 1975); Wilkinson v. Madera Comm. Hosp., 144 Cal. App. 3d 436, 192 Cal. Rptr. 593 (5th Dist. 1983) [hospital can require insurance to be with company approved by the state]; Annotation, *Propriety of hospital's conditioning physician's staff privileges on his carrying professional liability or malpractice insurance,* 7 A.L.R. 4TH 1238.

both the hospital and the physicians are generally sued. If one defendant is not adequately insured, the burden of any payment will fall disproportionately on the others. Thus, there is a legitimate business interest in assuring adequate malpractice protection. In the past, JCAHO recognized adequate professional liability insurance as an appropriate criterion but is now silent on the issue.[97] Some courts have required flexibility in enforcing such rules because they can become unreasonable when, for example, no malpractice insurance is available.[98] Some states have imposed statutory requirements for coverage,[99] but generally hospitals are still free to impose more strict requirements.

In a few states, hospitals can be liable to malpractice claimants when they fail to check on the physician's insurance status.[100]

Staff Size Limitations. Hospitals may limit the size of the medical staff in some circumstances. The limits should be adopted by the board with documentation of the reasons. Courts are concerned that these limits not be used to protect the economic interests of present medical staff members. Limitations on the number of staff members in certain specialties have been upheld in several court decisions.[101] However, a New Jersey court invalidated a moratorium on new staff appointments because inadequate evidence had been presented that the moratorium was needed to assure appropriate patient care.[102] The New Jersey Supreme Court disapproved closed staff arrangements that permitted only new physicians who associated with current members[103] or who had not practiced in the area for the past two years.[104] A North Carolina appellate court ruled that a hospital could close a part of its medical staff if the moratorium was reasonable for the hospital and community and was fairly

---

[97] *E.g.,* 1995 JCAHO CAMH, at 488.

[98] *E.g.,* Holmes v. Hoemako Hosp., 117 Ariz. 403, 573 P.2d 477 (1977).

[99] *E.g.,* FLA. STAT. § 458.320.

[100] *E.g.,* Megrelishvili v. Our Lady of Mercy Med. Ctr., 291 A.D.2d 18, 739 N.Y.S.2d 2 (1st Dep't 2002); Mercy Hosp. v. Baumgardner, 2003 Fla. App. LEXIS 19533 (3d Dist.); *but see* President v. Jenkins, 357 N.J. Super. 288, 814 A.2d 1173 (App. Div. 2003) [hospital has no duty to assure MD has insurance, even when bylaws require such insurance].

[101] *E.g.,* Hackett v. Metropolitan Gen. Hosp., 465 So. 2d 1246 (Fla. 2d DCA 1985); Guerrero v. Burlington County Hosp., 70 N.J. 344, 360 A.2d 334 (1976); Davis v. Morristown Mem. Hosp., 106 N.J. Super. 33, 254 A.2d 125 (Ch. Div. 1969); *see also* Oliver v. Board of Trustees, 181 Cal. App. 3d 824, 227 Cal. Rptr. 1 (4th Dist. 1986) [requirement of specialty not represented on staff or renowned reputation].

[102] Walsky v. Pascack Valley Hosp., 145 N.J. Super. 393, 367 A.2d 1204 (Ch. Div. 1976), *aff'd,* 156 N.J. Super. 13, 383 A.2d 154 (App. Div. 1978).

[103] Desai v. St. Barnabas Med. Ctr., 103 N.J. 79, 510 A.2d 662 (1986).

[104] Berman v. Valley Hosp., 103 N.J. 100, 510 A.2d 673 (1986).

administered but that the challenging podiatrist was entitled to a trial in which he could attempt to show the moratorium was unreasonable.[105] The South Dakota Supreme Court permitted a private hospital to close its medical staff for some procedures.[106]

In the past, JCAHO recognized the appropriateness of criteria related to the ability of the hospital to provide facilities and support services but is now silent on the issue.[107]

When a hospital enters an exclusive contract with one physician or group for a specialty or procedure, others are not eligible to be granted privileges for that specialty or procedure. Courts generally permit hospitals to start a new exclusive contract and terminate the privileges of other physicians to perform the specialty or procedure.[108] In 1994, Illinois passed a law that requires notice and a hearing before privileges of others are terminated due to an exclusive contract.[109]

One of the factors that the IRS uses for determining whether a hospital qualifies for tax exemption is whether it has an open medical staff.[110] Such factors are not enforceable by private parties, such as other applying physicians. However, the IRS could use the absence of this factor as the basis for considering revocation of the hospital tax exemption. The minimum characteristics necessary to assure tax exemption remain unclear (see discussion in Chapter 9). The purpose behind the open staff requirement was to demonstrate that the hospital was "operated to serve a public rather than a private interest." The focus appears to have been on assuring that the general public could gain access to the hospital, not to assure that physicians could use the hospital for their private practices. There was also a concern that a closed staff could result in insider benefit to the physicians on the staff.[111] Again, the focus appears to be on avoiding benefit to insiders, not on providing benefit to other

---

[105] Claycomb v. HCA-Raleigh Comm. Hosp., 76 N.C. App. 382, 333 S.E.2d 333 (1985), *rev. denied*, 315 N.C. 586, 341 S.E.2d 23 (1986).

[106] Mahan v. Avera St. Luke's, 621 N.W.2d 150 (S.D. 2001).

[107] *E.g.*, 1995 JCAHO CAMH, at 480.

[108] *E.g.*, Ann Arundel Gen. Hosp. v. O'Brien, 49 Md. App. 362, 432 A.2d 483 (1981) [even when the bylaws are viewed as a contract]; Holt v. Good Samaritan Hosp. & Health Ctr., 69 Ohio App. 3d 439, 590 N.E.2d 1318 (1990) [employee of former exclusive provider of emergency medical services not entitled to hearing when clinical privileges lost due to awarding of contract to new group].

[109] *Governor signs bill that requires fair hearing for excluded providers*, 3 H.L.R. 1330 (1994).

[110] Rev. Rul. 69-545, 1969-2 C.B. 117.

[111] Sound Health Ass'n v. C.I.R., 71 T.C. 158 (1978), *acq.* 1981-2 C.B.2.

physicians. Thus, it is possible that the IRS would accept a closed staff if there were contractual commitments and hospital policies that assured public access and effective nonphysician control of the benefits received by those on the closed staff. Such an arrangement could provide the public with better access than an open staff. Tax exemption has been approved for entities that include closed departments in other contexts without addressing the impact on hospital tax exemption.[112]

Sometimes states attempt to challenge closed staffs in other ways. In 2002, Maine threatened a hospital with loss of a certificate of need for heart surgery unless it opened its staff.[113]

Economic Credentialing. Several different criteria are lumped together under the label of economic credentialing. Three of these criteria are (1) promoting efficient practice, (2) requiring participation in hospital managed care and related arrangements, and (3) avoiding economic competition with the hospital. Some persons also apply the economic credentialing label to exclusive contracts, but exclusive contracts are addressed separately in this book. Although still controversial, many of these criteria have been upheld by courts.

Hospitals have generally not required participation in managed care plans as a condition of medical staff membership, except in hospital-based specialties. The requirement for hospital-based specialists to participate is usually found in a contract between the physician and hospital, rather than in the medical staff requirements.

Efficient practice issues usually arise in the context of review of performance, and economic competition issues usually arise in the context of nonrenewal or termination of clinical privileges. They will be discussed in those sections of this chapter. One case of economic competition arose in the application context. In 1992, a Florida court upheld denial of surgical privileges to the head of the open heart surgery program at the competing hospital.[114]

---

[112] *E.g.,* B.H.W. Anesthesia Found., Inc. v. C.I.R., 72 T.C. 681 (1979), *nonacq,* 1980-2 C.B.2 [closed anesthesia department granted tax exemption]; *see also* Rev. Rul. 73-417, 1973-2 C.B. 332 [pathologist/hospital laboratory director with apparently exclusive contract was found to be an employee of hospital]; Kiddie v. C.I.R., 69 T.C. 1055 (1978) [pension plan issues concerning pathologist who apparently had exclusive contract with hospital].

[113] *Concannon warns Central Maine to open doors to outside heart doctors,* AP, Apr. 12, 2002.

[114] Rosenblum v. Tallahassee Mem. Reg. Med. Ctr., No. 91-589 (Fla. Cir. Ct. June 18, 1992), *as discussed in* 26 J.HEALTH & HOSP.L. 61 (1993).

Health Status. JCAHO requires that health status be used as a criterion to the extent permitted by the Americans with Disabilities Act.[115] The ADA regulates when inquiries can be made concerning health status in situations related to employment (see Chapter 4). Even though most physicians are not employees, the ADA restrictions may apply to some medical staff applicants due to the impact of the medical staff membership decision on their other employment relationships.[116] If a hospital determines that the ADA applies, it should limit application inquiries concerning health status to questions permitted by the ADA. Any offer of membership can then be contingent on ascertainment of health status. The ADA permits consistently applied inquiries and examinations after the employment-related decision has otherwise been made.

Background Check. Some states require a criminal background check for all persons who have direct patient contact, including medical staff members, and bar persons with certain convictions from any direct patient contact. Even when it is not required, some health care providers require a background check.[117] Background checks are discussed in Section 4-3.1.

UNACCEPTABLE CRITERIA. Some criteria are unacceptable, including (1) violations of nondiscrimination laws, (2) citizenship, (3) required kickbacks and other illegal contracts, (4) medical society membership, and (5) nonstandardized tests.

Violation of Nondiscrimination Laws. Hospitals cannot base their refusal to appoint a physician on the applicant's race, creed, color, sex, national origin, or handicap. Alleged violations are often addressed under the antidiscrimination laws discussed in Chapter 4.[118] These laws generally apply to all institutions receiving federal funds, whether the institutions are public or private. Some of these laws also apply to some entities not receiving federal funds.

---

[115] 2005 JCAHO CAMH, Element of Performance 10 and Note 2, MS.4.20.

[116] *E.g,* Chadha v. Hardin Mem. Hosp., 2000 U.S. App. LEXIS 439 (6th Cir.) [unpub] [Title I of ADA not apply to physician who was not employee]; Elbrecht v. HCA Health Servs. of Fla., Inc., 1994 U.S. Dist. LEXIS 18877 (N.D. Fla.) [neurologist sought exemption from emergency call on disability grounds, but ADA did not apply because hospital was not employer; employment relationship between physician, her patients not sufficient to trigger coverage].

[117] *E.g.,* WIS. STAT. § 48.685, 50.065; D. Adams, *Criminal checks increasingly a fact of life for physicians,* AM. MED. NEWS, Dec. 20, 2004, 1.

[118] *E.g.,* Chowdhury v. Reading Hosp., 677 F.2d 317 (3d Cir. 1982), *cert. denied,* 463 U.S. 1229 (1983).

Some of the nondiscrimination laws apply only to employees;
they generally do not apply to nonemployee medical staff members.[119] However, it is advisable to avoid discrimination based on the
grounds encompassed in the employment laws because in some circumstances nonemployment nondiscrimination laws may apply.[120]

Citizenship. Citizenship can probably not be used as a criterion.[121] Thus, legal aliens with appropriate licenses and an immigration status permitting medical practice probably cannot be
excluded on the basis of lack of citizenship. Exclusion of undocumented aliens is permitted and in some circumstances required.[122]

Illegal Contracts. In most states, there are limits on the contracts that facilities can require physicians to enter. In 1986, a New
York appellate court questioned a nursing home that had required a
physician to enter a fee-splitting arrangement before allowing practice in the facility.[123]

Medical Society Membership. Hospitals cannot require membership in a medical society.[124] Courts view such requirements as an
abdication of the hospital's responsibility to screen applications and
are concerned that medical society membership could be denied for
discriminatory reasons. A few older court decisions accepted this
criterion for private hospitals,[125] but it is doubtful that courts will

---

[119] *E.g.,* Alexander v. Rush North Shore Med. Ctr., 101 F.3d 487 (7th Cir. 1996) [no Title VII claim for revocation of privileges, not hospital employee applying common law agency test]; Shah v. Deaconess Hosp., 355 F.3d 496 (6th Cir. 2004) [no ADEA age or Title VII national origin claim for revocation of privileges, not hospital employee].

[120] *E.g.,* Menkowitz v. Pottstown Mem. Med. Ctr., 154 F.3d 113 (3d Cir. 1998) [medical staff member can claim disability discrimination under Rehabilitation Act and Title III of ADA]; Rubin v. Chilton, 359 N.J. Super. 105, 819 A.2d 22 (App. Div. 2003) [independent contractor pathologists can challenge change in pathology contractors based on age discrimination complaint under state law contract discrimination law, but not under employment law].

[121] Duane v. Government Employees Ins. Co., 37 F.3d 1036 (4th Cir. 1994), *cert. dismissed,* 515 U.S. 1101 (1995) [42 U.S.C. § 1981 prohibits private discrimination against aliens in making contracts]; *contra,* Bhandari v. First Nat'l Bank, 829 F.2d 1343 (5th Cir. 1987) (en banc), *vacated,* 429 U.S. 901 (1989), *reinstated on remand,* 887 F.2d 609 (5th Cir. 1989), *cert. denied,* 494 U.S. 1061 (1990) [with dissent by Justices White, O'Connor], but note *Bhandari* was decided before 1991 amendment to § 1981 (see discussion of amendment in Chapter 9); Annotation, *Application of 42 USCS § 1981 to private discrimination against aliens,* 99 A.L.R. FED. 835; *see also,* 8 U.S.C. § 1324b [prohibition of employment discrimination against protected noncitizens]; Espinoza v. Farah Mfg. Co., 414 U.S. 86 (1973) [Title VII does not prohibit discrimination on the basis of citizenship]; *accord,* Fortino v. Quasar Co., 950 F.2d 389 (7th Cir. 1991).

[122] 8 U.S.C. § 1324a [prohibition of employment of unauthorized aliens, with subsection (a)(4) including contracts for labor in the definition of employment].

[123] Hauptman v. Grand Manor Health Related Facility, Inc., 121 A.D.2d 151, 502 N.Y.S.2d 1012 (1st Dep't 1986).

[124] *E.g.,* Greisman v. Newcomb Hosp., 40 N.J. 389, 192 A.2d 817 (1963).

[125] *E.g.,* Natale v. Sisters of Mercy, 243 Iowa 582, 52 N.W.2d 701 (1952).

permit this criterion today except in states that do not review any private hospital criteria.

Nonstandardized Tests. A California public hospital adopted a requirement that applicants be given "such tests, oral and written, as the credentials committee shall in its discretion determine." A California appellate court invalidated the requirement because it was vague and ambiguous and provided no standards for what the examinations would be.[126] The Alaska Supreme Court also found an oral examination to be prohibited where there was no disclosure of the standards or what was inadequate in the answers.[127] Courts will probably uphold a reasonable, relevant examination uniformly given to all applicants for certain clinical privileges.

WAITING PERIOD. Hospitals may impose a reasonable waiting period before accepting another application from a person who has lost membership or privileges or had a prior application denied. In 1989, a federal appellate court upheld a hospital rule that a physician must wait one year after a summary suspension before reapplying for staff membership.[128] An Oklahoma court ruled that a public hospital could refuse to consider the application of a physician previously removed for good cause until he offered evidence that the past problems no longer existed.[129] In 2005, a federal appellate court upheld the refusal of a hospital to accept an application from a physician who had permanently resigned from the staff as part of a prior settlement.[130]

5-3 Delineation of Clinical Privileges

Hospitals must also determine the scope of practice for each physician on the medical staff. A licensed physician can act within the entire scope of medical practice without violating the medical licensing laws of some states. However, no physician is actually competent to perform all medical procedures. The hospital protects

---

[126] Martino v. Concord Comm. Hosp. Dist., 233 Cal. App. 2d 51, 43 Cal. Rptr. 255 (1st Dist. 1965).

[127] Kiester v. Humana Hosp. Alaska, Inc., 843 P.2d 1219 (Alaska 1992).

[128] Leach v. Jefferson Parish Hosp. Dist., 870 F.2d 300 (5th Cir.), *cert. denied*, 493 U.S. 822 (1989); *accord*, Huellmantel v. Greenville Hosp. Sys., 303 S.C. 549, 402 S.E.2d 489 (Ct. App. 1991) [one-year wait].

[129] Theissen v. Watonga Mun. Hosp. Bd., 550 P.2d 938 (Okla. 1976).

[130] Khouw v. Methodist Hosp., 126 Fed. Appx. 657, 2005 U.S. App. LEXIS 4206 (5th Cir. 2005) (unpub).

patients and physicians by examining physician credentials and granting clinical privileges limited to a defined scope of clinical practice. The board usually looks to the organized medical staff for expert advice in delineating clinical privileges.

A physician who acts outside the granted scope, except in an emergency, is subject to medical staff discipline, including termination of medical staff membership. However, the lack of clinical privileges is generally not negligence per se in malpractice cases. The lack of privileges may be evidence of negligence, but this determination is not automatic.[131]

There are many ways to delineate clinical privileges. The key element is that they be well-defined. Some hospitals grant clinical privileges for individual procedures. Some hospitals group broad categories of patient conditions and procedures into levels, and physicians are granted clinical privileges to perform everything in the appropriate group. Other hospitals grant clinical privileges by specialty, defining what each specialty is permitted to do. Combinations of these approaches are also used.

Some hospitals require documentation of prior performance of a specified number of certain procedures before privileges are granted for those procedures. Such requirements are generally acceptable if the numbers are reasonably attainable. In 1992, New York adopted official guidelines requiring surgeons to perform at least fifteen laparoscopies under supervision before hospitals could credential them to perform the operation independently.[132]

Hospitals should require appropriate licensure. Licensing can vary depending on the privileges sought. For example, it is appropriate for hospitals to require dentists to have a medical license before permitting them to provide anesthesia services for nondental patients.[133]

Hospitals may condition clinical privileges for certain procedures on such requirements as having (1) a consultation, (2) assistants, or (3) supervision. Physicians may be disciplined for violating these conditions. Hospitals may change their requirements so that all physicians must begin to meet new conditions. Generally, such universal changes would not be viewed as a reduction in clinical

---

[131] *E.g.,* Lingle v. Dion, 776 So. 2d 1073 (Fla. 4th DCA 2001).

[132] *Surgical injuries lead to new rule,* N.Y. TIMES, June 14, 1992, at 1.

[133] *E.g.,* Paravecchio v. Memorial Hosp., 742 P.2d 1276 (Wyo. 1987), *cert. denied,* 485 U.S. 915 (1988).

privileges; so no right to hearing or report to a data bank would be triggered. However, in the past, some courts have viewed such changes as a clinical privilege reduction, requiring that each affected staff member be given the same opportunity for a hearing as offered for other reductions.[134] When establishing a consultation requirement, hospitals should consider that at least one court has ruled that a hospital with a consultation requirement must assist physicians in obtaining consultations.[135]

5-4 Periodic Review and Reappointment

After physicians are appointed to the medical staff and granted clinical privileges, their performance should be reviewed periodically as part of the process to determine whether to grant reappointment. Both JCAHO and Medicare conditions of participation require review and reappointment.[136]

OBSERVATION DURING PROVISIONAL APPOINTMENT. The initial appointment period for most medical staffs is provisional. JCAHO authorizes, but no longer requires, a provisional period for the initial appointment.[137] During this period, the practice of the new medical staff member is observed.[138] A federal appellate court ruled that a holder of provisional privileges in an army hospital did not have a property interest in obtaining full privileges.[139] A federal district court decided that a terminated physician's initial provisional appointment did not create a property interest in the appointment.[140]

PERIODIC REVIEW. After the provisional period, hospitals and their medical staffs use several different methods to review

---

134 *E.g.*, Fahey v. Holy Family Hosp., 32 Ill. App. 3d 537, 336 N.E.2d 309 (1st Dist. 1975), *cert. denied*, 426 U.S. 936 (1976).

135 Johnson v. St. Bernard Hosp., 79 Ill. App. 3d 709, 399 N.E.2d 198 (1st Dist. 1979).

136 2005 JCAHO CAMH, Element of Performance 4, MS.4.20; 42 C.F.R. § 482.22(a)(1).

137 2005 JCAHO CAMH, Element of Performance 11, MS.4.20.

138 One court ruled that a patient cannot sue a monitoring physician who is proctoring surgery during the probationary period, Clark v. Hoek, 174 Cal. App. 3d 208, 219 Cal. Rptr. 845 (1st Dist. 1985). For use of unfavorable proctor report, *see* Nicholson v. Lucas, 21 Cal. App. 4th 1657, 26 Cal. Rptr. 2d 778 (5th Dist. 1994); Payne v. Harris Methodist H-E-B, 2000 U.S. Dist. LEXIS 21776 (N.D. Tex. magistrate recommendation), *adopted* 2001 U.S. Dist. LEXIS 815, (N.D. Tex. 2001) [probationary privileges terminated due to observations during proctoring; summary judgment for defendants based on HCQIA immunity from damages and lack of evidence of antitrust conspiracy to support injunction].

139 Randall v. United States, 30 F.3d 518 (4th Cir. 1994), *cert. denied*, 514 U.S. 1007 (1995).

140 Draghi v. County of Cook, 991 F. Supp. 1055 (N.D. Ill. 1998).

performance of individual medical staff members. Ongoing review is conducted by medical staff committees or by an administrative process established to replace the committees.

JCAHO requires hospitals to have an approach to improving organizational performance,[141] sometimes called a *performance improvement* program. JCAHO requires that relevant findings of the assessment process be considered in peer review and periodic evaluations of licensed independent practitioners.[142]

If problems are discovered through this formalized review or through day-to-day interaction, hospitals have a responsibility to determine what action is appropriate and to initiate that action. Educational efforts will often be adequate, but sometimes steps such as suspension or termination of all or some clinical privileges may be necessary.

Periodic individual review is also necessary to determine whether each medical staff member is still fulfilling the responsibilities of membership and any clinical privileges granted. Medical staff appointments are for a limited time period, usually one or two years.[143] Before appointment expiration, each member is reviewed. The review includes clinical performance, judgment, and skills; licensure; health status; compliance with hospital and medical staff policies; and fulfillment of other medical staff responsibilities, such as active involvement in assigned committees.[144] An Ohio appellate court confirmed that review and denial of reappointment could be based on factors other than patient care, such as disruptive behavior and conflicting business interests.[145] A federal appellate court confirmed that review did not have to be limited to the period after the previous review; so denial of reappointment could be based on prior misconduct.[146] Based on this review, a decision is made whether to reappoint the person to the medical staff and whether to maintain present clinical privileges or to modify them.

ECONOMIC CREDENTIALING. The aspect of economic credentialing that is most likely to arise in the periodic review context is the promotion of efficient practice.

---

[141] 2005 JCAHO CAMH, PI.1.10 - PI.3.20.

[142] *Id.*, MS.4.20, 4.40, 4.70.

[143] *Id.*, Element of Performance 4, MS.4.20 [no longer than two years].

[144] *Id.*, MS.4.20.

[145] Siegel v. St. Vincent Charity Hosp., 35 Ohio App. 3d 143, 520 N.E.2d 249 (1987).

[146] Yashon v. Hunt, 825 F.2d 1016 (6th Cir. 1987), *cert. denied*, 486 U.S. 1032 (1988); *accord* Bhatnagar v. Mid-Maine Med. Ctr., 510 A.2d 233 (Me. 1986).

Most hospitals attempt to promote cost-effective practices by physicians. One California hospital tried financial incentives in 1985,[147] but the reaction led to a federal law that forbids the use of financial incentives to control services to Medicare or Medicaid patients.[148]

Some hospitals use efficiency criteria in clinical privilege decisions. Courts have generally upheld these criteria if they are properly developed and fairly applied.[149]

ACTIVITY REQUIREMENTS. Some hospitals require medical staff members to meet minimum utilization requirements in order to be reappointed.[150] Some commentators have expressed a concern that this could be construed as a referral requirement in violation of Medicare antikickback provisions.[151] Others have pointed out that unless there is a base line of clinical activity at the hospital that it is impossible to conduct a meaningful review of the physician's continuing performance. Thus, there are good quality reasons for requiring minimum utilization. Some hospitals have adopted an activity requirement that can be satisfied by either clinical utilization or other activities, such as consultations, committee work, and teaching. In 1998, the United States Supreme Court denied review of a federal appeals court decision that upheld judgment for a hospital in an antitrust suit brought by physicians whose surgical privileges were terminated because they failed to meet surgery volume requirements.[152]

---

147 *Kickback plan by hospital hit*, AM. MED. NEWS, June 28-July 5, 1985, at 1 [Paracelsus Corp. cash reward for minimizing services to Medicare patients]; *Investigation into hospital pledged*, AM. MED. NEWS, June 28-July 5, 1985, at 34; *Plan to cut costs by rewarding doctors assailed*, N.Y. TIMES, Sept. 24, 1985, at 12; *For-profit chain admits mail fraud*, AM. MED. NEWS, Dec. 12, 1986, at 2 [mail fraud plea unrelated to physician bonus, but arose out of IG bonus investigation].

148 42 U.S.C. § 1320a-7a(b).

149 *E.g.*, Freidman v. Delaware County Mem. Hosp., 672 F. Supp. 171 (E.D. Pa. 1987), *aff'd without op.*, 849 F.2d 600, 603 (3d Cir. 1988) [overutilization of bronchoscopies]; Knapp v. Palos Comm. Hosp., 125 Ill. App. 3d 244, 465 N.E.2d 554 (1st Dist. 1984) [termination of privileges for overutilization of lung scans, other tests]; J.D. Blum, *Evaluation of medical staff using fiscal factors: Economic credentialing*, 26 J. HEALTH & HOSP. L. 65 (1993); *see also* Hassan v. Independent Practice Assocs., P.C., 698 F. Supp. 679 (E.D. Mich. 1988) [upholding decision of IPA to exclude physicians because of indications of unjustified use of tests; cost containment objectives procompetitive].

150 *E.g.*, Jackaway v. Northern Dutchess Hosp., 139 A.D.2d 496, 526 N.Y.S.2d 599 (2d Dep't 1988); *see also*, St. Louis v. Baystate Med. Ctr., Inc., 30 Mass. App. Ct.393, 568 N.E.2d 1181 (1991) [group lost exclusive contract, terminated for lack of admissions].

151 *E.g.*, J.D. Blum, *Evaluation of medical staff using fiscal factors: Economic credentialing*, 26 J. HEALTH & HOSP. L. 65, 70 (1993).

152 Kerth v. Hamot Health Found., 989 F. Supp. 691 (W.D. Pa. 1997), *aff'g without op.* 159 F.3d 1351 (3d Cir. 1998), *cert. denied*, 525 U.S. 1055 (1998).

ABUSIVE BEHAVIOR. Some physicians are occasionally physically or verbally abusive of staff, patients, or visitors.[153] Hospitals need to take prompt action to investigate reports of such actions and take appropriate action when the reports are substantiated. Sometimes peer counseling is effective. Sometimes it is necessary to terminate membership on the medical staff. In some circumstances, hospitals can be liable for harassment of hospital staff by medical staff members.[154]

DECLINING CAPABILITY. Difficult situations sometimes arise when a physician does not recognize declining capabilities. Often physicians will recognize changes when they are approached tactfully and will agree to adjust their scope of practice to fit their capabilities. Often this can be done at the time of reappointment. Some hospitals have an emeritus staff category. If the physician will not agree to needed adjustments, the hospital and medical staff have the duty to protect patients by reducing the physician's clinical privileges to the appropriate scope.

LIABILITY. Failure to review performance and take appropriate action can result in hospital liability. For example, a California appellate court ruled that a hospital could be liable for failing to review periodically the performance of those persons granted clinical privileges.[155] However, at least one state has passed a statute that bars hospital liability for professional services of professionals who are not employees or agents; so there is no hospital liability in that state for negligent review.[156]

In an unusual case in 2003, a Michigan hospital pled guilty to a federal criminal charge of fraud for failing to take credentialing actions against a physician who was performing many unnecessary procedures.[157]

---

[153] *E.g.,* Ross v. Beaumont Hosp., 687 F. Supp. 1115 (E.D. Mich. 1988) [verbal abuse by physician]; *Nurse gets $65,000 for a pulled ponytail,* N.Y. TIMES, July 24, 1988, 10 [out of court settlement with doctor]; D. Adams, *Staff less tolerant of rude doctors,* AM. MED. NEWS, Sept. 20, 2004, 1.

[154] *E.g.,* Dunn v. Washington County Hosp., 2005 U.S. App. LEXIS 24660 (7th Cir.); K. Hattie, *Nurses accuse doc; Eight say he sexually harassed them at B'klyn hospital,* NEWSDAY (New York, N.Y.), Aug. 16, 2001, A5 [EEOC filed lawsuit against hospital].

[155] Elam v. College Park Hosp., 132 Cal. App. 3d 332, 183 Cal. Rptr. 156 (4th Dist. 1982); *see also,* Annotation, *Hospital liability for negligence in failing to review or supervise treatment given by doctor, or to require consultation,* 12 A.L.R. 4TH 57.

[156] McVay v. Rich, 255 Kan. 371, 874 P.2d 641 (1994), *aff'g,* 18 Kan. App. 2d 746, 859 P. 2d 399 (1993).

[157] U.S. v. United Mem. Hosp., No. 1:01-CR-238 (W.D. Mich. pleas entered Jan. 8, 2003).

5-5 Modification and Termination of Privileges

Clinical privileges must sometimes be modified or terminated because of changes in the physician's capabilities, violation of hospital or medical staff policies, changes in hospital standards, or other reasons. When physicians challenge modification or termination of privileges, they challenge the adequacy of procedures followed and the reasons given for the action. Procedural issues are discussed in the due process section of this chapter.

Evidence of poor performance or violation of policies should be carefully reviewed before deciding to take adverse action. The hospital should be prepared to justify the action in court.

MEDICAL RECORDS. Clinical privileges are frequently temporarily suspended when physicians fail to complete medical records properly within time limits established by hospital policy.[158] Suspension of admitting privileges usually continues until overdue records are completed. Physicians who do not have time to complete records do not have time to accept responsibility for additional patients. Courts have generally upheld disciplinary actions for failure to complete records.[159] In 1998, a federal appellate court upheld suspending privileges of a physician who had removed a portion of the medical record of her own care until she returned it.[160]

STANDARDS. Some physicians have challenged adverse actions by claiming that the standards by which they were judged were too vague. Vague standards can violate due process by failing to give notice of what conduct is expected or prohibited. However, courts have generally upheld actions taken on the basis of subjective standards when the standards are applied in a reasonable way.[161] For example, the Nevada Supreme Court upheld a clinical privilege termination based on the general standard of "unprofessional conduct."[162] The court recognized that it was not feasible to specify the variety of unprofessional conduct. The physician had not used gloves when touching a spinal needle before using it and had appeared for surgery in no condition to perform it, requiring cancellation of the

---

158 *E.g., Hospital suspends 300 Tampa doctors slow on paperwork*, MIAMI [FL] HERALD, May 18, 1988, 1A.
159 *E.g.,* Peterson v. Tucson Gen. Hosp., 114 Ariz. 66, 559 P.2d 186 (Ct. App. 1976).
160 Wayne v. Genesis Med. Ctr., 140 F.3d 1145 (8th Cir. 1998).
161 *E.g.,* Jackson v. Fulton-DeKalb Hosp. Auth., 423 F. Supp. 1000 (N.D. Ga. 1976), *aff'd without op.,* 559 F.2d 1214 (5th Cir. 1977).
162 Moore v. Board of Trustees, 88 Nev. 207, 495 P.2d 605, *cert. denied,* 409 U.S. 879 (1972).

surgery. The court found that the standard was properly applied. A New Jersey appellate court affirmed a physician's suspension based on a bylaws provision that permitted suspension "for cause."[163] The physician had negligently treated a patient. The court found sufficient evidence, so that "for cause" was not too vague. The situation leading to suspension demonstrated that all grounds for suspension could not be specified in advance.

In 1999, a federal appellate court ruled that it was necessary to have a specific rule addressing a particular deficiency before a hospital could take action against a physician.[164] The court reversed a lower court decision that had enjoined limitations in clinical privileges of a surgeon with a high mortality rate based on the absence of hospital rule setting a mortality rate as a standard.

MODIFYING STANDARDS. When hospitals modify standards, clinical privileges of some physicians may be reduced. Reasonable changes will generally be upheld. The Ohio Supreme Court upheld a hospital's new requirement that a physician be board certified, be board eligible, be a fellow in the American College of Surgeons, or have ten years experience to qualify for major surgical privileges.[165] An Illinois appellate court refused to enjoin a hospital's new requirement that surgeons with general surgery clinical privileges consult with a gynecologist before doing major gynecological surgery. The court ruled that the physician was entitled to a hearing concerning the reasonableness of the rule.[166] Some courts have permitted suits concerning the application of new rules.[167]

When a New Mexico hospital adopted a new rule forbidding all hip-pinning procedures because it lacked the proper equipment, the New Mexico Supreme Court ruled against a physician who lost his hip-pinning privileges.[168]

CHANGING TO A FULL-TIME OR EXCLUSIVE STAFF ARRANGEMENT. Generally, courts have been supportive of hospitals that change staffing arrangements. When a full-time staff approach is adopted, generally the privileges of those who choose not to be full-

---

[163] Pagliaro v. Point Pleasant Hosp., No. A-3932-75 (N.J. Super. Ct. App. Div. Jan. 19, 1979), *as discussed in* 12 Hosp. L., Apr. 1979, at 5.

[164] Sokol v. Akron Gen. Med. Ctr., 173 F.3d 1026 (6th Cir. 1999); *see also* Yashon v. Hunt, 825 F.2d 1016 (6th Cir. 1987) [state hospital not limited to previously memorialized standards to review physician].

[165] Khan v. Suburban Comm. Hosp., 45 Ohio St. 2d 39, 340 N.E.2d 398 (1976).

[166] Fahey v. Holy Family Hosp., 32 Ill. App. 3d 537, 336 N.E.2d 309 (1975).

[167] *E.g.*, Cooper v. Delaware Valley Med. Ctr 539 Pa. 620, 654 A.2d 547 (1995).

[168] Clough v. Adventist Health Sys., 780 P.2d 627 (N.M. 1989).

time can be terminated.[169] When an exclusive contract approach is adopted, generally the privileges of those who do not get the full-time contract can be terminated, especially if they had a fair opportunity to get the exclusive contract. The Maine Supreme Court upheld a hospital that terminated an emergency medicine contract with a group, offered the physicians individual direct contracts, and terminated those who chose not to sign.[170]

There are exceptions where substantial amounts have been awarded to physicians who are excluded,[171] but generally there are extenuating circumstances of misconduct beyond the termination of privileges.[172] These changes in staffing arrangements need to be carefully planned to minimize the risk of successful legal challenge.

ECONOMIC CREDENTIALING. Some hospitals try to remove physicians who are competing economically with the hospital.[173] Examples of such competition include investing in a competing specialty hospital or ambulatory surgery center. There have been a few cases where trial courts have enjoined removal during litigation, but generally the right of the hospital to exclude competing physicians has been upheld.[174]

In one of the few cases where physicians obtained a temporary injunction, an Arkansas hospital had adopted a policy not to grant privileges to physicians who had an ownership interest in a competing

---

169 *E.g.,* Katz v. Children's Hosp. Corp., 33 Mass. Ct. App. 574, 602 N.E.2d 598 (1992).
170 Bartley v. Eastern Me. Med. Ctr., 617 A.2d 1020 (Me. 1992).
171 *E.g,* B. McCormick, *Hospital loses over economic credentialing,* AM. MED. NEWS, Mar. 28, 1994, at 4 [radiologist awarded $12.7 million due to exclusive contract].
172 *E.g.,* American Med. Int'l v. Scheller, 590 So. 2d 947 (Fla. 4th DCA 1991), *rev. denied,* 602 So. 2d 533 (Fla. 1992).
173 *See* R. Abelson, *Hospitals battle for-profit groups for patients,* N.Y. TIMES, Oct. 30, 2002, C1 [doctors who invest in other hospitals losing privileges]; *Idaho doctors who own specialty facility sue over lost privileges at other hospital,* H.L.R., Mar. 11, 2004, 363 [Biddulph v. HCA Inc., No. CV-04-1219 (Idaho Dist Ct. filed Mar. 2004)]; K. Vogt, *Doctor-investors could lose Ohio hospital privileges,* AM. MED. NEWS, Jan. 12, 2004, 18 [community hospitals terminating privileges for doctors who invested in specialty hospital].
174 Huhta v. Children's Hosp. of Phila., 1994 U.S. Dist. LEXIS 7327 (E.D. Pa.) [dismissal of antitrust suit by former chief of division of pediatric cardiology who had resigned to open a multispecialty group practice at competing hospital after denied access to certain hospital-owned pediatric cardiology equipment, facilities]; Tarabishi v. McAlester Reg. Hosp., 951 F.2d 1558 (10th Cir. 1991), *cert. denied,* 505 U.S. 1206 (1992) [rejecting antitrust challenge to termination after attempted to open outpatient surgical clinic]; Katz v. Children's Hosp. Corp., 33 Mass. App. Ct. 574, 602 N.E.2d 598 (1992) [hospital may restrict subspecialties to persons who practice full time at hospital]; Walborn v. UHHS, No. CV-02-479572 (Ohio Com. Pl. June 16, 2003) [court upheld policy forbidding material financial relationship with competing hospital]; Berasi v. Ohio Health, No. 04CVA-03-2406 (Ohio County Ct. Com. Pl. Mar. 3, 2004) [court denied restraining order to physicians who lost privileges for investing in competing specialty hospital].

hospital. Cardiologists who had an ownership interest in a competing heart hospital were denied renewal of their privileges. They first sued in federal court, but the court found it had no jurisdiction and dismissed the case. A similar case was then filed in state court. The trial judge issued a temporary injunction, and the hospital could not enforce its policy against the suing doctors. On appeal the Arkansas Supreme Court reversed, finding the trial court had not adequately evaluated the likelihood of the physicians succeeding on the merits, which is one of the criteria for a temporary injunction. However, the court left the injunction in place while the trail court performs the required evaluation.[175]

Hospitals have taken action against physicians for economic issues other than competition. In one case, a federal court rejected an antitrust challenge to removal of a physician from the emergency on-call schedule allegedly for charging excessive fees.[176]

HUMAN IMMUNODEFICIENCY VIRUS (HIV) AND ACQUIRED IMMUNE DEFICIENCY SYNDROME (AIDS). Hospitals have generally been upheld in restricting privileges of surgeons who test positive for HIV.[177] The Pennsylvania Supreme Court permitted a hospital to inform patients they may have been exposed to the virus in surgery by a HIV-positive surgeon.[178]

SUBSTANCE ABUSE. The difficult situation of a physician impaired by substance abuse has become easier to address because

---

[175] *E.g., Baptist Hospital temporarily enjoined from using economic credentialing policy*, H.L.R, Apr. 1, 2004, 455 [Murphy v. Baptist Health, No. CV2004-2002 (Ark. Cir. Ct. Pulaski County temp. injunction Mar. 22, 2004)]; Baptist Health v. Murphy, 2005 Ark. LEXIS 354 (reversing trial court, remanding for further evaluation, but allowing temporary injunction to stay in place).

[176] Mamakos v. Huntington Hosp., 653 F. Supp. 1447 (E.D. N.Y. 1987).

[177] *E.g.,* Estate of Behringer v. Medical Ctr. at Princeton, 249 N.J. Super. 597, 592 A.2d 1251 (1991) [upholding suspension of surgical privileges of physician with AIDS]; Scoles v. Mercy Health Corp., 887 F. Supp. 765 (E.D. Pa. 1994) [HIV-positive surgeon's practice justifiably restricted]; *Court: Hospital may bar HIV-positive doctor from surgery*, AM. MED. NEWS, Jan. 16, 1995, at 11 [Scoles may pursue claims of wrongful removal from occupational programs where he did not perform invasive procedures]; Doe v. University of Md. Med. Sys. Corp., 50 F.3d 1261 (4th Cir. 1995) [affirming judgment in favor of hospital on claims under Rehabilitation Act, ADA by resident suspended from surgery when tested HIV positive; was offered nonsurgical residency which he refused; court ruled he posed significant risk to patients that could not be eliminated by reasonable accommodation; hospital may elect to restrict activities of only those known to be HIV positive].

[178] *In re* Milton S. Hershey Med. Ctr., 535 Pa. 9, 634 A.2d 159 (1993); *but see* Tolman v. Doe, 988 F. Supp. 582 (E.D. Va. 1997) [former medical partner liable for defamation for letters sent to patients warning them of HIV status of physician].

of the availability of state or medical society programs for rehabilitation[179] and the growing awareness that the first approach should be to promote rehabilitation. Most physicians attempt to cooperate with these efforts, including temporary reductions in clinical privileges as necessary, to protect patients. Unfortunately, it is sometimes extremely difficult to remain rehabilitated; so the hospital must decide how many rehabilitation opportunities to give. If rehabilitation fails, permanent action must eventually be taken to preserve acceptable standards of patient care.

OTHER HEALTH ISSUES. When health status interferes with the ability to practice or perform other medical staff functions, appropriate action needs to occur. There is still some disagreement on the extent to which the ADA applies to nonemployee medical staff members.[180] However, even where the ADA applies, suspension or termination of physicians has been upheld for resulting behaviors that threaten patient care or institutional operations.[181] In 1998, a federal appellate court ruled that it was not an ADA violation to fire a physician with attention deficit disorder. His short-term memory problems led to problems in patient records, and he could not perform the administrative task of his job.[182] Another federal appellate court upheld denial of reinstatement of the terminated clinical privileges of an internist who had been stealing and tampering with internal mail in other physicians' mailboxes.[183] His diagnosis was a bipolar disorder, and his physician stated that his conduct was a symptom of his disorder. The intolerable conduct and continuing concerns with his behavior and honesty justified the denial of reinstatement.

---

179 *E.g.,* Fla. Stat. § 455.261; Goetz v. Noble, 652 So. 2d 1203 (Fla. 4th DCA 1995) [absolute immunity from state law claims, qualified immunity from federal civil rights claims for medical director of program under § 455.261].

180 *E.g.,* Menkowitz v. Pottstown Mem. Med. Ctr., 154 F.3d 113 (3d Cir. 1998) [nonemployee physician permitted to sue under public accommodations provisions of ADA].

181 *E.g.,* Hong v. Temple University, 2000 U.S. Dist. LEXIS 7301 (E.D. Pa.) [employer did not violate ADA by terminating anesthesiologist who was unable to concentrate or focus due to pain behind his eye, no reasonable accommodation would allow performing essential functions of job].

182 Robertson v. Neuromedical Ctr., 161 F.3d 292 (5th Cir. 1998), *cert. denied,* 526 U.S. 1098 (1999); *see also* Brohm v. JH Properties, Inc., 947 F. Supp. 299 (D. Ky. 1996), *aff'd,* 149 F.3d 517 (6th Cir. 1998) [no state law disability discrimination claim for physician discharged for sleeping during surgical procedures, notwithstanding claim of sleep apnea].

183 Landefield v. Marion Gen. Hosp., 994 F.2d 1178 (6th Cir. 1993).

The ADA may apply in some cases to limit otherwise permissible actions.[184] Thus, it is prudent to consider reasonable accommodations even where they may not be legally required.

FREE SPEECH IN PUBLIC HOSPITALS. Public hospitals usually cannot terminate clinical privileges because of a physician's public criticism of the quality of care. Federal courts have found such criticism to be protected by the First Amendment right of free speech.[185] However, physicians cannot insulate themselves from adverse action by public criticism. In 1986, a federal appellate court upheld the dismissal of a physician who had criticized the hospital.[186] The hospital convinced the court the dismissal was due to patient care concerns, not the public criticism.

Public criticism can also exceed the bounds of protected speech. In 1989, a federal appellate court ruled that a physician's caustic personal attacks were disruptive and unprotected; so termination was justified.[187] In a 1992 hospital case, a federal appellate court applied the general rule that public speech is protected only when it addresses a matter of public concern.[188]

REPORTING REQUIREMENTS. The Health Care Quality Improvement Act of 1986 (HCQIA) requires that all hospitals that want the benefit of the liability limitation provisions of HCQIA must report many of their adverse medical staff actions to the National Practitioner Data Bank (NPDB).[189] The first physician challenge to

---

[184] *E.g.,* Mark v. Burke Rehab. Hosp., 1997 U.S. Dist. LEXIS 5154 (S.D. N.Y. 1997) [deny dismissal of ADA claim that cardiac physician with cancer was fired for refusal to postpone chemotherapy session]; Hennefent v. Mid Dakota Clinic. P.C., 164 F.3d 419 (8th Cir. 1998) [dismissal of challenge to termination of employed physician where he refused to report for evaluation of his present disability].

[185] *E.g.,* Ulrich v. San Francisco, 308 F.3d 968 (9th Cir. 2002) [physician resigned to protest layoffs while under investigation; permitted to challenge denial of request to rescind resignation; possible retaliation for protected speech]; Malak v. Associated Physicians, Inc., 784 F.2d 277 (7th Cir. 1986); Schwartzman v. Valenzuela, 846 F.2d 1209 (9th Cir. 1988) [jury question whether discharge was retaliation]; Cohen v. County of Cook, 677 F. Supp. 547 (N.D. Ill. 1988).

[186] Zaky v. Veterans Admin., 793 F.2d 832 (7th Cir.), *cert. denied,* 479 U.S. 937 (1986); *accord* Setliff v. Memorial Hosp., 850 F.2d 1384 (10th Cir. 1988).

[187] Smith v. Cleburne County Hosp., 870 F.2d 1375 (8th Cir.), *cert. denied,* 493 U.S. 847 (1989).

[188] DeMarco v. Rome Hosp., 952 F.2d 661 (2d Cir. 1992).

[189] 42 U.S.C. § 11133; 45 C.F.R. pt. 60; U.S. Dep't of HHS, National Practitioner Data Bank Guidebook (1990); I.S. Rothschild, *Operation of National Practitioner Data Bank,* 25 J. Health & Hosp. L. 225 (1992); American Dental Ass'n v. Shalala, 303 U.S. App. D.C. 231, 3 F.3d 445 (1993) [HCQIA does not require reports of payments by individual practitioners]; N.J. Schendel, *Banking on confidentiality: Should consumers be allowed access to the National Practitioner Data Bank?* 27 J. Health & Hosp. L. 289 (1994); OIG Report: *Hospital reporting to the National Practitioner Data Bank,* Feb. 1995.

the data bank was dismissed in 1994.[190] A federal appellate court reversed an injunction of reporting a medical staff action.[191]

When challenged, the U.S. Department of Health and Human Services must review the appropriateness of maintaining a report in the NPDB and its content. The NPDB has been ordered to remove at least one report.[192] In 2004, a federal district court ruled that the federal Privacy Act applied when the NPDB reviewed a challenge to the content of a report.[193]

There are separate state reporting requirements that are sometimes different from HCQIA requirements.[194]

In 1985, a federal court of appeals ruled that a hospital could not be sued for defamation for filing a required report of suspension of a medical staff member.[195] The hospital was found immune because the report was mandated. In 1994, another federal appellate court decided that a hospital could be liable for defamation for submitting a report that it knew to be false. In that case, a medical chart had been submitted as evidence of a patient incident with knowledge that the reported physician had not been involved in the care of the patient. The court found that bad faith destroyed the qualified immunity.[196] Similarly, in 1996, a federal appellate court found that a hospital and its staff were not entitled to HCQIA immunity when a physician's privileges were revoked based on a review of the med-

190 Doe v. United States D.H.H.S., 871 F. Supp. 808 (E.D. Pa. 1994) [no private right of action under HCQIA, no liberty or property interest in having mail fraud conviction excluded from data bank]; *see also* Randall v. United States, 30 F.3d 518 (4th Cir. 1994), *cert. denied*, 514 U.S. 1107 (1995) [entry in national data base that physician's privileges had been restricted due to incompetence did not deprive of constitutional liberty interest].
191 Sokol v. Akron Gen. Med. Ctr., 173 F.3d 1026 (6th Cir. 1999).
192 Simkins v. Shalala, 999 F. Supp. 106 (D. D.C. 1998).
193 Doe v. Thompson, 332 F. Supp. 2d 124 (D. D.C. 2004).
194 *E.g.*, FLA. STAT. §§ 395.011(7), 395.0115(4); Weirton Med. Ctr., Inc. v. West Va. Bd. of Med., 450 S.E.2d 661 (W. Va. 1994) [hospital must report disciplinary action against physician within sixty days of completion of formal disciplinary proceedings, again after completion of legal action, if any, but hospital fine of $7,500 reversed due to ambiguity in statute]; Medical Society of N.J. v. Mottola, 320 F. Supp. 2d 254 (D. N.J. 2004).
195 Cuatico v. Idaho Falls Consol. Hosps., Inc., 753 F.2d 1081 (9th Cir. 1985) (mem.), *as described in* 18 HOSP. L., Mar. 1985, at 6; *accord* Dorn v. Mendelzon, 196 Cal. App. 3d 933, 242 Cal. Rptr. 259 (1st Dist. 1987).
196 Purgess v. Sharrock, 33 F.3d 134 (2d Cir. 1994); *MD gets $5.1 million from hospital in defamation suit*, AM. MED. NEWS, Sept. 12, 1994, at 13; *see also* Wheeler v. Methodist Hosp., 95 S.W.3d 628 (Tex. App. 2002) [reversing hospital summary judgment in defamation claim for NPDB report, MD allowed more discovery to establish malice].

ical records of only two patients, and an incorrect report, based on that review, was submitted to the NPDB.[197]

Almost any voluntary or involuntary adverse action that is taken while a physician is under investigation, other than exoneration, must be reported. This has resulted in physicians challenging the determination that they were under investigation. Courts have generally rejected such challenges and found that reports were properly made.[198] However, in one case a federal judge found that a physician had not been under the investigation at the time of the reported event and that the Department of Health and Human Services should not have accepted the report.[199] The judge ordered the report to be removed from the NPBD.

When reports are required, the hospital no longer has the option of entering an agreement that the physician will resign and the hospital will not disclose the circumstances. The enforceability of such agreements is questionable anyway. In 1989, a federal appellate court ruled that a hospital was not liable for disclosure because the nondisclosure agreement was against public policy.[200] However, it is best not to make any statements concerning nondisclosure. In 1993, the West Virginia Supreme Court ruled that a physician could sue a hospital for reporting to another hospital that his privileges had been summarily suspended, even though they had been so suspended.[201] The physician claimed that he had voluntarily resigned after the suspension pursuant to a promise that his privileges would be reinstated, the suspension would be expunged, and no reports

---

[197] Brown v. Presbyterian Healthcare Servs., 101 F.3d 1324 (10th Cir. 1996), *cert. denied*, 520 U.S. 1181 (1997); *see also* Christenson v. Mount Carmel Health, 112 Ohio App. 3d 161, 678 N.E.2d 255 (1996) [abuse of discretion to deny privileges, report denial without notice of concerns, opportunity to respond].

[198] *E.g.*, Azmat v. Shalala, 186 F. Supp. 2d 744 (W.D. Ky. 2001), *aff'd sub nom.*, Azmat v. Thompson, 49 Fed. Appx. 521 (6th Cir. 2002) [unpub]; Omar v. Jewish Hosp. Healthcare Servs., 2004 Ky. App. LEXIS 50 [physician not entitled to declaratory judgment that he was not under investigation; committee review of five cases due to quality concerns was an investigation].

[199] Simkins v. Shalala, 999 F. Supp. 106 (D. D.C. 1998).

[200] Walton v. Jennings Comm. Hosp., 875 F.2d 1317 (7th Cir. 1989), *appeal after remand*, 999 F.2d 277 (7th Cir. 1993) [affirming judgment for defendants]; *accord* Taylor v. Kennestone Hosp, Inc., 266 Ga. App. 14, 596 S.E.2d 179 (2004) [agreement not to report to NPDB against public policy]; Mills v. Rhode Island Hosp., 828 A.2d 526 (R.I. 2003) [confidentiality agreement with MD cannot bar disclosure of application pursuant to subpoena from medical licensing board]; Salaymeh v. St. Vincent Mem. Hosp. Corp., 706 F. Supp. 643 (C.D. Ill. 1989).

[201] Garrison v. Herbert J. Thomas Mem. Hosp. Ass'n, 190 W.Va. 214, 438 S.E.2d 6 (1993); *see also* Keszler v. Memorial Med. Ctr., 105 S.W.3d 122 (Tex. App. 2003) [hospital can be sued for breach of contract to expunge records of medical staff matters].

would be made to anyone. The court ruled (1) the agreement would not be against public policy if it were in recognition that the initial suspension was improper and (2) the physician should have an opportunity to prove that was the basis for the agreement.

It is not uncommon to consult with the physician concerning the content of the NPDB report.[202] This is acceptable as long as the final report is accurate and contains the required information.

There is a procedure for updating and correcting reports. In some jurisdictions, there may be liability to the physician for failure to submit timely updates and corrections.[203]

5-6 Review Procedures for Adverse Actions

Public hospitals are generally required to provide review procedures that satisfy due process requirements. In most states, private hospitals are not required to provide the review processes that public hospitals must provide. States that require private hospitals to provide a fair procedure may not include all elements discussed in this section.

EXCEPTIONS TO FULL REVIEW PROCEDURES. In some circumstances, full review procedures are not required.

Applicants. In many jurisdictions, applicants are not entitled to the same review procedures as medical staff members.

Some courts find that the physician's rights are derived from medical staff membership. Because an applicant is not yet a member, the applicant does not have a legal right to make claims on the organization. In these jurisdictions, only actions during the appointment period are viewed as interfering with the rights of physicians, triggering a right to internal procedural review.

The rights of applicants for reappointment also vary, with some jurisdictions treating them the same as applicants for initial appointment and some recognizing entitlement to some review but not the full procedures available to physicians who are being disciplined during an appointment period. The scope of rights often depends on whether the hospital has created an entitlement to reappointment. Some jurisdictions will find that some acts of the

---

202 *E.g.,* Khouw v. Methodist Hosp., 126 Fed. Appx. 657, 2005 U.S. App. LEXIS 4206 (5th Cir. 2005) (unpub).

203 *E.g.,* Wuchenich v. Shenandoah Mem. Hosp., 2000 U.S. App. LEXIS (4th Cir.) (unpub).

hospital have created an entitlement to reappointment, so that there is a right to a review process when reappointment is denied. Absent such an entitlement, in some jurisdictions, hospitals may not be as vulnerable to challenges under federal law when they deny reappointment rather than modify or terminate privileges during an appointment term.[204] In those jurisdictions, hospitals may wait until the reappointment process to address problems with physicians that do not involve immediate risks to patients.

JCAHO requires a fair hearing for applicants and members but does not require the procedures to be identical.[205]

Some medical staff bylaws specify that applicants do not have procedural rights. Unless a hospital is in a state that recognizes this difference and the difference is specified in the bylaws, it is prudent to follow the same procedures for both applicants and members.

Substantial Compliance. Most courts do not require technical compliance with every detail of the bylaws procedure. Substantial compliance is usually sufficient.[206] However, it is best practice to seek to achieve technical compliance with the bylaws to reduce the number of issues that need to be addressed when adverse actions are challenged.

Informal Reviews. Most courts recognize that review procedures do not have to be provided during the informal reviews of potential medical staff problems that precede the decision whether to initiate formal proceedings.[207] Although seeking information from the affected physician early in the review is almost always helpful, the physician does not have a legal right to notice and an opportunity to present information until formal action is initiated.

It is best not to call these preliminary reviews "investigations" because this can create confusion concerning whether the physician is "under investigation" for purposes of National Practitioner Data Bank reporting requirements.

---

[204] *E.g.,* Jit Kim Lim v. Central DuPage Hosp., 871 F.2d 644 (7th Cir. 1989).

[205] 2005 JCAHO CAMH, MS.1.20; Element of Performance 1, MS.4.50.

[206] *E.g.,* Houston v. Intermountain Health Care, Inc., 933 P.2d 403 (Utah App. 1997); Owens v. New Britain Gen. Hosp., 229 Conn. 592, 643 A.2d 233 (1994); Everhart v. Jefferson Parish Hosp. Dist., 757 F.2d 1567 (5th Cir. 1985); *see also* Evans v. Perry, 944 F. Supp. 2 (D. D.C. 1996) [failure to follow Army regulation, no prejudice to gynecologist whose privileges were restricted at Army community hospital].

[207] *E.g.,* Bryant v. Tenet, Inc., 969 S.W.2d 923 (Tenn. App. 1997) [no right to attorney during informal review]; Setliff v. Memorial Hosp., 850 F.2d 1384 (10th Cir. 1988); Mathews v. Lancaster Gen. Hosp., 87 F.3d 624 (3d Cir. 1996) [not necessary to follow HCQIA during informal review to qualify for immunity].

Seriousness of Actions. The full scope of review procedures is usually required only for actions that directly affect the physician's practice, such as decisions concerning the scope of clinical privileges. A New York court ruled that removal from an administrative position and termination of blocked operating room time did not entitle the physician to review.[208] A federal district court held that a change in an anesthesiologist's case assignments did not trigger a right to review.[209] However, in some states, less serious actions may trigger review rights. For example, a California court ruled that being on the call roster was a clinical privilege, so that removal entitled the physician to a hearing.[210]

Censure usually does not entitle the physician to a hearing.[211]

Waiver by Contract. Even in public hospitals, procedural rights can be waived by contract. Thus, exclusive and other contracts can provide for termination of privileges without a hearing when the contract terminates or other specified events occur.[212]

Arbitration. An alternate procedure that some physicians and hospitals may consider is arbitration.[213] HCQIA authorizes the alternative of using an arbitrator.[214] Some state laws limit the use of arbitration. The Federal Arbitration Act preempts these state laws when the contract affects interstate commerce. Some courts have found that some contracts with physicians affect interstate commerce and have applied federal law to enforce arbitration agreements.[215]

HEALTH CARE QUALITY IMPROVEMENT ACT. HCQIA[216] describes procedures for hospital medical staff decisions. HCQIA is a defense from liability. It does not provide a new basis for private suits against the hospital or peer review committees.[217] Hospitals are not required to follow HCQIA procedures, but if the procedures

---

208 Hanna v. Board of Trustees, 243 A.D.2d 362, 663 N.Y.S.2d180 (1st Dept. 1997).
209 Vakharia v. Swedish Covenant Hosp., 987 F. Supp. 633 (N.D. Ill. 1997).
210 Bergeron v. Desert Hosp. Corp., 221 Cal. App. 3d 146, 270 Cal. Rptr. 397 (4th Dist. 1990).
211 *E.g.,* Chaudhry v. Prince George's County, 626 F. Supp. 448 (D. Md. 1985); Hoberman v. Lock Haven Hosp., 377 F. Supp. 1178 (M.D. Pa. 1974) [hearing not required for censure]; *contra* Grodjesk v. Jersey City Med. Ctr., 135 N.J. Super. 393, 343 A.2d 489 (Ch. Div. 1975) [censure requires notice, opportunity to respond].
212 *E.g.,* Bloom v. Hennepin County, 783 F. Supp. 418 (D. Minn. 1992).
213 *E.g.,* International Med. Ctrs., Inc. v. Sabates, 498 So. 2d 1292 (Fla. 3d DCA 1986) [confirming arbitrator award for physician].
214 42 U.S.C. § 11112(a).
215 *E.g.,* Thornton v. Trident Med. Ctr., L.L.C., 357 S.C. 91, 592 S.E.2d 50 (App. 2003).
216 Pub. L. No. 99-660, 100 Stat. 3784 (1986) (*codified at* 42 U.S.C. §§ 11101-11152).
217 *E.g.,* Wayne v. Genesis Med. Ctr., 140 F.3d 1145 (8th Cir. 1998); Bok v. Mutual Assurance, 119 F.3d 927 (11th Cir. 1997); Hancock v. Blue Cross-Blue Shield, 21 F.3d 373 (10th Cir. 1994).

are followed, HCQIA provides protection from monetary liability in private suits, except under civil rights laws. There is no protection from suits seeking injunctions or from civil rights suits. The antitrust immunity is only from private suits; the state or federal attorney general may still sue. However, most suits concerning medical staff matters are private suits; so this protection can be significant. HCQIA states that the "immunity" applies only when the peer review action was taken "in the reasonable belief that the action was in furtherance of quality health care" and "after a reasonable effort to obtain the facts of the matter." There is a statutory presumption that this standard is met,[218] and most courts apply an objective standard to determine whether the reasonableness standards have been met.[219] So it is not easy for a physician to defeat HCQIA immunity.[220]

In 1996, a federal appellate court held that HCQIA procedures were needed only for "professional review actions" that affected clinical privileges in order to qualify for HCQIA immunity; "professional review activities," such as fact-finding or decisions to monitor, did not have to follow the HCQIA procedures.[221]

In 2003, a District of Columbia court ruled that if HCQIA procedures were followed when conditions were imposed that it was not necessary to follow them again when automatically terminating the physician for violating the conditions.[222]

HCQIA protects hospitals from monetary liability, not from suit. Thus, a refusal by a trial judge to dismiss such a suit cannot be appealed. The hospital must wait until after there is a final judgment against the hospital to obtain appellate review.[223]

---

[218] 42 U.S.C. § 11112(b)(3)(A)(i).

[219] *E.g.,* Meyers v. Columbia/HCA Healthcare Corp., 341 F.3d 461 (6th Cir. 2003); Mathews v. Lancaster Gen. Hosp., 87 F.3d 624 (3d Cir. 1996) [since test is objective, bad faith is immaterial]; Bryan v. James E. Holmes Reg. Med Ctr., 33 F.3d 1318 (11th Cir. 1994), *cert. denied,* 514 U.S. 1019 (1995) [judge, not jury, determines immunity; jury verdict for physician reversed based on HCQIA immunity].

[220] *E.g.,* Meyers v. Columbia/HCA Healthcare Corp., 341 F.3d 461 (6th Cir. 2003); Brader v. Allegheny Gen. Hosp., 167 F.3d 832 (3d Cir. 1999); Wayne v. Genesis Med. Ctr., 140 F.3d 1156 (8th Cir. 1998); Imperial v. Suburban Hosp. Ass'n, Inc., 37 F.3d 1026 (4th Cir. 1994); Smith v. Ricks, 31 F.3d 1478 (9th Cir. 1994), *cert. denied,* 514 U.S. 1035 (1995) [peer review proceedings need not be like trial]; Meyer v. Sunrise Hosp., 22 P.3d 1142 (Nev. 2001).

[221] Mathews v. Lancaster Gen. Hosp., 87 F.3d 624 (3d Cir. 1996).

[222] Ali v. Medstar Health, 2003 (D.C. Super. LEXIS 32).

[223] *E.g.,* Decker v. IHC Hosp., Inc., 982 F.2d 433 (10th Cir. 1992), *cert. denied,* 509 U.S. 924 (1993); Manion v. Evans, 986 F.2d 1036 (6th Cir. 1993), *cert. denied,* 510 U.S. 818 (1993).

Many hospitals have availed themselves of the protection of HCQIA. In 1988, an Indiana court authorized a hospital to substitute HCQIA procedures for the procedures in its bylaws without first amending the bylaws.[224] It is not clear whether other courts will allow this substitution. However, hospitals and affected physicians can agree to change procedures, and some physicians may agree to HCQIA procedures. Refusal to agree may be a waiver by the physician in some contexts.

SUMMARY ACTION. Restrictions on clinical privileges may be imposed without prior due process procedures when there is potential immediate risk to patient well-being.[225] Although review procedures must usually be followed before adverse action is taken, courts recognize that summary action can be necessary and appropriate. For example, the Alaska Supreme Court ruled that the fair hearing could be conducted within a reasonable time after the summary suspension of clinical privileges when there was immediate risk to patients.[226]

Courts have issued injunctions prohibiting summary suspension when the risk is not sufficiently immediate.[227] Courts will reconsider an injunction if the physician's conduct during the injunction indicates that summary suspension is needed.[228]

Summary suspension without a hearing is also appropriate when a physician ceases to be licensed to practice medicine, ceases to have a valid DEA registration to prescribe controlled substances, or ceases to meet other objective prerequisites to the appointment.[229]

THE REGULAR REVIEW PROCESS. This section discusses the elements that need to be considered when conducting a full fair hearing for a medical staff member. Not all of these elements are required in

---

[224] Van Kirk v. Trustees of White County Mem. Hosp., No. 91C01-8809-CP-128 (Ind. Cir. Ct. White County Nov. 9, 1988), *as discussed in* 16 HEALTH L. DIG., Dec. 1988, at 67.

[225] *E.g.,* Caine v. Hardy, 943 F.2d 1406 (5th Cir. 1991), *cert. denied,* 503 U.S. 936 (1992); Medical Staff of Sharp Mem'l Hosp. v. Superior Court, 121 Cal. App. 4th 173, 16 Cal. Rptr. 3d 769 (4th Dist. 2004); Gureasko v. Bethesda Hosp., 116 Ohio App. 3d 724, 689 N.E.2d 76 (1996).

[226] Storrs v. Lutheran Hosps. & Homes Soc'y, 609 P.2d 24 (Alaska 1980), *aff'd after remand,* 661 P.2d 632 (Alaska 1983); *accord* Darlak v. Bobear, 814 F.2d 1055 (5th Cir. 1987).

[227] *E.g.,* Poe v. Charlotte Mem. Hosp., 374 F. Supp. 1302 (W.D. N.C. 1974) [two-year-old incidents were insufficient basis for summary action]; *Calif. physicians' summary suspension overturned,* AM. MED. NEWS, Feb. 23, 2004, 10 [hospital summarily suspended physician on voluntary leave of absence].

[228] *E.g.,* Conley v. Brownsville Med. Ctr., 570 S.W.2d 583 (Tex. Civ. App. 1978) [injunction dissolved after mistreatment of patient].

[229] *E.g.,* Paskon v. Salem Mem. Hosp., 806 S.W.2d 417 (Mo. Ct. App.), *cert. denied,* 502 U.S. 908 (1991).

every jurisdiction or for every type of facility. It is prudent to consider these elements and either include them or understand why they are not being followed. The elements are (1) reasonable notice, (2) hearing, (3) physician presence, (4) legal counsel, (5) composition of the hearing body, (6) discovery, (7) opportunity to present information, (8) opportunity to cross-examine witnesses, (9) record, (10) report, (11) internal review process, and (12) final institutional decision.

Reasonable Notice. The first step of due process is to give reasonable written notice of the reasons for the proposed action and of the time and place where the physician may present information. Reasonable notice must include sufficient information to permit preparation of a response,[230] but a detailed and exhaustive listing of each perceived deficiency is not required in most states.[231] In 1999, a federal appellate court ruled that it was not necessary to identify records with specific complaints when the proposed action was based on a statistical overview of cases.[232] The case involved proposed limitations on performing coronary artery bypass surgery based on a statistically high mortality rate.

The hospital does not have to cater to the idiosyncrasies of the physician in giving notice.[233] Standard methods such as personal delivery or registered mail are appropriate.

Hearing. The second step is to provide the physician with an opportunity to present information. Often the physician will have had one or more opportunities to present information during the informal investigative steps that precede formal action. However, a formal opportunity to present information is usually required after the formal recommendation of adverse action. Courts vary on the degree of the formality that they require. It is generally agreed the physician is entitled to only one hearing unless the bylaws specify additional hearings.[234]

An opportunity is all that is required. Health care entities may and usually do require physicians to request a hearing within a specified time. Failure to make such a request waives the right to a hearing and generally waives objections to the process. In 1996, a

---

[230] *E.g.,* Christenson v. Mount Carmel Health, 112 Ohio App. 3d 161, 678 N.E.2d 255 (1996).

[231] *E.g.,* Woodbury v. McKinnon, 447 F.2d 839 (5th Cir. 1971).

[232] Sokol v. Akron Gen. Med. Ctr., 173 F.3d 1026 (6th Cir. 1999).

[233] Arizona Osteopathic Med. Ass'n v. Fridena, 105 Ariz. 291, 463 P.2d 825, *cert. denied*, 399 U.S. 910 (1970).

[234] *E.g.,* Sywak v. O'Connor Hosp., 199 Cal. App. 3d 423, 244 Cal. Rptr. 753 (6th Dist. 1988), *op. withdrawn*, 1988 Cal. LEXIS 177 (May 19, 1988).

federal appellate court ruled that a physician could not deprive a hospital of HCQIA immunity by failing to request or participate in the hearing required by HCQIA.[235]

Physician Presence. Hospitals may require that the physician attend the hearing. Unexcused failure to appear can waive the right to the hearing and the right to object to other defects in the proceedings.[236]

Legal Counsel. There is disagreement on whether the physician should be represented by legal counsel at the hearing. Some attorneys can assist in assuring that information is provided in an orderly fashion and can help the physician understand the outcomes that can be reasonably expected. Some attorneys cannot adapt to the informality of the medical staff hearing and, thus, are disruptive, for example, by attempting to apply formal court rules. As a result, some hospitals do not permit attorneys to be involved; others encourage their involvement.

Courts have disagreed on whether there is a legal right to legal representation. New Jersey requires hospitals to permit representation by an attorney.[237] A federal court ruled that in army hospital proceedings the attorney can be limited to providing advice to the physician and not questioning witnesses or providing argument.[238] California hospitals do not have to permit representation by an attorney, especially when the hospital is not represented by an attorney.[239] Hospitals will have a difficult time convincing any court of the fairness of their procedures if only one side is permitted legal representation.

The safe harbor for HCQIA immunity specifies that the physician be given an opportunity to be represented by a lawyer.[240] This does not create a legal right to an attorney, but denial of an attorney may make it more difficult to maintain HCQIA immunity.

---

[235] Mathews v. Lancaster Gen. Hosp., 87 F.3d 624 (3d Cir. 1996).

[236] *E.g.,* Randall v. United States, 30 F.3d 518 (4th Cir. 1994), *cert. denied,* 514 U.S. 1107 (1995); *In re* Corines, 149 A.D.2d 591, 540 N.Y.S.2d 273 (2d Dep't 1989), *appeal dismissed,* 75 N.Y.2d 850, 522 N.Y.S.2d 923, 552 N.E.2d 171 (1990); Suckle v. Madison Gen. Hosp., 499 F.2d 1364 (7th Cir. 1974).

[237] Garrow v. Elizabeth Gen. Hosp., 79 N.J. 549, 401 A.2d 533 (1979).

[238] Randall v. United States, 30 F.3d 518 (4th Cir. 1994), *cert. denied,* 514 U.S. 1107 (1995).

[239] Anton v. San Antonio Comm. Hosp., 19 Cal. 3d 802, 140 Cal. Rptr. 442, 567 P.2d 1162 (1977); *accord* Yashon v. Hunt, 825 F.2d 1016 (6th Cir. 1987); Wright v. Southern Mono Hosp. Dist., 631 F. Supp. 1294 (E.D. Cal. 1986), *aff'd without op.,* 924 F.2d 1063 (9th Cir. 1991).

[240] 42 U.S.C. § 11112(b)(3)(C)(i).

In 2004, the Wisconsin Supreme Court ruled that only attorneys who were admitted to practice in Wisconsin could represent physicians at medical staff hearings; so an out-of-state attorney was not permitted to participate.[241]

Composition of the Hearing Body. The committee or individual conducting the hearing should not be biased against the physician. The South Carolina Supreme Court found that a physician's due process rights were violated when three of the original accusing physicians were members of the joint conference committee that made the final recommendation to the governing board.[242] A California appellate court ruled that a physician had been denied due process because the committee that recommended his suspension was not impartial.[243] Two committee members depended on the obstetrical expertise of the physician who brought the charges. The HCQIA safe harbor requires that the hearing committee not include physicians who are economic competitors.[244] State law may specify composition. An Indiana court ruled that under state law only physicians could serve on a hearing committee.[245]

Courts have recognized the virtual impossibility of complete impartiality because all physicians in a hospital have a collaborative relationship. Some courts require a demonstration of actual bias before a due process violation can be found.[246] A California appellate court ruled that the physician should be given an opportunity to examine committee members for possible bias before the hearing.[247] A New Jersey appellate court overturned a lower court ruling that had found that all internal bodies were disqualified and had ordered the county medical society (a private unrelated corporation) to make the final decision on renewal of clinical privileges.[248] The appellate court ruled that participation in prior investigations and preliminary decisions did not disqualify the internal bodies; the institution could combine investigative, charging, and adjudicative functions in the same body. Some courts find that review and

---

[241] Seitzinger v. Community Health Network, 2004 WI 28, 676 N.W.2d 426.

[242] *In re* Zaman, 285 S.C. 345, 329 S.E.2d 436 (1985).

[243] Applebaum v. Board of Directors, 104 Cal. App. 3d 648, 163 Cal. Rptr. 831 (3d Dist. 1980).

[244] 42 U.S.C. § 11112(b)(3)(A).

[245] Mann v. Johnson Mem. Hosp., 611 N.E.2d 676 (Ind. Ct. App. 1993).

[246] *E.g.,* Laje v. R.E. Thomason Gen. Hosp., 564 F.2d 1159 (5th Cir. 1977).

[247] Lasko v. Valley Presbyterian Hosp., 180 Cal. App. 3d 519, 225 Cal. Rptr. 603 (2d Dist. 1986).

[248] Ende v. Cohen, 296 N.J. Super. 350, 686 A.2d 1239 (App. Div. 1997).

approval by an unbiased appeal committee can correct earlier bias,[249] while other courts find no corrective effect.[250]

One federal appellate court ruled that when the applicant falsified his application any bias in the review process was irrelevant because this applicant would have been denied privileges anyway.[251]

Persons with known biases should be excluded from the hearing body. Persons in the same specialty should generally also be excluded because they may appear to be motivated to remove a competitor. Physicians do not have a right to have persons in the same specialty on a hearing body.[252] To the extent feasible, it is helpful to also exclude those who were involved in earlier stages of the investigation and review process, but this is not essential in all jurisdictions. These steps will assure fairness and minimize the risk of successful challenge. In some cases, hospitals with a smaller medical staff may have to arrange for someone from outside the hospital to conduct the hearing.

Discovery. Courts have disagreed on which hospital records of patient care and peer review the physician may obtain to prepare the presentation.[253] The Missouri Supreme Court permitted broad discovery with only redaction of identifying characteristics of patients who were not patients of the physician challenging his loss of staff privileges.[254]

In 1998, a California appellate court ruled that a peer review committee's policy of not disclosing the sources that had triggered the review did not deprive a physician of fair procedure.[255]

Opportunity to Present Information. The purpose of the hearing is to give the physician an opportunity to present information on his or her own behalf. One issue is whether the physician is entitled to an opportunity to present witnesses. Some courts have ruled that the bylaws can require all submissions to the hearing body to be in writing.[256] The HCQIA safe harbor includes an opportunity to present

---

[249] *E.g.,* Ladenheim v. Union County Hosp. Dist., 76 Ill. App. 3d 90, 394 N.E.2d 770 (5th Dist. 1979).

[250] Applebaum v. Board of Directors, 104 Cal. App. 3d 648, 163 Cal. Rptr. 831 (3d Dist. 1980).

[251] Pariser v. Christian Health Care Sys., 859 F.2d 78 (8th Cir. 1988).

[252] Ezpeleta v. Sisters of Mercy Health Corp., 800 F.2d 119 (7th Cir. 1986).

[253] *E.g.,* Rosenblit v. Superior Court, 231 Cal. App. 3d 1434, 282 Cal. Rptr. 819 (4th Dist. 1991) [new medical staff hearing ordered for several reasons including failure to give physician copies of thirty charts].

[254] State *ex rel.* Health Midwest Dev. Group, Inc. v. Daugherty, 965 S.W.2d 841 (Mo. 1998).

[255] Goodstein v. Cedars-Sinai Med. Ctr., 66 Cal. App. 4th 1257, 78 Cal. Rptr. 2d 577 (2d Dist. 1998).

[256] *E.g.,* Ezekiel v. Winkley, 20 Cal. 3d 267, 142 Cal. Rptr. 418, 572 P.2d 32 (1977).

witnesses.[257] However, one federal court has ruled that HCQIA does not require an opportunity for the physician to introduce evidence concerning the performance of other physicians.[258]

Opportunity to Cross-examine Witnesses. Courts have recognized that hospitals do not have the power to compel witnesses to attend hearings. Due process usually does not require an opportunity to cross-examine all those who have complained about the physician's conduct.[259] However, a few courts have found a right to cross-examine some witnesses.[260] Many hospitals permit cross-examination of witnesses who actually provide information at the hearing. The HCQIA safe harbor includes an opportunity to cross-examine the witnesses who testify.[261]

Record. It is prudent to make a record of hearing proceedings. If the final decision is appealed to the courts, a record will be necessary to prove fairness of the proceedings and evidence of the basis for the decision. A court reporter's transcript of the proceedings is expensive and may not be necessary. However, if the physician requests a court reporter and is willing to share the cost appropriately, a court reporter should be considered. Sometimes a tape recording or, in some situations, detailed notes will be sufficient. In some states, permission of all participants may be required for a tape recording. In 1998, the highest court of Massachusetts held that a hospital had violated the state wiretap law by tape-recording a meeting.[262] The HCQIA safe harbor includes a record of the hearing, but the physician can be required to pay reasonable charges to obtain a copy.[263]

Report. The hearing committee should make a substantive report of its findings, especially when such a report is required by the bylaws. A District of Columbia court ruled that a physician who was denied privileges could base a suit on the lack of an adequate hearing report.[264] The bylaws required the medical executive com-

---

257 42 U.S.C. § 11112(b)(3)(C)(iii); *see also* Poliner v. Texas Health Sys., 2003 U.S. Dist. LEXIS 17162 (N.D. Tex.) [no HCQIA immunity when physician not given opportunity to explain].

258 Smith v. Ricks, 798 F. Supp. 605 (N.D. Cal. 1992), *aff'd,* 31 F.3d 1478 (9th Cir. 1994), *cert. denied,* 514 U.S. 1035 (1995).

259 *E.g.,* Woodbury v. McKinnon, 447 F.2d 839 (5th Cir. 1971); Kaplan v. Carney, 404 F. Supp. 161 (E.D. Mo. 1975).

260 *E.g.,* Poe v. Charlotte Mem. Hosp., 374 F. Supp. 1302 (W.D. N.C. 1974).

261 42 U.S.C. § 11112(b)(3)(C)(iii).

262 Birbiglia v. St. Vincent Hosp., 427 Mass. 80, 692 N.E.2d 9 (1998).

263 42 U.S.C. § 11112(b)(3)(C)(ii).

264 Balkisson v. Capital Hill Hosp., 558 A.2d 304 (D.C. 1989).

mittee to consider a fact-finding report from the hearing committee. Without an adequate report, it could not do so; so the bylaws were violated. The HCQIA safe harbor includes a written recommendation by the hearing entity and a written decision by the hospital, with each to include a statement of the basis for the recommendation or decision.[265]

Internal Review Process. JCAHO requires an internal review process.[266] Some hospitals seek to comply with this requirement by permitting the practitioner to make a written and/or oral presentation to the board or a board committee after an adverse medical executive committee recommendation, but before the board's decision. This first approach can provide the board with useful information. Other hospitals interpret appellate review to require that an appellate process occur after the board makes an adverse decision. Because the board has the acknowledged authority to make the final decision, such internal appellate review is in essence reconsideration by the board. It is not clear what useful function this second approach performs that justifies the burden on the board.

One physician sought to disqualify the board from acting as its own appellate tribunal. A Colorado court rejected the challenge.[267]

Final Institutional Decision. The final decision in medical staff disciplinary matters is made by the board of directors of the institution after consideration of the findings and recommendations that have been generated by the internal review process. The board is not required to endorse the medical staff's recommendations. This was again recognized in a 2005 decision by the Alabama Supreme Court that held that the corporation was not required to adopt the hearing panel's recommendation.[268]

JUDICIAL APPEAL. Courts have permitted only the affected physician to seek judicial review of adverse decisions. Courts have not permitted other medical staff members,[269] patients,[270] or families

265 42 U.S.C. § 11112(b)(3)(D).
266 2005 JCAHO CAMH, Element of performance 5, MS.4.50.
267 Leonard v. Board of Directors, Prowers County Hosp. Dist., 673 P.2d 1019 (Colo. Ct. App. 1983).
268 Radiation Therapy Oncology, P.C. v. Providence Hosp., 2005 Ala. LEXIS 10 (Jan. 14, 2005).
269 *E.g.,* Ad Hoc Exec. Comm v. Runyan, 716 P.2d 465 (Colo. 1986) [committee cannot challenge governing board rejection of suspension it recommended]; Forster v. Fisherman's Hosp., Inc., 363 So. 2d 840 (Fla. 3d DCA 1978) [chief of hospital staff cannot challenge privileges granted after he recommended denial].
270 *E.g.,* Brindisi v. University Hosp., 131 A.D.2d 667, 516 N.Y.S.2d 745 (2d Dep't 1987) [patient cannot challenge denial of privileges to use laser]; Bello v. South Shore Hosp., 384 Mass. 770, 429 N.E.2d 1011 (1981).

of patients to challenge decisions to grant or deny medical staff membership or clinical privileges. The spouse of the physician also lacks standing, even when the family has to move causing the spouse to lose his job.[271]

Courts generally require the physician to pursue all procedures available within the hospital before allowing appeal to the courts. If a physician refuses to participate in the hospital hearing, courts will usually not allow an appeal based on denial of procedural due process.[272] However, hospital procedures usually do not have to be exhausted before court review when the hospital procedures clearly do not satisfy applicable due process or fair hearing requirements.[273]

When courts review a hospital action, they usually show great deference to the judgment of the hospital and its medical staff.[274] They limit their review to a determination of whether appropriate procedures were followed[275] and whether the action appears arbitrary or capricious. If credible evidence supports the action and proper procedures have been followed, the judiciary will almost always approve hospital actions. A few states do not follow this principle. For example, in 2003, Maryland rejected deference to hospitals.[276] Missouri applies deference to private hospitals, but not public hospitals.[277] Florida has a statutory prohibition of injunctions or damages against hospitals and those who participate in the disciplinary process unless actual fraud is demonstrated.[278] In some states, courts refuse to review the decisions of governing boards of private hospitals.[279]

In states with statutory requirements, courts will review whether there has been compliance with the statutes.[280]

---

[271] Hurst v. Beck, 771 F. Supp. 118 (E.D. Pa. 1991).

[272] *E.g.,* Yaeger v. Sisters of St. Joseph, 1988 U.S. Dist. LEXIS 8835 (D. Or.); Suckle v. Madison Gen. Hosp., 499 F.2d 1364 (7th Cir. 1974); *but see* Quasem v. Kozarek, 716 F.2d 1172 (7th Cir. 1983) [failure to pursue hospital procedures does not bar suit seeking only payment of damages by credentials committee member].

[273] *E.g.,* Christhilf v. Annapolis Emergency Hosp. Ass'n, Inc., 496 F.2d 174 (4th Cir. 1974).

[274] *E.g.,* University Health Servs., Inc. v. Long, 274 Ga. 829, 561 S.E.2d 77 (2002).

[275] *E.g.,* Pepple v. Parkview Mem. Hosp., Inc., 511 N.E.2d 467 (Ind. Ct. App. 1987), *aff'd,* 536 N.E.2d 274 (Ind. 1989).

[276] Sadler v. Dimensions Healthcare Corp., 378 Md. 509, 836 A.2d 655 (2003).

[277] Madsen v. Audrian Health Care, Inc., 297 F.3d 694 (8th Cir. 2002) [private hospital, applying Cowan v. Gibson, 392 S.W.2d 307 (Mo. 1965)]; Long v. Bates County Mem. Hosp., 667 S.W.2d 419 (Mo. Ct. App. 1983) [public hospital].

[278] FLA. STAT. § 395.0191(7).

[279] *E.g.,* Hottentot v. Mid-Maine Med. Ctr., 549 A.2d 365 (Me. 1988); Barrows v. Northwestern Mem. Hosp., 123 Ill. 2d 49, 525 N.E.2d 50 (1988); Lakeside Comm. Hosp. v. Levenson, 101 Nev. 777, 710 P.2d 727 (1985).

[280] *E.g.,* Medical Ctr. Hosps. v. Terzis, 235 Va. 443, 367 S.E.2d 728 (1988) [review limited to determination whether written reasons for adverse action are in list of permitted reasons in statute].

Injunction. Some physicians seek injunctions to require hospitals to keep them on or reinstate them to the medical staff. Generally, any person seeking an injunction must prove at least four elements: (1) substantial likelihood of ultimately winning the lawsuit on the merits, (2) irreparable injury, (3) the threatened injury without the injunction outweighs the injury to the opposing party from an injunction, and (4) the injunction will not be adverse to the public interest.[281] An injury is usually not irreparable if it can be compensated by monetary remedies.[282]

In most states, injunctions are seldom issued concerning medical staff privileges.[283] When they are issued, they are generally overturned on appeal.[284] Often this is because (1) money damages are available or (2) potential injuries to the hospital and patients generally outweigh injuries to the physician.

Occasionally, injunctions have been issued requiring reinstatement until the bylaws procedures can be completed.[285] Some state courts are more prone to issue injunctions.

In 1989, a physician was assessed over $50,000 in damages by an Illinois court for wrongfully obtaining an injunction to restore clinical privileges.[286]

In one very unusual case in 2004, community citizens obtained a temporary restraining order from a Nebraska trial judge without notice to the hospital. When the hospital became involved, the judge realized that the patients did not have standing to seek such an order and dissolved the order.[287]

Mandamus. In California, a writ of administrative mandamus can be issued by a court to compel a hospital to reinstate a physician to

---

281 *E.g.,* United States v. Jefferson County, 720 F.2d 1511 (11th Cir. 1983).

282 *E.g.,* Deerfield Med. Ctr. v. Deerfield Beach, 661 F.2d 328 (5th Cir. 1981).

283 *E.g.,* Prakasam v. Popowski, 566 So. 2d 189 (La. Ct. App.), *cert. denied,* 569 So. 2d 986 (La. 1990) [error to issue injunction]; J. Sternberg, S. Schulman & Assocs., M.D., P.A. v. Hospital Corp. of Am., 571 So. 2d 1334 (Fla. 4th DCA 1989) [affirming denial of injunction]; Rdzanek v. Hospital Serv. Dist., 2004 U.S. Dist. LEXIS 503 (E.D. La.) [deny injunction of reduction in privileges to consulting privileges].

284 *E.g.,* University Health Servs., Inc. v. Long, 274 Ga. 829, 561 S.E.2d 77 (2002).

285 *E.g.,* Porter Mem. Hosp. v. Malak, 484 N.E.2d 54 (Ind. Ct. App. 1985); Lawler v. Eugene Wuesthoff Mem. Hosp. Ass'n, 497 So. 2d 1261 (Fla. 5th DCA 1986); *see also,* notes 191-192, *supra.*

286 Knapp v. Palos Comm. Hosp., 176 Ill. App. 3d 1012, 531 N.E.2d 989 (1989), *cert. denied,* 493 U.S. 947 (1989).

287 *Citizens obtain restraining order to keep Ord doctor at hospital,* AP, Feb. 19, 2004; *Judge dissolves restraining order for Ord doctor,* AP, Mar. 12, 2004.

medical staff membership and privileges.[288] California courts generally require physicians to pursue a mandamus proceeding before permitting a tort suit concerning medical staff decisions.[289] In other states, a *writ of mandamus*[290] is generally not available to private individuals unless they have obligations in the nature of a public or quasi-public duty[291] nor is it available to enforce private rights or to enforce contractual obligations.[292] Employment contracts, even with public entities, are generally not enforceable by mandamus unless a statute sets the terms of the employment.[293] In 1994, Wisconsin adopted the contrary position, permitting mandamus to be used in some medical staff matters.[294] Thus, a writ of mandamus will generally not be available outside California and Wisconsin in medical staff matters.

5-7 Potential Liability of Those Involved in the Process of Making Medical Staff Appointment and Clinical Privilege Decisions

When physicians challenge adverse hospital actions, they often seek payment of money in addition to reversal of the hospital action. They base their claims on several grounds, including breach of contract; interference with business relationships; lost earnings or emotional distress during the proceedings;[295] defamation; antitrust violations; and discrimination. Some legal doctrines provide those involved in these determinations with limited immunity from some of these claims.

---

[288] *E.g.,* Rosenblit v. Superior Court, 231 Cal. App. 3d 1434, 262 Cal. Rptr. 819 (4th Dist. 1991) [writ granted], *rev. denied*, 1991 Cal. LEXIS 4251 (Sept. 19, 1991); Bollenger v. Doctors Med. Ctr., 222 Cal. App. 3d 1115, 272 Cal. Rptr. 273 (5th Dist. 1990) [writ denied for failure to exhaust administrative remedies within hospital]; Bonner v. Sisters of Providence Corp., 194 Cal. App. 3d 437, 239 Cal. Rptr. 530 (1st Dist. 1987) [writ reversed because evidence supported finding that doctor did not meet hospital's reasonable standards]; Hay v. Scripps Mem. Hosp., 183 Cal. App. 3d 753, 228 Cal. Rptr. 413 (4th Dist. 1986) [affirming denial of writ because reasonable to require Ob-Gyn residency for D & C privileges].

[289] Westlake Comm. Hosp. v. Superior Court, 17 Cal. 3d 465, 131 Cal. Rptr. 90, 551 P.2d 410 (1976) [physician whose privileges are terminated cannot sue hospital or involved individuals in tort without first having hospital action overturned in mandamus proceeding].

[290] See also Fed. R. Civ. P. 81(b) [writ of mandamus abolished in federal courts].

[291] AM. JUR. 2D, *Mandamus* § 104.

[292] AM. JUR. 2D, *Mandamus* § 104; Green v. Board of Directors of Lutheran Med. Ctr., 739 P.2d 872 (Colo. Ct. App. 1987) [physician denied privileges not entitled to mandamus relief]; State *ex rel.* St. Joseph Hosp. v. Fenner, 726 S.W.2d 393 (Mo. Ct. App. 1987) [mandamus not appropriate relief for contract dispute between physician and hospital, not appropriate for breach of contract]; Lawnwood Med. Ctr. v. Cassimally, 471 So. 2d 1346 (Fla. 4th DCA 1985) [not appropriate to use mandamus to compel election of medical staff officers].

[293] AM. JUR. 2D, *Mandamus* § 69.

[294] Keane v. St. Francis Hosp., 522 N.W.2d 517 (Wis. Ct. App. 1994) [mandamus available to reinstate medical staff officer, but denied due to circumstances].

[295] *E.g.,* Laje v. R.E. Thomason Gen. Hosp., 665 F.2d 724 (5th Cir. 1982).

Refusing to take necessary actions also exposes the medical staff and hospital to liability; so inaction does not avoid liability.

WAIVER. Many hospitals require all applicants to sign a waiver protecting those involved from liability. Through 2003, JCAHO recognized this common practice by requiring applicants to sign such waivers but is silent on the issue in its 2004 and 2005 standards.[296] Several courts have upheld these waivers,[297] but some courts have declined to enforce them.[298]

BREACH OF CONTRACT. When a physician has a contract with the hospital, termination or other breach of the contract can result in an assessment of monetary damages for the breach. Some courts view the bylaws as such a contract, permitting a breach of contract claim for violation of the bylaws.[299] A federal court in California held that a hospital's bylaws create a binding contract and a physician whose privileges were terminated when the hospital entered a new exclusive contract could sue for breach of contract.[300] However, the Mississippi Supreme Court rejected breach of contract claims by physicians whose privileges were ended when a hospital signed an exclusive contract.[301] Similarly, a Texas appeals court addressed a physician whose privileges were terminated for failure to enter into the hospital's new exclusive contract and found that he could not sue for breach of contract based on the bylaws.[302] In 2000, the Illinois Supreme Court reversed a lower court finding that the bylaws were a contract and left the issue open. The court concluded that the bylaws had not been violated when a physician lost his privileges due to a new exclusive contract with another physician.[303]

---

[296] 2003 JCAHO CAMH, MS.5.10.3.

[297] *E.g.*, Everett v. St. Ansgar Hosp., 974 F.2d 77 (8th Cir. 1992); DeLeon v. St. Joseph Hosp., 871 F.2d 1229 (4th Cir.) *cert. denied*, 493 U.S. 825 (1989) [application release barred defamation claim]; Stizell v. York Mem. Osteopathic Hosp., 768 F. Supp. 129 (M.D. Pa. 1991); King v. Bartholomew County Hosp., 476 N.E.2d 877 (Ind. Ct. App. 1985) [immunity provision on application upheld].

[298] *E.g.*, Westlake Comm. Hosp. v. Superior Court, 17 Cal. 3d 465, 131 Cal. Rptr. 90, 551 P.2d 410 (1976); Keskin v. Munster Med. Research Found., 580 N.E.2d 354 (Ind. Ct. App. 1991) [release signed as part of application for privileges did not preclude action challenging exclusive anesthesia contract, but hospital found to be within its rights in entering contract]; Rees v. Intermountain Health Care, Inc., 808 P.2d 1069 (Utah 1991) [immunity provisions in bylaws only precluded defamation action, not action for violating bylaws].

[299] *E.g.*, Bass v. Ambrosius, 185 Wis. 2d 879, 520 N.W.2d 625 (Ct. App. 1994).

[300] Janda v. Madera Comm. Hops., 16 F. Supp. 2d 1181 (E.D. Cal. 1998).

[301] Sullivan v. Baptist Mem. Hosp., 722 So. 2d 675 (Miss. 1998).

[302] East Tex. Med. Ctr. Cancer Inst. v. Anderson, 1998 Tex. App. LEXIS 6442.

[303] Garibaldi v. Applebaum, 194 Ill. 2d 438, 742 N.E.2d 279 (2000).

INTERFERENCE WITH BUSINESS RELATIONSHIPS. Physicians claim that the actions of the hospital or its staff tortiously interfered with their business relationships with patients, other physicians, hospitals, and others. Generally, merely denying or terminating privileges or professional service contracts does not constitute tortious interference. Although tort liability for such action is possible,[304] the greatest exposure of hospitals and their staffs occurs when they take additional steps, such as when they try to deny access to billing information or other records,[305] discriminate in access to equipment or staff necessary to exercise remaining privileges,[306] or create or disseminate false information.[307]

Generally, a claim of tortious interference with a business relationship requires a showing of (1) an existing business relationship under which the plaintiff has legal rights,[308] (2) knowledge of that relationship by defendant, (3) an intentional and unjustified interference with the relationship, and (4) damage to the plaintiff as a result of the breach of the relationship.[309] In some jurisdictions, the business relationship does not need to be enforceable; so some expectancies are protected if there is an understanding that would have been completed if the interference had not occurred. The Florida Supreme Court ruled that this did not permit a claim based on the "mere hope that some of its past customers may choose to buy again" where there was no ongoing relationship with those customers.[310]

In assessing what interference is justified, some courts recognize a privilege of competition that permits efforts to convince others who are in business relationships that are terminable at will to shift their business, as long as certain prohibited means are not used.[311]

Generally, actions by a party to a business relationship cannot constitute tortious interference with that relationship. In general,

---

[304] See Annotation, *Liability in tort for interference with physician's contract or relationship with hospital*, 7 A.L.R. 4TH 572.

[305] *E.g.*, Scheller v. American Med. Int'l, Inc., 502 So. 2d 1268 (Fla. 4th DCA 1987), *rev. denied*, 513 So. 2d 1068 (Fla.), *appeal after remand*, 590 So. 2d 947 (Fla. 4th DCA 1991), *rev. dismissed*, 602 So. 2d 533 (Fla. 1992) [affirming punitive damage award of $19 million]; *Doctor, lawyer feud over $15.5 million settlement*, PALM BEACH [FL] POST, June 29, 1992, at 1B [case settled].

[306] *Id.*

[307] *E.g.*, Purgess v. Sharrock, 33 F.3d 134 (2d Cir. 1994); Chakrabarti v. Cohen, 31 F.3d 1 (1st Cir. 1994).

[308] *E.g.*, Scheller v. American Med. Int'l, 583 So. 2d 1047 (Fla. 4th DCA 1991), *rev. denied*, 598 So. 2d 78 (Fla. 1992) [no enforceable agreement for perpetual agreement].

[309] *E.g., id.*

[310] Ethan Allen, Inc. v. Georgetown Manor, 647 So. 2d 812 (Fla. 1994).

[311] *E.g.*, Greenberg v. Mount Sinai Med. Ctr., 629 So. 2d 252 (Fla. 3d DCA 1993).

only an individual or entity that is not a party to the relationship can tortiously interfere with a business relationship. Thus, a director, officer, or employee of a corporation cannot tortiously interfere with a contract between the corporation and someone else.[312] When these people cause a physician's contract with the hospital to be terminated, they generally cannot be sued personally for tortious interference with the physician's relationship with the hospital. In jurisdictions that recognize the medical staff to be within this intracorporate immunity, other medical staff members will generally also be immune from personal suit, except where they are acting out of person economic interests.

Some jurisdictions permit a claim for tortious interference with the relationship with patients or other physicians arising out of the termination of the relationship with the hospital. The intracorporate immunity may not apply to such claims. However, there are other barriers to prevailing with such claims, especially in jurisdictions that do not permit a claim for a mere expectancy.

In hospitals that have complex corporate structures, it is not clear whether the intracorporate immunity will apply to protect an action by one corporation that affects employment by or contracts with a parent, subsidiary, or other related corporation or entity.[313] Risk is minimized if communications and actions affecting employment and contractual relationships are kept in proper channels.

DEFAMATION. Wrongful injury to another person's reputation is *defamation*. Defamation is discussed in Chapter 11. One defense to a defamation claim is a qualified privilege, which means that there is no liability for certain privileged communications, even if they injure another's reputation, if the communications were not made with malice. Most courts apply a qualified privilege to communications during medical staff peer review activities, including hospital board review and action.[314] In 1982, a Pennsylvania court dismissed the portion of a defamation suit against the hospital because no malice had been shown but refused to dismiss the portion against

---

[312] Annotation, *Liability of corporate director, officer, or employee for tortious interference with corporation's contract with another*, 72 A.L.R. 4TH 492.

[313] *E.g.*, Hospital Corp. of Am. v. Jarvinen, 624 So. 2d 303 (Fla. 4th DCA 1993), *rev. denied*, 634 So. 2d 624 (Fla. 1994) [issue mentioned but not decided].

[314] *E.g.*, DeLeon v. St. Joseph Hosp., 871 F.2d 1229 (4th Cir.), *cert. denied*, 493 U.S. 825 (1989); Sibley v. Lutheran Hosp., 709 F. Supp. 657 (D. Md. 1988), *aff'd*, 871 F.2d 479 (4th Cir. 1989); Guntheroth v. Rodaway, 107 Wash. 2d 170, 727 P.2d 982 (1986); Spencer v. Community Hosp., 87 Ill. App. 3d 214, 408 N.E.2d 981 (1980).

the physicians.[315] It was asserted that the physicians had made their statements because they wanted the financial benefit of keeping a competitor from obtaining clinical privileges. If proved at trial, the financial motive could establish malice. The immunity statutes discussed later in this chapter may provide more protection than the qualified privilege.

ANTITRUST. Physicians frequently challenge medical staff actions by claiming the actions are a restraint of trade or an attempt to monopolize medical practice, thus violating federal antitrust laws. Four of the reasons for federal antitrust suits are: (1) if the physician wins, treble damages can be obtained, (2) suits are expensive to litigate, so hospitals may be more willing to compromise, (3) the suit can be tried in federal court, and (4) state laws that protect peer review documents from disclosure do not apply.

Prior to 1991, one of the major barriers that protected hospitals from medical staff antitrust suits was the difficulty in proving the impact on interstate commerce necessary for federal antitrust laws to apply. In 1991, the United States Supreme Court established a new standard so that impact on interstate commerce is easy to demonstrate in many medical staff cases.[316]

Antitrust cases against hospitals remain difficult for practitioners to win. HCQIA provides immunity from monetary liability based on antitrust claims for most credentialing actions, as discussed previously in this chapter. In the unusual cases where the physician can show failure to make reasonable efforts to comply with HCQIA, antitrust liability is still possible.[317]

There are other barriers to successful antitrust suits. Physicians frequently have difficulty showing antitrust standing,[318] antitrust injury,[319] or causation of their alleged injuries.[320] Other antitrust issues are discussed in Chapter 13.

DISCRIMINATION. Medical staff decisions should not be based on discriminatory criteria, such as race, creed, color, sex, national

---

[315] Baldwin v. McGrath, No. 76-5-336 (Pa. C.P. Ct. York County Mar. 18, 1982), *as discussed in* 10 HEALTH L. DIG., Apr. 1982, at 17.

[316] Summit Health, Ltd. v. Pinhas, 500 U.S. 322 (1991).

[317] *E.g.,* Brown v. Presbyterian Healthcare Srvcs., 101 F.3d 1324 (10th Cir. 1996), *cert, denied,* 520 U.S. 1181 (1997); *see also* Sisters of Providence v. A.A. Pain Clinic, Inc., 81 P.3d 989 (Alaska 2003) [upholding antitrust liability under state law].

[318] *E.g.,* Korshin v. Benedictine Hosp., 34 F. Supp. 2d 133 (N.D. N.Y. 1999).

[319] *E.g.,* Benjamin v. Aroostook Med. Ctr., 113 F.3d 1 (1st Cir. 1997), *cert. denied,* 522 U.S. 1016 (1997); Bocobo v. Radiology Consultants, 305 F. Supp. 2d 422 (D. N.J. 2004); Angelco v. Lehigh Valley Hosp., 984 F. Supp. 306 (E.D. Pa. 1997).

[320] *E.g.,* Read v. Medical X-ray Ctr., P.C., 110 F.3d 543 (8th Cir. 1997).

origin, and handicap. Sometimes medical staff actions are challenged on the basis that they violate federal and state statutes barring discrimination.[321] For example, an African-American physician in the District of Columbia claimed she had been terminated from her position in a health maintenance organization because of her race, violating the federal Civil Rights Act. In 1981, a federal court found sufficient evidence that her termination was based on complaints of African-American and Caucasian coworkers and on failure to improve her performance after being warned and not on her race; so no violation was found.[322]

Generally, staff privileges alone have not been sufficient to trigger coverage under discrimination laws that focus on employment because granting privileges is not employing.[323] However, some discrimination laws apply to interfering with employment opportunities. Thus, in some circumstances, physicians who have been denied or lost medical staff membership have been able to sue the hospital.[324] Appointments to compensated positions, such as director of a department, may be subject to employment protections.[325] Some discrimination laws are not based on employment. Courts have disagreed on whether laws that address discrimination in public accommodations can be applied to medical staff decisions.[326]

IMMUNITY. In some states, persons involved in medical staff review may be entitled to some immunity from liability for their statements or actions. The common law qualified privilege from liability for defamation previously discussed is an example. Some state statutes provide limited immunity from damages for actions in the peer review process.[327] An Arizona appellate court ruled that the

---

[321] *E.g.,* Fobbs v. Holy Cross Health Sys. Corp., 29 F.3d 1439 (9th Cir. 1994), *cert. denied,* 513 U.S. 1127 (1995) [race]; Johnson v. Hills & Dales Gen. Hosp., 40 F.3d 837 (6th Cir. 1994) *cert. denied,* 514 U.S. 1066 (1995) [race]; Gregory v. Georgia Dep't of Human Resources, 355 F.3d 1277 (11th Cir. 2004) [affirming jury award of $10,000 for race discrimination].

[322] Harris v. Group Health Ass'n, Inc., 213 U.S. App. D.C. 313, 662 F.2d 869 (1981).

[323] *E.g.,* Cilecek v. Inova Health Sys. Srvcs., Inc., 115 F.3d 256 (4th Cir. 1997), *cert. denied,* 522 U.S. 1049 (1998); Alexander v. Rush North Shore Med. Ctr., 101 F.3d 487 (7th Cir. 1996), *cert denied,* 522 U.S. 811 (1997).

[324] *E.g.,* Zaklama v. Mt. Sinai Med. Ctr., 842 F.2d 291 (11th Cir. 1988) [resulted in another hospital discharging physician]; Doe on behalf of Doe v. St. Joseph's Hosp., 788 F.2d 411 (7th Cir. 1986) [Title VII claim for interference with employment by others]; *but see* Bender v. Suburban Hosp., 159 F.2d 186 (4th Cir. 1998) [relationship with patient not employment for Title VII purposes].

[325] *E.g.,* Betkerur v. Aultman Hosp., 78 F.3d 1079 (6th Cir. 1996) [reliance on search committee recommendation was nondiscriminatory reason for selection, insufficient showing of pretext].

[326] *E.g.,* Menkowitz v. Pottstown Mem. Med. Ctr., 154 F.3d 113 (3d Cir. 1998) [suit permitted under public accommodation provisions of ADA].

[327] *E.g.,* Ariz. Rev. Stat. Ann. § 36-445.02; Harris v. Bellin Mem. Hosp., 13 F.3d 1082 (7th Cir. 1994).

chief of staff and the hospital administrator could not be sued for summarily suspending a surgeon's clinical privileges unless there was a showing that the primary purpose of the action was other than safeguarding patients.[328] Because a patient had died following "serious errors in judgment" by the surgeon and the surgeon had scheduled another patient for the same type of surgery, the court found the primary purpose was safeguarding patients.

Some states have enacted statutes that grant broader immunity for peer review participants. For example, in Florida there is no liability unless intentional fraud is proved.[329] However, the Florida Supreme Court declared unconstitutional an additional requirement that before suing that a physician must post a bond to pay the defendants' defense costs if liability is not found.[330] In Illinois, there is statutory absolute immunity.[331] The immunity statutes of Louisiana and California have been interpreted to protect only individuals, not institutions.[332] Tennessee's immunity statute has been interpreted to apply to hospitals, even though the term "hospital" does not appear in the statute.[333]

State statutes that prohibit the use of certain peer review records as evidence may make it impossible to prove certain claims, effectively granting immunity. For example, the Florida prohibition on introducing testimony and records concerning peer review proceedings effectively bars nearly all defamation claims for statements made in the peer review process.[334]

5-8   Relationship with Physicians Outside the Medical Staff Relationship

Most physicians who work in horpitals are not hospital employees or agents. However, many physician relationships with the hospital are based on and defined by a contract, either as an employee of the

---

[328] Scappatura v. Baptist Hosp., 120 Ariz. 204, 584 P. 2d 1195 (Ct. App. 1978); *accord* Rodriguez-Erdman v. Ravenswood Hosp. Med. Ctr., 163 Ill. App. 3d 464, 516 N.E. 2d 731 (1st Dist. 1987).

[329] FLA. STAT. §§ 395.011(8), (10), 395.0115(2), (5).

[330] Psychiatric Assocs. v. Siegel, 610 So. 2d 419 (Fla. 1992).

[331] Cardwell v. Rockford Mem. Hosp. Ass'n, 136 Ill. 2d 271, 555 N.E.2d 6, *cert. denied*, 488 U.S. 998 (1990).

[332] Smith v. Our Lady of the Lake Hosp., 639 So. 2d 730 (La. 1994); Axline v. St. John's Hosp. & Health Ctr., 63 Cal. App. 4th 907, 74 Cal. Rptr. 2d 385 (2d Dist. 1998).

[333] Eyring v. Fort Sanders Parkwest Med. Ctr., 991 S.W.2d 230 (Tenn. 1999).

[334] Holly v. Auld, 450 So. 2d 217 (Fla. 1984).

hospital or as an independent contractor or as an employee of an independent contractor or joint venturer with the hospital.

Physicians increasingly have other relationships with hospitals. Some examples include:

1. owning a limited partnership interest in the hospital or having other ownership interests in an entity that owns the hospital,
2. serving on the governing board,
3. contracting with the hospital or a related medical service organization for space, equipment, staff, and other support services, and
4. participating in organizations that may contract with managed care plans on behalf of the hospital and the physicians.

Some of these other relationships involve credentialing and review mechanisms that duplicate many of the medical staff functions. Procedures to centralize credentialing are developing. Sometimes other entities contract with hospitals to perform delegated credentialing. Sometimes third-party credentialing organizations are used.

The structuring of other aspects of these relationships is constrained by Medicare antikickback restrictions; Stark self-referral restrictions; federal tax exemption or other tax considerations; and state antikickback, self-referral, and other legal restrictions. Many of these restrictions are discussed in Chapters 9 and 12. The details concerning these relationships are beyond the scope of this book.

Most legal disputes between individual physicians and hospitals concern denial, restriction, or loss of clinical privileges or contracts. Frequently, contracts waive any rights that exist under the medical staff bylaws, so that the relationship can be predominantly defined by individual contract.

PHYSICIAN RECRUITMENT AND RETENTION. To attract and keep physicians, many hospitals in the past have offered loans, office space, practice assistance, liability protection, and income guaranties. There is increasing scrutiny of arrangements that tax-exempt hospitals make to recruit and retain physicians. Such arrangements must be properly limited and structured so that they are not (1) private inurement that could cause the loss of the hospital's tax-exempt status or (2) inducements or kickbacks for referrals that violate the Medicare and Medicaid fraud and abuse provisions. Private inurement and the fraud and abuse provisions are discussed in Chapters 9 and 12.

PHYSICIAN-HOSPITAL CONTRACTS. Hospitals and physicians often enter contracts concerning the performing of medical or administrative services in the hospital. Written contracts help to define the relationship to the mutual benefit of hospital and physician. Many questions must be considered in negotiating the contract. Will the contract be with an individual physician or a group of physicians? Will the physicians be hospital employees or independent contractors? The latter question will affect fringe benefits, applicability of personnel policies, potential liability, and responsibility for withholding taxes and paying workers' compensation. What qualifications must the physician meet? What services will the physician perform? In addition to providing direct patient care, the physician may also participate in professional review and other advisory capacities and may also have some administrative responsibilities, such as budgeting or preparing reports. Space, equipment, and supply issues may be addressed. Who will be responsible for selecting, training, supervising, scheduling, and disciplining professional and technical personnel who work with the physician? What insurance or indemnification agreements should the parties require? How will the physician be compensated? Salary, percentage, and fee-for-service arrangements or combinations of these arrangements are possible. Sometimes the physician is not compensated by the hospital and charges fees to the patient directly. How will the charges be established, and who will be responsible for billing them? How will changes in third-party payer requirements, such as the adoption of capitation or other global billing (one bill for both physician and hospital services), be addressed? Will the agreement include restrictions on competition during the term of the agreement or after termination? Some state laws and court decisions limit the scope of enforceable restrictions.[335] How can the agreement be amended or terminated? How are disagreements to be resolved? These and other questions must be considered in contracting with physicians.

The answers to these questions will be influenced by reimbursement policies of Medicare and other third-party payers and by tax

---

[335] *E.g.,* Vencor, Inc. v. Webb, 33 F.3d 840 (7th Cir. 1994) [when operator of long-term acute-care hospitals sought to enjoin competition by former employee contrary to noncompete agreement, agreement unenforceable under applicable Kentucky law].

implications, such as threats to tax exemption. For example, hospitals that desire to be eligible to raise funds from tax-exempt bonds must limit the length of many contracts with physicians.[336]

A clause concerning access to records should be included in all contracts for services that have a value of $10,000 or more over one year. Medicare will not pay the hospital for services under a contract that does not contain that clause.[337] The clause must allow the Secretary of Health and Human Services and the Comptroller General to have access to the subcontractor's books, documents, and records that are necessary to verify the costs of services furnished under the contract. The records must be retained for at least four years after the services are provided. This requirement will apply to many contracts with physicians.

EXCLUSIVE CONTRACTS. Hospitals frequently enter contracts with specialists that specify their exclusive right to provide certain types of care, such as radiology, pathology, emergency room services, and cardiac catheterization. These contracts can help hospitals to optimize patient care. Competing physicians have attacked these contracts as violations of equal protection, due process, and antitrust laws. Most courts have upheld these exclusive contracts when it is clear that they are intended to foster good quality patient care.[338]

In 1973, the Pennsylvania Supreme Court upheld a contract that granted exclusive cardiac catheterization privileges to the full-time director of the cardiology laboratory.[339] A physician who had been performing the procedure in the hospital challenged the contract. The court found the arrangement reasonable and related to the hospital's operation because it:

1. assured the best training and supervision of the catheterization team,
2. enabled the physician to maintain competence by performing more procedures,
3. centralized responsibility for use and maintenance of the equipment,

---

[336] Rev. Proc. 93-19, 1993-1 C.B. 526.
[337] 42 U.S.C. § 1395x(v)(1)(I); 42 C.F.R. §§ 420.300–420.304.
[338] *E.g.*, City of Cookeville v. Humphrey, 126 S.W.3d 897 (Tenn. 2004) [public hospital may enter exclusive contract].
[339] Adler v. Montefiore Hosp. Ass'n, 453 Pa 60, 311 A.2d 634 (1973), *cert. denied*, 414 U.S. 1131 (1974); *see also*, Annotation, *Validity and construction of contract between hospital and physician providing for exclusive medical services*, 74 A.L.R. 3D 1268.

4. reduced scheduling problems for patients,
5. improved the ability to monitor quality of care, and
6. assured the presence of a physician in the event of complications.

Antitrust attacks on exclusive contracts have generally been unsuccessful. However, in 1982, one federal appellate court declared an exclusive contract for anesthesia services to be a violation of the antitrust laws and ordered the hospital to permit the physician recommended for appointment by the medical staff to provide anesthesia services.[340] The court found the use of the operating room and the use of anesthesia services to be two separate products that were illegally "tied" by the exclusive contract. An agreement to sell one product only on the condition that the buyer also purchase a different product is a tying arrangement and, thus, a per se violation of antitrust laws if the seller has sufficient market power to coerce purchase of the tied product. The court defined the market area as so small that the hospital had sufficient market power. The court focused on the fact that anesthesia services were predominantly being provided by nurse anesthetists employed by the hospital and supervised by the anesthesiologists; so the court believed the "actual basis for the hospital's actions in this case" was "increasing the hospital's profit." The court rejected the other "business justifications" for the contract because it believed there were less restrictive ways to accomplish the same ends.

The 1982 decision led many to question the viability of exclusive contracts. Then, in 1984, the United States Supreme Court reversed the decision with an opinion that refined the definition of tying arrangements considered to be per se antitrust violations.[341] The Court concluded that the arrangement did not force purchases that would not otherwise have been made; so it was not a tying arrangement. Applying the rule of reason, the Court found the contract did not unreasonably restrain competition.

The Court's decision was not an endorsement of all exclusive contracts. Exclusive contracts may still be successfully attacked in some circumstances. However, the decision has made it possible in

---

[340] Hyde v. Jefferson Parish Hosp. Dist., 686 F.2d 286 (5th Cir. 1982).
[341] Jefferson Parish Hosp. Dist. No. 2 v. Hyde, 466 U.S. 2 (1984). On remand the appellate court rejected Dr. Hyde's other challenges to the denial of his application, 764 F.2d 1139 (5th Cir. 1985).

most settings to structure exclusive arrangements that have survived antitrust attack.[342] One of the few successful antitrust attacks was in a suit by nurse anesthetists challenging an exclusive contract with anesthesiologists.[343]

At least one hospital has tried to use antitrust laws as an excuse to break an exclusive contract. In 1989, a federal district court ruled that a hospital was not permitted to seek a declaration that a 35-year radiology contract violated the Sherman Act.[344]

In some states, state law may be more restrictive than federal law. For example, when a Texas hospital sought a court determination that it could legally have an exclusive radiology contract, the state counterclaimed on the basis of violation of state law.[345] The hospital entered a consent judgment agreeing to abandon the exclusive arrangement.

State law in Illinois requires notice and a hearing for physicians adversely affected by an exclusive contract.[346]

The Iowa Supreme Court ruled that a hospital could close its anesthesia department but affirmed jury verdicts in favor of two excluded anesthesiologists against the contracting anesthesia group.[347] The verdict was not based on an antitrust violation but on breach of contract. The group had promised to grant extensions to existing anesthesiologists who wanted to continue outside the group, but the group did not honor the promise.

CORPORATE PRACTICE OF MEDICINE. Some states have statutes or court decisions that forbid corporations from employing physicians.[348] This is called the *corporate practice of medicine* doctrine. Most states do not have or do not enforce the doctrine. In the states that do have the doctrine, frequently there are exceptions that permit employment by some types of corporations, such as nonprofit corporations,[349] physician-controlled corporations,

---

342 *E.g.,* White v. Rockingham Radiologists, 820 F.2d 98 (4th Cir. 1987); Collins v. Associated Pathologists, 676 F. Supp. 1388 (C.D. Ill. 1987), *aff'd,* 844 F.2d 473 (7th Cir.), *cert. denied,* 488 U.S. 852 (1988).

343 Oltz v. St. Peter's Comm. Hosp., 861 F.2d 1440 (9th Cir. 1988).

344 Community Hosp. v. Tomberlin, 712 F. Supp. 170 (M.D. Ala. 1989).

345 Medical Ctr. Hosp. v. Texas, No. 374,830 (Tex. Dist. Ct. Travis County Oct. 17, 1985), *as discussed in* 18 HOSP. L., Dec. 1985, at 4.

346 210 Ill. Comp. Stat. 85/10.4.

347 Tredrea v. Anesthesia & Analgesia P.C., 584 N.W.2d 276 (Iowa 1998); *accord,* Major v. Memorial Hosps. Ass'n, 71 Cal. App. 4th 1380, 84 Cal. Rptr. 2d 510 (5th Dist. 1999) [hospital may close anesthesia department without offering positions to incumbents].

348 *E.g.,* Cal. Bus. & Prof. Code § 2400.

349 *E.g.,* Mich. Op. Att'y Gen. No. 6770 (1993).

HMOs, or hospitals.[350] Some physicians attempt to use the doctrine to void contracts with hospitals and other entities, so that they can avoid noncompetition agreements and other duties in the contracts. These attempts are usually unsuccessful. For example, in 1997, the Illinois Supreme Court rejected an attempt by a physician to avoid a noncompetition agreement with a hospital by finding that the doctrine did not apply to contracts with hospitals. [351]

There are a few states that aggressively enforce the doctrine, especially California, Colorado, and Texas.[352] In those states, unusual business structures are frequently required to achieve integration without violating the doctrine. Hospitals in other states can usually avoid these unusual business structures.

FEE SPLITTING. Some states have laws against fee splitting that have been interpreted to bar some contractual arrangements with physicians. Florida courts have applied its law to invalidate some physician contracts.[353]

PHYSICIAN UNIONS. Some physicians have sought to form unions to collectively bargain their relationships with employers and others. This has been a controversial issue.[354] Employed physicians have the same scope of rights to collectively bargain as other employees,[355] including the exclusion of supervisory personnel from such rights[356] and the right to end union representation.[357]

---

[350] *E.g.,* St. Francis Reg. Med. Ctr. v. Weiss, 254 Kan. 728, 869 P.2d 606 (1994).

[351] Berlin v. Sarah Bush Lincoln Health Ctr., 179 Ill. 2d 1, 688 N.E.2d 106 (1997).

[352] *Id.*; Tex. Rev. Civ. Stat. Ann. art. 4495b; Garcia v. Texas State Bd. of Med. Exam'rs, 384 F. Supp. 434 (W.D. Tex. 1974), *aff'd*, 421 U.S. 994 (1974) [constitutional]; Parker v. Board of Dental Exam'rs, 216 Cal. 285, 14 P.2d 67 (1932); People *ex rel.* State Bd. of Med. Exam'rs v. Pacific Health Corp., 12 Cal. 2d 156, 82 P.2d 429 (1938), *cert. denied*, 306 U.S. 633 (1939); Pediatric Neurosurgery, P.C., v. Russell, 44 P.3d 1063 (Colo. 2002); *see also* American Chiropractic Clinic v. Saunders, 2001 Wash. App. LEXIS 1499 [unpub] [barred chiropractic corporation]; *Hanford medical provider sues company that wins new contract*, AP, Apr. 14, 2004 [losing bidder claims winner violates doctrine].

[353] Fla. Stat. §§ 458.331, 817.505; *e.g.*, Gold, Vann & White, P.A. v. Friedenstab, 831 So. 2d 692 (Fla. 4th DCA 2002).

[354] *E.g., Right to organize endorsed by AMA, but work stoppages are off limits*, 7 H.L.R. 1012 (1998); S. Klein, *AMA to establish national collective bargaining unit*, Am. Med. News, July 5, 1999, 1; T. Albert, *PRN separates from AMA, keeps no-strike policy*, Am. Med. News, Apr. 5, 2004, 12.

[355] *E.g.,* Thomas-Davis Med. Ctrs., 324 NLRB No. 15 (1997) [HMO ordered to bargain with physician union].

[356] *E.g.,* National Union of Hosp. & Health Care Employees v. Cook County, 295 Ill. App. 3d 1012, 692 N.E.2d 1253 (1st Dist. 1998) [attending physicians employed by county hospital are supervisors, not eligible for union representation]; *but see* New York Univ. Med. Ctr. v. NLRB, 156 F.3d 405 (2d Cir. 1998) [physicians not supervisors]; Occupational Health Ctrs. v. Physicians for Responsible Negotiation, Case 22-RC-11944 (NLRB Reg. Dir. 2002) [physicians not supervisors].

[357] *E.g.,* S. Hymon, *Los Angeles County doctors vote decisively to leave union; Hardball tactics and loss of a key benefits package are cited. Labor group defends its record and says it may seek more balloting later*, L.A. Times, June 20, 2003, pt. 2, 3.

Some physicians who are not employees have sought to collectively bargain. Their efforts have been challenged as not authorized under labor laws[358] or as violations of antitrust laws.[359] There were unsuccessful attempts to pass federal legislation to permit physician collective bargaining with HMOs.[360] At least three states have enacted a law to authorize and oversee such bargaining by some physicians, so that they are protected from federal antitrust law as state action.[361]

Discussion Points

1. What are the responsibilities of the board of directors and the medical staff concerning patient care?
2. What are Medical Staff Bylaws, and how are they changed?
3. What is the structure of the medical staff, and how are officers selected and removed?
4. What legal constraints are there on medical staff rules and processes?
5. What criteria may institutions consider in determining medical staff membership? What criteria are prohibited?
6. What are the issues involved in restricting membership by physicians who compete with the institution?
7. How should the institution determine which clinical privileges to grant?
8. What factors can the institution consider in making reappointment decisions?
9. What are the permitted grounds for modifying or terminating clinical privileges?
10. What are the issues involved in establishing closed staffs or exclusive arrangements for certain specialties?

---

[358] *E.g.*, M. Jaklevic, *Unions pursue new venture*, MOD. HEALTHCARE, Nov. 3, 1997, 33 [N.J. union sought to represent private practice physicians in negotiations with HMO]; *NLRB rejects New Jersey physician's union bid*, AM. MED. NEWS, June 7, 1999, 4 [regional office ruled physicians were independent contractors]; Amerihealth Inc./Amerihealth HMO v. United Food & Commercial Workers Union, 4-RC-19260 (NLRB Reg. Dir. May 29, 1999).

[359] *E.g.*, S. Klein, *Justice slaps Fla. physicians with antitrust charges*, AM. MED. NEWS, Feb. 15, 1999, 1; E. Hirshfield, *Physicians, unions and antitrust*, 32 J. HEALTH L. 39 (Wint. 1999).

[360] *E.g.*, R.D. Blair & J.B. Herndon, *Physician cooperative bargaining ventures: an economic analysis*, 71 ANTITRUST L.J. 989 (2004).

[361] *E.g.*, Tex. S.B. 1468 (1999), *codified as* TEX. INS. CODE §§ 29.01 – 29.14; *Gov. Bush signs first-ever law letting doctors bargain with HMOs*, 8 H.L.R. 1017 (1999); ALASKA STAT. §§ 23.50.010 – 23.50.099; N.J. STAT. §§ 52:17B-196 – 52:17B-208.

11. When must medical staff actions be reported to the National Practitioner Data Bank?
12. What steps are usually followed in medical staff review of adverse actions committed by medical staff? Which steps are required in order to have immunity under the Health Quality Improvement Act?
13. When will courts enjoin medical staff actions?
14. What are the grounds for potential liability for medical staff actions?
15. What are some of the potential contractual relationships between medical staff and institutions outside of the medical staff structure? What are some of the legal restrictions on such relationships?

CHAPTER SIX

Relationship of Patient and Provider

Objectives

The objective of this chapter is to provide an overview of the relationship between patients and providers. The reader will learn how the relationship starts and ends and what some of the legal limits are on the decision whether to start a relationship and when to end the relationship.

Health care services are delivered within the relationship of individual patients and individual providers. The relationship with the individual provider can be established with the individual provider or through a provider organization. Due to the clinical and administrative complexities of health care services, few health care services can be provided by individual providers without the collaboration and support of an organization and other providers. Thus, for most services a patient must have a relationship with an organization and with individual providers.

This chapter focuses on how the relationship starts and ends. The following questions are addressed:

6-1. How does a relationship with a physician begin?
6-2. How does a relationship with a hospital begin?
6-3. What are the special rules concerning emergency cases?
6-4. What are the effects of nondiscrimination laws?
6-5. How does a relationship with a physician end?
6-6. How does a relationship with a hospital end?

6-1 How Does a Relationship with a Physician Begin?

The relationship between a patient and a physician begins by an express or implied agreement. The creation of the relationship between the provider and individual patient is important because (a) it is not possible to access health care services without a relationship, (b) it is one of the ways providers control their workload and lifestyle, and (c) it commences professional and legal duties from the provider to the patient.

Providers and patients have considerable latitude in deciding whether or not to start a relationship, but this latitude is increasingly subject to constraints. For example, as discussed later in Section 6-4, neither provider nor patient can discriminate on the basis of race or other forbidden criteria. Economic realities can also constrain choices. For example, in many hospitals, physicians must agree to be on-call in order to practice in the hospital. Nurses and employed professionals generally must agree to care for all patients assigned to their service.

Generally, a physician or other independent practitioner has the right to accept or decline to establish a professional relationship with any person.[1] A physician does not have a legal responsibility to diagnose or treat anyone unless there is an express or implied agreement to do so. Likewise, an individual does not have an obligation to accept diagnosis or treatment from any particular physician unless the situation is one in which the law authorizes the person to be cared for involuntarily.

Of course, there are many situations where an individual's freedom of choice is limited economically. A government or private health plan, such as a HMO or other managed care plan, might cover services from only one physician or a panel of physicians. If the patient declines the covered services, the patient forfeits all or part of coverage. It might not be economically feasible for the patient to seek alternatives.

There are three ways in which a physician can establish a physician-patient relationship: (1) by contracting to care for a certain population and to have one of that population seek care, (2) by entering an express contract with a patient or the patient's representative by mutual agreement, or (3) by engaging in conduct from which a contract can be implied.

---

[1] *E.g.*, Sala v. Gamboa, 760 S.W.2d 838 (Tex. Ct. App. 1988).

CONTRACTS TO CARE FOR A CERTAIN POPULATION. A physician who enters a contract to care for members of a certain population must provide care for them to the extent required by the contract. For example, physicians enter contracts with hospitals to care for emergency patients or to provide certain services, such as radiology or pathology. Usually, these contracts do not permit the physician to refuse to care for individual hospital patients requiring those services.[2] Physician contracts with HMOs and other managed care entities are often of this type. Physicians frequently enter contracts with other institutions and organizations (such as athletic teams, schools, companies, prisons, jails,[3] and nursing homes) that include an agreement to provide certain kinds of care to all members of certain populations who seek care. In unusual circumstances other agreements can be interpreted to impose these duties.

Even when a physician has a contract to care for a certain population, in some circumstances a physician can decline to accept a nonemergency patient when it is known that a therapeutic relationship cannot be established due, for example, to threats or abuse by the patient, unreasonable patient expectations, or the patient's refusal to cooperate with treatment.

EXPRESS CONTRACT. A physician-patient relationship can begin by mutual agreement of the physician and the patient or the patient's representative.

Limits on Scope of Contract. The physician usually limits the scope of the contract and does not assume responsibility for all the patient's medical needs. For example, the contract with a specialist is generally limited to the services in that specialty; for example, a contract with an internist does not require the internist to perform surgery.[4] An obstetrician can refuse to participate in home deliveries.[5] Physicians can limit the geographic area in which they practice. A California court ruled that a patient who became ill while visiting out of town could not sue her physician for refusing to come to the other town to see her.[6] A consulting physician who examines a patient at the request of the primary physician can

---

[2] *E.g.*, Hongsathavij v. Queen of Angels/Hollywood Presbyterian Med. Ctr., 62 Cal. App. 4th 1123, 73 Cal. App. 2d 695 (2d Dist. 1998) [hospital board removed physician from on-call panel after refusal to deliver high-risk patient in labor].

[3] *E.g.*, Carswell v. Bay County, 854 F.2d 454 (11th Cir. 1988).

[4] *E.g.*, Skodje v. Hardy, 47 Wash. 2d 557, 288 P.2d 471 (1955).

[5] *E.g.*, Vidrine v. Mayes, 127 So. 2d 809 (La. Ct. App. 1961).

[6] McNamara v. Emmons, 36 Cal. App. 2d 199, 97 P.2d 503 (4th Dist. 1939).

limit involvement with the patient to the consultation and refuse continuing responsibility.

In 2000, a New York court ruled that an ophthalmologist could not be sued for abandonment because conducting an initial consultation to confirm the need for the surgery did not constitute agreement to undertake the actual surgical care.[7]

Some limitations on the scope of the contract are not permissible. An admitting physician assumes responsibility to examine the patient and offer appropriate treatment until the physician-patient relationship is terminated. In a Florida case, a physician who was at home recovering from an illness agreed to admit a patient as a favor to a friend but attempted to limit his contract solely to the act of admission by making it clear that he could not treat the patient.[8] The patient died of an undiagnosed brain abscess within a few days. The physician never saw her. The court ruled that there was a physician-patient relationship that included a duty to see the patient; so the patient's father was permitted to sue the physician for malpractice.

State-mandated Contracts. States have considered requiring all licensed physicians to accept certain patients. In 1994, Tennessee proposed a rule that would have required all licensed physicians who were accepting new patients to accept patients in the TennCare program, the state's Medicaid program. If TennCare patients were declined, all new patients would have had to be declined. In response to the strong reaction from physicians, the rule was withdrawn.[9]

IMPLIED CONTRACT. Sometimes a physician-patient relationship is inferred from physician conduct. When a physician commences treatment, courts will generally find a physician-patient relationship. Some courts have found a relationship from lesser contact. In an Iowa case, a relationship was established when a physician told a patient he would perform surgery.[10] A New York court found an implied contract when a physician listened to a recital of

---

[7] Heraud v. Weissman, 276 A.D.2d 376, 714 N.Y.S.2d 476 (1st Dept. 2000).

[8] Giallanza v. Sands, 316 So. 2d 77 (Fla. 4th DCA 1975); *see also* Maltempo v. Cuthbert, 504 F.2d 325 (5th Cir. 1974) [physician liable for failing to examine jailed patient after agreeing with his parents to do so even though patient was under care of jail physician].

[9] *Rule to ban physicians from limiting their Tenncare patient loads rescinded*, 4 HEALTH L. RPTR. [BNA] 372 (1995) [hereinafter HEALTH L. RPTR. cited as H.L.R.]; *but see also*, Catanzano v. Wing, No. 89-CV-1127L (W.D. N.Y. Feb. 4, 1998), *as discussed in* 7 H.L.R. 291 (1998) [freedom of choice in Medicaid law does not preclude state from compelling home health agencies to accept Medicaid patients who establish necessity in administrative proceedings].

[10] McGulpin v. Bessmer, 241 Iowa 1119, 43 N.W.2d 121 (1950).

the patient's symptoms over the telephone.[11] Physicians who do not wish to risk assuming the responsibility of a relationship should limit telephone calls to advising the caller to seek medical assistance elsewhere.

It is often difficult to predict what conduct will create a relationship. Courts have disagreed on whether an on-call consultant can establish a relationship with a patient by answering a telephone call from the attending physician.[12] In 2003, a Utah appellate court addressed a case where an endodontist had discovered that a patient could not pay and refused to perform a root canal procedure. The patient claimed abandonment. The court ruled that patient needed expert testimony to establish whether treatment had started.[13]

Although some specialists, such as pathologists and diagnostic radiologists, seldom see their patients, a physician-patient relationship is still established. This relationship does not usually include the responsibility for continuing care that is one of the elements of most relationships, but it does include responsibility for the consequences of intentional or negligent errors in providing pathology or radiology services.

6-2 How Does a Relationship with a Hospital Begin?

This section discusses the general rules for nonemergency patients. The special rules for emergency patients are discussed later in Section 6-3.

Under common law, a person who does not need emergency care usually does not have a right to be admitted to a hospital. The hospital can legally refuse to admit any person unless one of three exceptions applies: (1) common law exceptions, (2) contractual exceptions, or (3) statutory exceptions. Several statutes forbid discriminatory admission policies but generally do not grant a right to be admitted. These discrimination statutes are discussed in section

---

[11] O'Neil v. Montefiore Hosp., 11 A.D.2d 132, 202 N.Y.S.2d 436 (1st Dept. 1960); *contra*, Buttersworth v. Swint, 53 Ga. App. 602, 186 S.E. 770 (1936) [answers to questions in hallway not enough].

[12] *Compare* St. John v. Pope, 901 S.W.2d 420 (Tex. 1995) [no relationship created] *with* Kelley v. Middle Tenn. Emergency Physicians, P.C., 133 S.W.2d 587 (Tenn. 2004) [jury question whether relationship created].

[13] Newman v. Sonnenberg, 81 P.3d 808 (Utah Ct. App. 2003).

6-4. Rights to be admitted are also contingent on necessity for hospitalization, appropriateness of the hospital for the patient's needs, and availability of space.

COMMON LAW RIGHT TO ADMISSION. A person generally has a right to be admitted when the hospital is responsible for the original injury that caused the need for hospitalization. In some circumstances, a person who becomes ill or injured in hospital buildings or on hospital grounds has a right to be admitted even if the hospital is not otherwise responsible for the illness or injury. If a hospital begins to exercise control of a person by examining or beginning to provide care, a hospital-patient relationship can be started, entitling the patient to be admitted.

CONTRACTUAL RIGHT TO ADMISSION. When a hospital contracts to accept members of a certain population, those persons have a right to be admitted when they need care the hospital is able to provide. Some hospitals have contracts with employers agreeing to provide services to their employees or contracts with managed care entities, such as health maintenance organizations, agreeing to accept patients covered by the entity. An Alabama court found a hospital liable for breach of a contract to furnish hospital services to employees of a company because the jury concluded that a decision that hospitalization was unnecessary was not made in good faith.[14] When entering such contracts, hospitals should assure that the contract provides that patients will be entitled to admission only when admitted by a physician with clinical privileges at the hospital.

HILL-BURTON COMMUNITY SERVICE. Hospitals that accepted Hill-Burton construction grants or loans agreed to a "community service" obligation. The regulations defining this obligation specify that no person residing in the area serviced by the hospital will be denied admission to the portion of the hospital financed by Hill-Burton funds on any grounds other than the individual's lack of need for services, availability of the needed services in the hospital, or individual's ability to pay.[15] Inability to pay cannot be a basis for denial when the person needs emergency services or when the facility still has a Hill-Burton uncompensated care obligation. Emergency patients who are unable to pay and for whom services are not available under the uncompensated care obligation can be discharged or transferred

---

[14] Norwood Hosp. v. Howton, 32 Ala. App. 375, 26 So. 2d 427 (1946).
[15] 42 C.F.R §§ 124.601–124.607.

to another facility that is able to provide necessary services. However, there must be a medical determination that the discharge or transfer does not substantially risk deterioration of the patient's medical condition. Advance deposits can be required if the hospital permits alternative arrangements when patients who are able to pay do not have the necessary cash. Hospitals can require admission by a physician with clinical privileges only if sufficient physicians on the staff are willing to admit the patients who must be admitted under the community service obligation. If insufficient physicians on the medical staff will admit certain types of patients, such as Medicaid patients, the hospital must hire physicians who will admit them; condition appointments to the medical staff on an agreement to admit some of them;[16] or grant temporary admitting privileges to the patient's personal physician. Any hospital that received construction funds after the 1974 amendments must provide this access to persons who work in the area served by the facility, in addition to those who reside in the area. In 1988, one court ruled that the community service obligation only applies to direct admissions, not to attempted transfers from other hospitals.[17]

Hospitals also accepted an "uncompensated care obligation" which most have satisfied.[18] The community service obligation does not end when the uncompensated care obligation is satisfied.

STATUTORY RIGHT TO ADMISSION. Some hospitals, especially governmental hospitals, are obligated by statute to accept all patients from a certain population, which can be defined by geographic area of residence, inability to pay for care, or a combination of both. For example, county hospitals in Iowa are required to provide care and treatment to any resident of the county who is sick or injured and observes the rules of conduct adopted by the governing board.[19]

REASONS FOR NONADMISSION. Even when a person otherwise has a right to be admitted to a hospital, several reasons are generally recognized as justifying nonadmission.

Medical Necessity. If hospitalization is not medically necessary, there is no right to admission. A hospital is not a hotel; it is an institution for the provision of necessary medical services.

---

16 *E.g.*, Clair v. Center Comm. Hosp., 317 Pa. Super. 139, 463 A.2d 1065 (1983) [hospital can suspend physician who does not comply with rule requiring indigent care].
17 Ritter v. Wayne County Gen. Hosp., 174 Mich. App. 490, 436 N.W.2d 673 (1988).
18 For a list of hospitals that still have an obligation, *see* http://www.hrsa.gov/osp/dfcr/obtain/hbstates.htm (accessed June 10, 2005).
19 Iowa Code Ann. § 347.16.

Scope of Service. If the hospital does not provide the services the patient needs, it does not have to admit the patient. However, hospitals need to provide reasonable accommodations to permit the disabled to have the benefit of their services. Sometimes it might not be clear whether what is needed is a new service that is not required to be provided or an accommodation that must be provided. Even when the hospital cannot provide the needed definitive diagnosis or treatment, if the patient needs emergency care to prepare for transfer to an appropriate facility, the hospital must provide such care to the extent of its capability.

Capacity. Generally, when space or staffing is not available, the hospital can refuse to admit the patient but still must provide the emergency care necessary to prepare for transfer.[20] This rule usually applies even when a court orders admission. For example, the South Dakota Supreme Court ruled that the lower court had exceeded its jurisdiction when it ordered a state training school to accept a juvenile when no space was available.[21] Therefore, the superintendent's disobedience was not punishable as contempt. However, not all courts adopt this realistic position; so such court orders should be reviewed with legal counsel when compliance is not contemplated. In 1982, the Washington Supreme Court interpreted state law to require a mental hospital to accept all patients presented to the hospital by mental health professionals within its allocated area even though they would exceed the institutional capacity.[22] It based its analysis in part on the need of these patients for immediate treatment, so perhaps this case should be viewed as an example of the hospital's responsibility for emergency patients.

Disruptive Patients. In some circumstances, it is possible to avoid admitting disruptive patients. In 1998, the highest court of Massachusetts ruled that a methadone program could not be sued

---

[20] Davis v. Johns Hopkins Hosp., 86 Md. App. 134, 585 A.2d 841 (1991), *aff'd in pertinent part*, 330 Md. 53, 622 A.2d 128 (1993) [no duty to admit emergency pediatric patient when PICU full]; Ritter v. Wayne County Gen. Hosp., 174 Mich. App. 490, 436 N.W.2d 673 (1988) [no duty to admit patient when no bed available]; *but see* People v. Flushing Hosp., 122 Misc. 2d 260, 471 N.Y.S.2d 745 (Crim. Ct. 1983) [hospital found guilty of misdemeanor, fined when patient died after emergency care refused because hospital full].

[21] People in the Interest of M.B., 312 N.W.2d 714 (S.D. 1981); *see also* Rhode Island Dep't of Mental Health v. Doe, 533 A.2d 536 (R.I. 1987) [trial court cannot specify facility for commitment; department places patients based on resources, priorities]; Dennis v. Redouty, 534 So. 2d 756 (Fla. 1st DCA 1988) [hospital administrator, not hearing officer, decides whether committed patient should be discharged early].

[22] Pierce County Office of Involuntary Commitment v. Western State Hosp., 97 Wash. 2d 264, 644 P.2d 131 (1982).

for refusing to admit a patient discharged from another clinic after an argument with that clinic's staff members.[23]

6-3 What Are the Special Rules Concerning Emergency Cases?

In the past, the general rule was that persons did not have a right to emergency hospital care except under the circumstances discussed earlier in this chapter in which they would be entitled to any necessary hospital services.

THE EMERGENCY MEDICAL TREATMENT AND ACTIVE LABOR ACT. Part of the 1986 Medicare amendments, the Emergency Medical Treatment and Active Labor Act (EMTALA) required that all hospitals that participate in Medicare provide certain services to all patients who seek emergency care.[24] This law was often called either COBRA or the "anti-dumping" statute until the 1989 amendments modified the law and changed its name to the Emergency Medical Treatment and Active Labor Act (EMTALA).[25] EMTALA applies only to hospitals, not to medical clinics[26] or utilization review entities.[27]

Since the enactment of this requirement, there has been a phenomenal growth in the use of hospital emergency departments. The National Center for Health Statistics reported that between 1993 and 2003, visits to emergency departments rooms in U.S. hospitals increased by 26 percent to a total of 114 million visits. During the same time, the U.S. population increased by only 12.3 percent.[28]

Eligibility. All patients who seek emergency medical services, whether or not they are eligible for Medicare, must be given an appropriate medical screening to determine if they have an emergency medical condition or are in active labor. When the Act first

---

[23] Loffredo v. Center for Addictive Disorders, 426 Mass. 541, 689 N.E.2d 799 (1998).

[24] Pub. L. No. 99-272, § 9121(b) (1986) (*codified as amended at* 42 U.S.C. § 1395dd); 42 C.F.R. §§ 489.20, 489.24–489.27.

[25] Pub. L. No. 101-239, § 6211 (1989); *see* Annotation, *Construction and application of Emergency Medical Treatment and Active Labor Act*, 104 A.L.R. FED. 166.

[26] *E.g.*, King v. Ahrens, 16 F.3d 265 (8th Cir. 1994); Acosta v. Pelican State Outpatient Clinic, 2004 U.S. Dist. LEXIS 3788 (E.D. La.); Rivera v. Medical & Geriatric Admin. Servs., 254 F Supp 2d 237 (D. P.R. 2003).

[27] *E.g.*, Bangert v. Christian Health Servs., No. 92 613 WLB (S.D. Ill. Dec. 17, 1992), *as reprinted in* M.M.G. ¶ 41,081.

[28] NATIONAL HOSPITAL AMBULATORY MEDICAL CARE SURVEY: 2003 EMERGENCY DEPARTMENT SUMMARY (2005) [www.cdc.gov/nchs/data/ad/ad358.pdf].

went into effect, the patient had to come to the hospital to be covered by EMTALA,[29] although not necessarily through the emergency room.[30] In 1998, it was announced that EMTALA applied to hospital-owned ambulances and to hospital-operated clinics.[31] In 2000, more formalized requirements were adopted for off-site hospital-operated clinics, and EMTALA extended the requirements to certain areas outside of the hospital.[32] In 2003, the rules were clarified, and the requirements were somewhat simplified.[33] For example, it is now clear that EMTALA does not apply to persons who develop emergency conditions after they are admitted.[34] In 2003, a federal district court ruled that EMTALA did not apply to a patient who went directly to the unit and never sought emergency care.[35]

In 1999, the United States Supreme Court ruled that EMTALA is not limited to cases where there is an improper motive for the treatment of the patient; EMTALA applies to all patients who seek emergency services at the hospital.[36]

The federal government does permit one form of discrimination in the provision of emergency services. In 2001, a federal appellate court ruled that hospitals operating under the Indian Health Act can deny emergency treatment to non-Indians.[37]

Screening. Most courts have ruled that EMTALA is not a federal malpractice act; so misdiagnosis is not a violation of EMTALA provided that an appropriate screening is given.[38] Courts generally examine whether the standard screening for the patient's symptoms was provided.[39] Minor deviations from standard screening protocols

---

[29] *E.g.*, Miller v. Medical Ctr., 22 F.3d 626 (5th Cir. 1994) [no EMTALA violation to tell doctor over phone not to send child to hospital]; Johnson v. University of Chicago Hosps., 982 F.2d 230 (7th Cir. 1992) [no EMTALA violation from diversion by radio before reaching emergency room].

[30] *E.g.*, McIntyre v. Schick, 795 F. Supp. 777 (E.D. Va. 1992).

[31] State Operations Manual, Transmittal No. 2 (May 1998); *New guidelines no cause for panic but necessitate hospital review, compliance*, 7 H.L.R. 1265 (1998).

[32] 65 FED. REG. 18434 (Apr. 7, 2000).

[33] 68 FED. REG. 53221 (Sept. 9, 2003); OIG Supplemental Compliance Guidelines, 69 FED. REG. 32012 (June 8, 2004).

[34] 42 C.F.R. 489.24(d)(2)(ii); *see also* Lopez-Soto v. Hawayek, 988 F. Supp. 41 (D. P.R. 1997) [does not apply to baby born in hospital].

[35] Dollard v. Allen, 260 F. Supp. 2d 1127 (D. Wyo. 2003).

[36] *E.g.*, Roberts v. Galen of Va., Inc., 525 U.S. 249 (1999), *rev'g*, 111 F.3d 405 (6th Cir. 1997).

[37] Williams v. United States, 242 F.3d 169 (4th Cir. 2001).

[38] *E.g.*, Marshall v. East Carroll Parish Hosp. Serv. Dist., 134 F.3d 319 (5th Cir.1998); Summers v. Baptist Med. Ctr., 91 F. 3d 1132 (8th Cir. 1996) (en banc); *see also* Repp v. Anadarko Mun. Hosp., 43 F.3d 519 (10th Cir. 1994) [minor deviations from institutional policies concerning screening do not establish EMTALA liability].

[39] *E.g.*, Crystal Star Phillips v. Hillcrest Med. Ctr., 244 F.3d 790 (10th Cir. 2001); Harry v. Marchant, 237 F.3d 1315 (11th Cir. 2001).

do not constitute violations.[40] Generally courts recognize that an appropriate screening can result in a misdiagnosis.[41]

Stabilization. If the screening determines that an emergency medical condition or active labor is present, the hospital must provide services to stabilize the patient or arrange for an appropriate transfer. The responsibility to provide stabilization services and transfers does not apply until the emergency condition is determined.[42] The Act is satisfied if the patient is stabilized at discharge.[43]

Not every injury is an emergency medical condition. For example, a federal court ruled that a patient with a head laceration received the required screening and the injury did not constitute an emergency medical condition under EMTALA.[44]

At least one federal appellate court has ruled that the stabilization requirement applies only to patients who are transferred.[45] Another federal appellate court ruled that all patients with emergency medical conditions must be stabilized prior to discharge.[46]

Patients with chronic conditions have attempted to use EMTALA to require longer term treatment. There was some concern that courts were going to use EMTALA to mandate long-term treatment when a federal appellate court ruled in 1994 that a hospital could not discontinue the use of a respirator on an anencephalic baby that had been brought to the hospital as an emergency transfer even if the treatment was futile.[47] However, in

---

[40] *E.g.,* Kilroy v. Star Valley Med. Ctr., 237 F. Supp. 2d 1298 (D. Wyo. 2002).

[41] *E.g.,* Crystal Star Phillips v. Hillcrest Med. Ctr., 244 F.3d 790 (10th Cir. 2001) [misdiagnosis does not violate EMTALA]; Gerber v. Northwest Hosp. Ctr., Inc., 943 F. Supp. 571 (D. Md. 1996) [failure to address psychiatric symptoms while treating physical complaints in emergency room failed to state claim under EMTALA, at most state law claim for failure to diagnose].

[42] *E.g,* Bryant v. Adventist Health System/West, 289 F.3d 1162 (9th Cir. 2002); Jackson v. E. Bay Hosp., 246 F.3d 1248 (9th Cir. 2001); Urban v. King, 43 F.3d 523 (10th Cir. 1994).

[43] *E.g.,* Holcomb v. Monahan, 30 F.3d 116 (11th Cir. 1994); Green v. Youro Infirmary, 992 F.2d 537 (5th Cir. 1993).

[44] Taylor v. Dallas County Hosp. Dist., 959 F. Supp. 373 (D. Tex. 1996).

[45] *E.g.,* Harry v. Marchant, 291 F.3d 767 (11th Cir. 2002); *contra* Preston v. Meriter Hosp., 2005 WI 122, 700 N.W.2d 158 [EMTALA applies to baby born, died in hospital].

[46] Thomas v. Christ Hosp. & Med. Ctr., 328 F.3d 890 (7th Cir. 2003) [psychiatric emergency involving threat to self or others requires stabilization of hospitalization]; *see also, Hospital fined for refusing medical care to uninsured patient,* AP, Mar. 25, 2004 [$40,000 fine for refusing care to emergency psychiatric patient].

[47] *In re* Baby K, 16 F.3d 590 (4th Cir. 1994), *cert. denied,* 513 U.S. 825 (1994); *see* G.J. Annas, *Asking the courts to set the standard of emergency care - The case of Baby K,* 330 NEW ENG. J. MED. 1542 (1994).

1996, the same federal appellate court clarified the scope of its earlier ruling by holding that EMTALA did not require indefinite treatment; EMTALA applies only to immediate emergency stabilizing treatment.[48]

Transfers. The patient can be transferred only if (1) the patient requests the transfer or qualified medical personnel certify that benefits outweigh risks and (2) qualified personnel and equipment are used to transfer the patient to a hospital that has accepted the patient and that has space and staff to treat the patient. If a patient is transferred without approval of the receiving hospital, the sending hospital can be required to reimburse the receiving hospital for the care of the patient. In some limited circumstances, transfers by private car can satisfy the requirements.[49]

There are also requirements that documentation accompany the patient. Some federal courts have refused to premise liability on violations of some of these documentation requirements.[50] However, federal regulators still seek strictly to enforce the requirements.

The 1989 Medicare amendments and some state laws require hospitals to accept emergency transfers when the sending hospital is unable to care for the patient and the receiving hospital is able to benefit the patient.[51] In 1993, HCFA distributed a letter stating that Medicare hospitals do not have to accept transfers from foreign hospitals.[52]

Penalties. When a patient is refused a screening or emergency services, the hospital can be fined, lose its entitlement to participate in Medicare, and be sued by the patient for resulting injuries.[53]

---

[48] Bryan v. Rectors of Univ. of Va., 95 F.3d 349 (4th Cir. 1996); *see also* Greenery Rehabilitation Group v. Hammon, 150 F.3d 226 (2d Cir. 1998) [statute authorizing Medicaid payments for treatment of undocumented aliens for emergency medical conditions applied only to "sudden, serious and short-lived physical injury or illness that require immediate treatment to prevent further harm"; "emergency medical condition" does not include continuing care for stable but chronic debilitating conditions].

[49] *E.g.*, Wey v. Evangelical Comm. Hosp., 833 F. Supp. 453 (M.D. Pa. 1993).

[50] *E.g.*, Vargas v. Del Puerto Hosp., 98 F.3d 1202 (9th Cir. 1996) [certification requirement]; Hart v. Riverside Hosp., 899 F. Supp. 264 (D. Va. 1995) [requirement of written consent before transferring patient in active labor].

[51] 42 U.S.C. § 1395dd(g), *as added by* Pub. L. No. 101-239, § 6211(f) (1989); *e.g.*, FLA. STAT. § 395.0142 ; 25 TEX. ADMIN. CODE Ch. 11, §133.21.

[52] Letter from Acting HCFA Administrator Toby to Senator Lloyd Benson (Jan. 19, 1993), M.M.G. ¶ 41,049.

[53] 42 U.S.C. § 1395dd(d).

Generally, courts have applied state law procedures[54] and liability limits[55] to claims under EMTALA.

Physicians cannot be sued by private individuals for violations of EMTALA,[56] but they can be sanctioned by federal government officials.[57] When hospitals are found liable due to the acts of a physician, at least one court has permitted the hospital to sue the physician for reimbursement.[58]

STATE LAW. In nearly all states, a hospital is liable for injuries due to refusal of emergency treatment even if the hospital is one of the rare non-Medicare hospitals unaffected by federal law.[59] In Texas it is also a crime for any officer or employee of a general hospital supported with public funds to deny a person emergency services available in the hospital on the basis of inability to pay if a physician has diagnosed that the patient is seriously ill or injured.[60] In some states, it is crime for a physician to refuse to provide emergency services.[61]

---

[54] *E.g.*, Hardy v. New York City Health & Hosps. Corp., 164 F.3d 789 (2d Cir.1999) [state 90-day notice of claim requirement applies]; Draper v. Chiapuzio, 9 F.3d 1391 (9th Cir. 1993) [must comply with state one-year notice requirement]; *contra*, Root v. New Liberty Hosp. Dist., 209 F.3d 1068 (8th Cir. 2000) [state law procedures unrelated to damages do not apply]; Hewett v. Inland Hosp., 39 F. Supp. 2d 84 (D. Me. 1999) [state prelitigation, screening procedure not applicable].

[55] *E.g.*, Power v. Arlington Hosp. Ass'n, 42 F.3d 851 (4th Cir. 1994); Barris v. Los Angeles County, 2 Cal. 4th 101, 83 Cal. Rptr. 2d 145, 972 P.2d 966 (1999); Diaz v. CCHC-Golden Glades Ltd., 696 So. 2d 1346 (Fla. 3d DCA. 1997), *cert denied*, 523 U.S. 1119 (1998); Valencia v. St. Francis Hosp., 2004 U.S. Dist. LEXIS 7929 (S.D. Ind.); *but see* Root v. New Liberty Hosp. Dist., 209 F.3d 1068 (8th Cir. 2000) [sovereign immunity not applicable because it eliminated all liability]; *see also* Drew et al. v. University of Tenn. Reg. Med. Ctr., 211 F.3d 1268 (6th Cir 2000) [unpub] [governmental entities protected by the 11th Amendment cannot be sued for monetary damages by private entities under EMTALA].

[56] *E.g.*, Binkley v. Edwards Hosp., 2004 U.S. Dist. LEXIS 5539 (N.D. Ill.) [dismissing EMTALA suit against physician]; Palmer v. Hospital Auth., 22 F.3d 1559 (11th Cir. 1994) [although physician cannot be sued individually under EMTALA, can be sued under state law as part of suit against hospital under EMTALA]; Almond v. Town of Massena, 246 A.D.2d 697, 667 N.Y.S.2d 475 (3d Dept. 1998).

[57] Burditt v. U.S. DHHS, 934 F.2d 1362 (5th Cir. 1991) [affirming assessment of $20,000 penalty against individual physician]; Cherukuri v. Shalala, 175 F.3d 446 (6th Cir. 1999) [reversing civil money penalty against physician; wrong standard for stabilization applied by agency].

[58] McDougal v. LaForche Hosp. Serv., No. 92-2006, M.M.G. ¶ 41,542 (E.D La. May 25, 1993) (case dismissed in June 1993 pursuant to settlement).

[59] *E.g.*, Guerrero v. Copper Queen Hosp., 112 Ariz. 104, 537 P.2d 1329 (1975); Stanturf v. Sipes, 447 S.W.2d 558 (Mo. 1969); Wilmington Gen. Hosp. v. Manlove, 54 Del. 15, 174 A.2d 135 (1961); *see* Annotation, *Liability of hospital for refusal to admit or treat patient*, 35 A.L.R. 3D 841.

[60] TEX. REV. CIV. STAT. ANN. Art. 4438a.

[61] *E.g.*, People v. Anyakora, 236 A.D.2d 216, 656 N.Y.S.2d 253 (1st Dept. 1997) [affirming conviction of physician].

Patients are still free to decline treatment. A federal appellate court ruled that a hospital was not liable for the death of patient who left the emergency room after he called his insurance company and was told he was not covered at that hospital.[62] The family had settled with the insurance company. The court ruled that the insurance company could not compel the hospital to contribute toward the settlement. The hospital had made it clear to the patient that it would provide emergency treatment irrespective of his insurance coverage.

CONTINUING CARE. When care is provided under the emergency care obligation to patients the hospital would not otherwise accept, the hospital generally does not have a duty to provide continuing care if arrangements can be made for an appropriate transfer without substantial danger to the patient. This is recognized by the Hill-Burton community service regulations discussed earlier in this chapter. The Alabama Supreme Court ruled that a hospital has no obligation to admit a patient after providing proper emergency care.[63] The hospital fulfilled its responsibility by arranging for transfer to a charitable hospital. However, if the emergency care had created a dangerous condition requiring further care, the hospital would have had a duty to admit the patient under the general common law responsibility that everyone has to assist persons they have put in peril. In some states, financial transfers are permitted in a smaller range of circumstances.[64] If the hospital cannot provide the needed care, it has a duty to attempt to arrange a transfer. A California court found a hospital and the treating physician liable for negligent care of a severely burned patient, in part because the hospital did not have facilities to care for severe burns.[65] However, the hospital is not required to be the best facility providing the needed care. In a New York case, the patient was upset with a scar from a skin graft and sued the physician for failure to transfer the patient to a burn center. The court found no liability because although the hospital might not be the best that it could give adequate care for burn patients.[66]

---

[62] Consumer Health Found. v. Potomac Hosp., 172 F.3d 43, 1999 U.S. App. LEXIS 537 (4th Cir.) (unpub).

[63] Harper v. Baptist Med. Ctr.-Princeton, 341 So. 2d 133 (Ala. 1976).

[64] *E.g.*, Thompson v. Sun City Comm. Hosp., 141 Ariz. 597, 688 P.2d 605 (1984).

[65] Carrasco v. Bankoff, 220 Cal. App. 2d 230, 33 Cal. Rptr. 673 (2d Dist. 1963).

[66] Kenigsberg v. Cohn, 117 A.D.2d 652, 498 N.Y.S.2d 390 (2d Dept. 1986).

6-4 What Are the Effects of Nondiscrimination Laws?

Several statutes forbid discrimination in all aspects of patient care but generally do not grant a right to be admitted.

TITLE VI. Title VI of the Civil Rights Act of 1964[67] forbids discrimination on the basis of race, color, or national origin in any institution that receives federal financial assistance. Hospitals that receive Medicare or Medicaid reimbursement or other federal funds must comply with this statute and the implementing regulations.[68] There are few published court decisions concerning patient claims under this statute.[69] Prior to 1988, Title VI applied only to the portion of the hospital and its programs that were supported by federal financial assistance. In 1988, the law was amended so that it applied to the entire hospital if any part receives federal financial assistance.[70]

Title VI has been interpreted to require providers to arrange for language interpreters and translation of some documents for persons with limited English proficiency. Failure to arrange for this service is considered national origin discrimination.[71]

THE AMERICANS WITH DISABILITIES ACT. Title III of the Americans with Disabilities Act (ADA)[72] prohibits discrimination based on disability in the full enjoyment of the goods, services, facilities, privileges, and accommodations of any privately owned place of public accommodation. Hospitals and professional offices of health care providers are in the list of public accommodations

---

[67] 42 U.S.C. §§ 2000d–2000d-7.
[68] 45 C.F.R. pt. 80.
[69] *E.g.*, Ibarra v. Bexar County Hosp. Dist., 624 F.2d 44 (5th Cir. 1980) [abstention in suit concerning treatment of aliens]; Bryan v. Koch, 627 F.2d 612 (2d Cir. 1980) [hospital closing]; NAACP v. Medical Ctr., Inc., 657 F.2d 1322 (3d Cir. 1981) [hospital relocation]; *see also* Fobbs v. Holy Cross Health Sys. Corp., 29 F.3d 1439 (9th Cir. 1994), *cert. denied*, 513 U.S. 1127 (1995) [physician challenging summary suspension of clinical privileges lacked standing to assert rights of his minority patients].
[70] 42 U.S.C. § 2000d-4a(3)(A)(ii), *as added by* Pub. L. No. 100-259, § 6, 102 Stat. 31 (1988).
[71] *See* DOJ, Guidance to Federal Financial Assistance Recipients Regarding Title VI Prohibition Against National Origin Discrimination Affecting Limited English Proficient Persons (Apr. 12, 2002); DHHS, Guidance to Federal Financial Assistance Recipients Regarding Title VI Prohibition Against National Origin Discrimination Affecting Limited English Proficient Persons, 68 Fed. Reg. 47311 (Aug. 8, 2003); ProEnglish v. Bush, 70 Fed. Appx. 84 (4th Cir. 2003) [challenge to guidance rejected due to lack of standing]; *Brooklyn: Hospitals agree to provide interpreters*, N.Y. Times, Mar. 4, 2003, B4 [settlement with state attorney general]; *see also* G. Flores et al., *Errors in medical interpretation and their potential clinical consequences in pediatric encounters*, 111 Pediatrics 6 (2003).
[72] 42 U.S.C. §§ 12181–12189; *see*, M.A. Dowell, *The Americans with Disabilities Act: The responsibilities of health care providers, insurers and managed care organizations*, 25 J. Health & Hosp. L. 289 (1992).

covered.[73] There is an exemption for insurers and hospitals concerning some underwriting, classifying, and administering of risks.[74] Otherwise, the reach of Title III has been interpreted broadly.[75]

A disability means having a "physical or mental impairment" that "substantially limits" one or more "major life activities." Each of these terms is further defined by regulations and court decisions. In 1998, the United States Supreme Court ruled that reproduction was a major life activity that was substantially impaired by being HIV-positive, so that a nonsymptomatic HIV-positive person qualified as being disabled.[76] Different treatment of a disabled person can be justified when there is a direct threat to the health and safety of others. The assessment of the risk must be based on objective, scientific information.[77]

The ADA applies to individual physicians for their acts in their professional offices. In 1998, the United States Supreme Court applied the ADA to a case in which a dentist declined to provide office treatment to a HIV-positive patient.[78] In 1995, a federal court decided that a HIV-positive patient could sue his primary care physician in his managed care program for allegedly failing to treat him or refer him to another physician who would treat him.

A Colorado clinic and physician were sued for declining to provide fertility services to a single deaf woman who refused to cooperate in assuring appropriate arrangements were made for parenting. The woman claimed the refusal was discriminatorily based on her deafness. The clinic and physician defended on the basis that the decision was not based on disability, but on her failure to cooperate with parenting planning. In 2003, a federal jury found in favor of the providers. In 2005, the ruling was affirmed by a federal appellate court.[79]

---

[73] 42 U.S.C. § 12181(7)(F).

[74] 42 U.S.C. § 12201(c).

[75] *E.g.,* Carparts Distrib. Ctr., Inc. v. Automotive Wholesaler's Ass'n of N. Eng., 37 F.3d 12 (1st Cir. 1994) [not limited to physical structures; can apply to services]; *In re* Baby K., 832 F. Supp. 1022 (E.D. Va. 1993) [may require futile respiratory support of anencephalic baby], *aff'd on other grounds,* 16 F.3d 590 (4th Cir.), *cert. denied,* 513 U.S. 825 (1994); Mayberry v. Von Valtier, 843 F. Supp. 1160 (E.D. Mich. 1994) [interpreter for deaf patient]; Aikins v. St. Helena Hosp., 843 F. Supp. 1329 (N.D. Cal. 1994) [interpreter for deaf patient].

[76] Bragdon v. Abbott, 524 U.S. 624 (1998).

[77] *Id.;* School Bd. of Nassau County v. Arline, 480 U.S. 273 (1987); Chevron v. Echazabal, 536 U.S. 73 (2002) [direct threat can be to self].

[78] Bragdon v. Abbott, 524 U.S. 624 (1998).

[79] Chambers v. Melmed, No. 00-RB-1794 (CBS) (D. Colo. jury verdict Nov. 21, 2003), *aff'd* 2005 U.S. App. LEXIS 14270 (10th Cir.) (unpub).

There have been several cases where patients sought sign language interpreters. There have been several settlements in which hospitals have agreed to make better arrangements for such interpreters.[80]

The ADA permits individuals to seek an injunction but does not permit private claims for monetary damages.[81] The federal government can seek payments in its enforcement actions.[82]

The ADA does not guarantee a level of medical care; it only prohibits discrimination in care provided. In 1998, a federal appellate court ruled that the ADA could not form the basis for challenging the closure of a specialized health care facility that treated children with developmental disabilities.[83]

Similarly, discrimination by public programs and facilities is prohibited by Title II.[84] In 1999, the United States Supreme Court ruled that in some circumstances states must provide mentally disabled persons with community-based treatment rather than institutional placement.[85]

It remains an open question as to when state entities protected by the Eleventh Amendment can be sued by private individuals for ADA violations. In 2004, the United States Supreme Court ruled that private suits could be brought against state entities for violations of the ADA that interfered with access to the courts but declined to rule on other applications of Title II.[86]

THE REHABILITATION ACT OF 1973. The Rehabilitation Act of 1973[87] forbids discrimination on the basis of handicap in any institution that receives federal financial assistance. A hospital that

---

[80] *E.g.,* Connecticut Ass'n of the Deaf v. Middlesex Mem. Hosp., No. 3-95-CV-2408 (AHN) (D. Conn. settlement approved Aug. 20, 1998), *as discussed in* 7 H.L.R. 1065, 1378 (1998); *Oroville hospital settles federal disability suit,* AP, July 31, 2002.

[81] 42 U.S.C. §§ 12188(a)(2), 12188(b)(2)(B); Jairath v. Dyer, 154 F.3d 1280 (11th Cir. 1998); Access Now, Inc. v. AMH CGH, Inc., 2001 U.S. Dist. LEXIS 12876 (S.D. Fla.) [approval of consent decree concerning disability access to defendant's hospitals]; *California medical facility agrees to settle case alleging access denial,* DISABILITY COMPLIANCE BULLETIN, Mar. 10, 2000 [wheelchair user claimed rest rooms not accessible].

[82] *E.g.,* United States v. Morvant, 843 F. Supp. 1092 (E.D. La. 1994) [federal government could sue dentist for refusing to treat HIV-positive patients in office]; United States v. Jack H. Castle, D.D.S., Inc., No. H-93-31450 (S.D. Tex. Sept. 23, 1994), *as discussed in* 3 H.L.R. 1343 (1994) [dental clinic required to pay $100,000 for refusing to treat HIV patient].

[83] Lincoln CERCPAC v. Health & Hops. Corp., 147 F.3d 165 (2d Cir.1998).

[84] 42 U.S.C. §§ 12131–12134.

[85] Olmstead v. L.C., 527 U.S. 581 (1999).

[86] Tennessee v. Lane, 124 S. Ct. 1978 (U.S. 2004); *see also* Board of Trustees of Univ. of Ala. v. Garrett, 531 U.S. 356 (2001) [private ADA, Title I, suits barred by Eleventh Amendment].

[87] 29 U.S.C. § 794.

receives Medicare and Medicaid reimbursement must comply with this statute and the implementing regulations.[88]

In 1994, a federal district court ruled that a nursing facility did not violate the act by refusing to admit an Alzheimer's patient with psychotic tendencies where the facility did not provide psychiatric services for those with disruptive psychotic disorders.[89] In 1995, a federal appellate court reversed that decision and ruled that the facility had failed to show that accommodating the patient would require fundamental changes in its programs or be an undue burden where the patient was largely immobile so that a jury could determine the patient posed little harm to others.[90] The nursing facility is reported to have sought the transfer of the patient based on a change in medical opinion concerning the patient's status that coincided with expiration of the patient's insurance benefits; so perhaps this is just a case of the court not believing the diagnosis.[91] However, more broadly read, this case could be a troublesome precedent for forcing providers to initiate new services for handicapped patients whenever a jury concludes that the new service does not constitute a "fundamental change" in the program or an undue burden. However, in 1995, another federal district court ruled that a nursing home that did not offer subacute care did not have to accept a patient seeking that level of care.[92] Thus, most courts still appear reluctant to force providers to initiate new levels of services.

In 1992, another federal court ruled that the Act did not require a nursing home to keep a violent and aggressive patient who abused the staff and struck another patient. The court refused to enjoin the facility from discharging the patient after eight days notice to leave.[93]

Individual physicians can also be sued under this law.[94] In 1994, a federal court decided that a physician could be sued by a deaf patient for allegedly refusing to provide an interpreter in her

---

[88] 45 C.F.R. pt. 84.

[89] Wagner v. Fair Acres Geriatric Ctr., 859 F. Supp. 776 (E.D. Pa. 1994).

[90] Wagner v. Fair Acres Geriatric Ctr., 49 F.3d 1002 (3d Cir. 1995).

[91] *See also* N. Hershey, *Patient's discharge linked to end of insurance coverage*, 12 HOSP. L. NEWSLETTER (July 1995), at 1 [describing Muse v. Charter Hosp., 117 N.C. App. 468, 452 S.E.2d 589, *rev. denied*, 340 N.C. 114, 455 S.E.2d 663 (1995) [in which hospital was held liable for suicide of patient allegedly discharged pursuant to a hospital policy to discharge when insurance coverage expired].

[92] Grubbs v. Medical Facilities of Am., Inc., 879 F. Supp. 588 (W.D Va. 1995).

[93] Nichols v. St. Luke Ctr., 800 F. Supp. 1564 (S.D. Ohio 1992).

[94] *E.g.*, Woolfolk v. Duncan, 872 F. Supp. 1381 (E.D. Pa. 1995).

office.[95] However, this Act cannot be used to force unnecessary care that a handicapped person desires. In a 1993 federal case, a HIV-positive patient claimed he had not been seen frequently enough by a physician and HMO. The court found no violation of the Act because he had been seen nine times in ten months and had been referred to specialists three times.[96]

In 1996, a federal court ruled that an obstetrician violated the Act by refusing to provide prenatal care to a deaf woman.[97] However, in 2001, a federal appellate court ruled that an obstetrician had not violated the Act by referring a pregnant woman with HIV to another hospital for treatment when he had a reasonable medical basis for his determination that he was not competent to treat her properly.[98]

Most substance abusers are considered handicapped under this law and the ADA; so hospitals cannot discriminate against alcoholics and drug abusers in the providing of services.

THE AGE DISCRIMINATION ACT OF 1975. The Age Discrimination Act of 1975[99] forbids discrimination on the basis of age in federally assisted programs. In some circumstances, reasonable factors other than age can be used even when they have a disproportionate effect on persons of different ages.[100] Also, in some circumstances, entities can reasonably take into account age as a factor when it is necessary to the normal operation or achievement of the statutory objective of the program or activity.[101] Special benefits to children and elderly persons are permitted.[102]

STATE LAW. State nondiscrimination laws can also apply equally to hospitals and physicians. Refusal of individual practitioners to treat HIV-positive patients has also been punished under state law.[103] However, a New York court ruled that it was not discrimination to take

---

[95] Mayberry v. Von Valtier, 843 F. Supp. 1160 (E.D. Mich. 1994).

[96] Tony v. U.S Healthcare, Inc., 838 F. Supp. 201 (E.D. Pa. 1993), 840 F. Supp. 357 (E.D. Pa. 1993) [summary judgment granted for other defendants].

[97] Sumes v. Andres, 938 F. Supp. 9 (D. D.C. 1996) [pregnant deaf woman denied prenatal care by obstetrician could recover under Rehabilitation Act of 1973, local law].

[98] Lesley v. Chie, 250 F.3d 47 (1st Cir. 2001).

[99] 42 U.S.C. §§ 6101 – 6107; 45 C.F.R. pts. 90 [general], 91 [HHS].

[100] 45 C.F.R. § 91.14.

[101] 45 C.F.R. § 91.15.

[102] 45 C.F.R. § 91.17.

[103] *E.g.*, State by Beaulieu v. Clausen, 491 N.W.2d 662 (Minn. Ct. App. 1992); *CA surgeon slapped with $166,000 verdict for refusing surgery*, AIDS LITIGATION REPORTER, Mar. 22, 1999, 8; *Panel sides with HIV-positive patient who accused surgeon of bias*, AP, June 18, 2002 [Maine Human Rights Comm'n]; *Dentist suspended for refusing to treat lesbian patient*, AP, July 18, 2003 [N.H. Board of Dental Exam'rs].

extra precautions during dental work on a HIV-positive patient.[104] This reversed a state administrative ruling that such treatment had exposed the patient to public humiliation.

In 1993, the highest court of New York ruled that it was a violation of the state Human Rights law for a hospital to exclude all pregnant women from its inpatient drug detoxification program. The lack of equipment to treat pregnant women, lack of obstetricians on its staff, and lack of a license to provide obstetrical care did not justify excluding all pregnant women. These services did not have to be provided, but a case-by-case determination had to be made whether each pregnant woman could be treated safely without the availability of these services on-site or through arrangements with nearby off-site facilities.[105]

REQUIRED DISCRIMINATION. In 1994, California voters adopted Proposition 187, which required health care providers to refuse certain services to undocumented aliens and to report the aliens to authorities. A federal court enjoined implementation, and in 1999, the state dropped its appeal.[106]

6-5 How Does a Relationship with a Physician End?

A physician has a duty to continue to provide medical care until the relationship is legally terminated. A physician who discontinues care before the relationship is legally terminated can be liable for abandonment.[107] The physician-patient relationship can be ended if (1) medical care is no longer needed, (2) the patient withdraws from the relationship, (3) the care of the patient is transferred to another physician, (4) ample notice of withdrawal is given by the physician to the patient, or (5) the physician is unable to provide care.

PATIENT WITHDRAWAL. If the patient withdraws from the relationship, the physician has a duty to attempt to warn the patient if

---

[104] *E.g.*, Syracuse Comm. Health Ctr. v. Wendi A.M., 198 A.D.2d 830, 604 N.Y.S.2d 406 (4th Dept. 1993).

[105] Elaine W. v. Joint Diseases North Gen. Hosp., 81 N.Y.2d 211, 597 N.Y.S.2d 617, 613 N.E.2d 523 (1993), *rev'g*, 180 A.D.2d 525, 580 N.Y.S.2d 246 (1st Dept. 1992).

[106] Gregorio T. v. Wilson, No. 94-7652 (C.D. Cal. Nov. 22, 1994) [temporary restraining order], *as discussed in* 3 H.L.R. 1731 (1994); Gregorio T. v. Wilson, 54 F.3d 599, 59 F.3d 1002 (9th Cir. 1995); League of United Latin Am. Citizens v. Wilson, 1998 U.S. Dist. LEXIS 3418 (C.D. Cal.) [Proposition 187 preempted by federal law]; E. Nieves, *California calls off effort to carry out immigrant measure*, N.Y. TIMES, July 30, 1999, A1.

[107] *See* Annotation, *Liability of physician who abandons case*, 37 A.L.R. 2D 432.

further care is needed, but there is no duty to provide further fol-low-up.[108] Upon request, the physician should advise the successor physician, if any, of information necessary to continue treatment. When an episode of treatment is completed, the patient can termi-nate the relationship by not returning for future treatment.[109]

TRANSFER. A patient's care can be transferred to another physician. Physicians attend meetings, take vacations, and have other valid reasons they cannot be available. A physician can fulfill the duties of the physician-patient relationship by providing a quali-fied substitute.[110]

Transfer of a patient to another hospital can terminate the physi-cian-patient relationship with physicians at the first hospital.[111]

PHYSICIAN WITHDRAWAL. A physician can withdraw from the relationship without providing a substitute by giving the patient reasonable notice in writing with sufficient time for the patient to locate another physician willing to accept the patient if continuing care is required.[112] Some of the reasons for withdrawal are non-cooperation and failure to pay bills when able to do so.

Another reason for withdrawal is when the patient abuses, harasses, or is violent toward the physician or other health care ser-vice providers.

Some providers withdraw from relationships with patients who file malpractice suits. It is controversial when providers withdraw from relationships with patients who have sued others. However, it is sometimes appropriate to withdraw when the suit is directed against the withdrawing physician. It is difficult and sometimes not possible to maintain a professional relationship. In 2003, a California court ruled that a medical group could terminate its relationship with patients who had sued the group for malpractice.[113] However, even a malpractice suit does not justify a withdrawal without adequate

---

[108] *E.g.*, East v. United States, 745 F. Supp. 1142 (D. Md. 1990).
[109] *E.g.*, Bruske v. Hille, 1997 SD 108, 567 N.W.2d 872 (1997).
[110] *E.g.*, Rosen v. Greifenberger, 257 Va. 373, 513 S.E.2d 861 (1999) [doctor has no duty person-ally to provide continuous care; doctor may make arrangements for another physician to pro-vide care in his absence; care by group satisfied duty]; Kearns v. Ellis, 18 Mass. App. Ct. 923, 465 N.E.2d 294 (1984).
[111] *E.g.*, Bosel v. Babcock, 153 Mich. App. 592, 596, 396 N.W.2d 448 (1986) [physician-patient relationship terminated when patient transferred to another hospital for treatment by differ-ent doctor].
[112] *E.g.*, Miller v. Greater Southeast Comm. Hosp., 508 A.2d 927 (D.C. 1986).
[113] *E.g.*, Scripps Clinic v. Superior Court, 108 Cal. App. 4th 917, 134 Cal. Rptr. 2d 101 (4th Dist. 2003).

notice. In 2003, a Michigan court addressed a case where a surgeon had agreed to perform surgery related to delivery and after admission of the patient refused to perform the surgery when he discovered that the patient had sued his officemate. The court concluded that the refusing surgeon could be sued for abandonment.[114]

UNABLE TO PROVIDE CARE. A physician can be excused from the responsibilities of the relationship when unable to provide care. A physician who is ill should not accept additional responsibilities and should attempt to arrange for a substitute.[115] Sometimes physicians become too ill to be able to arrange a substitute. Also, a physician cannot be with two patients simultaneously. The necessity for attending another patient can provide a valid excuse if the physician has exercised prudence in determining the priority.[116] The physician cannot entirely give up one patient to attend another. The frequency of attendance to each patient will be an important factor in assessing whether one patient has been abandoned.

ABANDONMENT. A physician who fails to see a patient with whom there is a physician-patient relationship without an acceptable reason can face liability for breach of contract or malpractice if the patient is injured as a result. Physicians do not have to be with the patient continuously to satisfy their responsibility.[117] Physicians can leave orders for others to administer medications or other care if they return at intervals appropriate to the patient's condition.

When hospital admission is not indicated, the patient can usually be sent home with instructions to call if further care is needed. The patient has the responsibility to call. However, when the patient and those responsible for the patient are unable to provide the needed care in the home, the physician usually should have arrangements made for other assistance or placement. The patient or representative can be told to follow certain instructions or to return at a certain time. It is not abandonment if the patient fails to return or follow instructions. However, in some cases, if the patient has a known debility, it can be prudent to attempt to follow up if the patient does not return.

---

[114] Tierney v. University of Mich. Regents, 257 Mich. App. 681, 669 N.W.2d 575 (2003).

[115] *E.g.*, Kenny v. Piedmont Hosp., 136 Ga. App. 660, 22 S.E.2d 162 (1975) [not abandonment for ill surgeon to permit associate to operate].

[116] *E.g.*, Young v. Jordan, 106 W. Va. 139, 145 S.E. 41 (1928) [another patient is not an excuse when physician induced labor in first patient].

[117] *E.g.*, Haidak v. Corso, 2004 D.C. App. LEXIS 34 (2004) [intermittent care to an inpatient is not abandonment].

A Massachusetts surgeon is reported to have left an operation for approximately thirty minutes while he cashed a check at a bank. His clinical privileges and medical license were suspended.[118]

In some circumstances, abandonment can be a criminal act. In 2000, a California court ruled that abandonment of a nursing home patient could constitute elder abuse under the state statute.[119] A Florida physician was charged with felony neglect for leaving an apparent stroke victim at a rescue mission. In 2003, the felony charges were dropped in a settlement with the state.[120]

Although the duties of most nurses to patients is somewhat different from physicians because in inpatient settings they generally provide continuous care but only for defined periods of time, nurses can also be liable for abandonment in some circumstances. This is clearly the case when they leave during their assigned shift without appropriate arrangements for coverage. In 2000, a New York court ruled that a visiting nurse could be sued for the consequences of a fire that occurred when the nurse abandoned a patient by leaving the site an hour before end of the shift.[121] There is controversy over the scope of a nurse's responsibility when no replacement is available at the end of a shift. Most states still recognize a duty to assist in arranging for an orderly transition and in some circumstances to continue to work into the next shift. Some nurses will voluntarily perform this overtime work. However, it is a hardship for some, and they object to being forced to perform this overtime. A few states have passed laws restricting involuntary overtime, but even these states generally recognize exceptions for bona fide emergencies. These laws are discussed in Chapter 4.

6-6 How Does a Relationship with a Hospital End?

The inpatient relationship with the institution usually ends with discharge of the patient. The outpatient relationship ends in a manner analogous to the ending of the physician relationship discussed in Section 6-5.

---

[118] R. O'Neill, *Patient abandoned by surgeon says he was left in dark about incident*, AP Aug. 15, 2002.

[119] Mack v. Soung, 80 Cal. App. 4th 966, 95 Cal. Rptr. 2d 830 (3d Dist. 2000).

[120] *Panhandle doctor avoids felony charge in patient neglect case*, AP, July 15, 2003.

[121] Villarin v. Onobanjo, 276 A.D.2d 479, 714 N.Y.S.2d 90 (2d Dept. 2000); *see also* Harrington v. St. Mary's Hosp., 280 A.D.2d 912, 720 N.Y.S.2d 693 (4th Dept. 2001) [allegation nurse in stroke rehab program left patient unattended raised question about judgment in assessing patient needs].

This section focuses on ending the inpatient relationship. There is a fundamental tension between the liability that can result from holding a patient too long and the liability that can result from releasing a patient too soon. There are at least five other problems related to ending the relationship.

6-6.1. What are the institution's responsibilities when planning consensual discharge?

6-6.2. When can the institution refuse to discharge a patient who wants to leave?

6-6.3. What can the institution do when a patient refuses to cooperate with discharge planning or refuses to leave?

6-6.4. When can the institution discharge a patient who needs additional inpatient treatment?

6-6.5. When can the institution permit temporary releases without discharge?

6-6.1 What Are the Institution's Responsibilities When Planning Consensual Discharge?

Hospitals that participate in Medicare are required to have a discharge planning process and to arrange for the initial implementation of the patient's discharge plan.[122]

When patients no longer need the level of care provided in a hospital, they can be transferred to a nursing home or discharged to home care. When they no longer need the level of hospital care in a referral center or begin to need the more specialized level of care in a referral center, interhospital transfer is appropriate.

Consensual discharges are generally arranged with the patient and the patient's family. However, the family does not have a right to be involved if the patient or the patient's legal guardian desires to exclude other family. In 1996, a Georgia court ruled that the wife could not sue a nursing home for discharging her husband to

---

[122] 42 U.S.C. § 1395x(ee); 42 C.F.R. § 482.43(c). Nursing homes have separate discharge requirements under Medicaid law, 42 U.S.C. § 1396r(c)(2); 42 C.F.R. §§ 483.12, 483.200–483.206; O'Bannon v. Town Court Nursing Ctr., 447 U.S. 773 (1980) [residents have no right to hearing before state revocation of Medicaid participation of nursing home]; Blum v. Yaretsky, 457 U.S. 991 (1982) [private nursing home decisions to transfer to lower level of care not state action, no constitutional right to hearing]; Nichols v. St. Luke Ctr., 800 F. Supp. 1564 (S.D. Ohio 1992) [no private cause of action under Medicaid to challenge discharge by private nursing home, cause of action under Rehabilitation Act, but danger to staff justified discharge].

his guardian, who had moved her husband to another state without her knowledge.[123]

Discharge planning has become an increasingly complex problem as more complex conditions are no longer viewed as requiring inpatient hospital care. More complex treatment must be provided in other health care facilities or the home. It is increasingly challenging to find health care facilities or the necessary family and professional support for home care within the resources available to the patient. Most patients and families cooperate in this process. Section 6-6.3 discusses some of the options when they do not.

Often nursing homes and hospitals have agreements concerning transfers to assure that patients can move to the appropriate level of care. In most cases, these agreements work well, but sometimes there are problems. In 1996, an Alabama court ruled that a nursing home could be liable to a hospital for violating an agreement by not reaccepting a nursing home patient who had been transferred to the hospital for 23-hour evaluation and had not met the hospital admission criteria.[124]

In some unusual cases, government authorities must be consulted concerning discharge plans. For example, it was reported that FDA approval was required for the discharge plans of the recipients of some of the experimental artificial hearts.[125]

Children, the infirm aged, and others who are unable to care for themselves should be discharged only to the custody of someone who can take care of them. A California physician was found liable for discharging an abused 11-month-old child to the abusing parents without first giving the state an opportunity to intervene.[126]

6-6.2 When Can the Institution Refuse to Discharge a Patient Who Wants to Leave?

In most circumstances, a patient can leave an institution against medical advice at any time. However, there are several circumstances where the institution can or even must refuse to discharge a patient who wants to leave.

---

[123] Fisher v. Toombs County Nursing Home, 223 Ga. App. 842, 479 S.E.2d 180 (1996).

[124] Haleyville Health Care Ctr. v. Winston Count Hosp. Bd., 678 So. 2d 789 (Ala. Civ. App. 1996).

[125] B. Schreiner, *Heart recipient may spend time home*, AP, Oct. 30, 2001.

[126] Landeros v. Flood, 17 Cal. 3d 399, 551 P.2d 389 (1976); *see* Annotation, *Validity, construction, and application of state statutes requiring doctor or other person to report child abuse*, 73 A.L.R. 4TH 782.

If an adult patient is neither disoriented nor committable, the patient generally has a right to leave unless it is one of the unusual situations in which courts will order treatment, as discussed in Chapter 7. Interfering with this right can lead to liability. Honoring the patient's wishes to leave can cause the patient care staff great distress. For example, nearly all physicians and nurses are distressed when an oriented patient with a spinal fracture insists on leaving the hospital, risking paralysis or even death that could probably be prevented by appropriate care in the hospital. This distress does not change the patient's right to leave.

Patients who decide to leave against medical advice should be advised of the risks of leaving, if possible, and should be urged to reconsider if further care is needed. In some states, there is a duty to try to convince patients not to leave against medical advice. In 2003, a New York appellate court approved the revocation of the medical license of a physician where one of the reasons was failure to attempt to persuade a patient not to leave against medical advice.[127]

The explanation should be documented. Patients should be asked to sign a form that they are leaving against medical advice and that the risks have been explained to them. However, patients cannot be forced to sign. If patients refuse to sign, the explanation and refusal should be documented in the medical record by the involved staff.

There is a strange case from Ohio that illustrated the trouble that courts have in understanding the situation when patients leave against medical advice. The patient had not signed a form before leaving against medical advice. An expert and a hospital administrator were permitted to testify that the standard of care required the patient to sign a form before being discharged against medical advice. The court allowed the jury to determine whether such a form was required. The jury decided there was no liability and was upheld on appeal in 2003. The court did not address how a provider could have held the patient until a form was signed without committing false imprisonment and did not address why the legal issue of the need for a form could be a factual question for the jury to determine.[128]

---

[127] Ticzon v. N.Y. State Dept. of Health, 305 A.D.2d 816, 759 N.Y.S.2d 586 (3d Dept. 2003).
[128] Hampton v. Saint Michael Hosp., 2003 Ohio 1828, 2003 Ohio App. LEXIS 1743.

FALSE IMPRISONMENT. False imprisonment is holding a person against his or her will without lawful authority.[129] Health care institutions can be liable for false imprisonment when they do not permit patients to leave, absent one of the exceptions that permit delayed release. Physical restraints or physical barriers are not necessary. Threats leading to a reasonable apprehension of harm can provide enough restraint to establish false imprisonment.[130]

In the past, a few cases of false imprisonment arose when hospitals attempted to hold patients until their bills were paid.[131] There have been no reported cases in the United States concerning this situation in more than thirty years, which indicates that hospitals now understand this practice is unacceptable.

STATUTORY PROCEDURES. In many situations, it is appropriate for a hospital to detain or restrain a patient. All states have laws providing procedures for the commitment of persons who are seriously mentally ill, are substance abusers, or are a danger to the public health due to contagious disease.[132] They also have laws that provide procedures for taking custody of minors who are neglected or abused.[133] Generally, a hospital can hold these persons while reporting them to authorities and obtaining commitment or custody orders.

If parents try to discharge a child when removal presents an imminent danger to the child's life or health, most states either authorize the health care provider to retain custody of the child or provide an expeditious procedure for obtaining court authorization to retain custody.[134] Many parents will agree to acceptable treatment or postpone precipitous withdrawal when advised that these procedures will be invoked.

COMMON LAW DUTIES. When these laws do not apply, the hospital still has a common law duty to protect temporarily disoriented

---

129 *See False imprisonment in connection with confinement in nursing home or hospital*, 4 A.L.R. 4TH 449; *e.g.*, Alt v. John Umstead Hosp., 125 N.C. App. 193, 479 S.E.2d 800 (1997).

130 *But see* Williams v. Summit Psychiatric Ctrs., P.C., 185 Ga. App. 264, 363 S.E.2d 794 (1987) [threat of commitment if patient attempted to leave not sufficient to create false imprisonment where patient actually left without incident].

131 *E.g.*, Gadsden Gen. Hosp. v. Hamilton, 212 Ala. 531, 103 So. 533 (1925); *Baby held for hospital bill: Couple*, CHICAGO TRIBUNE, Nov. 29, 1974, 8.

132 *E.g.*, Jarrell v. Chemical Dependency Unit, 791 F.2d 373 (5th Cir. 1986) [chemical dependency]; *but see also* Collignon v. Milwaukee County, 163 F.3d 982 (7th Cir. 1998) [no constitutional right to be involuntarily detained; no liability when schizophrenic person committed suicide after release from jail]; Mottau v. State of N.Y., 174 Misc. 2d 884, 666 N.Y.S.2d 878 (Ct. Cl. 1997) [alcoholism treatment center owed no duty to protect voluntary patient from himself; struck by auto after discharge for violating rule prohibiting drinking].

133 *E.g.*, FLA. STAT. § 415.506; *In re* J.J., 718 S.W.2d 235 (Mo. Ct. App. 1986).

134 *E.g.*, Kempster v. Child Protective Servs., 130 A.D.2d 623, 515 N.Y.S.2d 807 (2d Dept. 1987).

patients. Physicians and hospitals generally have authority under the common law to temporarily detain and even restrain temporarily disoriented medical patients without court involvement. This authority is inferred from the cases in which hospitals have been found liable for injuries to patients who are not restrained during temporary disorientation.[135] However, there is no duty to restrain all disoriented patients; it is generally recognized that the decision whether to use restraints is a matter of professional judgment.[136]

The common law authority to restrain generally does not apply when the patient is being detained for treatment for mental illness or substance abuse. The applicable statutory procedures usually need to be followed in those cases. This common law authority does not apply when the patient is fully oriented, but the hospital can usually maintain custody long enough for the patient's status to be determined if there is reasonable doubt.

HABEAS CORPUS. Federal courts have the power under the Constitution to review the legality of the confinement of any person.[137] When a federal court issues a *writ of habeas corpus* concerning an individual, the person or entity holding that individual must present the individual to the court and prove the right to continue the confinement. If the right is not proven, the court orders release. This is most commonly used to challenge confinement of persons under the criminal law, but it is also used to challenge involuntary treatment of mentally ill persons[138] and others.[139] State courts also can issue writs of habeas corpus.

ESCAPE. In situations where hospitals have a duty to maintain custody of a patient, hospitals can be sued when patients escape and commit suicide, are injured or killed in accidents, or injure or kill others. The courts usually focus on (1) how much those involved in the care of the patient knew or should have known about the dangerousness of the patient to self or others and (2) the

---

[135] *E.g.*, Boles v. Milwaukee County, 150 Wis. 2d 801, 443 N.W.2d 679 (Ct. App. 1989) [county hospital may be liable for not detaining disoriented mentally ill person even when statutory procedure not available]; Smith v. Louisiana Health & Human Resources Admin., 637 So. 2d 1177 (La. Ct. App. 4th Cir. 1994) [liability for death of disoriented patient who took ambulance, crashed into construction barricade].

[136] *E.g.*, Gerard v. Sacred Heart Med. Ctr., 937 P.2d 1104 (Wash. App. Ct. 1997).

[137] U.S. Const., art. I, § 9, ¶ 2.

[138] *See* Pacelli v. deVito, 972 F.2d 871 (7th Cir. 1992) [civil rights action concerning failure to comply with class *writ of habeas corpus* ordered release].

[139] *E.g.*, United States *ex rel.* Siegel v. Shinnick, 219 F. Supp. 789 (E.D. N.Y. 1963) [dismissal of *habeas corpus* petition challenging isolation of person exposed to smallpox].

appropriateness of the precautions taken to prevent escape in light of that knowledge. Generally, if the injury was not foreseeable, there is little likelihood of liability for failure to take additional precautions. If the injury was foreseeable, courts will examine the reasonableness of the precautions, and liability will be more likely. However, many courts have recognized the therapeutic benefits of more open patient care units and have found them to be reasonable even for some patients at risk.[140] In other cases, the precautions have been found to be inadequate, and liability has been imposed.

One federal court ruled that there is no legal right to be involuntarily committed; so it is not a violation of 42 U.S.C. § 1983 for a mental health facility to fail to stop someone from leaving the facility who is later injured.[141]

6-6.3 What Can the Institution Do When a Patient Refuses to Cooperate with Discharge Planning or Refuses to Leave?

Patients and their representatives do not have the right to insist on unnecessary hospitalization. If patients refuse to leave or their representatives refuse to remove the patients after the physician's discharge order, the patients are trespassers, and the hospital can take appropriate steps to have the patients removed. If the delay in discharge is due to difficulties in arranging placement, the hospital will usually take reasonable steps to assist in making arrangements. However, if patients and their representatives will not cooperate, it can be necessary to use reasonable force to remove the patients or to obtain a court order.[142] In 1996, a New York court ordered a guardian to cooperate with discharge.[143] In 2002, a New York court

---

[140] *E.g.*, Lindsey v. United States, 693 F. Supp. 1012 (W.D. Okla. 1988).

[141] Wilson v. Formigoni, 42 F.3d 1061 (7th Cir. 1994); *see also* Collignon v. Milwaukee County, 163 F.3d 982 (7th Cir. 1998) [no liability for jail failing to seek commitment of released person who committed suicide].

[142] *E.g.*, Jersey City Med. Ctr. v. Halstead, 169 N.J. Super. 22, 404 A.2d 44 (Ch. Div. 1979); Lucy Webb Hayes Nat'l Training School v. Geoghegan, 281 F. Supp. 116 (D. D.C. 1967); *see also* W. Hoge, *Pinochet is shown the door by a vexed London hospital*, N.Y. Times, Dec. 2, 1998, A8 [left after threatened with legal action]; *Hospital sues to evict man on ventilator*, Miami Herald, Aug. 10, 1995; *Hospital drops eviction of paralyzed man*, Miami Herald, Aug. 26, 1995; *Move ends fight with hospital*, Miami Herald, Oct. 11, 1995; *Aventura hospital sues to force elderly patient to leave*, AP, Jan. 7, 2003 [patient and family refused discharge to nursing home]; *Robert Wood Johnson seeks to appoint guardian for heart attack patient*, AP, Feb. 2, 2001 [family of incapacitated patient did not cooperate with discharge].

[143] *In re* Claiman, 169 Misc. 2d 881, 646 N.Y.S.2d 940 (Sup. Ct. 1996); *see also In re* M.K., 284 Ill. App. 3d 449; 672 N.E.2d 271 (1st Dist. 1996) [neglect for state guardian to leave minor ward in psych hosp when ready for discharge].

issued an injunction requiring a patient to leave a hospital even though he did not like the nursing home that had accepted him and visiting nurses would not provide services due to violence.[144] Refusal to cooperate with discharge planning can result in personal liability for the cost of unnecessary hospital care.[145] In a few states, it is a crime to refuse to leave a hospital after discharge.[146]

When a patient who is refusing to leave is mentally ill, in some circumstances the patient can be involuntarily transferred to a mental facility if the patient meets the criteria for involuntary hospitalization.[147]

As with the discharge of noncooperative and disruptive patients discussed in Section 6-6.4, hospital administration should make decisions concerning forcible removal.

6-6.4 When Can the Institution Discharge a Patient Who Needs Additional Treatment?

Usually, a patient should be discharged only as a result of (1) a written order of a physician familiar with the patient's condition or (2) the patient's decision to leave against medical advice. This procedure helps to protect the patient from injury and the hospital from liability for premature discharge.

Patients do not have to be kept in the hospital until cured. Patients generally can be discharged when the hospital is no longer the appropriate level of care or when the patient becomes sufficiently disruptive. When there are capacity constraints, patients may need to be transferred to the care of other institutions. With appropriate notice, institutions or services can be closed.

Sometimes insurers and other third parties put pressure on physicians and hospitals to discharge or transfer patients. This will generally not be a defense to a premature discharge.

Any discharge of a patient in need of continued care without transfer to another provider could be controversial; so it should usually be limited to situations that interfere with the care of other patients or threaten the safety of staff members. Hospital adminis-

---

[144] *In re* Wyckoff Heights Med. Ctr., 191 Misc. 2d 207, 741 N.Y.S.2d 400 (Sup. Ct. 2002).
[145] *E.g.*, *In re* Estate of Bricker, 183 Misc. 2d 149, 702 N.Y.S.2d 535 (Sur. Ct. 1999) [Medicaid can recover additional hospital costs when patient refused discharge plan].
[146] *E.g.*, N.C. GEN. STAT. § 131E-90; *see also Man ends standoff at Miami hospital; demanded wife be kept there*, AP, Aug. 27, 2002.
[147] *E.g.*, Pruessman v. Dr. John T. MacDonald Found., 589 So. 2d 948 (Fla. 3d DCA 1991).

tration should review each case to minimize legal liability and other adverse effects on the hospital. When the attending physician desires an inappropriate discharge or refuses to cooperate with an appropriate discharge, it may be necessary to transfer the care of the patient to another physician.

CLOSURE OF THE INSTITUTION OR SERVICE. Generally, facilities can discontinue providing certain services and discharge patients who require the discontinued services.[148] In 1998, an Indiana court ruled that a nursing home that had closed its ventilator unit could transfer ventilator-dependant patients.[149] This was permitted under the state law that allowed transfers when a facility could not meet the patient's needs. In some jurisdictions, there are restrictions on closure of some institutions or services. This is discussed in Chapter 2.

Inpatients generally need to be transferred to the care of another institution. While most institutions assist patients in finding alternate outpatient providers, there is generally not a legal duty to make arrangements for a referral.

BEHAVIOR OF THE PATIENT. If a patient becomes sufficiently difficult or disruptive, it is permissible in some situations for the hospital to discontinue providing care. In 1982, a California court refused to order a physician and several hospitals to continue to provide chronic hemodialysis to a noncooperative, disruptive patient who had even refused to comply with the conditions of a court order that provided for continued treatment during the litigation.[150] The physician had given her due notice of his withdrawal from the physician-patient relationship with ample time for her to make other arrangements. The court was clearly troubled by the possibility that she would not be able to receive necessary care but concluded that several alternatives were available.

Courts are more comfortable with involuntary discharges when the patient's condition is not so severe. An Arizona court ruled that a physician and hospital were not liable for discharging a difficult

---

[148] *E.g.,* Lutwin v. Thompson, 361 F.3d 146 (2d Cir. 2004) [home health agencies must provide notice before service cuts].

[149] Bryant v. Indiana State Dep't of Health, 695 N.E.2d 975 (Ind. Ct. App. 1998).

[150] Payton v. Weaver, 131 Cal. App. 3d 38, 182 Cal. Rptr. 225 (1st Dist. 1982); *see also* Hall v. Bio-Medical Application, Inc., 671 F.2d 300 (8th Cir. 1982); *but see* M.S.D. Bosek, L.A. Burton & T.A. Savage, *The patient who could not be discharged: how far should patient autonomy extend?* JONA'S HEALTHCARE L., ETHICS, & REG., Dec. 1999, 23 [nursing perspective on what happens after every other dialysis facility refuses].

patient who had been admitted for the treatment of lesions on his lips.[151] The court observed that the patient was uncomfortable but not helpless and that the hospital staff had done nothing actively to retard his treatment or worsen his condition.

In 1992, a federal court refused to enjoin a nursing home from discharging a violent and aggressive patient who had abused staff and struck another patient. The court ruled that the discharge violated neither the Medicaid law nor the Rehabilitation Act.[152] In 1997, the Iowa Supreme Court upheld the involuntary discharge from a nursing home of a patient who abused staff and other residents.[153]

In some cases, it may be appropriate to pursue criminal charges or obtain a restraining order against a patient who is abusive, harassing, violent, or stalking.[154]

Some courts have found that employers can be liable for sexual harassment of staff by customers.[155] This has been applied to a health care office practice setting.[156] In 1997, former employees of a facility for mentally retarded and autistic adults were permitted to sue for harassment and violent assaults by a six foot tall, 200 pound, sixteen-year-old resident functioning at a two- to five-year-old level.[157] It is not clear how this trend will be applied in the inpatient or residential care setting when acute or chronic medical care is needed. In situations where the patient or resident can be safely discharged, this can provide another basis for involuntary discharge. This can also be the case when the patient or resident is able to control his or her behavior and refuses to do so, but courts are likely to be troubled by the loss of access to needed care unless

---

[151] Modla v. Parker, 17 Ariz. App. 54, 495 P.2d 494, *cert. denied*, 409 U.S. 1038 (1972); *but see* Morrison v. Washington County, 700 F.2d 678 (11th Cir.), *cert. denied*, 464 U.S. 864 (1983) [hospital could be liable for physician's discharge of unruly alcoholic patient].

[152] Nichols v. St. Luke Ctr., 800 F. Supp. 1564 (S.D. Ohio 1992).

[153] Robbins v. Iowa Dep't of Inspections & Appeals, 567 N.W.2d 653 (Iowa 1997).

[154] *E.g.*, People v. P.S., 189 Misc. 2d 71, 731 N.Y.S.2d 341 (Jus. Ct. 2001) [refusal to dismiss aggravated harassment charge against mother for telephone calls to hospital]; *Order bans harassment of abortion clinic owner*, STAR TRIBUNE (Minneapolis, MN), July 30, 1993, 7B; *but see* Scripps Health v. Marin, 72 Cal. App. 4th 324, 85 Cal. Rptr. 2d 86 (4th Dist 1999) [reversed because no showing of threat of future harm].

[155] *E.g.*, Lockard v. Pizza Hut, Inc., 162 F.3d 1062 (10th Cir. 1998); *see also* Ligenza v. Genesis Health Ventures, 995 F. Supp. 226 (D. Mass. 1998) [respiratory technician fired from nursing home for striking ventilator-dependent patient technician claimed looked up her blouse; no Title VII claim against employer because technician did not complain that patient's known inappropriate behavior had created a hostile working environment; court did not accept that facility could never be responsible for abuse by patient].

[156] *E.g.*, Anania v. Daubenspeck Chiropractic, 129 Ohio App. 3d 516, 718 N.E.2d 480 (1998).

[157] Crist v. Focus Homes Inc., 122 F.3d 1107 (8th Cir. 1997).

alternative care arrangements are possible. In cases where the self-control is not possible, it is possible this will be viewed as yet another behavior that the provider can and should take steps to control.[158] In some cases, transfer can be the appropriate response, if there is another facility with more expertise in handling the particular behavior that is willing to accept the patient.

A Minnesota court ruled that a nursing facility could not involuntarily discharge a patient with mental illness because she refused treatment by mental health professionals. The facility must first meet its obligations to assess the patient's needs and examine treatment alternatives, including a determination of decision-making incapacity, before forcing the medication.[159]

Disruptive behavior by the patient's parents, family, or friends is generally not grounds for refusing treatment to the patient.[160] The appropriate recourse is to address the behavior directly, if necessary to the point of excluding the disruptive individuals from the facility or legally changing who is the decisionmaker for the patient.[161]

In 2001, England authorized local regions to implement an innovative approach to violent patients. Modeled on the soccer penalty system, providers issue a "yellow card" as a warning to violent patients. Upon repetition of the problem, a "red card" is issued, banning the patient from hospital premises for a period of time.[162] Some areas in England have addressed the problem of what to do with banned patients by creating special centralized clinics for these patients.[163]

THIRD-PARTY PRESSURE TO DISCHARGE. The need for a treating physician's discharge order is especially important to remember

---

[158] *E.g.*, Turner v. Jordan, 957 S.W.2d 815 (Tenn. 1997) [psychiatrist owed duty to protect hospital nurse from violent acts of mentally ill patient hospitalized with known prior attacks on staff].

[159] In the Matter of the Involuntary Discharge or Transfer of J.S. by Ebenezer Hall, 512 N.W.2d 604 (Minn. Ct. App. 1994).

[160] *E.g.*, *In re* Williams, 133 Misc. 2d 817, 508 N.Y.S.2d 371(Sup. Ct. 1986) [cannot terminate child benefits due to abuse of staff by parent].

[161] *See In re* Koenig, 2003 Ohio 1727, 2003 Ohio App. LEXIS 1634 [mother denied guardianship in part due to her interference with her son's care in hospital leading to behavior contract with hospital].

[162] J. Carvel, *Blair plans red cards for violent patients: Move to protect hospital staff after 65,000 incidents last year*, THE GUARDIAN (London), June 19, 2001, 9; J. von Radowitz, *Hospitals refuse to treat abusive patients*, PRESS ASSOCIATION, Dec. 27, 2001; T. Richardson, *Patient is imprisoned for attack*, EVENING HERALD [Plymouth, UK], Aug. 9, 2004, 9 [red card recipient assaulted staff member during permitted emergency visit].

[163] *See Special clinics for violent patients*, HEALTH MEDIA GROUP MEDIA WATCH SERVICES [UK], May 30, 2003 [clinics at police stations]; S. Blakemore, *Special clinic for violent patients*, BIRMINGHAM POST [UK], Oct. 16, 2003, 4.

when a utilization review committee or a third-party reviewer decides that a patient should be discharged, but the treating physician believes the patient should stay. While the decision of a physician reviewer may be given some weight, it will not insulate the physician or hospital from liability. An independent judgment must be made by the treating physician. For example, a state physician reviewer in California was sued for the complications a patient suffered when the reviewer authorized only half the additional hospital days requested by the treating physician.[164] The trial court found the reviewer could be liable, but the appellate court reversed its finding that the treating physician had the legal responsibility to make the actual discharge decision. In 1990, a California appellate court ruled that the earlier case applied only to Medi-Cal (California's Medicaid program) patients, so that it did not apply to patients insured under policies issued in the private sector.[165] The case arose when a utilization reviewer determined that hospitalization was not medically necessary and the patient committed suicide after discharge. The case was remanded for trial. If a jury found that the utilization reviewer's actions were a substantial factor in causing the suicide, the reviewer could be liable. Liability was not limited to the treating physician. The liability of managed care entities is discussed in Chapters 10 and 11.

6-6.5 When May the Institution Permit Temporary Releases without Discharge?

Sometimes children, incompetent adults, cooperative committed patients, or competent adults who need continuing supervision or care ask to leave the hospital for a short time. This is permissible in many situations and can assist in patient care. Because liability is a possible outcome, precautions should be taken. A written physician authorization should indicate the temporary release is not medically contraindicated. Written authorization from competent adult patients or from the parent or guardian of other patients should acknowledge that the hospital is not responsible for the care of the patient while out of hospital custody. Except for adult patients who are able to take care of themselves and are not a danger to others, patients should only be released to appropriate adults who have

---

[164] Wickline v. State, No. NWC 60672 (Cal. Super. Ct.), *rev'd*, 192 Cal. App. 3d 1630, 239 Cal. Rptr. 810 (2d Dist. 1986).

[165] Wilson v. Blue Cross of So. Cal., 222 Cal. App. 3d 660, 271 Cal. Rptr. 876 (2d Dist. 1990).

been instructed concerning patient needs (such as medications and use of necessary medical equipment) during the release and the way to contact the hospital for information or assistance if needed. If the necessary arrangements are then made for the patient's needs, the risks associated with temporary releases are minimized.

An overnight release can result in loss of Medicare or other insurance coverage for the day.

If patients who are a danger to themselves or others are temporarily released and are harmed or harm others, the hospital could be liable.[166] A Florida court ruled that a hospital could be sued by a person who was injured in an automobile accident caused by a patient on a temporary release because the hospital should have known she would attempt to operate an automobile and could not do so safely.[167] However, courts recognize that temporary releases are an appropriate part of many treatment plans; so there are many circumstances where providers have been found not to be liable for injuries during releases.[168]

A Minnesota hospital's policy concerning passes for the mentally ill was challenged as a violation of the state's commitment law. The Minnesota Supreme Court upheld the policy by ruling that passes were not discharges. The court reviewed the precautions, including monitoring and giving interested individuals an opportunity to comment before the pass was issued, and concluded they were appropriate.[169]

Special rules may apply to releases of persons who have been acquitted of crimes due to insanity.[170]

---

[166] *E.g.*, Foster v. Charter Med. Corp., 601 So. 2d 435 (Ala. 1992) [facility could be liable for suicide of voluntary mental patient on temporary unsupervised pass]; *but see* Leonard v. State, 491 N.W.2d 508 (Iowa 1992) [psychiatrist did not owe duty to general public for release of patient].

[167] Burroughs v. Board of Trustees, 328 So. 2d 538 (Fla. 1st DCA 1976).

[168] *E.g.*, Estate of Emmons v. Peet, 950 F. Supp. 15 (D. Me. 1996) [no liability for suicide by drowning of voluntary mental patient while on release]; Cox v. Willis-Knighton Med. Ctr., 680 So. 2d 1309 (La. Ct. App. 1996) [no liability for suicide by gunshot during twelve-hour pass from chemical dependency unit].

[169] County of Hennepin v. Levine, 345 N.W.2d 217 (Minn. 1984).

[170] *E.g.*, United States v. Hinckley, 984 F. Supp. 35 (D. D.C. 1997) [hospital required to prove lack of dangerousness before permitting six-hour release]; United States v. Hinckley, 163 F.3d 647 (D.C. Cir.1999) [six-hour outing to eat holiday dinner with family under line-of-sight supervision of hospital escort was not a conditional release, so court lacked jurisdiction to reject it]; D. Stout, *Appeals court lets Hinckley take day trips,* N.Y. TIMES, Jan. 16, 1999, A15; United States v. Hinckley, 292 F. Supp. 2d 125 (D. D.C. 2003) [permitting conditional, time-limited outings under the supervision of parents]; Barna v. Hogan. 964 F. Supp. 52 (D. Conn. 1997) [due process rights of person acquitted for insanity not violated by termination of off-ward privileges].

Discussion Points

1. How does a physician-patient relationship start?
2. What limits can a provider place on the scope of the relationship?
3. What legal constraints are there on a physician's decision whether to start a relationship?
4. When does a patient have a right to be admitted to a hospital?
5. What are some of the permitted reasons for denying admission?
6. What services does EMTALA require hospitals and physicians to provide?
7. What characteristics cannot be used as the basis for admission decisions due to nondiscrimination laws?
8. What are the permitted ways for a physician-patient relationship to end?
9. What are the permitted ways for a patient relationship with a health care institution to end?
10. What are the institution's responsibilities concerning discharge planning?
11. When can an institution detain an individual who wants to leave?
12. What can an institution do when a patient refuses to leave?
13. What can an institution do with a patient whose behavior is disruptive?

CHAPTER SEVEN

Decision-making Concerning Individuals

Objectives

The objective of this chapter is to provide an overview of the law concerning making decisions regarding the care of individuals. The reader will learn how to identify the appropriate decisionmaker; determine what information needs to be given to the decision-maker; and proof of the decision. The reader will also learn some of the limits on the range of permitted decisions, when involuntary treatment may be given, and what the consequences are of providing services without authorization.

Who makes the decision whether a medical procedure will be performed on a patient? The decision is usually made by the provider who is willing to perform the procedure and the patient or the patient's representative who is authorized to make such decisions. Health care providers must obtain appropriate authorization before examining a patient or performing diagnostic or therapeutic procedures. Usually authorization is through the express or implied consent of the patient or the patient's representative. The person giving consent must have sufficient information concerning available choices so that the consent is an informed consent. If the decision is not to consent, usually the examination or procedure cannot be performed. The law overrides some refusals and authorizes involuntary treatment, such as for some mental illness and substance abuse.

Making these decisions about the treatment of individuals presents several recurring problems of health care law that will be addressed in this chapter.

7-1. Who is the appropriate decisionmaker?

7-2. What information needs to be given to the decisionmaker?

7-3. Who has the responsibility to provide information?

7-4. What should be done to prove the decision?

7-5. What constitutes coercion that makes consent involuntary and invalid?

7-6. What limits are placed on the permitted range of decisions?

7-7. When can the law authorize involuntary treatment?

7-8. What are the consequences of stopping treatment or providing unauthorized treatment?

7-1 Who Is the Appropriate Decisionmaker?

The general rule is that adults with decision-making capacity make the decisions regarding their own treatment and that decisions continue to be effective after the adult loses capacity. This is derived from the long-standing commitment of U.S. law to personal *autonomy* and *self-determination*. In 1891, the United States Supreme Court said that "no right is held more sacred, or is more carefully guarded by the common law, than the right of every individual to the possession and control of his [or her] own person, free from all restraint or interference of others, unless by clear and unquestionable authority of law."[1] A major problem for health care law is the determination when the authority of law should be exercised contrary to autonomy for the protection of the patient or others or the accomplishment of other societal priorities.

Some minors with decision-making capacity are treated like adults for some treatments. For all others, someone else must be the decisionmaker.

Health care providers have an essential role in the decision-making process. They shape the scope of available options in four ways. First, the health care provider is a source of information concerning potential options. However, the provider is not the only source. Many patients gather information independently from other sources,

---

[1] Union Pac. Ry. Co. v. Botsford, 141 U.S. 250 (1891).

including the Internet. Information gathering is discussed in more detail in Section 7-2. Second, the health care provider has a professional duty not to provide medically inappropriate services. Third, there are limits on what each health care provider has the capability to provide. Thus, the provider can refuse to provide some services that the decisionmaker wants based on a determination that is inappropriate or outside the scope of the services provided. The decisionmaker generally has to choose between (a) accepting the judgment and/or limitations of the provider and (b) seeking another provider. Fourth, in some circumstances providers will not provide services within the scope of their capability based on an unwillingness to establish or continue a relationship with the particular patient; so the decisionmaker must seek another provider. The relationship with the patient is discussed in more detail in Chapter 6.

In applying the general rule, several problems arise.

7-1.1. When does an adult have decision-making capacity?

7-1.2. When an adult with decision-making capacity gives directions and later loses capacity, what is the effect of the prior direction?

7-1.3. Who makes decisions for adults without decision-making capacity?

7-1.4. When can minors make their own decisions?

7-1.5. Who makes decisions for minors who cannot decide for themselves?

7-1.1 When Does an Adult Have Decision-Making Capacity?

In the United States, individuals are *adults* for most purposes on their eighteenth birthday and are able to make their own medical decisions. Adults have *decision-making capacity* if (1) they have not been declared incompetent by a court and (2) they are generally capable of understanding the consequences of alternatives, weighing the alternatives by the degree to which they promote their desires, and choosing and acting accordingly. The standard is not the degree to which the person's decision agrees with the provider's recommendations. Individuals can refuse even lifesaving treatment as long as they understand and accept the consequences. The individual who must live or die with the outcome should usually make the decision.

Few, if any, decisions are made in the pristine analytical fashion that theoreticians postulate as the ideal. Virtually all decisions involve external and internal influences, denial of some factors, some misunderstandings, erroneous beliefs, beliefs that are not based on evidence, incomplete information, personal preferences and priorities, concern for the impact on others, and other factors that can be contrary to "ideal" decision-making. For example, many nonprofessionals use information concerning probabilities and lack of certainty differently than health care professionals.[2] These must be accepted as part of the reality of decision-making or it might be impossible to find anyone with decision-making capacity. It is possible to fashion a test of capacity that no one can meet. The legal test for capacity is not this strict.

The determination of capacity is not necessarily the function of psychiatrists. It is usually a practical assessment that should be made by the provider who obtains the consent or accepts the refusal. For most patients, the assessment of capacity is not difficult.

Sometimes assessment of capacity is more complex. Patients can have capacity to make some decisions and not have capacity to make other decisions. If there is suspicion of underlying mental retardation, mental illness, or disorders that affect brain functions, consultation with a psychiatrist or appropriate specialist is advisable.

In most states, there is a strong legal presumption of continued capacity. A *presumption* means that the law assumes that persons have capacity and anyone who disagrees must prove otherwise. For example, a Pennsylvania court found a woman capable of refusing a breast biopsy even though she was committed to a mental institution with a diagnosis of chronic schizophrenia and two of her three reasons for refusal were delusional.[3] She understood the alternatives and consequences and had a nondelusional reason for her decision. A Massachusetts court found a woman capable of refusing amputation of her gangrenous leg even though her train of thought sometimes wandered, her conception of time was distorted, and she was confused on some matters. The fact that her decision was medically irrational and would lead to her death did not demonstrate incapacity. The court believed she understood the alternatives and consequences of her decision.[4] The Ohio Supreme Court ruled that a psychiatric patient was competent to refuse cancer treatment

---

[2] R. Friedman, *Mix math and medicine and create confusion*, N.Y. TIMES, Apr. 26, 2005, D11; K. Sepkowitz, *Doctors do know things patients don't know*, N.Y. TIMES, May 10, 2005, D5 [physicians are more experienced with handling the lack of certainty].

[3] *In re* Yetter, 62 D. & C. 2d 619 (Pa. Cm. Pl. Ct. Northampton County 1973).

[4] Lane v. Candura, 6 Mass. App. Ct. 377, 376 N.E.2d 1232 (1978).

despite delusions concerning her relationship to a faith healer.[5] However, an Illinois court ruled that merely presenting a single non-delusional reason for refusing psychotropic medications did not preclude a finding of incapacity to make reasoned decisions, so that administration of medications could be ordered.[6]

A Florida case involved a patient whose breathing tube had become dislodged and who refused reintubation for four hours. When she finally consented, she died soon after reintubation. Her estate and her husband (who had also refused intubation for her) sued claiming she had not been competent to refuse. Their expert pointed out that she was acutely ill, in intensive care, on medication, sleep deprived, and hypoxemic (low oxygen levels in the blood). However, the undisputed evidence was that she was awake, alert, oriented, and asking appropriate questions when she refused. The court ruled that she was competent.[7]

One state appears to have adopted a substantially weaker commitment to autonomy by eliminating the presumption of competency whenever there is medical evidence of mental illness or defect. In 2002, a New York appellate court ruled that when there is such evidence, a presumption against capacity is created, so that the person claiming capacity must prove capacity. In a case involving a patient with Alzheimer's disease, the court ruled that an advance directive was not valid because there was a failure to show that the patient was competent when she signed it.[8]

Some patients who are unhappy with cosmetic surgery claim that they lacked capacity to consent because their desire to change their appearance was due to mental illness. The highest court of New York rejected such a challenge in 2001. The court determined that the patient had presented insufficient proof that she had a mental condition that would cause her to lack capacity to consent to elective cosmetic surgery.[9] Many cosmetic surgeons prepare to defend such suits by requiring a psychological evaluation before accepting consent to surgery.[10]

---

5   *In re* Milton, 29 Ohio St. 2d 20, 505 N.E.2d 255, *cert. denied*, 484 U.S. 820 (1987).
6   *In re* Jeffers, 239 Ill. App. 3d 29, 606 N.E.2d 727 (4th Dist. 1992), *appeal granted*, 158 Ill. 2d 552, 643 N.E.2d 839 (1994), *adhered to*, 272 Ill. App. 3d 44, 650 N.E.2d 242 (4th Dist. 1995).
7   Rodriguez v. Pino, 634 So. 2d 681 (Fla. 3d DCA 1994).
8   *In re* Rose S., 293 A.D.2d 619, 741 N.Y.S.2d 84 (2d Dept. Apr. 15, 2002).
9   Lynn G v. Hugo, 96 N.Y.2d 306, 752 N.E.2d 250, 728 N.Y.S.2d 121 (2001).
10 *See* B. Carey, *Obsession with perfection: Some plastic surgeons are conducting psychological tests on patients who fixate on the smallest of flaws*, L.A. Times, Dec. 17, 2001, S1.

It is generally not the primary responsibility of the hospital to raise the question of incapacity. Illinois courts have ruled that the hospital generally has no duty to inquire into the availability of a surrogate decisionmaker until the attending physician has determined the patient lacks decisional capacity.[11]

Some states have special rules for determining capacity in certain cases. For example, until 1999, New Jersey required three physicians to determine capacity before a decision to refuse life-sustaining treatment could be honored.

TEMPORARY CAPACITY. Persons who generally lack decision-making capacity might regain capacity for temporary periods. This has long been recognized by courts when they approve wills that are made during *lucid intervals* by persons who are otherwise generally confused.[12]

TEMPORARY INCAPACITY. Persons who generally have decision-making capacity might have impaired capacity for temporary periods. From example, some drugs can impair capacity; so treatment decisions generally should not be solicited from patients after such drugs have reduced capacity.[13] Not all sedatives render a patient incapacitated.[14]

Courts disagree on whether a woman in labor has decision-making capacity.[15]

When a decision must be made in an emergency while a patient is temporarily incapacitated, generally others can make the decisions. In some situations, close family or friends can make the decisions. When time does not permit this consultation, providers can make emergency lifesaving decisions that are not contrary to the patient's directions.

In nonemergency situations of temporary incapacity where capacity is likely to be reestablished soon without treatment, consent of others generally should not be relied on. A Utah case involved a patient who was incapacitated temporarily due to preoperative medications. During that temporary incapacity, the physi-

---

[11] Collins v. Lake Forest Hosp., 213 Ill. 2d 234, 821 N.E.2d 316 (2004); Ficke v. Evangelical Health Sys., 285 Ill. App. 3d 886, 674 N.E.2d 888 (1st Dist. 1996).

[12] *E.g.*, Estate of Sorensen, 87 Wis. 2d 339, 274 N.W.2d 694 (1979).

[13] *E.g.*, Herrington v. Herrington, 692 So. 2d 93 (Miss. 1996) [jury question whether medications rendered patient incapable of consent].

[14] *E.g.*, Grannum v. Berard, 70 Wash. 2d 304, 422 P.2d 812 (1967).

[15] *E.g.*, Hare v. Parsley, 157 Misc. 2d 277, 596 N.Y.S.2d 313 (1993) [patient unable to consent to sterilization during labor]; Schreiber v. PIC Wis., 223 Wis. 2d 417, 588 N.W.2d 26 (1999) [duty to obtain new consent when woman withdrew consent to vaginal delivery during labor].

cian obtained the wife's consent for surgery. The court ruled that the consent was not valid. The wife could only consent when there was longer incapacity or there was an emergency.[16]

CONSISTENCY. When providers have formally determined that a patient lacks capacity, they should treat the patient consistently as incapacitated until there is a determination that capacity is restored. In a 1984 case, the federal district court ruled that when the Veterans Administration issues a "statement of incapacity" and designates the patient's wife or another person to be the one to whom it will turn for decisions on the patient's behalf, the patient's consent is no longer sufficient authorization for treatment; the consent of the person designated must be sought.[17] If a provider intends to rely on a patient making a decision during a lucid interval of capacity after incapacity has been determined, there generally should be a determination with the same degree of formality as the determination of incapacity.

7-1.2 When an Adult with Decision-Making Capacity Gives Directions and Later Loses Capacity, What Is the Effect of the Prior Direction?

Directions that adults give while they have decision-making capacity generally should be followed after they lose capacity. Most persons lose decision-making capacity prior to death. The only way to preserve the right to direct personal treatment is to honor advance directives made while the person had decision-making capacity. Most states have addressed this situation through statutes. In situations in which either there is no applicable statute or the statutory procedures have not been followed, common law and constitutional principles generally require that the patient's directives be followed. *Advance directives* can be written or oral.

WRITTEN DIRECTIVES. Some states have statutes that recognize written advance directives that are in a certain format. When written advance directives are in that format, the directives generally present few legal problems. Even when advanced directives are not in the recognized format, they present few legal problems and should be followed. The primary advantage of directives in the recognized formats is that they usually have the protection of statutory

---

[16] Lounsbury v. Capel, 836 P.2d 188 (Utah Ct. App. 1992).
[17] Aponte v. United States, 582 F. Supp. 65 (D. P.R. 1984).

presumptions of validity; so they are somewhat harder to challenge. In the absence of a challenge, there is little or no difference.

One way an advance directive can fail to satisfy most statutes is by being unsigned or improperly signed. In a Virginia case, the patient had prepared an advance directive but before signing it became comatose in an automobile accident. Family initially disagreed on whether tube feeding should be discontinued in accordance with his wishes. On petition of the wife, the trial court authorized that tube feeding be discontinued in accordance with the advance directive. The other family decided not to contest the decision. The state intervened at the direction of the governor, but the Virginia Supreme Court refused to review the case. So the tube feeding was discontinued.[18]

In the absence of a challenge, one of the few circumstances is in Wisconsin where the statutory format is essential for placement in a nursing home. An incapacitated person can be admitted to a nursing home in Wisconsin only with (1) an advance directive in the Wisconsin statutory format authorizing admission or (2) a pending guardianship proceeding. Thus, a directive in the statutory format is the only way to avoid the expense and delay of a guardianship proceeding. Other states have not imposed this barrier to entry to nursing homes.

The need for interpretation is one of the legal problems that can occasionally arise with directives. This can occur whether or not the directive is in the statutory format. Usually, these can be solved without court involvement by careful reading.

Rarely, written advance directives are legally challenged. Generally, such challenges are unsuccessful unless the signature is a forgery or the person lacked decision-making capacity at the time the directive was signed. Providers generally do not have a duty to investigate the circumstances of the signing of a directive, but if they have reasonable suspicions regarding its validity, they should resolve those suspicions before acting on the directive.

At or near the time of admission, patients and families of incapacitated patients should be asked if there is a written directive so it can be documented, discussed, and implemented. Hospitals that participate in Medicare are required to make this inquiry.[19] The Joint Commission on Accreditation of Healthcare Organiza-

---

[18] *In re* Finn, No. 39711 (Va. Cir. Ct. Aug. 31, 1998); *Family will allow a comatose man to die*, N.Y. TIMES, Sept. 29, 1998, A21; Gilmore v. Annaburg Manor Nursing Home, No. 44386 (Va. Cir. Ct. Chancery Oct. 2, 1998), *rev. denied,* (Va. Oct. 2, 1998); See Gilmore v. Finn, 259 Va. 448, 527 S.E.2d 426 (2000) [denying sanctions].

[19] 42 C.F.R. 489.102.

tions (JCAHO) also requires accredited hospitals to make this inquiry.[20]

ORAL DIRECTIVES. Oral advance directives generally should also be followed. For example, in 2002, a Tennessee appellate court ruled that a patient's oral directions to withhold artificial nutrition should be followed. The lack of a written direction did not create a presumption against withdrawal. The mother and siblings of the patient could not compel a hospice to provide artificial nutrition; so the trial court order was reversed.[21]

The difficulty with oral directions is that they can be harder to prove and, thus, easier to contest. When time permits, it is best to write and sign the oral directions. Some persons are willing to discuss their directions but reluctant to write them. When patients do not have written directives, it is helpful for health care providers to document discussions with patients about these matters in the medical record. This contemporaneous documentation of oral directions is strong evidence of the patient's directions.

Oral directions given to family and friends can also be strong evidence, but they sometimes can be difficult to assess. Providers can generally rely on reports from family and friends in the absence of conflicting reports or a reasonable basis for suspecting their veracity. If there is no reason to suspect the authenticity of the directive, it should usually be followed. When oral directives are contested, courts place substantial weight on oral directives when they can be proved.

In 1990, the United States Supreme Court ruled that states can require that advance directives be proved by *clear and convincing evidence*.[22] This means that there needs to be stronger evidence than is required to meet the usual civil standard of *preponderance of the evidence*, which only requires proof that it is more likely than not that the directive is what the patient wanted. In states that apply the more restrictive standard, oral directives are sometimes hard to prove when contested.

It is preferable to sign a written advance directive. Oral directives leave open the opportunity for extended family, legal, and political controversies. The extent of potential controversy is best

---

[20] JCAHO, 2005 COMPREHENSIVE ACCREDITATION MANUAL FOR HOSPITALS (2005) [cited hereinafter as 2004 JCAHO CAMH], RI. 2.80 & PC. 12.40.

[21] San Juan-Torregosa v. Garcia, 80 S.W.3d 539 (Tenn. Ct. App. 2002).

[22] Cruzan v. Director, Mo. Dept. of Health, 497 U.S. 261 (1990), *aff'g*, 760 S.W.2d 408 (Mo. 1988) (en banc).

illustrated by the case of Terri Schiavo. In 2001, Florida courts determined after extensive hearings that there was clear and convincing evidence that she had stated a preference for termination of life support, and the court authorized her guardian/husband to end life support. This was reaffirmed in 2003 after a series of legal challenges by her parents. Life support was discontinued in 2004. When her parents continued to object, the Florida legislature quickly passed a special law authorizing the governor to order the tube feeding to be resumed. He issued the order, and the feeding was resumed. A Florida court determined that the special law violated the state constitutional right of privacy of the patient and the separation of powers of the legislature and judiciary. In September 2004, the Florida Supreme Court affirmed the decision, and the United States Supreme Court denied review in January 2005. After many additional court proceedings, treatment was discontinued on March 18, 2005. On March 20, Congress enacted a special law permitting federal court review of the case. The reviewing federal courts concluded that the state courts had followed appropriate procedures and refused to intervene. Ms. Schiavo died on March 30, 2005.[23]

INTERPRETING ADVANCE DIRECTIVES. Some advance directives direct that certain treatments be provided. Most advance directives address refusal of treatments. They specify what treatments are refused and under what circumstances. Many advance directives are written in very broad terms so that when a triggering condition occurs a broad range of treatments are refused. Some advance directives are complex, specifying different triggering conditions for spec-

---

[23] Schindler v. Schiavo (*In re* Guardianship of Schiavo), 780 So. 2d 176 (Fla. 2d DCA 2001), *cert. denied,* 789 So. 2d 348 (Fla. 2001); 792 So. 2d 551 (Fla. 2d DCA 2001); 800 So. 2d 640 (Fla. 2d DCA 2001), *rev. denied,* 816 So. 2d 127 (Fla. 2002); Case No. 90-2908-GB-003, 2002 WL 31817960 (Fla. 6th Jud. Cir. Ct. Nov. 22, 2002), *aff'd* 2003 Fla. App. LEXIS 8342 (2d Dist. 2003); Schindler v. Schiavo, 851 So. 2d 182 (Fla. 2d DCA. 2003), *rev. denied,* 855 So. 2d. 621 (Fla. 2003); *writ denied,* 865 So. 2d 500 (Fla. 2d DCA 2003); AP, Oct. 15, 2003 [tube withdrawn]; AP, Oct. 17, 2003 [other courts refused to intervene]; Fla. HB-35-E (signed Oct. 21, 2003); N.Y. Times, Oct. 21, 2003, A1 [governor orders tube reinstated]; NYTimes, Oct. 30, 2003, A16 [challenge to new law]; Bush v. Schiavo, 861 So. 2d 506 (Fla. 2d DCA 2003); Bush v. Schiavo, 885 So. 2d 321 (Fla. 2004), *cert. denied,* 125 S. Ct. 1086 (U.S. 2005); M. Stacy, *Feeding tube removed after last-ditch congressional effort fails,* AP, Mar. 19, 2005; Pub. L.109-3; M. Darymple, *White House: Schiavo bill not a precedent,* AP, Mar. 21, 2005; Schiavo v. Schiavo, 2005 U.S. Dist., 357 F. Supp. 2d 1378 (M.D. Fla. 2005), *aff'd,* 403 F.d 1223 (11th Cir. 2005), *stay denied,* 125 S. Ct. 1692 (U.S. 2005), *aff'g stay denial,* 403 F.3d 1289 (11th Cir. 2005), *stay denied,* 125 S. Ct. 1722 (U.S. 2005); A. Goodnough, *Schiavo dies, ending bitter case over feeding tube,* N.Y. TIMES, Apr. 1, 2005, A1; L.O. Gostin, *Ethics, the constitution, and the dying process: The case of Theresa Marie Schiavo,* J.A.M.A., May 18, 2005, 2403.

ified treatments. The more complex directives are sometimes more difficult to interpret and implement, especially when they are written by patients or their attorneys without medical input.

When reviewing written directives, attention should be focused on what condition triggers the refusal of treatment and what treatment is being refused. Some of the triggering conditions that have been used include (1) terminal illness, (2) imminence of death, (3) loss of capacity to care for self, (4) loss of capacity to make medical decisions, and (5) loss of capacity to recognize or communicate with family. Some of the treatments refused include (1) extraordinary procedures, (2) life-prolonging procedures, (3) artificial nutrition and hydration, and (4) all procedures except comfort care.

APPLYING ADVANCE DIRECTIVES WHEN INCAPACITY IS TEMPORARY. When a competent patient still is able to communicate or when there is a reasonable likelihood that the patient will again have decision-making capacity and be able to communicate, reliance usually should not be placed on directives made before the condition was known. The patient should be given an opportunity to recover the ability to communicate and express his or her present directive. The major exception is that providers in most jurisdictions should not wait for recovery before following directives based on religious or other strongly held views that are intended to transcend individual conditions. An example of such a directive is a religious-based refusal of blood transfusions.

When the patient was aware of the current condition when giving the advance directive, it is generally appropriate to act in accordance with the advance directive even when there is a possibility of return to capacity. The directive needs to be read carefully. For example, some advance directives use irreversible loss of capacity as the triggering condition; so there would be no refusal of treatment during temporary incapacity.

NO FAMILY VETO. Numerous courts have emphasized the concurrence of the family or the absence of family in their decisions.[24] This should not be interpreted to mean that the family could veto the directive of a competent adult. Courts that have addressed actual disagreements have ruled in favor of the patient's directive. For example, in 1981, a federal district court ordered a Veterans Administration hospital to honor a competent adult's directive to

---

[24] *E.g.*, John F. Kennedy Mem. Hosp. v. Bludworth, 452 A.2d 921 (Fla. 1984).

discontinue his respirator, despite the opposition of his wife and children.[25] In 1994, another federal district court ruled that there was no duty to contact the parents of an eighteen-year-old adult before performing an embolization procedure to which the patient had consented.[26] Similarly, in 1989, the Alabama Supreme Court ruled that there is no duty to inform the wife or daughters of the patient before obtaining informed consent. When a competent adult patient consents, the only legally relevant information is the information given to the patient.[27]

7-1.3 Who Makes Decisions for Adults Without Decision-Making Capacity?

When patients have not expressed their directions and are no longer able to do so, some individual or group must be able to make surrogate decisions for them. In most states, decisions are made by a guardian if one has been appointed by a court. In the absence of a guardian, the health care agent designated by the patient makes decisions. In the absence of a designated agent, close family, friends, and others who have assumed supervision of the patient usually make the decisions.

Usually, the goal of the decision-making process is to make the decision that the patient would make—substitute decision-making—and, when it is not possible to determine what the patient would want, to make the decisions that are in the best interests of the patient.

If the incapacity is temporary, the procedure should usually be postponed until the patient regains capacity and can make his or her own decision, unless the postponement presents a substantial risk to the patient's life or health.[28]

EMERGENCIES. In most emergencies, decisions are made by the providers. Consent is presumed to exist in medical emergencies unless the provider has reason to believe that consent would be

---

[25] Foster v. Tourtellottee, No. CV-81-5046-RMT (C.D. Cal. Nov. 18, 1981), *as discussed in* 704 F.2d 1109 (9th Cir. 1983) [denying attorneys' fees]; *accord In re* Yetter, 62 D.& C. 2d 619 (Pa. Cm Pl. Ct. Northampton County 1973) [disagreement between patient, brother]; Lane v. Candura, 6 Mass. App. Ct. 377, 376 N.E.2d 1232 (1978) [disagreement between patient, daughter]; *see also* Brooks v. United States, 837 F.2d 958 (11th Cir. 1988) [no duty to involve relatives].

[26] Lasley v. Georgetown Univ., 842 F. Supp. 593 (D. D.C. 1994).

[27] Dick v. Springhill Hosps., 551 So. 2d 1034 (Ala. 1989).

[28] *E.g.*, Eis v. Chesnut, 96 N.M. 45, 627 P.2d 1244 (App. Ct. 1981).

refused.[29] When treatment has been refused, there can be no implied consent even in life-threatening situations.[30] An immediate threat to life or health is clearly a sufficient emergency. In an Iowa case, implied consent to removal of a limb mangled in a train accident was presumed because amputation was necessary to save the patient's life.[31]

Courts have disagreed on whether pain is a sufficient emergency to imply consent.[32]

GUARDIAN. In most states, the *guardian of the person* can make decisions regarding medical care of the patient. Guardianship usually supersedes any advance directive appointing a health care agent. Some court orders appointing guardians limit the authority of the guardian or grant the guardian special powers.

Providers can generally rely on the representations of guardians of the person concerning the scope of their powers; so there is generally no duty to obtain a copy of the guardianship papers, unless there is reason to suspect the information from the guardian. Some providers request copies of guardianship papers and place them in the medical record. When this is done, it is important to review the papers so that limitations or special instructions can be addressed.

A *guardian of the estate* is granted powers over the person's property and has no authority to make medical decisions. Often a guardian serves as both guardian of the person and guardian of the estate.

A *guardian ad litem* is a person appointed to represent the patient in court proceedings and has no authority to make medical decisions, unless the court has granted this power. If a guardian ad litem asserts decision-making power, it is prudent to obtain a copy of the court order to confirm the power. Generally, the state law or the appointment order grants the guardian ad litem access to medical information concerning the patient. However, there can be restrictions on access to some information. In 2003, a Florida court ruled that a guardian ad litem did not have unrestricted to access to

---

[29] *E.g.*, Kozup v. Georgetown Univ., 271 U.S. App. D.C. 182, 851 F.2d 437 (1988) [jury question whether life-threatening emergency existed to justify transfusions that caused AIDS].

[30] *E.g.*, Rodriguez v. Pino, 634 So. 2d 681 (Fla. 3d DCA), *rev. denied*, 645 So. 2d 454 (Fla. 1994); Mulloy v. Hop Sang, [1935] 1 W.W.R. 714 (Alberta Sup. Ct.).

[31] Jacovach v. Yocum, 212 Iowa 914, 237 N.W. 444 (1931); *accord* Stafford v. Louisiana State Univ., 448 So. 2d 852 (La. Ct. App. 1984).

[32] *E.g.*, Sullivan v. Montgomery, 155 Misc. 448, 279 N.Y.S. 575 (City Ct. 1935) [pain is a sufficient emergency]; Cunningham v. Yankton Clinic, 262 N.W.2d 508 (S.D. 1978) [pain is not sufficient].

a fourteen-year-old patient's psychiatric records; so the patient could challenge such access.[33]

Many court decisions concerning terminally ill patients involve guardians because the appointment of a guardian is a procedure courts use to effectuate their judgments. However, generally courts have permitted family members to make these decisions without being legally designated guardians; so it is not necessary to routinely seek guardianship.

In some states, obtaining guardianship can substantially reduce the scope of permitted decisions. For example, in Wisconsin, guardians are not permitted to decide to end life-prolonging treatment unless the patient is in a persistent vegetative state or the decision is pursuant to directions from the patient; the only exception is that guardians can approve do not resuscitate orders.[34]

HEALTH CARE AGENT. In most states, a person can sign an advance directive designating one or more persons to serve as a *health care agent* to make medical decisions. Often this advance directive is called a *durable power of attorney for health care*. A *power of attorney* gives the designated agent the power to make decisions on the behalf of the person giving the power, called the *principal*. Powers of attorney have long been used to authorize agents to engage in business transactions for the principal. These traditional powers of attorney become invalid when the principal becomes incapacitated. To adapt this to health care decision-making, special forms authorizing health care decisions developed, and they were made *durable*, which means that they remain valid after the principal loses capacity.

In most states, the power to act as health care agent begins when the advance directive is *activated*. Activation occurs when health care providers document their determination that the patient lacks decision-making capacity.

SPOUSE, CLOSE FAMILY, FRIENDS, AND OTHERS. When decisions concerning treatment cannot be deferred until recovery of capacity, it is common practice to seek a decision from the spouse, other close family members, next of kin, or others who have assumed supervision of the patient.

---

[33] S.C. v. Guardian Ad Litem, 845 So. 2d 953 (Fla. 4th DCA 2003).
[34] Spahn v. Eisenberg (*In re* Edna M.F.), 210 Wis. 2d 558, 563 N.W.2d 485, *cert. denied sub nom*, Spahn v. Wittman, 522 U.S. 951 (1997); Wis. Stat. § 154.225.

In many states, laws or court decisions support this practice. For example, in 1990, a Utah appellate court ruled that a spouse may consent for a patient who is unable to consent.[35] In 2001, a Mississippi appellate court upheld consent by a niece.[36] An Ohio appellate court recognized consent by next of kin.[37] A Florida appellate court accepted decision-making by the parents of an incapacitated single adult.[38] In 1990, the Florida Supreme Court recognized that close family and friends could make decisions regarding termination of treatment in some situations.[39] In decisions in 1992 and 2003, the Wisconsin Supreme Court acknowledged the existence of the practice.[40]

Some state laws specify a priority list of who will be decisionmaker for some decisions.[41] In the absence of state statute or court decision, the most widely accepted order of priority of close family is spouse, adult children, parents, adult siblings, and others. When there is more than one close family member or other person with knowledge of the patient's desires seeking to make decisions, it is common practice to have a family conference to seek consensus. Often consensus can be reached. When consensus among the primary decisionmakers is not possible, it is sometimes necessary to seek guardianship, so that there can be one decisionmaker.

Some persons have established long-term and close relationships with other persons who are not legally recognized as family members. Most providers recognize a role for these partners in the decision-making process. In the absence of legal family, they generally serve as the decisionmaker. It is not clear what priority partners have when there are other close family members available. When consensus can be achieved, this is not a problem. In the absence of consensus, the partner often has an important role as a source of information of the patient's preferences that assists in achieving substituted judgment. The problem of the role of the partner can be avoided through an advance directive making the partner the health care agent.

---

[35] Lounsbury v. Capel, 836 P.2d 188 (Utah App. 1992).
[36] Marchbanks v. Borum, 806 So. 2d 278 (Miss. App. 2001).
[37] Greynolds v. Kurman, 91 Ohio App. 3d 389, 632 N.E.2d 946 (1993).
[38] Ritz v. Florida Patient's Compensation Fund, 436 So. 2d 987 (Fla. 5th DCA 1983).
[39] *In re* Guardianship of Browning, 568 So. 2d 4 (Fla. 1990).
[40] Guardianship of L.W., 167 Wis. 2d 53, 482 N.W.2d 60, 72 n.16 (1992); State v. Picotte, 2003 WI 42, P35, 261 Wis. 2d 249, 661 N.W.2d 381.
[41] *E.g.*, FLA. STAT. § 765.07.

In some states, physicians have been given the power to make some medical decisions for incompetents who have no other surrogate decisionmaker.[42]

SUBSTITUTED JUDGMENT AND BEST INTERESTS. Courts have developed two standards for surrogate decisionmakers to use. Most courts apply the *substituted judgment* standard, which requires the decisionmaker to strive to make the decision the patient would have made if able.[43] When the patient never had decision-making capacity, some courts apply the *best interests* standard, which focuses not on what the patient would want, but on what is best for the patient in the view of the decisionmaker.[44]

GIVING WEIGHT TO THE PATIENT'S WISHES. In making a treatment decision, appropriate weight should be given to what is known of the patient's wishes even if the wishes do not qualify as an advance directive. Patient wishes expressed after loss of capacity should also be considered. In 1984, a Massachusetts court considered the incapacitated patient's efforts to pull out tubes in deciding to permit termination of tube feeding.[45] In the same year, despite the guardian's preference for surgery, the Washington Supreme Court honored an incompetent's desire not to have surgery for cancer of the larynx that would have destroyed her ability to speak.[46]

INVOLUNTARY TREATMENT. In several circumstances, the law authorizes treatment without the consent and even over the opposition of the patient or the patient's representative. The authorizing laws specify who may exercise this decision-making power. Involuntary treatment is discussed in Section 7-7.

7-1.4 When Can Minors Make Their Own Decisions?

Minors may make their own medical decisions in four circumstances. First, many states have *statutes* that permit some minors to consent to some treatments. Second, in some circumstances, minors are considered *emancipated* and then have the same rights

---

[42] *E.g.*, CAL. HEALTH & SAFETY CODE § 1418.8; Rains v. Belshe, 32 Cal. App. 4th 157, 38 Cal. Rptr. 2d 185 (1st Dist. 1995) [constitutional to permit doctor to consent to treatment of incompetent in long-term care facility without legal surrogate].

[43] *E.g.*, Superintendent of Belchertown State School v. Saikewicz, 373 Mass. 728, 370 N.E.2d 417 (1977).

[44] *E.g.*, *In re* Guardianship of Hamlin, 102 Wash. 2d 810, 689 P.2d 1372 (1984).

[45] *In re* Hier, 18 Mass. App. Ct. 200, 464 N.E.2d 959 (1984).

[46] *In re* Ingram, 102 Wash. 2d 827, 689 P.2d 1363 (1984).

as adults to make medical decisions. Third, minors who are considered *mature minors* are permitted to consent to some treatments. Fourth, in many states, minors may contract for *necessaries*. Necessary medical services are usually considered necessaries.

STATUTES. Many states have treatment statutes for minors, empowering older minors to consent to medical treatment. The age limits and the scope of the treatments vary from state to state.[47] Many states have special consent laws for minors for venereal disease and substance abuse treatment that have no age limits.

Generally, these statutes are intended to expand the rights of minors. However, in 1993, a New York appellate court ruled that the state consent statute for minors abrogated all common law rights of minors to consent, so that the exclusive means for minors to consent were those listed in the statute.[48] This is probably an aberrant case. The court was addressing a program that was planning to provide condoms to minors at school without parental consent as part of an HIV/AIDS prevention program. The court reached its decision on minor consent in order to stop the program. It is likely that the court did not consider the other implications for delivery of medical services to adolescents when trying to respond to the public concerns about the role of the family and the school in addressing adolescent sexual behavior and disease prevention.

EMANCIPATED MINORS. Emancipated minors can consent to their own medical care. Minors are *emancipated* when they are no longer subject to parental control and are not supported by their parents. The specific factors necessary to establish emancipation vary from state to state.[49] Some states require that the parent and the child agree on the emancipation; so self-emancipation is not possible in those states.

MATURE MINORS. *Mature minors* may consent to some medical care under common law and constitutional principles and under the statutes of some states. In states that do not have an applicable minor consent statute, the risk associated with providing necessary treatment to mature minors with only their consent is minimal. The oldest

---

[47] *E.g.* 35 Pa. S. § 10101 [high school graduates, married persons, and persons who have been pregnant]; 35 Pa. S. § 1690.112 [controlled or harmful substances]; 35 Pa. S. § 521.14 [venereal disease]; N.Y. Public Health Law § 2504(1) [minor who has married or borne a child]; N.Y. Mental Health Law § 33. 21(c)(e) [outpatient mental health care and/or psychotropic medications]; N.Y. Public Health Law §§ 2780(5), 2781(1) [HIV testing].

[48] Alfonso v. Fernandez, 195 A.D. 2d 46, 606 N.Y.S.2d 259 (2d Dept. 1993).

[49] *E.g.*, Ind. Code § 16-36-1-3; Cal. Family Code §§ 7002, 7050.

minor who underwent a medical procedure with his personal consent and won a reported lawsuit based on lack of parental consent was fifteen[50] That 1941 case involved nontherapeutic removal of some skin for donation to another person for a skin graft operation.

When the age of adulthood was twenty-one, the English common law used the *Rule of Sevens* to assess the decision-making capacity of minors. Minors under age seven did not have capacity. From ages seven through thirteen, there was a rebuttable presumption of no capacity. A *rebuttable presumption* is the default rule that the court follows until it is proven not to apply in the case. Thus, in individual cases, capacity may be proved for this age group. From ages fourteen through twenty, there was a rebuttable presumption of capacity. Persons in this age group were assumed to have capacity, unless it was disproven. Thus, most persons of this age range had capacity, but in individual cases, capacity might be disproved. In 1987, the Tennessee Supreme Court recognized the continuing vitality of the Rule of Sevens and upheld the consent to medical treatment of a minor over age thirteen.[51] However, in 1989, when the Illinois Supreme Court ruled that a mature seventeen-year-old minor with leukemia could refuse transfusions and that it was not neglect for her mother to acquiesce,[52] the court required proof of maturity with clear and convincing evidence. Thus, it did not apply a rebuttable presumption of maturity.

Unless there are contrary laws or court decisions in the jurisdiction, the Rule of Sevens provides a good benchmark for evaluating whether a minor is a mature minor. From ages fourteen to twenty, a minor can be assumed to be mature unless it becomes clear during the consent process that the minor cannot understand the consequences of the particular decision that needs to be made. Below age fourteen, maturity cannot be assumed; so it is advisable to require an affirmative demonstration of ability to understand the consequences of the decision to be made.

The risks of relying on the decisions of mature minors can be minimized by the selection of the procedures for which minor consent is accepted. Procedures that are necessary and relatively low risk present the lowest probability of challenge. Procedures that are controversial on cultural, religious, and/or political grounds, such as

---

[50] Bonner v. Moran, 75 U.S. D.C. App. 156, 126 F.2d 121 (1941).
[51] Cardwell v. Bechtol, 724 S.W.2d 739 (Tenn. 1987).
[52] *In re* E.G., 133 Ill. 2d 98, 549 N.E.2d 322 (1989).

abortion and contraception, are more likely to lead to challenge; so careful review of local law and practice is prudent. In many states, statutes require court approval to accept the decisions of mature minors to have abortions without parental consent. There are more legal risks associated with permitting mature minors to make decisions that are more elective or higher risk. Thus, for example, it is usually advisable not to perform cosmetic surgery on mature minors who refuse to involve their parents in the decision.

In situations where life-prolonging treatment is refused, the issue is usually not whether the parent or guardian must be involved. In most cases, the parent or guardian is involved, and the issue is whether treatment can be refused when the parent and minor agree. Sometimes the issue is what to do when the parent and mature minor disagree.

Some courts have been reluctant to recognize minors as mature when they are refusing treatment that is likely to restore them to health. At least one court expressed this position by rejecting the mature minor doctrine in its entirety. In 1994, a federal court decided that a sixteen-year-old Jehovah's Witness could not refuse a transfusion in a situation where restoration to health was likely. To reach this conclusion, the court held that Georgia does not recognize any right of a mature minor to refuse medical care.[53] Another court rejected the mature minor doctrine in part. In 2000, the Pennsylvania Supreme Court addressed a case where a sixteen-year-old girl had died from untreated diabetes. She and her parents had relied on prayer in accordance with their religious beliefs. Her parents were convicted of involuntary manslaughter and endangering the welfare of a child because they had not sought medical care for her. The court ruled that their daughter's agreement with the approach was not a defense. The court discussed the mature minor doctrine and ruled that it could not be used as a defense by parents who failed to seek medical care.[54] While recognizing the mature minor exception, some courts are reluctant to find maturity in cases where the minor can be restored to health. In 1990, a New York court found that a seventeen-year-old Jehovah's Witness was not sufficiently mature to understand the fatal consequences of refusing a transfusion seven weeks before his eighteenth birthday.[55]

---

[53] *E.g.*, Novak v. Cobb County-Kennestone Hosp. Auth., 849 F. Supp. 1559 (N.D. Ga. 1994).
[54] Comm. v. Nixon, 563 Pa. 425, 761 A.2d 1151 (2000).
[55] *In re* Long Island Jewish Med. Ctr., 147 Misc. 2d 724, 557 N.Y.S.2d 239 (Sup. Ct. 1990).

Other courts have found that mature minors can refuse treatment that is likely to restore them to health. In 1999, a Massachusetts court found that a lower court had erred in ordering a transfusion for a seventeen-year-old Jehovah's Witness without assessing maturity. The court ruled that a mature minor could refuse a transfusion in these circumstances.[56]

In cases where the minor is terminally ill or otherwise unlikely to be restored to health by the proposed treatment, courts have generally respected minor refusals, especially when there is concurrence of the parents. For example, after a state agency forcibly removed a fifteen-year-old liver transplant patient from his home and placed him in a hospital to force him to take antirejection drugs, which could cause painful side effects, a Florida trial court authorized the refusal.[57]

There are practical limits to forcing treatment on an older minor. In 1994, a California court ordered a fifteen-year-old Hmong girl to submit to chemotherapy. She ran away. The court lifted the order in an effort to induce her to return for the treatment she would accept.[58]

Preferences of younger minors have been respected in some cases. In 1998, a Wisconsin juvenile court commissioner denied the state custody and refused to order a twelve-year-old Vietnamese girl to submit to chemotherapy that she opposed. She was in the custody of her grandfather, and they were obtaining alternative treatment for her cancer in accordance with advice of a Vovi Buddhist spiritual leader.[59]

Failure to include a mature minor in the decision-making process can lead to liability. In 1992, the West Virginia Supreme Court ruled that suit could be brought challenging a DNR order for a mature minor whose parents had consented to the DNR order without consulting the patient. After the child died, the father as executor brought the suit. The court remanded for a determination whether the son was a mature minor who was entitled to participate in the decision.[60]

The mature minor doctrine has been recognized by the United States Supreme Court in cases involving decisions to have an abor-

---

[56] *In re* Rena, 46 Mass. App. Ct. 335. 705 N.E.2d 1155 (1999).

[57] *Youth who refused a liver transplant drug dies,* N.Y. TIMES, Aug. 22, 1994, A7.

[58] Mark Arax, *Order for Hmong girl's cancer treatment dropped,* L.A. TIMES, Jan. 5, 1995.

[59] E. Brixley, *Ruling leaves Vietnamese girl with cancer smiling,* WIS. ST. J. (Madison WI), Apr. 21, 1998, 3B.

[60] Belcher v. Charleston Area Med. Ctr., 188 W.Va. 105, 422 S.E.2d 827 (1992).

tion. While states can mandate parental involvement in the decision for minors, states must provide an alternative process to bypass parental involvement in some situations when the minor is mature. Reproductive issues are discussed in Chapter 14.

NECESSARIES. Under the common law, minors have only limited capacity to enter valid contracts. Most contracts cannot be enforced against minors. Minors can disavow most contracts and get their money back. One of the few exceptions in the common law is that minors can enter binding contracts for *necessaries.* Necessary medical treatment has long been recognized as a necessary.[61] Necessary medical care is not limited to emergency care; for example, care for extended and chronic conditions can be included. Parents generally have the primary obligation to pay for these necessaries. However, the minor is generally also obligated to pay.[62]

This common law doctrine of necessaries provides precedent to support accepting consent of mature minors in states where courts have not yet expressly addressed consent by mature minors.

URGING PARENTAL INVOLVEMENT. When treating any unemancipated minor, the minor should be urged to involve his or her parents. When a mature minor refuses to permit parental involvement, the provider can provide necessary care without substantial risk unless there is likelihood of harm to the minor or others that requires adult involvement to avoid. When such harm is likely, parents should usually be involved unless state law forbids parental notification or there is reasonable suspicion that the parents can be a source of the risk of harm. When the parents are suspected to be a source of the risk of harm, other adults should be involved, and in many cases, the circumstances can require reporting to child abuse authorities.

7-1.5 Who Makes Decisions for Minors Who Cannot Decide for Themselves?

Consent of the parent or guardian should be obtained before treatment is given to a minor[63] unless it is (1) an emergency, (2) one of the situations in which the consent of the minor is sufficient, or (3) a situation in which a court order or other legal authorization is obtained.

---

61 *E.g.,* Wiley v. Fuller, 310 Mass. 597, 39 N.E.2d 418 (1942).
62 *E.g.,* Wilson v Knight, 26 Kan. App. 2d 226, 982 P.2d 400 (1999) [minor is liable for payment for necessaries, including medical treatment].
63 Annotation, *Medical practitioner's liability for treatment given child without parent's consent,* 67 A.L.R. 4TH 511.

EMERGENCIES. As with adults, consent is implied in medical *emergencies* when there is an immediate threat to life or health unless the provider has reason to believe that consent would be refused by the parent or guardian. In 1986, one New York trial court ruled that a hospital could not be liable for giving necessary emergency treatment over parental objections when a court would have ordered the treatment.[64] However, when time permits seeking a court order, most providers obtain court authorization when parents refuse necessary treatment. When time does not permit seeking a prior court order, most providers will do that which is necessary to preserve life until a court decision can be obtained. In some states, this is expressly authorized in child abuse statues.

GUARDIAN. When a guardian of the person of the minor has been appointed, the guardian makes medical decisions within the scope of the guardianship. It is not unusual for a guardian to be appointed with the limited authority to consent to only some medical treatments, such as transfusions, leaving all other medical decisions to the parents.

PARENT. When there is no applicable guardianship in effect, either parent can give legally effective consent except when there is legal separation or divorce. It is not necessary to seek the wishes of the other parent. When objections are known and consensus cannot be reached, either the treatment should not be given or court authorization should be obtained.[65] When the parents are legally separated or divorced, usually the consent of the custodial parent must be obtained, but sometimes the arrangements can be complex. So it is prudent to ask if the court has specified decision-making.[66] If inconsistent or unclear answers are given, it is prudent to obtain a copy of the court's order.

When both parents are available, it is prudent to seek consensus. It is appropriate for one parent to consult with the other. A New York court ruled that it was not neglect for one parent to briefly delay consenting to treatment for child in order to consult with the other parent.[67]

The provider generally has no duty to confirm the identity or parental status of persons who reasonably present themselves as

---

[64] Joswick v. Lenox Hill Hosp., 134 Misc. 2d 295, 510 N.Y.S.2d 803 (Sup. Ct. 1986).

[65] *E.g.*, *In re* Rotkowitz, 25 N.Y.S.2d 624 (Dom. Rel. Ct. 1941) [surgery ordered].

[66] *But see* Faust v. Johnson, 223 Wis. 2d 799, 589 N.W.2d 454, 1998 Wisc. App. LEXIS 1436 (unpub.) [joint legal custody after divorce, but sole custody for medical issues to one parent].

[67] *In re* Vulon, 56 Misc. 2d 19, 288 N.Y.S.2d 203 (Fam. Ct. 1968).

parents. When the circumstances create suspicions, then it is appropriate to confirm identity and status. Persons who misrepresent themselves can be subject to liability, but there is generally no liability for the provider. In 2003, a Wisconsin woman was accused of falsely giving parental consent for an abortion for her son's fifteen-year-old girlfriend. She was charged with the misdemeanor of intentionally falsifying a patient health care record.[68]

In some states, there may be a duty to check identification before some procedures. In 2004, Texas adopted a rule that requires identification checks before consent can be obtained for abortions.[69]

ADVANCE DIRECTIVES/AGENTS FOR THE PARENT. It is not uncommon for parents to leave their children in the care of others for hours, days, or weeks. This can include day care; summer camp; visits to grandparents; or living with relatives or others while parents are on active military duty, business trips, vacations, in legal custody, or incapacitated by substance abuse. When the time period becomes too long or the arrangements are not adequate, the parental absence can constitute abandonment under the laws of some states, triggering state intervention to formally modify parental rights and legal custody. In the many situations where these arrangements are acceptable, it is necessary for the persons who are taking care of the child to be able to arrange for necessary medical care. The emergency exception to the consent requirement is not broad enough to address all of the medical needs of children. For example, in some states, pain alone does not justify treatment under the emergency exception. Thus, someone needs to have authority to consent when the parents cannot be reached in order to mitigate the effects of the consent requirement on those who are not able to consent for themselves.

Two approaches have been used to address parental absence. One approach is for parents to sign forms consenting to medical care. Providers generally prefer to have a decisionmaker who has the power to make informed decisions concerning specific treatments. Thus, the other approach is for the parents to designate someone as the parent's agent to make decisions for the parents. In some circumstances, this agency can be implied by the arrangements, but it is better for one or both parents to grant express authority by signing a

---

[68] *Abortion consent brings charges*, Wis. St. J. (Madison WI), Dec. 26, 2003, G1.
[69] *Texas Board of Health institutes rule requiring proof of identification before getting an abortion*, All Things Considered (National Public Radio), Mar. 19, 2004.

document designating the agent. At least one state has enacted express statutory authority for such a written delegation.[70]

IN LOCO PARENTIS. Some states consider that persons can stand *in loco parentis* (in the place of a parent) to a minor by assuming the status and obligation of a parent without formal adoption or designation by the natural parent. In these states, the term "parent" in some legal contexts is construed to include persons who are *in loco parentis*.[71]

OTHER RELATIVES. Some states recognize that in the absence of a parent or guardian, the closest available relative has authority to consent without an express directive from the parent.[72]

PERSONS WITH CUSTODY. Many minors are in the custody of governmental agencies, public or private facilities, or foster parents designated by governmental agencies. Under the laws of some states, some of these custodians have the statutory power to make some medical decisions. In other states, custodians have no power to make medical decisions, unless a court specifically grants them the power or the parents make the custodian an agent for medical decision-making. In those states, the parent or parents generally retain parental rights to make medical decisions.

SUSPECTED CHILD ABUSE CASES. When health care providers see minor patients who they suspect have been abused or neglected, there is generally a duty to report this to child abuse authorities.[73] The definition of what constitutes reportable abuse and neglect varies. In some states, child abuse authorities have the power to authorize some treatments.[74] In some states, health care providers are authorized to provide some treatments, but curiously most states limit this to diagnostic procedures.[75] Thus, for example, in most states, when abused minors are not permitted to consent for themselves, providers technically are required to wait for administrative, judicial, or parental consent before providing treatment, including treatment for pain, unless the treatment falls within the emergency treatment exception to the consent requirement. However, as discussed in Section 7-1.3, in at least one state, South Dakota, pain alone is not a sufficient emergency to permit treatment without consent.

---

[70] 11 PA. STAT. § 2513.
[71] *E.g.*, Gritzner v. Michel R., 2000 WI 68, 235 Wis. 2d 781, 611 N.W.2d 906.
[72] *E.g.*, Cobbs v. Grant, 8 Cal. 3d 229, 502 P.2d 1, 104 Cal. Rptr. 505 (1972).
[73] *E.g.*, WIS. STAT. § 48.981.
[74] *E.g.*, FLA. STAT. § 39.304.
[75] *E.g.*, TENN. CODE ANN. § 37-1-406(f).

7-2 What Information Needs to Be Given to the Decisionmaker?

The general rule is that consent for most treatments must be an *informed consent*. This means that the treating provider is required to give to the decisionmaker several elements of information before the consent decision.

The common law has long recognized the right of persons to be free from harmful or offensive touching. The intentional harmful or offensive touching of another person without authorization is called *battery* (see the discussion in Chapter 11). When there is no consent or other authorization for a procedure, the physician or other practitioner doing the medical procedure can be liable for battery even if the procedure is properly performed, is beneficial, and has no negative effects.[76] The touching alone leads to liability. When consent is given but the person consenting does not have sufficient information for an informed decision, the provider can be liable for violating the duty to disclose such information. In some early cases, courts ruled that providing incorrect or insufficient information invalidated the consent, making the physician liable for battery. Today, in most jurisdictions, failure to disclose necessary information does not invalidate consent; so the procedure is not a battery.[77] There is still a minority position that a medical procedure without informed consent is a battery.[78] The majority rule is that failure to disclose is a separate wrong for which there can be liability based on principles applicable to negligent torts discussed in Chapter 11. Uninformed consent protects from liability for battery, but informed consent is necessary to protect from liability for negligence.

Although some providers view the obtaining of informed consent as simply an administrative burden, providers who actually engage in

---

[76] *E.g.*, Fox v. Smith, 594 So. 2d 596 (Miss. 1992) [removal of IUD during laproscopy could be battery after express directions not to remove]; Bommareddy v. Superior Court, 222 Cal. App. 3d 1017, 272 Cal. Rptr. 246 (5th Dist. 1990) [punitive damages allowable for battery, cataract surgery when consent only for tear duct surgery]; Gaskin v. Goldwasser, 166 Ill. App. 3d 996, 520 N.E.2d 1085 (4th Dist. 1988); Throne v. Wandell, 176 Wis. 97, 186 N.W. 146 (1922); *but see* Garcia v. Meiselman, 220 N.J. Super. 317, 531 A.2d 1373 (App. Div. 1987) [no damages when beneficial surgery properly performed without consent].

[77] *E.g.*, Batzell v. Buskirk, 752 S.W.2d 902 (Mo. Ct. App. 1988); Kohoutek v. Hafner, 383 N.W.2d 295 (Minn. 1986); Moser v. Stallings, 387 N.W.2d 599 (Iowa 1986).

[78] *E.g.*, Fox v. Smith, 594 So. 2d 596 (Miss. 1992); Marino v. Ballestas, 749 F.2d 162 (3d Cir. 1984) [battery action permitted]; Hales v. Pittman, 118 Ariz. 305, 576 P.2d 493 (1978) [battery action permitted]; Ariz. Rev. Stat. Ann. § 12-562(B) (1982) [battery action eliminated by statute]; Rubino v. DeFretias, 638 F. Supp. 182 (D. Ariz. 1986) [Arizona statute unconstitutional].

the intended communication with their patients find that it not only performs its intended function of respecting individual autonomy, but it also can improve compliance, outcomes, and satisfaction.[79]

In applying the general rule, several problems arise.

7-2.1. When is informed consent required?

7-2.2. What elements of information concerning the treatment should be given?

7-2.3. To what extent do alternatives have to be disclosed?

7-2.4. What elements of information concerning the provider should be given?

7-2.5. What is the effect of information that the decisionmaker obtains from other sources?

7-2.6. What is the effect of barriers to understanding the information?

7-2.7. When can information be withheld?

7-2.1 When Is Informed Consent Required?

Most courts apply the informed consent doctrine only to services that are provided. The focus is on whether there was adequate information to obtain consent for the services provided. In 1997, a New York court ruled that where there is no violation of the physical integrity of the patient, there could not be a claim for lack of informed consent.[80] States vary on which services require consent. In 1998, a New Jersey court decided that a surgeon could be liable for lack of informed consent to his prescription of conservative bed rest.[81]

There have been attempts to extend the informed consent doctrine. A person who was involuntarily committed to a Maine facility for mental health treatment claimed that the facility needed her informed consent to wake her in the morning. She wanted to sleep to 11 a.m. In 2001, the Maine Supreme Court ruled that the Commissioner of the Department of Mental Health had properly decided that consent was not required for waking the person since it did not constitute treatment or services, but was instead intended to give her opportunity to participate in treatment, to give clinical staff a chance to observe her, and for smooth hospital operation.[82]

---

[79] F.J. Skelly, *The payoff of informed consent*, AM. MED. NEWS, Aug. 1, 1994, at 11.

[80] Schel v. Roth, 242 A.D.2d 697, 663 N.Y.S.2d 609 (2d Dept. 1997).

[81] Matthies v. Mastomonaco, 310 N.J. Super. 572, 709 A.2d 238 (App. Div. 1998).

[82] Green v. Commissioner of Dep't of Mental Health, 776 A.2d 612 (Me. 2001).

A few courts have extended the informed consent doctrine to require informed refusal. The California Supreme Court ruled that a physician could be liable for a patient's death from cervical cancer because the physician did not inform the patient of the risks of not consenting to a recommended Pap smear.[83] The Pap smear probably would have discovered her cancer in time to begin life-extending treatment. A New Jersey court ruled that an obstetrician could be sued for failing to advise the patient sufficiently of the hazards of leaving the hospital against medical advice.[84]

There is an aberrant trend in some courts to reverse the thrust of the informed consent doctrine in cases involving refusal of transfusions in the emergency context. The complete reversal is from a duty of the provider to provide information to a duty of the patient to collect and understand the information. These courts then honor only informed refusals, using the reversal of the informed consent doctrine as the stated rationale for disregarding the patient's directions.

In 1987, the Pennsylvania Supreme Court upheld a court ordered transfusion of an adult Jehovah's Witness who had been in an accident and was unable to express his directions at the time.[85] The patient was carrying a card that stated that he was a Jehovah's Witness and directed that he should not be given blood. There was some question whether the card had accompanied the patient when he was transferred to the hospital where the transfusion order was obtained and the transfusion was administered. However, the court did not ground its decision on this uncertainty. It ruled that, even if there was a refusal, the refusal was invalid because it was uninformed in that the patient had not known that refusal of blood could threaten his life. The court stated that there had to be a contemporaneous refusal.

A few other states have adopted the same position. One case involved elective surgery where the patient had expressly conditioned her consent to the surgery on not using transfusions.[86] In another case, the court did not permit the patient to sue a doctor who had unilaterally disregarded the patient's expressed directions without seeking a court order.[87]

---

[83] Truman v. Thomas, 27 Cal. 3d 285, 165 Cal. Rptr. 308, 611 P.2d 902 (1980).
[84] Battenfeld v. Gregory, 247 N.J. Super. 538, 589 A.2d 1059 (App. Div. 1991).
[85] *In re* Dorone, 517 Pa. 3, 534 A.2d 452 (1987), *aff'g*, 349 Pa. Super. 59, 502 A.2d 1271 (1985).
[86] *E.g.*, *In re* Hughes, 259 N.J. Super. 193, 611 A.2d 1148 (App. Div. 1992).
[87] Werth v. Taylor, 190 Mich. App. 141, 475 N.W.2d 426 (1991).

In the past, the emergency exception to the consent requirement was limited to cases where the patient's directions were not
known. Here the courts had to go through the two-step process of
voiding the express refusals of these patients through the informed
refusal doctrine, so that the court could adopt the fiction that the
patient's directions were not known and then invoke the emergency
exception to the consent doctrine. These cases represent a significant retreat from the respect for religious and other beliefs of adults
that the law has demonstrated in other jurisdictions. Requiring
informed refusal stands the informed consent doctrine on its head.
The informed consent doctrine was designed (1) to preserve the
individual's right to autonomy and to be left alone by not permitting
treatment without informed consent and (2) to promote disclosure
of information by physicians to facilitate the exercise of that autonomy. This informed refusal doctrine removes the requirement that
providers obtain consent to treatment and permits the courts and
doctors to force emergency treatment on a person unless the person can meet a strict standard set by the court.

7-2.2 What Elements of Information Concerning the Treatment Should be Given?

DISCLOSURE STANDARDS. Courts have developed two standards
for determining whether disclosure is adequate: the reasonable
physician standard and the reasonable patient standard.[88]

Reasonable Physician. Some states apply the professional
(reasonable physician) standard of accepted medical practice. In
those states, the professional has a duty to make the disclosure that
a reasonable medical practitioner would make under the same or
similar circumstances.[89] Expert testimony is necessary to prove
what disclosure was required.

Reasonable Patient. The majority of states apply the reasonable
patient standard under which the duty to disclose is determined by
the patient's informational needs, not by professional practice.[90]

---

[88] *See* Annotation, *Modern status of views as to general measure of physician's duty to inform patient of risks of proposed treatment,* 88 A.L.R. 3D 1008.

[89] *E.g.,* Gorab v. Zook, 943 P.2d 423 (Colo. 1997); Natanson v. Kline, 186 Kan. 393, 350 P.2d 1093 (1960).

[90] *E.g.,* Korman v. Mallin, 858 P.2d 1145 (Alaska 1993); Largey v. Rothman, 110 N.J. 204, 540 A.2d 504 (1988); Pauscher v. Iowa Methodist Med. Ctr., 408 N.W.2d 355 (Iowa 1987).

Information that is "material" to the decision must be disclosed. A risk is material "when a reasonable person, in what the physician knows or should know to be the patient's position, would be likely to attach significance to the risk or cluster of risks in deciding whether or not to forgo the proposed therapy."[91] No expert testimony is required on the issue of whether specific information should have been disclosed, but expert testimony can sometimes be necessary to prove that a specific risk was present or a specific treatment was actually an alternative.[92]

Consumer Protection Laws. Some aggressive attorneys have tried to convince courts that the scope of disclosure should be subject to consumer protection laws. This has generally been unsuccessful.[93]

ELEMENTS OF DISCLOSURE. The usual elements to be disclosed under either standard are the patient's medical condition, the nature and purpose of the proposed procedure, its risks and consequences, and the feasible accepted alternatives, including the consequences of no treatment.

Patient's Medical Condition. The decisionmaker needs to be told about the patient's medical condition, so that the context and purpose of the treatment can be understood. However, in 1999, a New Jersey appellate court ruled that failure to give advice about the patient's medical condition was not an informed consent issue, when it was not connected to a decision regarding a proposed treatment.[94]

Nature and Purpose of the Treatment. The decisionmaker needs to be told what the proposed procedure is and what the purpose of the procedure is. Disclosure should include a realistic discussion of the likelihood of success from the proposed treatment. In 1995, a Louisiana court found lack of informed consent where there had been no disclosure that the bunion surgery would not restore the foot to normal.[95]

---

[91] Canterbury v. Spence, 150 D.C. App. 263, 464 F.2d 772, 787, *cert. denied*, 409 U.S. 1064 (1972).

[92] *E.g.*, Hapchuck v. Pierson, 495 S.E.2d 854 (W.Va. 1997) [affirming dismissal for absence of expert testimony as to risks, alternatives, and outcome without treatment]; Moure v. Raeuchle, 529 Pa. 394, 604 A.2d 1003 (1992).

[93] *E.g.*, Darviris v. Petros, 442 Mass. 274, 812 N.E.2d 1188 (2004); Lareau v. Page, 34 F.3d 384 (1st Cir. 1994); Foflygen v. Zemel, 420 Pa. Super. 18, 615 A.2d 1345 (1992); Benoy v. Simons, 66 Wash. App. 56, 831 P.2d 167 (1992); *but see*, Quimby v. Fine, 45 Wash. App. 175, 724 P.2d 403 (1986).

[94] Eagel v. Newman, 325 N.J. Super. 467, 739 A.2d 986 (1999).

[95] Hartman v. D'Ambrosia, 665 So. 2d 1206 (La. Ct. App. 1995).

Risks and Consequences. Knowledge of risk is an important part of thoughtful decision-making.[96] Only risks that are known or should be known by the physician to occur without negligence are required to be disclosed.[97] Nearly all courts recognize that not all risks can be disclosed. Rare risks are generally not considered material and need not be disclosed.[98] However, there is no bright line definition of what percentage constitutes rare. One useful guideline is to disclose the risks of the most severe consequences and the risks that have a substantial probability of occurring.

When risks are disclosed, it is generally not necessary to disclose percentage of risk. In 1993, the California Supreme Court decided that physicians did not need to disclose the odds of success of procedures.[99] However, if statistics are volunteered and significantly wrong, there could be liability for misstating the risks.

In 1992, one federal court decided no disclosure of risks needed to be made before a polio vaccine was given because under state law the vaccine was legally required, with the only permitted exception being for religious objections.[100]

Sometimes there are consequences that occur in virtually all cases. These consequences are technically not risks because risk usually implies that there is a chance that the event will not occur. Consequences can include follow-up regimens or changes in bodily functions that will continue for days or weeks or will be permanent. Generally, these consequences should be disclosed.

Alternatives. Known feasible accepted alternatives should be disclosed, including the option of no treatment. This is discussed in Section 7-2.3.

Regulatory Status. There are many accepted uses of drugs and devices that are not yet approved by the FDA. With few exceptions, physicians can use approved drugs for off-label uses. The scope of permitted off-label uses of devices is not as broad. However, many off-label uses do not violate the law. Off-label uses for individual

---

[96] *E.g.*, V.S. Elliott, *Communicating risk key step to good care,* AM. MED. NEWS, Oct. 20, 2003, 23 [patients cannot make best decisions when they misunderstand risks].

[97] *E.g.*, Tyndall v. Zaboski, 306 N.J. Super. 423, 703 A.2d 980 (App. Div. 1997) [plaintiff must prove by expert testimony risk was known to practitioners]; Gilmartin v. Weinreb, 324 N.J. Super. 367, 735 A.2d 620 (App. Div. 1999) [need not disclose risk of negligence].

[98] *E.g.*, Galvan v. Downey, 933 S.W.2d 316 (Tex. Ct. App. 1996).

[99] Arato v. Avedon, 5 Cal. 4th 1172, 23 Cal. Rptr. 2d 131, 858 P.2d 598 (1993).

[100] Snawder v. Cohen, 804 F. Supp. 910 (W.D. Ky. 1992), *aff'd on other grounds,* 5 F.3d 1013 (6th Cir. 1993).

patients outside of research protocols are generally not considered to be research. Some attorneys have tried to establish a duty to disclose such off-label uses. This has generally been rejected by courts. In 2002, a New York appellate court decided that the FDA status of an internal fixation device for the spine did not have to be disclosed.[101] In 1996, an Ohio court ruled that a physician need not disclose that an approved medical device was being used in an off-label manner.[102]

Medicare will not pay for some off-label uses of devices. Medicare law requires patients to be given an advance beneficiary notice (ABN) of these uses for financial reasons so that the patient can decide whether to incur the unreimbursed costs.

RESEARCH. There are federal and state requirements concerning consent for research.

Patients ordinarily expect physicians to use the drugs and procedures customarily used for their condition. When experimental methods are used or when established procedures are used for research purposes, the investigator must disclose this to the subject and obtain the consent of the subject or the subject's representative. Governmental regulations specify review procedures for many types of research and specify disclosures that must be made to obtain informed consent to such research.

All research supported by the U.S. Department of Health and Human Services (HHS) must comply with regulations for the protection of human subjects.[103] These regulations require that an institutional review board (IRB) approve the research before HHS can support the research. Each institution must submit an acceptable institutional assurance to HHS that it will fulfill its responsibilities under the regulations before HHS will accept the decisions of its IRB.

The HHS regulations require that consent be sought "only under circumstances that provide the prospective subject or the representative sufficient opportunity to consider whether or not to participate and that minimize the possibility of coercion or undue influence." The information must be in a language understandable to the subject or representative. Exculpatory wording cannot be included in the information given. Federal regulations specify

---

[101] Blazoski v. Cook, 346 N.J. Super. 256, 787 A.2d 910 (App. Div. 2002).
[102] Klein v. Biscup, 109 Ohio App. 3d 855, 673 N.E.2d 225 (1996).
[103] 45 C.F.R. pt. 46 [HHS].

numerous basic elements of information that must be included in the consent form.

Several kinds of studies are exempt from these regulations, such as the "collection or study of existing data, documents, records, pathological specimens, or diagnostic specimens, if these sources are publicly available or if the information is recorded by the investigator in such a manner that subjects cannot be identified. . . ." Expedited review is authorized for categories of research that HHS determines involve no more than minimal risk.[104] Examples of such categories are collection of small amounts of blood by venipuncture from certain adults and moderate exercise by healthy volunteers.

The HHS regulations do not preempt other federal, state, or local laws or regulations. Thus, proposals involving investigational new drugs or devices must also satisfy the regulations of the Food and Drug Administration.[105] State and local law must also be reviewed because several states have enacted laws regulating research with human subjects.[106]

Hospitals should take appropriate steps to review research involving human subjects, regardless of the sponsorship of the research, to protect patients and avoid liability. Some courts have decided that because federal regulations require institutional review of consent for certain research that the reviewing institution can be liable for lack of informed consent for such research.[107]

EFFECT OF PATIENT REQUESTS FOR ADDITIONAL INFORMATION. When a patient indicates a desire for additional information, there is usually a duty to provide it. For example, a patient told a physician that his ability to work was crucial; so the Arizona Supreme Court ruled that the physician should have provided information concerning risks affecting ability to work.[108] In 1992, a Louisiana appellate court ruled that where the patient's primary motivation for treatment was pain relief that the physician had a duty to disclose that the proposed surgery was unlikely

---

[104] 45 C.F.R. § 46.110; *see* 46 FED. REG. 8,392 (Jan. 26, 1981) [initial approved categories].
[105] 21 C.F.R. pts. 50, 56, 312, 314, 812.
[106] *E.g.*, N.Y. PUB. HEALTH LAW §§ 2440 – 2446.
[107] *E.g.*, Anderson v. George H. Lanier Mem. Hosp., 982 F.2d 1513 (11th Cir. 1993) [use of experimental intraocular lens]; Friter v. IOLAB Corp., 414 Pa. Super. 622, 607 A.2d 1111 (1992) [use of experimental intraocular lens]; Daum v. SpineCare Med. Group, 52 Cal. App. 4th 1285, 61 Cal. Rptr. 2d 260 (1st Dist. 1997) [spinal fixation device].
[108] Hales v. Pittman, 118 Ariz. 305, 576 P.2d 493 (1978).

to give such relief.[109] However, there are limits to the scope of information that must be provided even when requested. The California Supreme Court ruled that nonmedical concerns of the patient did not create a more extensive fiduciary duty for the physician; so the physician did not have to become the patient's financial advisor.[110]

OTHER ISSUES. Some states have passed statutes or created administrative processes that address what disclosure should be made.[111] In one state, Oregon, the statute requires the physician to ask the patient if a more detailed disclosure is desired. If the physician fails to ask, then the physician has a duty of full disclosure.[112]

Some states mandate that specific nonmedical information concerning abortions must be provided before consent can be obtained. Since 1993, these laws have generally been upheld.[113] However, a Florida appellate court found such a mandate to violate the state constitution.[114] There is no constitutional or common law duty to provide such information in the absence of a statutory mandate.[115]

7-2.3 To What Extent Do Alternatives Have to Be Disclosed?

Known feasible accepted alternatives should be disclosed, including the option of no treatment. This is not limited to alternatives that the provider would perform. If the decisionmaker selects an option that the provider does not perform, the decisionmaker is declining the services offered by the provider and needs to make arrangements for another provider. Options that are available only in research protocols generally do not have to be disclosed.

---

[109] Givens v. Cracco, 607 So. 2d 727 (La. Ct. App. 1992).

[110] Arato v. Avedon, 5 Cal. 4th 1172, 23 Cal. Rptr. 2d 131, 858 P.2d 598 (1993).

[111] *E.g.,* TEX. CIV. STATS., art. 4590i, subch. F; 25 TEX. ADMIN. CODE §§ 601.1 – 601.08; Jones v. Papp, 782 S.W.2d 236 (Tex. Ct. App. 1989) [form met statutory standard]; Tajchman v. Giller, 938 S.W.2d 95 (Tex. Ct. App. 1996) [statute required disclosure of risks, hazards when no state approved consent form; need for cutting vein was step in procedure, not a risk or hazard, so statutory disclosure standard met]; Eckmann v. Des Rosiers, 940 S.W.2d 394 (Tex. Civ. App. 1997) [consent form protected by statutory presumption even though medical disclosure panel had not updated requirements].

[112] ORE. REV. STAT. § 677.097(2); Zacher v. Petty, 312 Or. 590, 826 P.2d 619 (1992).

[113] Planned Parenthood v. Casey, 505 U.S. 833 (1992).

[114] State v. Presidential Women's Ctr., 707 So. 2d 1145 (Fla. 4th DCA 1998).

[115] Marie v. McGreevey, 314 F.3d 136 (3d Cir. 2002); D Adams, *N.J. OB wins informed consent case,* AM. MED. NEWS, Jan. 5, 2004, 11 [N.J. Superior Court ruled in *Acuna v. Turkish* not required to express moral, philosophical or religious judgments in advising about abortion].

The alleged failure to disclose alternatives is often the focus of informed consent cases.[116] Courts have not agreed on which alternatives must be disclosed.[117] This issue is also discussed in Section 7-6., which discusses limits on treatment that must be offered.

In 2001, the New Jersey Supreme Court ruled that there was no need to discuss a treatment that was not a medically reasonable alternative.[118] In 2002, an Iowa court found that the patient had not demonstrated that there was any alternative to a repeat cesarean section; so the physician had no duty to disclose alternatives.[119] Similarly, in 1997, an Illinois court decided that a physician could justify not disclosing any alternatives by showing there were no reasonable alternatives to disclose.[120] Experts testified that the wart removal surgery was necessary due to the size and depth of the warts.

Courts have disagreed on whether the availability of additional diagnostic tests should be considered an alternative. In 1999, a New Jersey court decided that an additional diagnostic test was not an alternative.[121] In 1996, a Wisconsin court decided that a jury could find lack of informed consent for failure to disclose availability of diagnostic CT scan.[122]

Some managed care organizations tried to impose "gag" clauses through their contracts, restricting the information physicians could provide to patients. These restrictions were widely attacked, and most were abandoned or modified.[123]

---

[116] *See* Annotation, *Medical malpractice: Liability for failure of physician to inform patient of alternative modes of diagnosis and treatment*, 38 A.L.R. 4TH 900; WIS. STAT. § 448.30 [statutory requirement to disclose alternatives].

[117] *E.g.*, Wachter v. United States, 689 F. Supp. 1420 (D. Md. 1988), *aff'd*, 877 F.2d 257 (4th Cir. 1989) [need not disclose alternative not in general use or subject of definitive study]; Smith v. Reisig, 686 P.2d 285 (Okla. 1984); Marino v. Ballestas, 749 F.2d 162 (3d Cir. 1984) [parents must be told alternatives to surgery for child]; Logan v. Greenwich Hosp. Ass'n, 191 Conn. 282, 465 A.2d 294 (1983) [feasible alternatives involving greater risks must also be disclosed].

[118] Sgro v. Ross, 166 N.J. 338, 765 A.2d 745 (2001).

[119] Taylor v. Brownlee, 2002 Iowa App. LEXIS 501.

[120] Ruperd v. Ryan, 292 Ill. App. 3d 22, 683 N.E.2d 166 (2d Dist. 1997); *but see* Caputa v. Antiles, 296 N.J. Super. 123, 686 A.2d 356 (App. Div. 1996) [nondisclosure of observation as alternative to surgery warranted directed verdict on failure to disclose, but jury to decide causation, whether reasonable person would have refused with disclosure].

[121] Farina v. Kraus, 333 N.J. Super. 165, 754 A.2d 1215 (App. Div. 1999).

[122] Kuklinski v. Rodriguez, 203 Wis. 2d 324, 552 N.W.2d 869 (App. 1996).

[123] *E.g.*, S. Klein, *Texas forces change in Aetna contracts*, AM. MED. NEWS, Jan. 19, 1998, at 3 [Aetna agreed to modify provider contract to omit gag clause after challenge by state Dept. of Ins.]; Weiss v. CIGNA Healthcare Inc., 972 F. Supp. 748 (S.D. N.Y. 1997) [plan participant can sue plan for breach of fiduciary duty under ERISA for limiting extent participating physicians may discuss medical treatments with plan members].

7-2.4 *What Elements of Information Concerning the Provider Should Be Given?*

It is generally recognized that the identity of the provider should be disclosed. There have been efforts to expand the scope of required information about the individual provider; so additional information is required in some states. When additional information is given, it needs to be accurate.

NAME OF PROVIDER. Patients generally have a right to know the identity of their providers. Undisclosed substitution of surgeons can result in liability.[124] For example, in 1983, the New Jersey Supreme Court ruled that there could be liability for undisclosed substitution of surgeons.[125] However, in 1984, the highest court of Massachusetts ruled that a substitute physician did not commit battery by performing a myelography because the patient had not directed postponement if the requested physician could not perform it.[126]

As long as the fact that assistants can be used is disclosed, there is generally no duty to disclose the identity of each assistant. A North Carolina court found that an attending physician did not have a duty to inform a patient of the identity and qualifications of the individuals who would be assisting him.[127] When residents or students are involved in procedures, it is prudent to disclose that residents or students will be involved.

When a patient directs that a specific physician not perform a procedure and the forbidden physician performs it, both the forbidden physician and those who let that physician perform the procedure can be liable.[128]

CHARACTERISTICS OF PROVIDER. Courts disagree on when physicians are required to disclose certain information about themselves as part of the consent process.

Substance Abuse. There is disagreement over whether substance abuse needs to be disclosed. A Louisiana court found that a surgeon had failed to obtain informed consent when he failed to disclose his chronic alcohol abuse.[129] However, in 1997, a federal court

---

[124] Annotation, *Recovery by patient on whom surgery or other treatment was performed by other than physician who patient believed would perform it*, 39 A.L.R. 4TH 1034.

[125] Perna v. Pirozzi, 92 N.J. 446, 457 A.2d 431 (1983).

[126] Forland v. Hughes, 393 Mass. 502, 471 N.E.2d 1315 (1984).

[127] Bowlin v. Duke Univ., 108 N.C. App. 145, 423 S.E.2d 320 (1992) [bone marrow harvest].

[128] *E.g.*, Johnson v. McMurray, 461 So. 2d 775 (Ala. 1984).

[129] Hidding v. Williams, 578 So. 2d 1192 (La. Ct. App. 1991).

in Hawaii ruled that there was no duty to disclose a past history of substance abuse.[130] In 2000, the Georgia Supreme Court decided that providers have no duty to disclose life factors that might subjectively be considered to adversely affect the performance, absent inquiry from the patient. This included no duty to disclose cocaine use outside of work when not on call.[131] In 2003, an Ohio court ruled that a surgeon did not have to disclose addiction to painkillers where there was no affect on the outcome of the surgery.[132]

Transmissible Disease. Despite the professional debate over the necessity of such disclosures, some courts have ruled that surgeons and some other health care professionals should disclose that they are HIV-positive, especially when the patient asks.[133] However, at least one state will permit suits based on nondisclosure only when actual exposure to the disease occurred.[134]

A New Jersey court ruled that a hospital could require a HIV-positive surgeon to disclose his condition as part of the consent process.[135] In 2002, the New York State Health Department ordered a heart surgeon with hepatitis C to obtain signed consent disclosing his infection before performing any surgery.[136]

Other Conditions. In 2002, an Iowa court ruled that a surgeon had no duty to disclose the herniated disc in her neck region where it had no impact on her performance of surgery.[137]

Experience. Courts have disagreed on whether a physician must disclose experience or competence with proposed procedures. Most courts have ruled that this is not an informed consent issue. For example, in 1997, the Hawaii Supreme Court ruled that the informed consent doctrine did not require physicians to disclose their qualifications.[138] In 2001, the Pennsylvania Supreme Court

---

[130] Domingo v. Doe, 985 F. Supp. 1241 (D. Hawaii 1997).

[131] Albany Urology Clinic, P.C. v. Cleveland, 272 Ga. 296, 528 S.E.2d 777 (2000).

[132] Schwaller v. Maguire, 2003 Ohio 6917, 2003 Ohio App. LEXIS 6227.

[133] *E.g.*, Faya v. Almarez, 329 Md. 435, 620 A.2d 327 (1993) [HIV-infected surgeon could be liable for failing to inform patients, even when they did not get infected]; Kerins v. Hartley, 17 Cal. App. 4th 713, 21 Cal. Rptr. 2d 621 (2d Dist. 1993) [patient asked about surgeon's health and conditioned consent on operation by healthy surgeon, so could sue for battery when HIV-positive status not disclosed], *transferred*, 28 Cal. Rptr. 2d 151, 868 P.2d 906 (Cal. 1994), *on transfer*, 27 Cal. App. 4th 1062, 33 Cal. Rptr. 2d 172 (2d Dist, 1994) [statistically insignificant chance of HIV exposure during surgery by infected doctor precluded recovery for emotional distress from fear of AIDS].

[134] Majca v. Beekil, 183 Ill. 2d 407, 701 N.E.2d 1084 (1998).

[135] Estate of Behringer v. Medical Ctr., 249 N.J. Super. 597, 592 A.2d 1251 (1991).

[136] B. Lambert, *Infected doctor told to get patient's consent*, N.Y. TIMES, Apr. 19, 2002, B4.

[137] Slutzki v. Grabenstetter, 2002 Iowa App. LEXIS 1028.

[138] Ditto v. McCurdy, 86 Haw. 84, 947 P.2d 952 (1997).

decided that the physician's personal characteristics and experience were never relevant to an informed consent claim; so even a misrepresentation of experience would not support an informed consent suit.[139] In 1996, the Wisconsin Supreme Court ruled that a physician had a duty to disclose lack of experience in some circumstances.[140] There has been no disagreement concerning the absence of a hospital duty to disclose concerns about competence.[141]

Some states post some information about physicians' experience on the Internet.[142] There have been efforts to expand this disclosure.[143]

License. An Iowa court ruled that a physician did not have to disclose the probationary status of his license where it was due to the activity of an assistant.[144] However, this may suggest that some restrictions on licenses may need to be disclosed.

Financial Interests. Disclosure of financial interests has been another issue. Generally, courts have not mandated disclosure of financial interests. In 2000, the United States Supreme Court ruled that managed care organizations were not required to disclose financial incentives for physicians to control expenditures.[145] One exception is a California Supreme Court ruling that decided a physician could have a fiduciary duty to disclose his economic interest in cells that would be extracted in a procedure, which the physician later developed into a commercially valuable product.[146]

INFORMATION GIVEN SHOULD BE ACCURATE. In 2002, the New Jersey Supreme Court addressed a case in which the physician had misrepresented his credentials. The court ruled that the provider could not be sued for fraud so that extra uninsured punitive damages could not be awarded, but did rule that the provider could be sued for lack of informed consent.[147] However, as previously noted, in 2001, Pennsylvania decided not to permit informed consent claims based on misrepresentation of experience.

---

[139] Duttry v. Patterson, 565 Pa. 130, 771 A.2d 1255 (2001).
[140] Johnson by Adler v. Kokemoor, 199 Wis. 2d 615, 545 N.W.2d 495 (1996).
[141] *E.g.*, Wachter v. United States, 877 F.2d 257 (4th Cir. 1989).
[142] *E.g.*, R. Perez-Pena, *Newly released data offer hints of doctors' experience*, N.Y. TIMES, Feb. 14, 2000, A20 [N.Y. report of number of times doctor/hospital has performed 21 surgeries].
[143] M. Melia, *Groups seek more information about surgeons' experience*, AP, Mar. 27, 2002 [NY].
[144] Bray v. Hill, 517 N.W.2d 223 (Iowa Ct. App. 1994).
[145] Pegram v. Herdrich, 530 U.S. 211 (2000).
[146] Moore v. Regents of Univ. of Cal., 51 Cal. 3d 120, 271 Cal. Rptr. 146, 793 P.2d 479 (1990), *cert. denied*, 499 U.S. 936 (1991).
[147] Howard v. University of Med. & Dentistry, 172 N.J. 537, 800 A.2d 73 (2002).

7-2.5 What Is the Effect of Information That the Decisionmaker Obtains from Other Sources?

When the informed consent doctrine was developed in the 1950s, patients had little access to accurate information about medical knowledge and available treatments. Their primary source of accurate information was their physicians. A few patients in big cities and college campuses did research in medical libraries. Some patients sought second opinions from other physicians. Occasionally, there were articles in newspapers or in television news stories about health care topics, especially when a celebrity experienced a particular disease or treatment. Drug companies advertised over-the-counter drugs but limited advertising of prescription drugs to medical journals. Hospitals seldom advertised their services except when they opened a new program or were conducting fund-raising.

This has all changed. The amount of health care information available has experienced explosive growth, and an ever-growing amount of the information is directly available to the public through the Internet. Advertising of health care services by providers has also experienced rapid growth. Direct advertising of prescription medicines has exploded—"Ask your doctor about . . ." Newspaper and other media coverage of health care topics have increased.

It is not unusual for some patients to arrive at their physician appointments with extensive information about their condition and treatment options.[148] In some cases, they will have information that the physician does not have. Despite the fiction of omniscience that some courts seem to ascribe to physicians, there is a limit to the ability to keep current on all information. Many physicians welcome this active involvement of patients in structuring their own care.

DEALING WITH ERRONEOUS OR MISUNDERSTOOD INFORMATION. The availability of medical information is a mixed blessing. There is evidence that a large percentage of the members of the public have difficulty distinguishing reliable medical information from unreliable and have difficulty understanding reliable medical information. There are also strongly held ethnic and cultural beliefs

---

[148] *See* D. Tuller, *On rare diseases, parents take hope into their own hands*, N.Y. Times, Nov. 17, 2003, 14 [support groups and the Internet]; L. Landro, *Internet use for medical data shifts doctor-patient roles*, Wall St. J., July 17, 2003, D3; G. Kolata, *Web research transforms visit to the doctor*, N.Y. Times, Mar. 6, 2000, A1.

that predate the Internet.[149] Thus, the provider may have to spend considerable time undoing beliefs that the patient has acquired with great effort or has held for a long time, before being able to convince the patient to accept accurate information.

Generally, the provider does not have a legal duty to undo the patient's mistaken beliefs. The provider's responsibility is to provide accurate information, not to assure that it is believed. However, it is unlikely that it will be possible to move forward with a therapeutic relationship when the provider and patient are not on the same page. Thus, providers will generally seek to deal with the erroneous or misunderstood information.

DEALING WITH PATIENT DEMANDS. In some cases, patients arrive demanding particular treatments or drugs. This might be based on advertising, recommendation of a friend, Internet research, or other sources. Providers then have the challenge of staying within professional standards for appropriate use, avoiding unnecessary expense to the patient and the health care system, and maintaining a relationship with the patient. As discussed in Section 7-6.1, patient demands do not justify inappropriate uses.

Some institutions have begun counterdetailing of expensive new drugs. Drug company promotion of new drugs is sometimes called detailing. Through counterdetailing, institutions educate physicians in ways to avoid the promotional pressure and to explain to patients who request the drug why it is not necessary or appropriate.

IMPACT ON DUTY TO DISCLOSE. In existing informed consent law, there is no requirement to tell decisionmakers information that they already have.[150] When the patient arrives already informed about alternatives and risks, the scope of the provider's duty to disclose can be reduced. Providers should not rely on this when the sources used by the patient are known to be unreliable. However, it will be helpful in an informed consent case to note in the providers' records that the patient had studied the treatment and its alternatives through particular Web sites.

---

149 *See* A. O'Connor, *Finding of fact: Myth about lung cancer can be deadly*, N.Y. TIMES, Oct. 7, 2003, D5 [some Americans refuse lifesaving surgery believing that exposing lung cancer tumors spread when exposed to air; survey found 61% of Afro-Americans believed this; 19% cited this as the reason to reject surgery, and 14% said a doctor could not convince them otherwise].

150 *E.g.,* Kaplan v. Simmons, 5 A.D.3d 321, 774 N.Y.S.2d 142 (1st Dept. 2004); Spano v. Bertocci, 299 A.D.2d 335; 749 N.Y.S.2d 275 (2d Dept. 2002); Ciarlariello v. Schacter, [1993] 2 S.C.R. 119 [patient undergoing second cerebral angiogram capable of consenting based on earlier disclosures].

Courts are apparently not yet willing to place any responsibility on the patient in this context. In 2003, a New Jersey appellate court addressed a case concerning the adequacy of genetic counseling. The family was given considerable information, and the physician claimed that the family should have had a duty to seek additional information from other sources. The court noted that the duty to provide information "presupposes essential ignorance on the part of the patient with respect to medical issues," and declined to revisit this supposition. The court found that the patient has no duty to seek information from another source, but acknowledged that when the patient does obtain information from other sources the scope of the physician's duty is reduced to a duty to "fill any informational gaps that preclude a meaningful exercise of the patient's self-determinative right."[151]

7-2.6 What Is the Effect of Barriers to Understanding the Information?

There are several barriers to understanding information presented in the consent process. These barriers can also apply to information that is given concerning the patient and familiy's role in ongoing care and monitoring.

ILLITERACY. A substantial portion of patients either cannot read or cannot read at the level that most health documents are written. Frequently, patients who cannot read or cannot read technical documents hide this fact from health care providers.

Persons are generally presumed to have read and understood documents they have signed. Sometimes courts will not apply this rule when the document is either too technical or in a language foreign to the person. Forms that require too high a level of reading ability have been criticized. It is advisable, when possible, to write so that the person signing can understand them. This is not always possible because the content of some forms is mandated by law.

When providers become aware that a patient cannot read or cannot read at the required level, it is advisable to use other means of communication to supplement the forms.[152]

---

[151] Geler v. Akawie, 358 N.J. Super. 437, 818 A.2d 402 (App. Div. 2003).

[152] *See* B. Weiss & C. Coyne, *Communicating with patients who cannot read,* 337 N. ENG. J. MED. 272 (July 24, 1997).

HEALTH ILLITERACY. Sometimes patients can read but cannot understand health care information. This is related to the problem of the reading level of the information, but there is a distinct problem with understanding the significance of health care information and how it is structured. This is an important issue that is receiving increasing attention.[153]

LANGUAGE AND INTERPRETERS. When the person has difficulty understanding English, the communications need to be in the language of the decisionmaker. When the provider is not fluently bilingual, an interpreter must be provided for key oral communications related to collecting medical history, making medical decisions, and providing directions related to care. This is required of any health care provider that receives federal funds, including reimbursement from Medicare, Medicaid, or other governmental programs.[154] When a patient is incapacitated and another person is acting as decisionmaker, an interpreter needs to be provided for decisionmakers who cannot communicate in English.[155] It is no longer adequate to rely on family or friends of the patient to interpret. National telephone services exist that provide interpretation on demand in virtually any language. This satisfies the requirement. Large providers often hire or contract with interpreters for languages that are frequently encountered.

These requirements also apply to providing sign language interpreters for deaf patients.[156]

Translation of forms into other languages is generally not required, with one exception. Providers are expected to have translations of key

---

[153] *See* L. Landro, *Tips to better understand those doctor's orders*, WALL ST. J., July 3, 2003, D2 [health literacy program sponsored by Partnership for Clear Health Communication]; S.J. Landers, *Low health literacy pervasive*, AM. MED. NEWS, Apr. 26, 2004, 23; Agency for Healthcare Research and Quality, LITERACY AND HEALTH OUTCOMES (2004); Institute of Medicine, HEALTH LITERACY: A PRESCRIPTION TO END CONFUSION.

[154] *See* DOJ, GUIDANCE TO FEDERAL FINANCIAL ASSISTANCE RECIPIENTS REGARDING TITLE VI PROHIBITION AGAINST NATIONAL ORIGIN DISCRIMINATION AFFECTING LIMITED ENGLISH PROFICIENT PERSONS (Apr. 12, 2002); DHHS, GUIDANCE TO FEDERAL FINANCIAL ASSISTANCE RECIPIENTS REGARDING TITLE VI PROHIBITION AGAINST NATIONAL ORIGIN DISCRIMINATION AFFECTING LIMITED ENGLISH PROFICIENT PERSONS, 68 FED. REG. 47311 (Aug. 8, 2003).

[155] *E.g.,* Aikins v. St. Helena Hosp., 843 F. Supp. 1329 (N.D. Cal. 1994).

[156] *See* Connecticut Ass'n of the Deaf v. Middlesex Mem. Hosp., No. 3-95-CV-2408 (AHN) (D. Conn. settlement approved Aug. 20, 1998), *as discussed in* 7 H.L.R. 1065, 1378 (1998) [agreement concerning sign language interpreters in hospitals]; *New York case explores role of sign language interpreter during exams*, AM. MED. NEWS, Feb. 22, 1999, 33 [New York Office of Professional Misconduct investigation of physician who rejected patient who insisted on sign language interpreter because uncomfortable using intermediary, other deaf patients used lipreading, writing on paper].

forms into languages of patient groups who speak a primary language other than English and who constitute a substantial portion of the provider's patients.[157] There is no requirement that all written materials be translated. It is usually sufficient to translate forms and other written materials orally. The involvement of the translator should be documented.

7-2.7 When Can Information Be Withheld?

Courts have recognized several situations in which information may be withheld from patients.

EMERGENCIES. In an emergency, when there is no time to obtain consent, consent is implied.[158] When there is time to obtain some consent but insufficient time for the usual disclosure, an abbreviated disclosure is sufficient.[159]

THERAPEUTIC PRIVILEGE. Most courts recognize a therapeutic privilege not to make disclosures that pose a significant threat of patient detriment.[160] Courts limit the privilege; so it is not applicable when a physician solely fears that the information might lead a patient to forgo needed therapy. Physicians should rely on the privilege only when they can document that a patient's anxiety is significantly above the norm. In some states, when the therapeutic privilege permits nondisclosure, the information must be disclosed to a relative and that relative must concur with the patient's consent before the procedure can be performed.[161] However, at least one court ruled that relatives did not need to be informed of withheld information.[162]

PATIENT WAIVER. A patient can waive the right to be informed.[163] However, courts will be skeptical of waivers initiated by providers; so prudent providers should not suggest waivers but instead should encourage reluctant patients to be informed.

---

[157] *See* Note 154, *supra; see also* Ramirez v. Plough, Inc., 6 Cal. 4th 539, 25 Cal. Rptr. 2d 97, 863 P.2d 167 (1993) [drug manufacturer not liable for labeling nonprescription drug only in English in accordance with FDA regulations].

[158] *E.g.*, Niklaus v. Bellina, 696 So. 2d 120 (La. Ct. App. 1997) [extension of tumor removal to hysterectomy justified by emergency during surgery].

[159] *E.g.*, Shinn v. St. James Mercy Hosp., 675 F. Supp. 94 (W.D. N.Y. 1987), *aff'd without op.*, 847 F.2d 836 (2d Cir. 1988); Crouch v. Most, 78 N.M. 406, 432 P.2d 250 (1967).

[160] *E.g.*, Schultz v. Rice, 809 F.2d 643 (10th Cir. 1986); Pardy v. United States, 783 F.2d 710 (7th Cir. 1986).

[161] Lester v. Aetna Casualty & Sur. Co., 240 F.2d 676 (5th Cir.), *cert. denied*, 354 U.S. 923 (1957).

[162] Nishi v. Hartwell, 52 Haw. 188, 296, 473 P.2d 116 (1970).

[163] Putenson v. Clay Adams, Inc., 12 Cal. App. 3d 1062, 91 Cal. Rptr. 319 (1st Dist. 1970).

7-3   Who Has the Responsibility to Provide Information?

INDIVIDUAL PROVIDER RESPONSIBILITY. Physicians have the responsibility to provide necessary information and to obtain informed consent; it is generally not a hospital responsibility. Other independent practitioners who order or perform procedures have the same responsibility concerning their procedures.

Physicians who order or perform procedures have the responsibility to obtain consent.[164] A referring physician generally does not have a duty to obtain informed consent for procedures ordered or performed by a specialist.[165] However, in some jurisdictions, when the referring physician retains a sufficient degree of participation in the ongoing treatment plan, the referring physician can have a duty to obtain informed consent to services provided by specialists.[166] The duty is discharged if the specialist obtains informed consent; there is no duty to obtain multiple consents.[167]

LIMITED INSTITUTIONAL RESPONSIBILITY. Hospitals are generally not liable for the failure of a physician or other independent practitioner to obtain informed consent unless the professional is the hospital's employee or agent. Both court decisions and state statutes have recognized this principle.[168] Plaintiffs have tried to convince courts to require hospitals to intercede in the professional-patient relationship by imposing institutional liability for inadequate disclosures. These efforts have not been successful except in a few cases.[169] Hospital responsibility for the content of the physician's disclosure would require monitoring that could destroy the physician-patient relationship.

The hospital can be liable for failing to intervene when it knows a procedure is being performed without authorization.[170] In some

---

164 *E.g.*, Nieves v. Montefiore Med. Ctr., 305 A.D.2d 161, 760 N.Y.S.2d 419 (1st Dept. 2003).

165 *E.g.*, Logan v. Greenwich Hosp. Ass'n. 191 Conn. 282, 465 A.2d 294 (1983).

166 *E.g.*, O'Neal v. Hammer, 87 Haw. 183, 953 P.2d 561 (1998); Nieves v. Montefiore Med. Ctr., 305 A.D.2d 161, 760 N.Y.S.2d 419 (1st Dept. 2003).

167 *E.g.*, O' Neal v. Hammer, *supra.*

168 *E.g.*, Bryant v. HCA Health Servs., 15 S.W.3d 804 (Tenn. 2000); Espalin v. Children's Med. Ctr. of Dallas, 27 S.W.3d 675 (Tex. App. 2000); Pauscher v. Iowa Methodist Med. Ctr., 408 N.W.2d 355 (Iowa 1987); Fiorentino v. Wenger, 19 N.Y.2d 407, 280 N.Y.S.2d 373, 227 N.E.2d 296 (1967).

169 *E.g.*, Keel v. St. Elizabeth Med. Ctr., 842 S.W.2d 860 (Ky. 1992) [hospital liable for failing to disclose risks of CT scan with contrast since hospital performed procedure]; Magana v. Elie, 108 Ill. App. 3d 1028, 439 N.E.2d 1319 (2d Dist. 1982); Creech v. Roberts, 908 F.2d 75 (6th Cir. 1990), *cert. denied*, 499 U.S. 975 (1991) [hospital liable for physician's failure to obtain consent where patient had no prior relationship with physician].

170 *E.g.*, Urban v. Spohn Hosp., 869 S.W.2d 450 (Tex. Ct. App. 1993); Schloendorff v. Society of N.Y. Hosp., 211 N.Y. 125, 105 N.E. 92 (1914).

states, this liability can be extended to situations in which the hospital should have known there was no authorization, but it is doubtful that liability will be imposed when the only way the hospital could have known is by monitoring physician-patient communications. In 1997, a Wisconsin appellate court ruled that when a nurse found no consent form for a tubal ligation and informed the surgeon of the absence of the form, this was not sufficient to conclude that the procedure was nonconsensual. Based on the surgeon's response, she could reasonably conclude that consent had been obtained and the absence of the form was no more than a clerical error.[171]

JCAHO provides that accredited hospitals must have policies concerning informed consent but makes it clear that the intent is to establish a "mutual understanding" between the patient and the physician or other licensed independent practitioner.[172]

Research. In addition, some courts have interpreted the federal rules governing research to impose hospital responsibility for informed consent for participation in research projects.[173]

Role of Hospital Staff. The role of nurses and other hospital staff in the consent process varies from hospital to hospital. In some hospitals, hospital staff members are permitted to act as agents of the physician in providing information. In some hospitals, hospital staff members are permitted to obtain signatures on forms after the physician has provided the required information. The other approach is for hospital staff not to be involved in either step. In some states, courts may use the nurses' involvement to shift responsibility for the consent process on the hospital. However, at least one court has ruled that performing the clerical function of obtaining signatures on the forms does not shift responsibility to the hospital.[174] Other courts have recognized that the physician may delegate the providing of information and still remain legally responsible for the informed consent.[175]

Under all these approaches, a hospital employee who becomes aware of a patient's confusion or change of opinion regarding a procedure should notify the responsible physician. If the physician does not respond, appropriate medical staff and hospital officials should be notified so that they can determine whether intervention is necessary.

---

[171] Mathias v. St. Catherine's Hosp., Inc., 212 Wis. 2d 540, 569 N.W.2d 330 (Ct. App. 1997).
[172] 2005 JCAHO CAMH, RI.2.40.
[173] *E.g.,* Anderson v. George H. Lanier Mem. Hosp., 982 F.2d 1513 (11th Cir. 1993).
[174] Ritter v. Delaney, 790 S.W.2d 29 (Tex. Ct. App. 1990).
[175] *E.g.,* Smoger v. Enke, 874 F.2d 295 (5th Cir. 1989) [cardiologist may delegate disclosure of risks to laboratory technician].

7-4 What Should Be Done to Prove the Decision?

Most malpractice cases claim lack of consent or informed consent; so it is important that providers be prepared to prove informed consent or the applicability of one of the exceptions.

Most hospitals require the use of a standard form before major procedures. This usually helps to reduce the liability exposure for lack of consent.[176] The battery consent form described in Section 7-4.2 is usually used. When the hospital requires consent for a procedure, hospital personnel generally should not participate in the procedure until consent is documented, alternative authorization has been obtained, or there is determination that an exception applies.[177]

This section addresses the following questions:

7-4.1. When is express consent required, and when is implied consent sufficient?

7-4.2. What information should be in consent forms?

7-4.3. For which procedures should a signed consent be obtained?

7-4.4. What can be done when a patient with capacity is physically unable to sign?

7-4.5. How can the signed consent requirement be met when the decisionmaker is not present?

7-4.6. How long is a consent form valid?

7-4.7. What are other ways to document consent?

7-4.1 When Is Express Consent Required, and When Is Implied Consent Sufficient?

Consent may be either express or implied.

EXPRESS CONSENT. Express consent is consent given by direct words, either oral or written. Express consent is generally required whenever consent is not implied and involuntary treatment is not authorized (see Section 7-1.5). Written consent is sometimes

---

[176] *E.g.*, Graham v. Ryan, 641 So. 2d 677 (La. Ct. App. 1994) [adult children of deceased surgery patient failed to rebut presumption of informed consent from written consent]; Jones v. United States, 720 F. Supp. 355 (S.D. N.Y. 1989) [documentation showed informed consent was obtained]; Blincoe v. Luessenhop, 669 F. Supp. 513 (D. D.C. 1987) [required disclosures made, documented in two consent forms].

[177] *But see* Mathias v. St. Catherine's Hosp., Inc., 212 Wis. 2d 540, 569 N.W.2d 330 (Ct. App. 1997) [no duty to intervene in the absence of consent form, surgeon's response that he had obtained consent sufficient].

required. For example, some states require written consent before most HIV tests may be performed. Otherwise, either oral or written consent can be legally sufficient authorization. However, oral consent is difficult to prove, so most providers seek written consent whenever express consent is needed.

IMPLIED CONSENT. Implied consent is (1) inferred from some patient conduct or (2) presumed in most emergencies. Consent is usually implied from voluntary submission to a procedure with apparent knowledge of its nature. In a Massachusetts case, a woman was ruled to have given her implied consent to being vaccinated by extending her arm and accepting a vaccination without objection.[178] In a Louisiana case, acceptance of preoperative medications without objection was viewed as implied consent.[179] Implied consent is why express consent is usually not obtained for physical examinations or minor procedures performed on competent adults.

Consent is presumed to exist in medical emergencies unless the provider has reason to believe that consent would be refused. When treatment has been refused, there can be no implied consent even in life-threatening situations. An immediate threat to life or health is clearly a sufficient emergency. In an Iowa case, implied consent to removal of a limb mangled in a train accident was presumed because amputation was necessary to save the patient's life.[180] Courts have disagreed on whether pain is a sufficient emergency to imply consent.

The existence of an emergency does not overcome the right of a patient with capacity to refuse treatment. When express refusals are ignored in emergencies, it is likely that courts will permit close examination of the circumstances. A New York court ruled that a jury should determine whether a patient had been sufficiently incapacitated to justify the providers' disregard of his refusals of surgery and, if so, whether there was a sufficient emergency to justify reliance on implied consent. He arrived in the emergency room with multiple stab wounds and a blood alcohol level later found to be more than twice the standard for driving intoxicated.[181]

When unexpected emergency conditions arise during surgery, especially life-threatening conditions, implied consent is sometimes found to extensions or modifications of surgical procedures beyond

---

[178] O'Brien v. Cunard S.S. Co., 154 Mass. 272, 28 N.E. 266 (1891).
[179] Busalacchi v. Vogel, 429 So. 2d 217 (La. Ct. App. 1983).
[180] Jacovach v. Yocum, 212 Iowa 914, 237 N.W. 444 (1931).
[181] Oates v. New York Hosp., 131 A.D.2d 368, 517 N.Y.S.2d 6 (1st Dept. 1987).

the scope expressly authorized. Many surgical consent forms include express consent to these extensions or modifications to preserve life or health. However, a federal appellate court ruled that when there is express consent to extensions in the consent form, such extensions should be limited to bona fide emergencies.[182]

7-4.2 What Information Should Be in Consent Forms?

CONSENT FORM TYPES. There are three types of consent forms: (1) blanket consent forms, (2) battery consent forms, and (3) detailed consent forms.

Blanket Consent Forms. Prior to the mid-1960s, many hospitals used blanket consent forms that authorized any procedure the physician wished to perform. Courts have ruled that these forms are not evidence of consent to major procedures because the procedure is not specified on the form.[183] Many attorneys recommend continued use of blanket admission consent forms to cover procedures for which individual special consent is not sought even though implied consent to most of these procedures is inferred from hospital admission and submission to the procedures. Admission forms can serve many other purposes unrelated to consent, such as assigning insurance benefits.[184]

Blanket consent forms are receiving new attention and use for the services of specialized units that use many procedures for which individual consent is often obtained in other settings, but is too burdensome on decisionmakers and providers due to the volume of consents that would be required. For example, some intensive care units use forms that authorize a wide range of their standard procedures. Although these forms have not yet been tested in the courts, it is anticipated that they will be more acceptable because they are focused on a specific list of types of procedures and because the practical need for prompt response in this setting makes the need for advance consent readily apparent.

Battery Consent Forms. For major procedures, nearly all hospitals now require consent forms that include the name and a description of

---

[182] Lipscomb v. Memorial Hosp., 733 F.2d 332 (4th Cir. 1984).
[183] *E.g.*, Cross v. Trapp, 170 W.Va. 459, 294 S.E.2d 446 (1982); Rogers v. Lumbermen's Mut. Casualty Co., 119 So. 2d 649 (La. Ct. App. 1960).
[184] *E.g.*, State Cent. Collection Unit v. Columbia Med. Plan, 300 Md. 318, 478 A.2d 303 (1984) [valid assignment in registration form].

the specific procedure. These forms usually also state that (1) the person signing has been told about the medical condition, consequences, risks, and alternatives; (2) all questions have been answered to the person's satisfaction; and (3) no guarantees have been made. These forms will almost always preclude a successful battery claim if the proper person signs the form and if the described procedure is performed.[185] These forms also provide support for the reasonableness of the hospital's lack of suspicion that the person who signed was uninformed, while providing some support for the physician's assertion that the patient was informed.[186]

However, courts can still be convinced that the information concerning consequences, risks, and alternatives was not actually given.[187] Because of this fact, prudent practitioners either use more detailed consent forms or supplement the battery consent form with a note in the medical record documenting disclosure of specific risks, benefits, and alternatives.

Detailed Consent Forms. Some physicians use forms that detail the medical condition, procedure, consequences, risks, and alternatives. Such forms have been mandated for federally funded sterilizations and research.[188] Plaintiffs can seldom prove that the information included in this form was not disclosed. One difficulty with detailed consent forms is the cost and time to prepare them for each individual procedure and to keep them updated. Some physicians use these forms only for procedures, such as cosmetic surgery, that carry a higher risk of misunderstanding and unacceptable results.

Detailed forms may not provide protection for risks not disclosed on the form,[189] except that detailed forms will make it more difficult for patients who accepted serious consequences to prove that disclosure of additional risks would have made them change their minds.[190]

---

[185] *E.g.*, Moser v. Stallings, 387 N.W.2d 599 (Iowa 1986).

[186] *E.g.*, Blincoe v. Luessenhop, 669 F. Supp. 513 (D. D.C. 1987).

[187] *E.g.*, Barner v. Gorman, 605 So. 2d 805 (Miss. 1992) [signed consent not specific to procedure insufficient to bar action]; MacDonald v. United States, 767 F. Supp. 1295 (M.D. Pa. 1991), *award of damages*, 781 F. Supp. 320, *aff'd without op.*, 983 F.2d 1051 (3d Cir. 1992) [failure to obtain informed consent notwithstanding consent form—no risks or alternatives ever described to patient]; Hansbrough v. Kosyak, 141 Ill. App. 3d 538, 490 N.E.2d 181 (4th Dist. 1986); Pegram v. Sisco, 406 F. Supp. 776 (W.D. Ark. 1976), *aff'd without op.*, 547 F.2d 1172 (8th Cir. 1976).

[188] 42 C.F.R. §§ 441.250–441.259 [sterilization]; 45 C.F.R. pt. 46 [research].

[189] *E.g.*, Bedel v. University OB-GYN Assoc., Inc., 76 Ohio App. 3d 742, 603 N.E.2d 342 (1991).

[190] *See* the discussion of the causation requirement in Section 7-8.2.

CONSENT STATUTES. Some states have statutes concerning consent forms.[191] These statutes should be considered when developing consent forms for use in those states. Several states provide that if the consent form contains certain information and is signed by the appropriate person that it is conclusive evidence of informed consent or creates a presumption of informed consent. For example, in Nevada if certain information is on the form, it is conclusive evidence of informed consent.[192] In Iowa, if certain information is on the form, informed consent is presumed.[193] Such statutes address how courts will consider forms that contain certain information. They do not address forms that do not contain the information. It is not a violation to use a form that contains different information or to forgo the use of a form. Serious consideration should be given to using forms that qualify, especially when such forms are conclusive evidence.

EXCULPATORY CLAUSES. Exculpatory clauses state that the person signing waives the right to sue for injuries or agrees to limit any claims to not more than a specified amount. Although courts have enforced these clauses in other contexts, courts have not enforced them in suits on behalf of patients against health care providers. For example, in 1979, a federal court refused to enforce a $15,000 limit on liability in an agreement the patient signed before surgery.[194]

7-4.3 For Which Procedures Should a Signed Consent Be Obtained?

There are several sources of requirements for signed consent. Federal and state statutes require signed consent for some procedures. Federal and state regulations also impose requirements. These are usually found in institutional and professional licensing requirements or in conditions of participation in payment programs, such as Medicare. Often these sources only require consent and leave the method of documentation to be determined by the provider, but in some cases, signed consent is mandated. There are some organizations that have virtually eliminated signed consent forms, relying

---

191 *E.g.*, Hondroulis v. Schumacher, 531 So. 2d 450 (La. 1988) [statute establishes rebuttable presumption of consent], *on remand*, 612 So. 2d 859 (La. Ct. App. 1992) [judgment against physician affirmed].

192 Nev. Rev. Stat. § 41A.110; Allan v. Levy, 109 Nev. 46, 846 P.2d 274 (1993) [consent form did not meet requirement of state statute].

193 Iowa Code Ann. § 147.137.

194 Tatham v. Hoke, 469 F. Supp. 914 (W.D .N.C. 1979), *aff'd without op.*, 622 F.2d 584, 587 (4th Cir. 1980); *see also* Emory Univ. v. Porubiansky, 248 Ga. 391, 282 S.E.2d 903 (1981) [dental school exculpatory clause invalid].

instead on a note in the medical record by the physician or other professional detailing the specific disclosures and the fact the patient or representative agreed to proceed.

Often requirements of signed consent are imposed without adequate consideration of the wide range of potential circumstances; so they become a barrier to access to care for persons who are unable to sign or have decisionmakers who are either not recognized by the requirements or not available. Some requirements, especially for abortions, appear to be intended to be a barrier to access certain services.

Accreditation bodies are another important source of requirements. While these are not legally mandated, providers who desire accreditation need to meet the standards. JCAHO accreditation standards provide that informed consent be obtained and documented in accordance with hospital policy.[195] JCAHO does not specify the procedures or treatments and does not specify how the consent must be documented, except for requiring "written consent" for electroconvulsive therapy.[196]

One list of procedures that can be used as a starting point for developing a policy includes:

1. Procedures performed in an operating room;
2. Other operative and diagnostic procedures requiring anesthesiology services regardless of location;
3. Radiotherapy;
4. Chemotherapy;
5. Dialysis;
6. Transfusions of blood or blood products (except albumin, plasma protein fraction (PPF), and recombinant products);
7. Electroconvulsive therapy;
8. All other *invasive procedures*, whether through an incision or natural body opening;
9. Experimental procedures; and
10. Other procedures that the medical staff determines require a specific explanation to the patient.

Many institutions exclude certain routine minor procedures from the invasive procedures requiring consent. Examples include venipuncture, peripheral intravenous line placement, insertion of a

---

[195] 2005 JCAHO CAMH, Elements of Performance for RI.2.40.
[196] 2005 JCAHO CAMH, Elements of Performance for PC.13.50.

nasogastric tube, or urinary catheter placement. This position is consistent with JCAHO's exclusion of these procedures from the scope of its Universal Protocol for Preventing Wrong Side, Wrong Procedure, Wrong Person Surgery.[197]

EXCEPTIONS. The actual process of providing information to the decisionmaker and of determining that person's decision is more important than the consent form. The form is evidence of the consent process, not a substitute for the process. Someone should have authority to determine that there is actual consent even when the form has been lost or inadvertently not signed prior to patient sedation or when other circumstances make it difficult to obtain the necessary signature.

7-4.4 What Can Be Done When a Patient with Capacity Is Physically Unable to Sign?

It is not necessary that patients be able to sign their normal signatures in order for a consent form, advance directive, or other document to be valid.

When the patient can make a mark, the mark constitutes the signature of the patient. The person witnessing the mark should document the fact that it was made by the patient.

When the patient is physically unable to make a mark, the document can be signed by another person at the direction of the patient. In most states, the other person signs the patient's name and then indicates that it is signed at the direction of the patient, signing their own name. Generally, it is advisable for a third party to document witnessing the direction and the signature.

7-4.5 How Can the Signed Consent Requirement Be Met When the Decisionmaker Is Not Present?

When the decisionmaker is not physically present and a written consent is required, there are solutions.

The information necessary for an informed consent can usually be provided by telephone. It is prudent to have another staff member listen to the conversation and document the role as witness. The information exchange can be by other means, including e-mail. However, care needs to be taken to assure the security of electronic exchanges.

---

[197] JCAHO, *Frequently asked questions,* www.jcaho.org/accredited+organizations/ patient+safety/ universal+protocol/faq_up.htm#5 [accessed May 24, 2004].

The documentation of consent can be transmitted by facsimile. Alternatively, telephonic consent should generally be accepted as written consent. The person hearing the consent signs the consent form at the direction of the decisionmaker, which is the same as the process that is used when the decisionmaker is physically unable to sign due to physical incapacity. It is prudent to have another staff member listen to the consent and document the role as witness. The actual documentation of the consent can probably not yet be done by e-mail, unless there have been advance arrangements to establish a unique code that qualifies as an electronic signature.

7-4.6 How Long Is a Consent Form Valid?

There is no limit on the period of validity of consent or the documentation of that consent. If the patient's condition or available treatments change significantly, earlier consents are no longer informed, and a new consent should be obtained.[198] Otherwise, the consent is valid until it is withdrawn. A claim that consent was withdrawn becomes more credible as time passes.[199] The guideline some hospitals follow is to recommend a new consent at each admission. Some hospitals use a guideline that consent forms should be signed no more than thirty days before the procedure. Hospitals are not legally required to have such guidelines, but they generally should follow their own rules. It is helpful for hospital guidelines to state that they are not requirements or that someone has authority to grant exceptions to deal with repetitive treatments for chronic disease, situations in which the person who gave consent now lacks capacity or is unavailable, and other unusual circumstances.

7-4.7 What Are Other Ways to Document Consent?

Some physicians supplement their explanations with other educational materials, such as booklets and videotapes.[200] When these

---

[198] *E.g.*, Kratt v. Morrow, 455 Pa. Super. 140, 687 A.2d 830 (1996) [preoperative fall created jury question whether there were new risks that should have been disclosed for an additional consent].

[199] *E.g.*, Busalacchi v. Vogel, 429 So. 2d 217 (La. Ct. App. 1983).

[200] Foard v. Jarman, 326 N.C. 24, 387 S.E.2d 162 (1990) [informed consent claim barred by admission of reading, understanding pamphlet]; *see also* G. Borzo, *CIGNA gives new life to patient empowerment initiative*, AM. MED. NEWS, Sept. 19, 1994, 1 [sent outcome-based videotapes to patients to educate about treatment options].

supplements are used, it is helpful to document the name of the educational material in the medical record.

Some physicians make audio and visual recordings of the consent process to supplement or substitute for written consent.

Some patients are given tests of knowledge or write their own consent forms to document their level of understanding.

These steps are not legally required and may not preclude malpractice suits,[201] but they can be helpful, especially for controversial procedures.

7-5 What Constitutes Coercion That Makes Consent Involuntary and Invalid?

A consent form can be challenged if the signature was not voluntary. The person signing would have to demonstrate that there had been some threat or undue inducement to prove the signature was not voluntary; so this challenge will apply in few hospital situations. However, there are limits to the extent which threats and inducements can be used to obtain consent.

In 2001, a federal circuit court found that consent to sterilization was not voluntary when it was coerced by the threat of losing custody of children.[202]

In 1992, a Canadian court found that a patient's consent to sex with a physician was not voluntary when she was an addict and he was providing her with pain-killing drugs. His exploitation of the power dependency relationship made her consent involuntary.[203] In most states, sexual relations between physicians and patients is forbidden so that consent is not relevant and whether the consent is voluntary is irrelevant.

Sometimes the personal circumstances of a patient will create pressure to make a particular decision. Impending loss of insurance coverage may cause patients to elect to undergo procedures they otherwise might delay. Providers are not accountable for these personal circumstances. They do not render the patient's decisions involuntary from a legal perspective.

---

201 *E.g.*, Hanson v. Parkside Surgery Ctr., 872 F.2d 745 (6th Cir.), *cert. denied*, 493 U.S. 944 (1989) [claim permitted despite videotape, but jury found for defendant physician].

202 Vaughn v. Ruoff, 253 F.3d 1124 (8th Cir. 2001).

203 Norberg v. Wyntrib, [1992] 2 S.C.R. 226.

In 2002, a Minnesota nursing home resident filed suit seeking to return home and claiming that her consent to admission had been coerced by the threat that a court order would compel admission. The suit was dismissed when the patient died; so the court did not rule on the question.[204] However, it is unlikely that the threat of a court order would constitute coercion.

7-6 What Limits Are Placed on the Permitted Range of Decisions?

There are many limits on the permitted range of decisions. This section will first review the differences in the limits on adults, incapacitated adults, and minors. It will then look at the case of withdrawal of consent during a course of treatment. The following questions will be examined:

7-6.1. What are the limits on the scope of decision-making by adults with decision-making capacity?

7-6.2. What are the limits on the scope of decision-making for adults without decision-making capacity?

7-6.3. What are the limits on the scope of decision-making for minors?

7-6.4. What limitations are there on withdrawal of consent?

7-6.1 What Are the Limits on the Scope of Decision-making by Adults with Decision-making Capacity?

In the past, there has been some concern about whether there are limits on the scope of life-sustaining treatment a patient may refuse. Books like this have devoted pages to proving that there is a right to refuse life-sustaining treatment. The right is now clearly established throughout the United States.[205] The remaining issues concerning withholding and withdrawing life-sustaining treatment now center on what others can decide when there are no directions from

---

204 W. Wolfe, *She fought to return home, and won; Josephine Bronczyk, right, wants a court ruling to protect others from being sent to nursing homes too soon*, STAR TRIBUNE (Minneapolis, MN), Dec. 9, 2002, 1A ; W. Wolfe, *Woman can't replace plaintiff who died*, STAR TRIBUNE (Minneapolis, MN), Feb. 20, 2003, 3B.

205 *E.g.*, Cruzan v. Director, Mo. Dep't of Health, 497 U.S. 261 (1990) [federal constitutional rights]; John F. Kennedy Mem. Hosp. v. Bludworth, 452 So. 2d 921 (Fla. 1984) [state constitutional right]; *In re* Storar, 52 N.Y.2d 363, 438 N.Y.S.2d 266, 420 N.E.2d 64, *cert. denied*, 454 U.S. 858 (1981) [common law right]; Annotation, *Living wills: Validity, construction, and effect*, 49 A.L.R. 4TH 812 [statutory rights].

the patient or the patient's directions are disputed. Refusal by others is discussed in Section 7-6.2.

There are some limits on the scope of decision-making by adults even when they clearly have decision-making capacity. First, patients cannot select assisted suicide, except in Oregon. Second, patients cannot select willful injury, such as amputation of a healthy limb. Third, patients cannot select inappropriate or medically unnecessary treatment. Fourth, generally patients do not have to be offered treatment that is unlikely to provide substantial therapeutic benefit and cannot insist that such treatment be provided. Fifth, patients cannot select the use of drugs, devices, or services prohibited by law. Sixth, there is no right to participate in medical experiments. Seventh, as discussed in Section 7-7, there are some circumstances where state interests override the patient's rights.

Sometimes when a patient selects a particular treatment, the individual provider cannot or will not provide it. The patient generally does not have a right to force the provider to change the way it provides services, although some practices can be challenged if they discriminate on prohibited grounds. In most cases, patients will not have a basis for a challenge and will need to make their own arrangement with an alternate provider.

ASSISTED SUICIDE. Providers cannot assist patient with suicide outside of Oregon. No constitutional right to assisted suicide has been recognized. The United States Supreme Court decided in 1997 that there was no federal constitutional right to physician aid in dying, leaving the issue to individual states.[206] Several state courts have ruled that state constitutions do not afford such a right.[207]

The Oregon law was adopted by a direct vote of the people and has survived numerous court challenges. In 1994, the voters of Oregon approved the Oregon Death with Dignity Act. A federal judge enjoined the law before it could take effect. In 1997, the Oregon voters again approved the law. The United States Ninth Circuit Court of Appeals removed the injunction, and the first assisted suicides occurred in 1998. The Oregon law permits actions only with the consent of the patient. In 1999, an Oregon court upheld suspending a physician's license for approving use of an agent to paralyze the patient's muscles resulting in death, where the patient's directions had only permitted

---

[206] Vacco v. Quill, 521 U.S. 793 (1997); Washington v. Glucksberg, 521 U.S. 702 (1997).
[207] *E.g.*, Krischer v. McIver, 697 So. 2d 97 (Fla. 1997).

discontinuing life support. In 2001, the federal Department of Justice published a ruling that controlled substances could not be dispensed for assisted suicide. In 2002, a federal court granted a permanent injunction against enforcement of this ruling in Oregon.[208]

In 1999, a Michigan physician was convicted for assisted suicide. He participated in many widely publicized assisted suicides. Some of the cases against him were dismissed on various grounds, but they were reinstated. Juries had acquitted him in several previous cases, but in 1999, he was convicted.[209]

WILLFUL INJURY/MAYHEM. Intentional maiming or disfiguring of a person without justification is the crime of *mayhem*, which now is sometimes called *willful injury*. Consent or even the request of the victim is not a defense when there is no medical justification. In a North Carolina case, a physician was convicted of aiding and abetting mayhem because, at the victim's request, he anesthetized the victim's fingers so they could later be removed by the victim's brother. [210]

INAPPROPRIATE OR UNNECESSARY TREATMENT. Physicians have a professional obligation to refuse to provide clearly inappropriate treatment despite patient insistence. Some court decisions in the nineteenth century ruled that patient insistence after being informed of the inappropriateness insulated the physician from liability.[211] Modern cases have consistently ruled that patient consent does not relieve a physician from the obligation to follow the usual standard of care. For example, a New York court upheld discipline of a physician for treating cancer patients solely with nutritional therapy despite their consent and even instance on the treatment.[212]

When patients or their families seek therapies outside the accepted range, the first response is often tactful communications

---

[208] ORE. REV. STAT. §§ 127.800–127.897; Lee v. State, 869 F. Supp. 1491 (D. Or. 1994), 891 F Supp. 1429 (D. Or. 1995) [injunction], *vacated*, 107 F.3d 1382 (9th Cir. 1997), *cert. denied subnom*, Lee v. Harcleroad, 522 U.S. 927 (1997); Gallant v. Board of Medical Examiners, 159 Ore. App. 175, 974 P.2d 814 (1999); 66 FED. REG. 56607 (2001); Oregon v. Ashcroft, 192 F. Supp. 2d 1077 (D. Ore. 2002), *aff'd*, 368 F.3d 1118 (9th Cir. 2004, *cert. granted*, 125 S. Ct. 1299 (U.S. 2005).

[209] People v. Kevorkian, 205 Mich. App. 180, 517 N.W.2d 293 (1994), *vacated & remanded*, 447 Mich. 436, 527 N.W.2d 714 (1994), *cert. denied*, 514 U.S. 1083 (1995); J. Lessenberry, *Jury acquits Kevorkian in common-law case*, N.Y. TIMES, May 15, 1996, A9; P. Belluck, *Kevorkian found guilty of murdering dying man*, N.Y. TIMES, Mar. 27, 1999, A1.

[210] State v. Bass, 255 N.C. 42, 120 S.E.2d 580 (1961); *see also*, R.M. Henig, *At war with their bodies, they seek to sever limbs*, N.Y. TIMES, Mar. 22, 2005, D6 [body integrity identity disorder].

[211] *E.g.*, Gramm v. Boener, 56 Ind. 497 (1877).

[212] Gonzalez v. New York State Dep't of Health, 232 A.D.2d 886, 648 N.Y.S.2d 827 (3d Dept. 1996).

to give them information and support to accept the limitations. It is becoming less economically feasible to give them long periods of time to adjust; so confrontation cannot always be avoided. Physicians have the responsibility and authority to refuse to provide illegal and inappropriate therapies. In 1997, the United States Supreme Court ruled that terminally ill persons have no special right to treatment that the government has declared illegal.[213]

A physician who provides a legal, but inappropriate, treatment can be liable for malpractice, notwithstanding patient consent. When reputable physicians disagree regarding the appropriateness of legal treatment, reasonable efforts should be made to transfer the treatment of the patient to a physician who concurs with the patient. If inappropriate treatment desired by the patient is neither illegal nor dangerous, sometimes it is prudent to acquiesce if the patient is willing to continue other accepted necessary therapy simultaneously.

Under the standards of Medicare and most third-party payers, physicians and hospitals are supposed to provide only medically necessary services. Billing the payer for unnecessary services can be a false claim subject to civil and criminal penalties. Inappropriate treatments can also raise billing issues. A federal appellate court ruled in 1994 that a physician had a duty to disclose the illegality of treatments in his bills to third-party payers; so billing without disclosure was fraud.[214]

These laws generally do not forbid providing additional services, but under Medicare and most managed care contracts, the patient cannot be billed for the additional services unless the patient has been given advance notice that the third-party payer will not pay. In most circumstances, a provider should also have the discretion to decide whether to offer or provide such additional services.

TREATMENT THAT IS UNLIKELY TO PROVIDE SUBSTANTIAL THERAPEUTIC BENEFIT. The more difficult question arises when a treatment could temporarily prolong life but is unlikely to improve the patient's condition. Sometimes this is called *futile treatment*, although there continues to be debate concerning the use of the term and the practice of not providing futile treatment.[215]

---

[213] United States v. Rutherford, 442 U.S. 544 (1979).

[214] Trustees of the Northwest Laundry & Dry Cleaners Health & Welfare Trust Fund v. Burzynski, 27 F.3d 153 (5th Cir. 1994), *cert. denied*, 513 U.S. 1155 (1995).

[215] *E.g.*, J.R. Curtis, et al., *Use of the medical futility rationale in do-not-attempt-resuscitation orders*, 273 J.A.M.A. 124 (1995); A. Alpers & B. Lo, *When is CPR futile?* 273 J.A.M.A. 156 (1995); R.D. Truog et al., *The problem with futility*, 326 N. Eng. J. Med. 1560 (1992).

There are indications that physicians forgo futile treatment without involvement of the patient or the patient's representatives in some circumstances. Some institutions have developed policies. In 1999, the AMA Council on Ethics and Judicial Affairs recommended that institutional processes be developed to address these issues.

There are also indications that government agencies accept, expect, or require such behavior in some circumstances when examining the issue from an insurance coverage or regulatory perspective. The highest court of Massachusetts ruled that an undocumented alien who had died at the end of a seven-week hospitalization was not eligible for Medicaid. Her care was considered covered treatment for an emergency medical condition since she was so compromised at time of admission that lack of immediate attention would not place her in more serious jeopardy.[216] Another example is that Medicare covers lung transplant programs only when a program has patient selection criteria for determining suitable candidates based on critical medical need and "strong likelihood of a successful clinical outcome."[217] A federal appellate court upheld denial of a liver transplant on grounds it was not medically appropriate in light of patient's history, including hepatitis B which made success unlikely.[218]

When courts are confronted with this question, there is still some disagreement. There are two types of cases—those seeking court authorization and those examining decisions that have already been carried out.

Court Cases Seeking Approval. In 1991, Minnesota providers sought court permission to remove the respirator that they believed to be futile for the brain-damaged patient. The family opposed the petition. The court rejected the petition. The patient died a few days later still on the respirator.[219] In 2004, Massachusetts providers sought court permission to remove the ventilator from a patient with Lou Gehrig's disease who had been in the hospital for four

---

[216] Norwood Hospital v. Commissioner of Pub. Welfare, 417 Mass. 54, 627 N.E.2d 914 (1994).

[217] 60 FED. REG. 6537 (Feb. 2, 1995).

[218] Barnett v. Kaiser Found. Health Plan, 32 F.3d 413 (9th Cir. 1994).

[219] *Judge rejects request by doctors to remove a patient's respirator*, N.Y. TIMES, July 2, 1991, A13 [Helga Wanglie]; *Brain-damaged woman at center of lawsuit over life-support dies*, N.Y. TIMES, July 6, 1991, 8; *Helga Wanglie's ventilator*, HASTINGS CENTER RPT. (July-Aug. 1991), at 23.

years. The daughter (who was the health care agent) opposed the petition. The court rejected the petition.[220]

A 1994 decision by the United States Fourth Circuit Court of Appeals appeared to prohibit withholding futile life-prolonging treatment from patients covered by EMTALA.[221] In 1996, the Fourth Circuit made it clear that it did intend this interpretation, ruling that EMTALA did not require indefinite treatment; EMTALA applies only to immediate emergency stabilizing treatment.[222]

More recently there have been several cases where parents refused to terminate futile treatment for abused children in circumstances where the parents could be charged with murder upon the child's death. Trial courts in some states have authorized the withdrawal of treatment in these circumstances.[223] In other cases, courts have permitted the parent who is not charged to withdraw treatment over the objection of the charged parent.[224] Many of these cases do not result in a court decision because either the provider waits so long before applying to the court that the patient dies before a decision or the family agrees to terminate treatment when they learn that a lawsuit has or will be filed.[225]

Court Cases after Action Taken. In 1995, a Massachusetts jury decided that providers were not liable for discontinuing the respirator for a terminally ill patient after consultation with the hospital Optimal Care Committee, but without patient or family

---

[220] L. Kowalczyk, *Judge rules Mass. General can't end life support for Gehrig's disease patient,* BOSTON GLOBE, Mar. 24, 2004, C3.

[221] *In re Baby "K,"* 16 F.3d 590 (4th Cir.), *cert. denied,* 513 U.S. 825 (1994); EMTALA is discussed in Section 6-3.

[222] Bryan v. Rectors of Univ. of Va., 95 F.3d 349 (4th Cir. 1996); *see also* Greenery Rehabilitation Group v. Hammon, 150 F.3d 226 (2d Cir.1998) [statute authorizing Medicaid payments for treatment of undocumented aliens for emergency medical conditions applied only to "sudden, serious and short-lived physical injury or illness that require immediate treatment to prevent further harm;" "emergency medical condition" does not include continuing care for stable but chronic debilitating conditions].

[223] *E.g., Shaken baby taken off life support,* AP, Dec. 12, 2002 [Guardian appointed and Ohio court approved guardian's recommendation]; *Abused baby dies after court ends life support,* AP Nov. 10, 1998 [Wisconsin]; *but see In re* Guardianship of Stein, 157 Ohio App. 3d 417, 2004 Ohio 2948, 811 N.E.2d 594 (2004) [upholding decision to appointing guardian with authority to withdraw treatment], *stay granted,* 102 Ohio St. 3d 1475, 2004 Ohio 2995, 810 N.E.2d 441 (2004), *rev'd,* 105 Ohio St. 3d 30, 2004 Ohio 7114, 821 N.E.2d 1008 [court must terminate parental rights before it can let guardian withdraw life support].

[224] *E.g., In re* Christopher I., 106 Cal. App. 4th 533, 131 Cal. Rptr. 2d 122 (4th Dist. 2003) [affirming order to withdraw treatment from abused child. Reject appeal of perpetrator father]; *see also* R. Chase, *Woman's agonizing decision leaves baby dead, husband charged with murder,* AP, Nov. 15, 2001.

[225] *E.g., Boy in 2-1/2-year coma dies after respirator stopped,* N.Y. TIMES, June 25, 1990, A11 [parents refused termination in fear mother would face murder charge; when hospital announced plans to sue, father agreed to termination].

consent, because the treatment was futile.[226] However, in 1998, the Iowa Supreme Court ruled that a physician could be liable for failure to attempt resuscitation, in the absence of either patient or family agreement, even though there was an estimate of only a 10 percent chance of survival.[227] In 1992, a federal court ruled that failure to obtain informed consent from a mother prior to deciding to administer only supportive care to her son did not cause any injury because due to the child's anencephaly it would not have survived with vigorous treatment.[228] In 1995, a Tennessee court decided that providers were not liable for extubating (removing breathing tubes) an infant believed to be too premature to survive.[229]

DRUGS OR DEVICES OR SERVICES PROHIBITED BY LAW. The government has broad power to regulate, license, and prohibit medical services. Some court decisions would appear to permit the prohibition of virtually all health care services. In 1889, the United States Supreme Court upheld the power of the state to prohibit all physician practice that was not licensed.[230] In 1966, the Supreme Court held that states did not have to create a license for naturopaths but could require them to qualify for a full medical license.[231] In 1997, a federal appellate court decided that there was no right to have midwives recognized or licensed.[232] Most of the uses of this power have been limited and broadly accepted; so there has been little political or judicial exploration of the limits, if any, to this power.

The federal government, through the Food and Drug Administration (FDA), has restricted the use of new drugs and devices until their safety and effectiveness are proved. Drugs and devices generally cannot be used legally outside approved testing projects until they are approved by the FDA, even when requested by terminally ill patients who believe they have no alternative.[233]

---

[226] Gilgunn v. Massachusetts Gen. Hosp., No. 92-4820-H (Mass. Super. Ct. Suffolk County jury decision Apr. 21, 1995), *as discussed in* 4 H.L.R. 698 (1995).
[227] Wendland v. Sparks, 574 N.W.2d 327 (Iowa 1998).
[228] Johnson v. Thompson, 971 F.2d 1487 (10th Cir. 1992), *cert. denied*, 507 U.S. 910 (1993); Smith v. Shalala, 954 F. Supp. 1 (D.D.C. 1996).
[229] Hartsell v. Fort Sanders Reg. Med. Ctr., 905 S.W.2d 944 (Tenn. Ct. App. 1995).
[230] Dent v. West Virginia, 129 U.S. 114 (1889).
[231] Beck v. McLeod, 382 U.S. 454 (1966).
[232] Lange-Kessler v. Department of Educ. of N.Y., 109 F.3d 137 (2d Cir. 1997).
[233] *E.g.*, Rutherford v. American Medical Ass'n, 379 F.2d 641, 1967 U.S. App. LEXIS 5870 (7th Cir.), *cert. denied*, 389 U.S. 1043 (1967).

In 2001, the United States Supreme Court ruled that there was no medical necessity defense to prosecution for violating federal laws prohibiting possession and use of marijuana.[234]

After drugs are approved for general distribution, many can be distributed only by prescription. A physician or other authorized health professional can write a prescription only for appropriate medical uses. Inappropriate prescriptions can subject the professional to licensing discipline and to criminal prosecution. Consent of the patient to the prescription is not a defense.

The government cannot punish physicians for discussing prohibited drugs. The federal government attempted to bar physicians from discussing the use of marijuana for medicinal purposes. In 2002, a federal appellate court ruled that physicians were protected by the constitutional freedom of speech when they recommended marijuana as medical treatment of their patients; so the federal government could not investigate, threaten, or punish physicians for these recommendations.[235]

MEDICAL EXPERIMENTS. There is no right to participate in research protocols. They generally do not constitute an available alternative that providers must disclose or offer. Thus, decision-makers cannot select this option when it is not offered. Even when the option is offered and accepted, an individual still may not be able to participate. Most protocols have inclusion and exclusion criteria as part of the study design and required precautions. Individuals who do not satisfy these criteria cannot be included.

THERE ARE FEW LIMITS ON THE POWER TO REFUSE TREATMENT. In the past, there was some question whether patients could refuse life-prolonging treatment. It is now clear that adults with decision-making capacity can decide to withhold or withdraw virtually any treatment even if it will result in their death. The only exceptions are the situations where involuntary treatment is authorized as discussed in Section 7-7.

The following cases demonstrate the scope of the right. In 1986, a California appellate court ruled that a competent adult could refuse tube feeding even when she was not terminally ill.[236] The

---

234 United States v. Oakland Cannabis Buyers' Coop., 532 U.S. 483 (2001).

235 Conant v. Walters, 309 F.3d 629 (9th Cir. 2002), *cert. denied,* 540 U.S. 946 (2003).

236 Bouvia v. Superior Court (Glenchur), 179 Cal. App. 3d 1127, 225 Cal. Rptr. 297 (2d Dist. 1986); *Elizabeth: quadriplegic with cerebral palsy decides to live after winning court case to remove food-induced food supply so that she may starve herself to death,* CBS 60 MINUTES, Sept. 7, 1997 [interview].

case involved a woman who was born in 1957 with severe cerebral palsy and was almost completely paralyzed for most of her life.

The right to withdraw treatment includes assistance in the withdrawal. Such assistance in withdrawal is not considered assisting suicide. In the 1986 California case previously discussed, the hospital withdrew painkillers from the patient after she got the order authorizing discontinuing tube feeding. A supplemental court order was obtained requiring that the painkillers be reinstated. In 1989, the Georgia Supreme Court ruled that a quadriplegic's right to refuse included the right to have sedatives before the ventilator was disconnected.[237] In the same year, a quadriplegic in Michigan found a physician who was willing to provide him with sedatives so that his respirator could be turned off. He sought a court order to protect the physician. The judge said that there was no one opposing the action and the right was clear; so she did have jurisdiction to issue an order.[238]

Individual providers generally may refuse to participate in carrying out these decisions, but this does not permit them to thwart the decision. They must transfer the care to other providers. In most jurisdictions, private institutions can enforce policies that prohibit carrying out some decisions, but this does not permit them to thwart the decision. They must transfer the patient to another institution. In cases, where transfer is impossible, some courts will bar the institution from enforcing the policy in the individual case.

The enforcement of such institutional polices can create hardship for patients who live in areas where there are no competing institutions that do not have the restrictive polices. It is an open question whether a state can permit some restrictive polices in the only hospital that the state permits to function in a service area. States might have to permit the creation of competing facilities or mandate that institutions not restrict patient decisions to withhold or withdraw treatment.

Nutrition and Hydration. Withholding and withdrawing artificial nutrition and hydration (tube feeding) continues to receive special attention. There have been several widely publicized controversies

---

[237] State v. McAfee, 259 Ga. 579, 385 S.E.2d 651 (1989); *An angry man fights to die, then tests life*, N.Y. TIMES, Feb. 9, 1990, A1 [McAfee decided not to exercise right he had established].

[238] M. Williams, *Michigan quadriplegic earns right to die*, AM. MED. NEWS, Aug. 4, 1989, 3; *See also After three decades on ventilator, man dies*, NEWSDAY, Apr. 15, 1999 [on request of patient and after consulting with local prosecutor, N.Y. hospital turned off ventilator that had kept patient alive in the hospital since 1967].

over individual cases. Nearly all appellate courts that have addressed the issue have agreed that artificial nutrition and hydration (tube feeding) are medical treatments that can be refused in the same situations in which other medical treatments can be refused.[239] While acknowledging the symbolic importance of feeding, which has led some groups to seek to preclude refusal of these treatments, courts have ruled that there is no legal difference between artificial breathing with a respirator and artificial feeding with a tube. Some groups who have opposed refusal of tube feeding have asserted that such feeding is necessary for comfort care. Medical studies tend to show that tube feeding does not contribute to comfort.[240]

The Missouri Supreme Court is the only state Supreme Court that has suggested that artificial feeding may be a mandatory procedure that cannot be refused.[241] However, Missouri later permitted withdrawal of artificial nutrition and hydration for the same patient, Nancy Cruzan. After the United States Supreme Court affirmed the Missouri decision on other grounds, the Cruzan family initiated new proceedings to prove Nancy's wishes. The state withdrew from the case. A lower court found clear and convincing evidence of Nancy Cruzan's intent and approved withdrawal of her feeding tube. The Missouri Supreme Court declined to review the decision. The feeding tube was withdrawn. Despite protests at the hospital that led to arrests of protestors and despite the protectors' unsuccessful attempts to obtain intervention from several different state and federal courts, the feeding tube was not replaced, and Nancy Cruzan died.[242]

In 2001, the Attorney General of New York intervened to stop the withdrawal of artificial nutrition and hydration of a profoundly mentally and physically handicapped person. The family had

---

239 *E.g.*, Brophy v. New Engl. Sinai Hosp., Inc., 398 Mass. 417, 497 N.E.2d 626 (1986); *In re Tavel*, 661 A.2d 1061 (Del. 1995).

240 R.M. McCann et al., *Comfort care of terminally ill patients: The appropriate use of nutrition and hydration*, 272 J.A.M.A. 1263 (1994); *Terminally ill should be allowed to refuse artificial sustenance, report says*, N.Y. TIMES, Oct. 26, 1994, A7.

241 Cruzan v. Harmon, 760 S.W.2d 408 (Mo. 1988) (en banc), *aff'd on other grounds*, Cruzan v. Director, Mo. Dep't of Health, 497 U.S. 261 (1990).

242 *State asks to quit right-to-die case*, N.Y. TIMES, Oct. 12, 1990, A9; *Missouri family renews battle over right to die*, N.Y. TIMES, Nov. 2, 1990, A12; *Judge allows removal of woman's feeding tube*, N.Y. TIMES, Dec. 15, 1990, 1; *Ordeal ending for Nancy Cruzan with removal of feeding tube*, AM. MED. NEWS, Dec. 28, 1990, 1; *Protestors thwarted in effort to feed comatose woman*, N.Y. TIMES, Dec. 19, 1990, A14; *Missouri high court upholds right to die in Cruzan case*, N.Y. TIMES, Dec. 21, 1990, A16; *For Missouri's Webster, '92 gubernatorial race appears likely to be a life-and-death campaign*, WALL ST. J., Dec. 20, 1990, A18; *Cruzan's condition worse; court rejects 7th appeal*, PALM BEACH [FLA.] POST, Dec. 26, 1990, 4A; *Nancy Cruzan dies, outlived by debate over right to die*, N.Y. TIMES, Dec. 27, 1990, A1.

directed the withholding in consultation with the institution's ethics committee. A court eventually ordered the withdrawal and denied the Attorney General's request for a stay of the order to permit appeal. The patient died. The family sued the Attorney General seeking to recover the costs of defending his intervention. In 2002, a federal court ruled that the Attorney General had immunity.[243]

In 2003, the legislature and governor in Florida intervened to postpone withdrawal of artificial feeding of Terri Schiavo. In 2005, the United States Congress also passed a law intervening in the case. However, after extensive legal proceedings, nutrition and hydration were discontinued, and Ms. Schiavo died. For a detailed discussion of this case, see Section 7-1.2.

The American Medical Association has recognized that refusal of artificial nutrition and hydration is appropriate in some cases.[244]

Courts have enforced refusals of this treatment by competent patients[245] and by patient representatives on behalf of patients who are terminally ill[246] or irreversibly unconscious.[247] Courts have had difficulty in defining when substituted decisions to refuse any treatment, including artificial nutrition, should be permitted on behalf of other patients. In 1985, the New Jersey Supreme Court addressed a patient who was neither terminally ill nor unconscious.[248] After ruling that tube feeding was a treatment like a respirator that could be discontinued in appropriate cases, the court stated that discontinuance would be appropriate pursuant to the clearly articulated wishes of an elderly nursing home patient with severe and permanent mental and physical impairments and a life expectancy of a year or less. Without adequate proof of the patient's wishes, the feeding could be discontinued when either (1) there was trustworthy evidence of the patient's wishes and unavoidable pain caused patient suffering that markedly outweighed any physical pleasure,

---

[243] Blouin v. Spitzer, 213 F. Supp. 2d 184 (N.D. N.Y. 2002).

[244] American Medical Association, Council on Ethical and Judicial Affairs, *Withholding or Withdrawing Life-Prolonging Medical Treatment* (Mar. 15, 1986), *quoted in* Corbett v. D'Alessandro, 487 So. 2d 368, 371, n.1 (Fla. 2d DCA 1986).

[245] *E.g.*, Bouvia v. Superior Court, 179 Cal. App. 3d 1127, 225 Cal. Rptr. 297 (2d Dist. 1986); Application of Plaza Health & Rehab. Ctr. (N.Y. Sup. Ct. Onondaga County Feb. 2, 1984); N.Y. TIMES (Feb. 3, 1984), at A1 [describing Plaza case]; Williams, *Michigan quadriplegic earns right to die*, AM. MED. NEWS, Aug. 4, 1989, 3.

[246] *E.g.*, *In re* Guardianship of Grant, 109 Wash. 2d 545, 747 P.2d 445 (1987), *corrected*, 757 P.2d 534 (Wash. 1988).

[247] *E.g.*, Brophy v. New Engl. Sinai Hosp., Inc., 398 Mass. 417, 497 N.E.2d 626 (1986).

[248] *In re* Conroy, 98 N.J. 321, 486 A.2d 1209 (1985); *see also In re* Guardianship of Browning, 568 So. 2d 4 (Fla. 1990).

emotional enjoyment, or intellectual satisfaction the patient still derived from life or (2) there was no trustworthy evidence of the patient's wishes, the net burdens of the patient's life with treatment markedly outweighed the benefits the patient derived from life, and recurring, unavoidable, and severe pain with treatment made the administering of treatment inhumane. The emphasis that this decision places on pain can be questioned, but it is an important contribution to the legal responses to nutritional technologies.

In 1984, in the only prosecution of physicians for withholding artificial nutrition and hydration from a terminally ill patient, a California appellate court ordered the dismissal of homicide indictments against two physicians.[249] The court ruled that artificial means of feeding are treatment, not natural functions; so there is no duty to continue the treatment when it becomes ineffective. The physicians could not be criminally liable for their professional decision made in concert with the patient's family when the individual was incompetent and terminally ill, with virtually no hope of significant improvement.

7-6.2 What Are the Limits on the Scope of Decision-making for Adults Without Decision-making Capacity?

Any person acting on behalf of an incapacitated adult or a minor does not have the same latitude for consent as in self-treatment decisions. Decisionmakers cannot authorize two procedures— organ donation and sterilization—for incompetent adults or minors without prior court approval. The issue of sterilization of minors and incompetent adults is discussed in Chapter 14. Decisionmakers do not have the same broad scope to refuse all treatments in the absence of an advance directive from the patient. The limits on consents by adults for their own treatment discussed earlier in this chapter also apply to surrogate decisions.

ORGAN DONATION. Courts in a few states will not approve kidney donations by minors and incompetents,[250] but courts in other states have authorized them.[251] Bone marrow donations have been

---

249 Barber v. Superior Court, 147 Cal. App. 3d 1006, 195 Cal. Rptr. 484 (2d Dist. 1984).
250 *E.g.*, *In re* Guardianship of Pescinski, 67 Wis. 2d 4, 266 N.W.2d 180 (1975) [incompetent adult]; *In re* Richardson, 284 So. 2d 185 (La. Ct. App.), *application denied*, 284 So. 2d 338 (La. 1973) [minor]; *see* Annotation, *Propriety of surgically invading incompetent or minor for benefit of third party*, 4 A.L.R. 5TH 1000.
251 *E.g.*, Strunk v. Strunk, 445 S.W.2d 145 (Ky. 1969) [incompetent adult]; Hart v. Brown, 29 Conn. Supp. 368, 289 A.2d 386 (Super. Ct. 1972) [minor].

approved.[252] The courts that have approved kidney donations have usually based their approval on the close relationship between the donor and the proposed recipient and on the emotional injury to the donor if the recipient was to die.

SCOPE OF PERMITTED REFUSALS. Nearly all state appellate courts that have addressed treatment refusal have decided that surrogate decisionmakers may refuse treatment for some incapacitated patients without an advance directive.[253] At least one state, Missouri, has rejected this position and allows refusals only when there is an advance directive.[254] New York initially adopted this more restrictive view but has modified its position to permit some surrogate refusals.[255]

The discretion to refuse is generally limited to situations in which the treatment is elective or not likely to be beneficial. Life prolongation is not always viewed as beneficial. States that allow surrogate refusals generally agree that they are permitted when the patient is irreversibly unconscious[256] or terminally ill.[257]

Some states are more restrictive. For example, in the absence of an advance directive, Wisconsin permits guardians to authorize orders not to resuscitate and, when the patient is in a permanent vegetative state, to refuse other treatment.[258] Other surrogate decisionmakers who act without judicial appointment are apparently not subject to these restrictions.

There is no widely accepted definition of terminal illness; it remains a diagnosis based on medical judgment. One element is that no available course of therapy offers a reasonable expectation of remission or cure of the condition. Another element is that death is imminent, but there is no consensus on the time period, largely

---

[252] *E.g.*, *In re* Doe, 104 A.D.2d 200, 481 N.Y.S.2d 932 (4th Dept. 1984).
[253] *E.g.*, John F. Kennedy Mem. Hosp. v. Bludworth, 452 So. 2d 921 (Fla. 1984).
[254] *E.g.*, Cruzan v. Harmon, 760 S.W.2d 408 (Mo. 1988) (en banc), *aff'd*, 497 U.S. 261 (1990).
[255] *In re* Storar, 52 N.Y.2d 363, 438 N.Y.S.2d 266, 420 N.E.2d 64, *cert. denied*, 454 U.S. 858 (1981); *New York rule compounds dilemma over life support*, N.Y. TIMES, May 12, 1992, A1 [no surrogate decision-making in N.Y.]; NY CLS PUB HEALTH § 2965 [priority list for who can consent to DNR order]; Blouin v. Spitzer, 213 F. Supp. 2d 184 (N.D. N.Y. 2002) [dismiss suit against NY attorney general for challenging case where court authorized withdrawal of hydration at family direction]; Matter of Christopher, 177 Misc. 2d 352, 675 N.Y.S.2d 807 (Sup. Ct. 1998) [refuse to allow feeding tube over son's objections].
[256] *E.g.*, John F. Kennedy Mem. Hosp. v. Bludworth, 452 So. 2d 921 (Fla. 1984); *In re* Quinlan, 70 N.J. 10, 355 A.2d 647 (1976), *cert. denied*, 429 U.S. 922 (1976).
[257] *E.g.*, FLA. STAT. § 765.07.
[258] Spahn v. Eisenberg (*In re* Edna M.F.), 210 Wis. 2d 558, 563 N.W.2d 485 (1997), *cert. denied sub nom.* Spahn v. Wittman, 522 U.S. 951 (1997).

because it is not possible to predict time of death precisely.[259] Some courts have accepted patients as being terminally ill with predicted lives of one to five years.[260] Thus, the range of medical opinion concerning terminal illness appears to be legally acceptable. It is prudent to avoid establishing a specific time period. Some widely publicized institutional systems for classifying patients have not included a definition of terminal illness, but instead have focused on the appropriate therapeutic effort.[261]

A few courts have addressed refusals on behalf of patients who are incapacitated, conscious, and not terminally ill, but there is no consensus.[262] In 2001, the California Supreme Court decided that nutrition and hydration could be withheld from a patient only when the patient is terminally ill, comatose, or in a persistent vegetative state or has left formal instructions or appointed a health care agent.[263] Hospitals should generally take these cases to court unless the issue has been adequately addressed in their state.

7-6.3 What Are the Limits on the Scope of Decision-making for Minors?

All limits on consents by adults for their own treatment and for the treatment of incapacitated adults discussed earlier in this chapter apply when parents and guardians make decisions concerning the treatment of minors.

In addition, courts tend to require that decisions on behalf of minors be in their best interests. Because minors have never had decision-making capacity, substituted judgment seldom applies even though courts do often give weight to minors' preferences. In addition to the state interests which the state asserts concerning adults, the state asserts an interest in minors and some incapacitated adults under its *parens patriae* power, the general power as "parent" to protect the welfare of incompetent persons.

---

259 *E.g., Survival predictions found imprecise for hospice patients*, AM. MED. NEWS, Dec. 9, 1988, 40 [predictions tend to be overly optimistic].

260 *E.g., In re* Spring, 380 Mass. 629, 405 N.E.2d 115, 118 (1980) [five years].

261 *E.g.,* Wanzer et al., *The physician's responsibility toward hopelessly ill patients*, 310 N. ENG. J. MED. 955 (1984); Grenvik et al., *Cessation of therapy in terminal illness and brain death*, 6 CRITICAL CARE MED. 284 (1978); *Optimal care for hopelessly ill patients*, 295 N. ENG. J. MED. 362 (1976).

262 *E.g., In re* Guardianship of Conroy, 98 N.J. 321, 486 A.2d 1209 (1985); *In re* Guardianship of Browning, 568 So. 2d 4 (Fla. 1990).

263 Conservatorship of Wendland, 26 Cal. 4th 519, 28 P.3d 151, 110 Cal. Rptr. 2d 412 (2001).

Parents do still have considerable latitude in decision-making concerning their minor children's care.[264]

REFUSALS FOR MINORS. Courts tend to find that because adults with decision-making capacity have the right to refuse treatment that those making decisions on behalf of minors have a right to refuse on their behalf in some situations.[265] However, because the decisionmakers have an obligation to act in the best interest of the minor, they must provide necessary treatment. Their discretion to decline treatment is generally limited to situations in which the treatment is elective or not likely to be beneficial. The duty to provide necessary treatment to minors is reinforced in all states by legislation concerning abused or neglected minors. This legislation facilitates state intervention to provide needed assistance.

The duty to provide necessary treatment is illustrated by a 2003 Texas Supreme Court case that ruled providers could not be liable for resuscitating a newborn without parental consent because the parents had no right to refuse.[266] In 2002, a Wisconsin appellate court reached the same decision.[267] This is not a new position. In 1987, a New Jersey appellate court also ruled that providers have no duty to inform parents of the alternative of withholding treatment in cases where withholding is illegal.[268]

However, the state has no constitutional duty to protect children in this fashion; so it is not liable for failing to intervene.[269] The state's responsibilities are limited to those it assumes under its statutes.

Courts have generally permitted the refusal of treatment for irreversibly comatose minors[270] and some terminally ill minors. For example, in 1982, the highest court of Massachusetts approved a decision not to attempt resuscitative efforts if a terminally ill child

---

[264] *E.g.*, Grecco v. University of Med. & Dentistry, 345 N.J. Super. 94, 783 A.2d 741 (App. Div. 2001) [parents have immunity for negligent exercise of parental authority or provision of customary child care unless their behavior is willful and wanton; refusal of a liver transplant was not willful and wanton].

[265] *E.g.*, Ball v. Hamilton County Emergency Med. Servs., 1999 Tenn. App. LEXIS 149 [emergency team has no duty to transport to hospital child who appears healthy when mother signs service refusal, so no liability for child's death when breathing problems recurred].

[266] Miller v. HCA. Inc., 118 S.W.3d 758 (Tex. 2003).

[267] Montalvo v. Borkovec, 2002 WI App 147, 256 Wis. 2d 472, 647 N.W.2d 413.

[268] Iafelice v. Zarafu, 221 N.J. Super. 278, 534 A.2d 417 (App. Div. 1987).

[269] DeShaney v. Winnebago County Dept. of Social Servs., 489 U.S. 189 (1989).

[270] *E.g.*, *In re* L.H.R., 253 Ga. 439, 321 S.E.2d 716 (1984); *In re* Guardianship of Barry, 445 So. 2d 365 (Fla. 2d DCA 1984), *approved*, John F. Kennedy Mem. Hosp. v. Bludworth, 452 So. 2d 921 (Fla. 1984).

less than one year of age experienced cardiac or respiratory arrest.[271] In 1992, a Michigan appellate court authorized parents to terminate the life support of an eleven-year-old in a persistent vegetative state.[272] These decisions are being made on a regular basis without court involvement. One study of care decisions in pediatric intensive care units (PICUs) in sixteen hospitals reported 119 patients who had their care limited in 1990 and 1991. Ninety-four of the patients died in the PICU.[273]

Courts have declined to override parental refusals in several situations in which the benefit did not clearly outweigh the risk. Surgery that is not lifesaving is frequently not compelled because there is a risk of death from the surgery itself. While parents can decide to take this risk, courts are reluctant to compel it. For example, the Washington Supreme Court refused to authorize the amputation of an eleven-year-old girl's arm, which was so abnormally large that it was useless and interfered with her association with other people.[274] In 1972, the Pennsylvania Supreme Court refused to authorize transfusions that would permit an operation to correct the severe spinal curvature of the sixteen-year-old son of a Jehovah's Witness.[275]

Risk of death is not the only risk that is considered. Pain and other side effects of the proposed treatment are important, as is the probability of success. In 1991, the Delaware Supreme Court ruled that a three-year-old child with Burkitt's syndrome was not neglected when his Christian Science parents refused to consent to radical chemotherapy that had only a 40 percent chance of success; so the court reversed the trial court order that had awarded custody to the state. The Supreme Court applied the "best interests" test and concluded:

> The egregious facts of this case indicate that Colin's proposed medical treatment was highly invasive, painful, involved terrible temporary and potentially permanent side effects, posed an unacceptably low chance of success, and a high risk that the treatment itself would cause death. The State's authority to intervene in this case,

---

[271] Custody of a Minor, 385 Mass. 697, 434 N.E.2d 601 (1982).
[272] *In re* Rosebush, 195 Mich. App. 675, 491 N.W.2d 633 (1992).
[273] M. Levetown et al., *Limitations and withdrawals of medical intervention in pediatric critical care*, 272 J.A.M.A. 1271 (1994).
[274] *In re* Hudson, 13 Wash. 2d 673, 126 P.2d 765 (1942).
[275] *In re* Green, 448 Pa. 338, 292 A.2d 387 (1972).

therefore, cannot outweigh the Newmark's parental prerogative and Colin's inherent right to enjoy at least a modicum of human dignity in the short time that is left for him.[276]

Some courts do give substantial weight to the integrity of the parent-child relationship. In 1994, a Florida court reversed an order that a child be treated with chemotherapy and transfusions for acute mono-cytic leukemia despite the religious objections of the parents. The court found that the state must show a compelling interest to override the liberty interest in the parent-child relationship. The state's interest in preservation of life could provide that interest, but that "interest diminishes as the severity of an affliction and the likelihood of death increase." It was not clear that the trial court had weighed the compet-ing interests of the parents in making such decisions for their children and of the child's right of privacy under the state constitution; so the court ordered further consideration of the case.[277]

Courts will generally decline to intervene when parents or guardians are following the advice of a licensed physician in good standing even if the advice is unorthodox. In 1979, the highest court of New York refused to authorize chemotherapy for a child with leukemia because the parents were following the advice of a physi-cian who had prescribed laetrile even though laetrile was not proven to be effective.[278] In 1998, the Maine Supreme Court affirmed denial of a state application to compel aggressive drug therapy for a HIV-positive four-year-old.[279] The mother had gone through similar treat-ment with another child who had eventually died, and she had found a licensed physician who supported her approach.

Courts do not have unbridled authority to compel treatment of minors. In 1993, an Illinois court voided a juvenile court order giv-ing police authority to consent to medical exams of minors taken into custody when parents or guardians were unavailable or willing to consent because the order was beyond the juvenile court's authority.[280] Courts must follow the proper procedures for their orders to be valid. In 1994, a federal appellate court upheld a $1.95

---

[276] Newmark v. Williams/DCPS, 588 A.2d 1108, 1118 (Del. 1991).

[277] M.N. v. Southern Baptist Hosp., 648 So. 2d 769 (Fla. 1st DCA 1994).

[278] *In re* Hofbauer, 47 N.Y.2d 648, 419 N.Y.S.2d 936, 393 N.E.2d 1009 (1979).

[279] *In re* Nickolas E., 720 A.2d 562, 1998 ME 243; *Woman wins the right to deny son AIDS drug,* N.Y. Times, Sept. 15, 1998, A20; *Mother wins right to stop H.I.V. drugs for her son,* 4, N.Y. Times, Sept. 20, 1998, 17.

[280] *In re* General Order of October 11, 1990, 256 Ill. App. 3d 693, 628 N.E.2d 786 (1st Dist. 1993).

million award against a physician for the death of a minor after the insertion of a Hickman catheter over the objection of the father.[281] A court order had been obtained but was found to be invalid.[282]

There are practical limits on the ability of the state to intervene. There have been several highly publicized cases in which the state has initiated efforts to compel treatment and has eventually chosen to drop its efforts or compromise with the family. In 2003, a Michigan prosecutor sought to compel brain surgery to remove a tumor from a two-year-old but dropped the effort when it was discovered the child was unlikely to live to age five even with the surgery.[283] In 2003, Utah obtained a court order placing a twelve-year-old in state custody for chemotherapy when his parents denied that he had cancer and refused the treatment. His parents took him out of state. In the face of strong public reaction and an assessment that it was not feasible to force a twelve-year-old and his parents to submit to eleven months of chemotherapy, authorities dropped the custody and chemotherapy orders. Kidnapping charges were dropped in exchange for a guilty plea to custodial interference. The state later dropped the remaining charges.[284]

Parents who fail to obtain necessary medical care have been convicted of child abuse and even homicide,[285] but criminal liability has generally not been imposed when there are questions concerning (1) the parent's knowledge of the seriousness of the child's condition or (2) the necessity for or net benefit from the proposed services.[286]

INFANTS. The treatment of infants with severe deformities that are inconsistent with prolonged or sapient life has been controversial.[287]

---

[281] Bendiburg v. Dempsey, 19 F.3d 557 (11th Cir. 1994).

[282] Bendiburg v. Dempsey, 909 F.2d 463 (11th Cir. 1990), *cert. denied*, 500 U.S. 932 (1991); *but see*, Novak v. Cobb County-Kennestone Hosp. Auth., 849 F. Supp. 1559 (N.D. Ga. 1994) [*Bendiburg* does not mean that ex parte orders are invalid in bona fide emergencies].

[283] L.L. Brasier, *Oakland County, Mich., drops case to force surgery for girl with tumor*, DETROIT FREE PRESS, May 13, 2003.

[284] P. Foy, *Jensens surrender to state authorities on kidnapping charges*, AP, Sept. 10, 2003; P. Foy, *Bill would block state from interfering in "competent" parents' medical decisions*, AP, Oct. 1, 2003; P. Foy, *Parents who fled with son over chemotherapy order face medical neglect trial*, AP, Oct. 8, 2003; P. Foy, *Utah drops case against parents who refused to give son chemotherapy*, AP, Oct. 23, 2003.

[285] *E.g.*, K. Auge, *Mom sentenced to 6 years in death of diabetic son*, DENVER POST, July 17, 1999 B3 [did not provide insulin].

[286] *E.g.*, Martineau v. Angelone, 25 F.3d 734 (9th Cir. 1994) [in *habeas corpus* action court found insufficient evidence to support convictions for child abuse for delay in seeking medical attention; state court had affirmed convictions, King v. State, 105 Nev. 373, 784 P.2d 942 (1989)].

[287] *E.g.*, Lantos et al., *Survival after cardiopulmonary resuscitation in babies of very low birth weight. Is CPR futile therapy?* 318 N. ENG. J. MED. 91 (1988).

It has been accepted practice in many hospitals, upon the concurrence of the parents and the treatment team, to provide only ordinary care to these infants so that their suffering is not prolonged through extraordinary efforts. If parents wish heroic measures, they generally are attempted. If parents refuse treatment when the attending physician believes treatment provides a reasonable likelihood of benefit, child neglect laws are invoked to obtain court authorization for treatment.

Health care professionals disagree on whether some conditions are sufficiently severe that treatment offers no reasonable likelihood of benefit. There has been general acceptance of withholding treatment when the condition is anencephaly (the absence of the higher brain) or other conditions that preclude development of sapient life or are inconsistent with prolonged life.[288] In the past, surgical treatment for spina bifida was frequently withheld. With improvements in treatments and outcomes, surgery can now be withheld only in the most severe cases. A New York hospital obtained a court order authorizing surgical repair of a newborn with several of the complications associated with spina bifida.[289]

Neither mental retardation at a sapient level nor physical deformities consistent with prolonged survival are considered to justify withholding treatment from newborns. This is illustrated by the refusal of a Massachusetts probate court in 1978 to approve parental refusal of respiratory support and cardiac surgery, in spite of some degree of mental retardation and multiple medical problems, because the condition was not terminal and the degree of mental retardation had not been established.[290]

The Department of Health and Human Services (HHS) began an effort in 1982 to force aggressive treatment of virtually all severely deformed newborns. HHS sent a letter to many hospitals threatening to withhold federal funding from any hospital that permitted medically indicated treatment to be withheld from a handicapped newborn.[291]

---

[288] *E.g.*, *In re* Guardianship of Barry, 445 So. 2d 365 (Fla. 2d DCA 1984), *approved*, John F. Kennedy Mem. Hosp. v. Bludworth, 452 So. 2d 921 (Fla. 1984) [approval of termination of ventilator support of infant who had only minimal brain stem function; court review not required when diagnosis confirmed by two physicians]; *In re* Baby "K," 16 F.3d 590 (4th Cir.), *cert. denied*, 513 U.S. 825 (1994) [treatment for anencephalic baby after emergency admission required until parents agreed to termination].

[289] *In re* Cicero, 101 Misc. 2d 699, 421 N.Y.S.2d 965 (Sup. Ct. 1979); *but see* Johnson v. Thompson, 971 F.2d 1487 (10th Cir. 1992), *cert. denied*, 507 U.S. 910 (1993) [no cause of action stated under Rehabilitation Act for treatment of infant with myelomeningocele].

[290] *In re* McNulty, 4 Fam. L. Rptr. 2255 (Mass. P. Ct. Essex County Feb. 15, 1978).

[291] HHS letter reprinted in Hastings Center Rpt. (Aug. 1982), at 6.

This letter was a reaction to a widely publicized case in Indiana in which an infant with Down syndrome, (which usually results in mental retardation), was permitted to starve to death when relatively minor surgery would have permitted the newborn to live. A court order was sought to authorize the surgery, but the Indiana courts refused to intervene.[292]

In 1983, HHS published rules (1) creating a hotline in Washington, D.C., for the reporting of suspected violations and (2) requiring notices to be posted in hospitals announcing the hotline.[293] A federal court enjoined the rules[294] that were widely criticized.[295] HHS published revised rules in 1984 that continued the hotline, required notices to be posted, and recommended the creation of institutional ethics committees.[296] The revised rules were also declared to be beyond the authority of HHS.[297]

In 1983, New York's highest court upheld parental refusal of corrective surgery for a newborn with spina bifida and hydrocephalus.[298] The federal government sought access to the child's medical records, and the parents and the hospital refused to grant access. A federal appellate court refused to order access and ruled that the federal government did not have authority under existing handicapped rights laws to investigate the case.[299] Congress then passed legislation that required states to implement programs within their child abuse prevention and treatment systems to address the withholding of medically indicated treatment from infants with life-threatening conditions.[300] The HHS implementing regulations recommended institutional infant care review committees.[301]

---

[292] *In re* Infant Doe, No. GU 8204-00 (Ind. Cir. Ct. Monroe County Apr. 12, 1982), *writ of mandamus dismissed sub nom.* State *ex rel.* Infant Doe v. Baker, No. 482 S 140 (Ind. May 27, 1982). For a description of the medical status of Infant Doe, *see* 309 N. ENG. J. MED. 664 (1983). The records of the case are not public records, Marzen v. Department of HHS, 825 F.2d 1148 (7th Cir. 1987).

[293] 48 FED. REG. 9630 (Mar. 7, 1983).

[294] American Acad. of Pediatrics v. Heckler, 561 F. Supp. 395 (D. D.C. 1983).

[295] *E.g.*, President's Commission for the Study of Ethical Problems in Medicine and Biomedical and Behavioral Research, DECIDING TO FORGO LIFE-SUSTAINING TREATMENT 227 (Mar. 1983).

[296] 49 FED. REG. 1622 (Jan. 12, 1984).

[297] Bowen v. American Hosp. Ass'n, 476 U.S. 610 (1986).

[298] Weber v. Stony Brook Hosp., 60 N.Y.2d 208, 469 N.Y.S.2d 63, 456 N.E.2d 1186, *cert. denied*, 464 U.S. 1026 (1983); *parents later authorized limited surgery,* N.Y. TIMES, Apr. 12, 1984, 12.

[299] United States v. University Hosp., 729 F.2d 144 (2d Cir. 1984).

[300] Child Abuse Amendments of 1984, Pub. L. No. 98-457, 98 Stat. 1753.

[301] 50 FED. REG. 14,878 (Apr. 15, 1985); *see* Kopelman et al., *Neonatologists judge the "Baby Doe" regulations*, 318 N. ENG. J. MED. 677 (1988).

These decisions will continue to be controversial, but the real exposure to potential legal sanctions is minimal if refusals are carefully limited to appropriate cases. Withholding treatment is acceptable only when the deformities are inconsistent with prolonged or sapient life. When these cases are taken to court, courts approve refusal in appropriate cases.[302] It is important to obtain consultations regarding diagnosis, prognosis, and treatment decisions. Documenting the reasons for the decisions and the decision-making process is essential to ensure that decisionmakers give principled consideration to all relevant information.

7-6.4 What Limitations Are There on Withdrawal of Consent?

In most circumstances, a patient has the right to withdraw consent to treatment, unless the law authorizes involuntary treatment as discussed in Section 7-7. Consent, including signed consent forms, can be challenged by claiming that the consent was withdrawn after it was signed but before the procedure was performed.[303]

For example, many patients elect to stop dialysis and died of their kidney disease.[304] Adult patients can elect to stop taking their insulin and die of their diabetes.[305] Generally, in these cases, there is an opportunity to assess the patient's capacity and understanding of the effect of the decision. When this has occurred, providers generally should accept the patient's decision.

Withdrawal of consent in the middle of procedures can be problematic. For example, in 1993, the Canadian Supreme Court addressed a case in which a patient undergoing a second cerebral angiogram had withdrawn her consent.[306] The procedure was properly stopped. On calming down, the patient instructed that the test be finished. She had a rare reaction that caused quadri-

---

[302] *E.g.*, Hillsborough County Hosp. Auth. v. Muller, No.88-1073 (Fla. Cir. Ct. 13th Cir. Feb. 9, 1988) [ventilator removal authorized for semicomatose infant]; *In re* Steinhaus, No.J-8692 (Minn. Dist. Ct. Redwood County Oct. 13, 1986) [treatment removal authorized for comatose infant], *as discussed in* AM. MED. NEWS, Oct. 24/31, 1986, 1.

[303] *E.g.*, Fox v. Smith, 594 So. 2d 596 (Miss. 1992); Mullany v. Eiseman, 125 A.D.2d 457, 509 N.Y.S.2d 387 (2d Dept. 1986); *see also* Cook v. Highland Hosp., 168 N.C. 250, 84 S.E. 352 (1915) [patient did not waive right to change his mind by signing agreement to abide by hospital rules, so free to leave].

[304] *See* L.M. Cohen et al., *Dying well after discontinuing the life-support treatment of dialysis*, 160 ARCH. INTERNAL MED. 2513 (2000).

[305] *See* Commonwealth v. Konz, 498 Pa. 639, 450 A.2d 638 (1982) [no duty to intervene when competent diabetic husband discontinued insulin].

[306] Ciarlariello v. Schacter, [1993] 2. S.C.R. 119.

plegia. She challenged the consent to the continuation. The court concluded that the patient was capable of consenting based on the earlier disclosures and there was no duty to make additional disclosures where there had been no significant change in risks since the prior disclosure. In 2000, the Kentucky Supreme Court ruled that a patient could revoke her consent to use of an automatic blood pressure cuff during surgery and a jury should decide whether she had done so.[307]

Some courts have indicated that women can withdraw their consent to certain management techniques during labor. In 2002, an Iowa court found that during delivery a woman could withdraw consent to the use of forceps, but in the case, the jury properly found that she had not done so.[308]

At some stages of some procedures, it is not possible to stop without serious injury to the patient. In the past, most of these procedures were performed under general anesthetic; so there was no opportunity to withdraw consent. With the increased use of local anesthetics and conscious sedation, the opportunities have increased. Although there are few cases on the issue, it is likely that when a patient withdraws consent the patient must give the physician an opportunity to sew up the surgical site, withdraw endoscopic instruments, and take other steps to wind up the procedure safely. This should be implicit in the consent to the procedure. This was recognized in a 2004 federal appellate court decision that upheld dismissing a case against an abortion doctor. Complications arose during the procedure. The patient withdrew her consent and demanded transfer to a hospital. The physician restrained her while he took steps to stabilize her and then transferred her to the hospital.[309]

7-7 When Can the Law Authorize Involuntary Treatment?

In some cases, state interests outweigh the right to refuse; so involuntary treatment is authorized.[310] Courts have traditionally used an analysis that focuses on four state interests: (1) preservation of life, (2) prevention of irrational self-destruction, (3) protection of

---

[307] Coulter v. Thomas, 33 S.W.3d 522 (Ky. 2000).
[308] Even v. Bohle, 2002 Iowa App. LEXIS 1256.
[309] Roe II v. Aware Woman Ctr., 357 F.3d 1226 (11th Cir. 2004).
[310] *See* Annotation, *Power of courts or other public agencies, in the absence of statutory authority, to order compulsory medical care for adult*, 9 A.L.R. 3D 1391.

dependent third parties, and (4) protection of the ethical integrity of health professionals. However, in practice, few of these interests ever apply to outweigh the right to refuse. The analysis of the involuntary treatment cases in this section is based on the grounds courts have actually used to justify involuntary treatment. The questions addressed are:

7-7.1. When do threats to the community justify involuntary treatment?

7-7.2. When does impaired capacity justify involuntary treatment?

7-7.3. When do the lives of others justify involuntary treatment?

7-7.4. When does criminal law enforcement justify involuntary treatment?

7-7.5. When does civil law discovery justify involuntary treatment?

7-7.6. When do the needs of the management of governmental institutions justify involuntary treatment?

7-7.7. When do the other traditional state interests justify involuntary treatment?

7-7.1 When Do Threats to the Community Justify Involuntary Treatment?

CONTAGIOUS DISEASE. Courts have long recognized the power of the state to require individuals to submit to medical treatment when refusal threatens the community. In 1905, the United States Supreme Court upheld the power of the state to require an adult to submit to vaccination to help prevent the spread of disease.[311] In 1973, a federal appellate court upheld a Denver ordinance that required prostitutes to accept treatment for venereal disease.[312] In 1988, a federal district court ruled that a prisoner could not sue for the forcible administration of a diphtheria-tetanus inoculation.[313]

---

[311] Jacobson v. Massachusetts, 197 U.S. 11 (1905).

[312] Reynolds v. McNichols, 488 F.2d 1378 (10th Cir. 1973); *see also* Love v. Superior Court, 226 Cal. App. 3d 736, 276 Cal. Rptr. 660 (1st Dist. 1990) [upholding HIV testing of prostitutes]; *but see* Hill v. Evans, 1993 U.S. Dist. LEXIS 19878 (M.D. Ala.) [state law allowing physician to test patient for AIDS without consent when physician thinks patient at risk violates equal protection, but other exceptions to consent upheld where necessary to protect other health workers or may be necessary to change treatment].

[313] Zaire v. Dalsheim, 698 F. Supp. 57 (S.D. N.Y. 1988), *aff'd without op.*, 904 F.2d 33 (2d Cir. 1990).

With the resurgence of tuberculosis in the 1990s, states returned to holding noncompliant patients against their will.[314]

The severe acute respiratory syndrome (SARS) outbreak in 2003 required extensive quarantines in Canada, Hong Kong, and China.[315] Smaller scale quarantines occurred in the United States,[316] focusing new attention in the United States on the containment and treatment of contagious disease.

DANGEROUSNESS TO OTHERS. Courts have also recognized the power of the state to hospitalize persons who have demonstrated dangerousness to the community due to mental illness or substance abuse.[317]

7-7.2 When Does Impaired Capacity Justify Involuntary Treatment?

When adults have sufficient impairment of their decision-making capacity due to mental illness or substance abuse, the state authorizes involuntary hospitalization and treatment but requires that

---

[314] *Woman arrested for failing to seek TB treatment*, AP, Feb. 8, 2005 [NC]; *Some hospitals reviving quarantine to fight spread of new TB strain*, MOD. HEALTHCARE, Nov. 28, 1992, 4A [holding patients against their will in Mass., N.Y., Cal.]; *Tuberculosis spreads civil rights concerns*, WALL. ST. J., Feb. 16, 1993, B10 [NYC quarantined over 90 people in 2 years]; L.O. Gostin, *Controlling the resurgent tuberculosis epidemic: A 50-state survey of TB statutes and proposals for reform*, 269 J.A.M.A. 255 (1993); *Confinement for TB: Weighing rights vs. health*, N.Y. TIMES, Nov. 21, 1993, 1 [15 people held in NYC under guard]; *San Joaquin County officials resort to arrests in TB treatment crackdown*, 3 H.L.R. 1702 (1994); *TB control act quarantine provisions include adequate procedural protection*, 4 H.L.R. 58 (1995) [Tenn]; T. Flowers, *Quarantining the noncompliant TB patient: Catching the "red snapper"*, 28 J. HEALTH & HOSP. L. 95 (1995); C. Chaulk & V. Kazandjian, *Directly observed therapy for treatment completion of pulmonary tuberculosis: Consensus statement of the Public Health Tuberculosis Guidelines Panel*, 279 J.A.M.A. 943 (1998).

[315] *See* D. Beveridge, *Hong Kong will move SARS victims from apartment block to quarantine camps; New deaths reported*, AP, Apr. 1, 2003; J. Kahn, *Quarantine set in Beijing areas to fight SARS*, N.Y. TIMES, Apr. 25, 2003, A1; *Toronto hospitals hunker down for possible new SARS outbreak*, AP WORLDSTREAM, May 24, 2003.

[316] *E.g.*, *Possible SARS victim quarantined in North Texas*, AP, June 18, 2003; S. Russell, *Signs of SARS quarantine Bay Area man; He violated voluntary isolation order*, SAN FRANCISCO CHRONICLE, June 6, 2003, A21; *see also Bush authorizes quarantine for mystery illness*, AP, Apr. 5, 2003.

[317] *E.g.*, O'Connor v. Donaldson, 422 U.S. 563 (1975); Addington v. Texas, 441 U.S. 418 (1979) [mental illness must be proved by clear, convincing evidence]; Schell v. State Dep't of Mental Health & Mental Retardation, 606 So. 2d 1149 (Ala. Civ. App. 1992) [patient mentally ill, dangerous despite control of behavior by drugs, where patient would not comply without supervision]; Glass v. Mayas, 984 F.2d 55 (2d Cir. 1993) [qualified immunity for doctors, nurses in 42 U.S.C.A. § 1983 challenge to involuntary commitment; objectively reasonable belief in dangerousness]; *In re* Blodgett, 510 N.W.2d 910 (Minn.), *cert. denied*, 513 U.S. 849 (1994) [state may authorize commitment of persons with "psychopathic personality" even if not medically recognized as "mentally ill"].

specific procedures be followed and that the person's condition be proven to a court by clear and convincing evidence. Under the common law, providers may involuntarily treat some temporarily disoriented patients without judicial approval.

INVOLUNTARY HOSPITALIZATION/COMMITMENT. Most states have statutory procedures for involuntarily committing persons to institutions for treatment for mental illness or substance abuse.[318] In 1975, the United States Supreme Court ruled that the Constitution permitted involuntary confinement of mentally ill persons, but that they must be treated when their confinement is not based on dangerousness.[319] In 1997, the United States Supreme Court clarified that mental illness was not required in all cases.[320] It upheld a statute that permitted commitment of dangerous persons with mental abnormalities. Commitment procedures vary from state to state. For adults, a judicial hearing is generally required, after which the judicial officer decides whether the evidence is sufficient to justify commitment. Many states do not permit involuntary commitment unless the person is found to be dangerous to self or others.[321]

Courts have generally upheld reasonable police procedures, including force, to take such persons into custody.[322] Most states permit adults to be held temporarily on an emergency basis until the judicial officer can act. In 1979, the United States Supreme Court ruled that states could permit parents to admit their minor children involuntarily for mental treatment without court authoriza-

---

[318] *E.g.*, Dudley v. State, 730 S.W.2d 51 (Tex. Ct. App. 1987) [involuntary alcoholism treatment].

[319] O'Connor v. Donaldson, 422 U.S. 563 (1975).

[320] Kansas v. Hendricks, 521 U.S. 346 (1997).

[321] *E.g.*, Morgan v. Rabun, 128 F.3d 694 (8th Cir. 1998) [need not wait for someone to suffer injury, swinging pool cue at persons, tearing up ping pong table sufficient demonstration of dangerousness]; *In re* Clark, 700 A.2d 781 (D.C. App. 1997) [assault on hospital employee can demonstrate dangerousness]; Thompson v. State Dep't of Mental Health & Mental Retardation, 620 So. 2d 25 (Ala. Civ. App. 1992) [dangerousness to self proved by setting fires and assaultive behavior when not taking drugs, which she refused to do outside facility due to lack of insight into illness, and by refusal to stop smoking, comply with diet, or learn to self-administer insulin, despite diabetes and precancerous throat lesion]; *In re* E.J.H., 493 N.W.2d 841 (Iowa 1992) [mere status as untreated substance abuser did not justify commitment without evidence of dangerousness to self or others].

[322] *E.g.*, Estate of Phillips v. Milwaukee, 123 F.3d 586 (7th Cir. 1997) [affirming summary judgment for defendants, individual died as result of police force used to remove him from hotel room after strange, disorderly behavior, force used was objectively reasonable response to escalating situation]; S.P. v. City of Takoma Park, 950 F. Supp. 705 (D. Md. 1997) [police involuntarily transported, detained person for psychiatric evaluation; summary judgment for defendant city, "reason to believe" imminent danger sufficient]; *see also* McCabe v. Life-Line Ambulance Serv., Inc., 77 F.3d 540 (1st Cir. 1996), *cert. denied*, 519 U.S. 911 (1996) [city policy permitting forcible, warrantless entries into private residences to enforce involuntary civil commitment order does not violate Fourth Amendment].

tion if the admission is approved as necessary by a qualified physician after adequate inquiry.[323] However, many states require judicial involvement in the commitment of minors.

Commitment is not the same as a court determination of incompetency. In 1986, the Texas Supreme Court ruled that a mentally ill person must be informed of the risks of treatment that would influence the decision of a reasonable person.[324] An involuntarily committed person is still competent to be involved in some or all medical decisions unless a court has determined otherwise. Commitment laws usually authorize involuntary treatment that is necessary to preserve the patient's life or to avoid permanent injury to the patient or others.[325] However, there is variation in the extent to which commitment laws authorize the use of antipsychotic drugs or electroconvulsive therapy for purposes of nonemergency treatment of mental illness.[326] Thus, familiarity with local law is important. Most courts have ruled that the constitutional rights to privacy and due process are violated if medication or electroconvulsive therapy is given involuntarily without a judicial finding of incompetency.[327] Some states have resolved this issue by requiring that the judicial officer find the person unable to make treatment decisions as part of the commitment process.[328] In states that authorize involuntary treatment of committed patients without a judicial determination of inability to make treatment decisions, hospitals should give consideration to this evolving standard in developing their treatment policies.

Some courts have required a judicial determination of the need for antipsychotic medications when a patient who has been adjudicated incompetent refuses the medications in a nonemergency situation.[329]

---

[323] Parham v. J.L. & J.R., 442 U.S. 640 (1979); Secretary of Public Welfare v. Institutionalized Juveniles, 442 U.S. 640 (1979).

[324] Barclay v. Campbell, 704 S.W.2d 8 (Tex. 1986).

[325] *See* Sherman v. Four County Counseling Ctr., 987 F.2d 397 (7th Cir. 1993) [qualified immunity protected hospital for involuntary medication during emergency commitment].

[326] *See In re* C.E., 161 Ill. 2d 200, 641 N.E.2d 345 (1994) [law authorizing court ordered involuntary psychotropic drugs is constitutional], *cert. denied*, 514 U.S. 1107 (1995), *see also* Annotation, *Nonconsensual treatment of involuntarily committed mentally ill persons with neuroleptic or antipsychotic drugs as violative of state constitutional guaranty*, 74 A.L.R. 4TH 1099.

[327] *E.g.*, *In re* B., 609 P.2d 747 (Okla. 1980); State *ex rel.* Jones v. Gerhardstein, 141 Wis. 2d 710, 416 N.W.2d 883 (1987).

[328] *E.g.*, IOWA CODE ANN. § 229.1(2).

[329] *E.g.*, Jarvis v. Levine, 418 N.W.2d 139 (Minn. 1988); *In re* Guardianship of Roe, 383 Mass. 415, 421 N.E.2d 40 (1981); Rogers v. Commissioner of Dep't of Mental Health, 390 Mass. 489, 458 N.E.2d 308 (1983); *contra* United States v. Charters, 863 F.2d 302 (4th Cir. 1988), *cert. denied*, 494 U.S. 1016 (1990).

DISORIENTATION. Disoriented patients are frequently restrained temporarily. Physicians and hospitals have authority under common law to detain and restrain temporarily disoriented medical and surgical patients without court involvement. This authority derives from the hospital's duty to use such reasonable care as the patient's known mental and physical condition requires.[330] Hospitals have been found liable for injuries to patients because they were not restrained during temporary disorientation. This common law authority should not be relied on when a patient is being detained for mental illness or substance abuse. The statutory commitment procedures should be followed for those patients. This common law authority also does not apply when a patient is fully oriented, although custody can be maintained temporarily while the patient's status is adequately determined.

7-7.3 When Do the Lives of Others Justify Involuntary Treatment?

Courts ordered treatment for pregnant women to protect the lives of their unborn children but have disagreed on when such orders are permitted. Courts have refused to order persons to donate tissue to save the lives of others. Courts have disagreed on whether the need of dependents for support justifies ordering parents to submit to treatment.

PREGNANCY. Some courts will authorize treatments for pregnant women to preserve the life of the unborn child, especially immediately before and during birth.[331] In 1964, the New Jersey Supreme Court authorized transfusions for a woman if necessary to save the life of either the unborn child or herself.[332] Other courts have limited their authorizations to transfusions necessary to save the life of the unborn child. In 1981, the Georgia Supreme Court authorized a caesarean operation because it was informed of a near certainty the child would not survive a vaginal delivery.[333] In 1999, a federal court in Florida rejected a challenge to a state court-ordered caesarean operation.[334]

---

[330] *E.g.*, Boles v. Milwaukee County, 150 Wis. 2d 801, 443 N.W.2d 679 (1989).

[331] *See* D. Ridley, *Treatment refusals by pregnant women*, HOSP. L. NEWSLETTER (July 1998), at 1.

[332] Raleigh Fitkin-Paul Morgan Mem. Hosp. v. Anderson, 42 N.J. 421, 201 A.2d 537, *cert. denied*, 377 U.S. 985 (1964); *accord* Crouse-Irving Mem. Hosp., Inc. v. Paddock, 127 Misc. 2d 101, 485 N.Y.S.2d 443 (Sup. Ct. 1985).

[333] Jefferson v. Griffin Spalding County Hosp. Auth., 247 Ga. 86, 274 S.E.2d 457 (1981); *see also* L. J. Nelson & N. Mulliken, *Compelled medical treatment of pregnant women: Life, liberty, and law in conflict*, 259 J.A.M.A. 1060 (1988).

[334] Pemberton v Tallahassee Mem. Hosp. Med. Ctr., 66 F. Supp. 2d 1247 (N.D. Fla. 1999).

Other courts have refused to authorize treatment for pregnant women even when necessary to preserve the life of the unborn child. In 1997, an Illinois appellate court refused to authorize such a transfusion of a pregnant woman.[335] In 1983, the highest court of Massachusetts refused to order a pregnant woman to submit to an operation to help postpone premature delivery.[336] In 1987, three judges of the District of Columbia appellate court upheld a court order of a caesarean operation on a terminally ill pregnant woman in extremis, which resulted in the death of the mother and the child.[337] There was widespread criticism of the decision. The full appellate court vacated the 1987 decision and reversed finding that the order should not have been issued.[338] In 1993, the Illinois courts ruled that a mentally competent pregnant woman could refuse a caesarian operation even when this might harm her child.[339]

In 1997, the Wisconsin Supreme Court ruled that the child abuse law did not apply prior to birth; so a drug-using woman could not be taken into custody to protect her unborn child.[340] The legislature then enacted a law expressly authorizing custody of a pregnant woman to protect her unborn child.[341]

In 2000, Massachusetts placed a pregnant member of a religious group in custody. The state became involved due to suspicion that a prior child had died due the group's opposition to medical treatment. Initially, the court refused to order custody, giving her an opportunity to cooperate with home nursing. She was taken into custody when she refused to cooperate with home nursing. She

---

[335] *In re* Brown, 294 Ill. App. 3d 159, 689 N.E.2d 397 (1st Dist. 1997).

[336] Taft v. Taft, 388 Mass. 331, 446 N.E.2d 395 (1983).

[337] *In re* A.C., 533 A.2d 611 (D.C. 1987), *vacated for reh'g* en banc, 539 A.2d 203 (D.C. 1988).

[338] *In re* A.C., 573 A.2d 1235 (D.C. 1990) (en banc); H. Neale, *Mother's rights prevail: In re A.C. and the status of forced obstetrical intervention in the District of Columbia*, 23 J. HEALTH & HOSP. L. 208 (1990)

[339] Baby Boy Doe v. Mother Doe, 260 Ill. App. 3d 392, 632 N.E.2d 326 (1st Dist. Dec. 14, 1993 with formal opinion Apr. 5, 1994) [mentally competent pregnant woman has right to refuse cesarean operation even if refusal will harm her child], *cert. denied*, 510 U.S. 1168 (1994); *Illinois is seeking to force woman to have caesarean*, N.Y. TIMES, Dec. 14, 1993, A11; *Baby whose mother refused C-section appears healthy*, MIAMI HERALD [FL], Dec. 31, 1993, 6A.

[340] State *ex rel.* Angela M.W. v. Kruzicki, 209 Wis. 2d 112, 561 N.W.2d 729 (1997); *accord*, Winnipeg Child & Family Servs. v. G.(D.F.), [1997] 3 S.C.R. 925 [cannot detain mother to prevent harm to unborn child]; *but see* State v. Whitner, 328 S.C. 1, 492 S.E.2d 777 (1997) [affirming criminal neglect conviction of mother for causing baby to be born with cocaine metabolites in its system due to her use of crack cocaine during her pregnancy].

[341] WIS. STAT. §§ 48.193, 48.203, 48.205, 48.213, 48.345, 48.347; S.B. Lalwani, *Pregnant painkiller addict released; She was held under law meant to protect fetus*, MILWAUKEE [Wis.] JOURNAL SENTINEL, May 25, 2005, 6.

gave birth in custody, and the newborn and a child born in 2002 after her release were placed in state custody.[342]

Some mothers do decide to take significant medical risks for the benefit of their unborn children in situations where courts clearly could not order such behavior. For example, in 1994–1995, a mother delayed chemotherapy for leukemia so that it would not harm her twins. After they were born, it was too late for her to be treated for her leukemia, and she died.[343]

MANDATORY DONATION. Courts have refused to order involuntary donation of tissue to save the life of another.[344] In 1978, a Pennsylvania court refused to order a relative of a patient to donate bone marrow necessary to attempt to save the life of the patient.[345] A similar result has been reached in cases where courts have refused to disclose to patients the names of persons with matching tissues who refuse to be donors.[346]

In 1990, the noncustodial father of three-year-old twins sought an order compelling them to submit to a blood test and bone marrow donation for the benefit of his other son, who was their half brother and had leukemia. The custodial mother of the twins opposed the procedures. The trial court denied the order.[347] The Illinois Supreme Court ordered the trial court to appoint two guardians ad litem, one for the twins and one for the other child, and to permit them to present additional evidence.[348] After a hearing, the trial court again denied the order, and the Illinois Supreme Court affirmed.[349]

---

[342] D. Abel, *Pregnant sect member in state custody*, BOSTON GLOBE, Sept. 1, 2000, A1; D. Wedge, *SJC nixes suit aimed at freeing cult mom*, BOSTON HERALD, Sept. 15, 2000, 4; B. MacQuarrie & R. Higgins, *Attleboro sect member gives birth state custody seen; court hearing is set*, BOSTON GLOBE, Oct. 17, 2000, B1; D. Wedge, *Attleboro cult mom believed to have given birth again*, BOSTON HERALD, Jan. 5, 2002, 7; *Judge holds sect parents in contempt after failing to deliver baby*, AP, Jan 17, 2002; L. Miller, *Appeals court upholds state custody for Attleboro sect children*, AP, Apr. 11, 2002.

[343] *A mother loses life so twins can be born*, N.Y. TIMES, Feb. 13, 1995, A14.

[344] *See Propriety of surgically invading incompetent or minor for benefit of third party*, 4 A.L.R. 5TH 1000.

[345] McFall v. Shimp, 10 D.& C. 3d 90 (Pa. Cm. Pl. Ct. Allegheny County 1978); A. Meisel & L. Roth, *Must a man be his cousin's keeper?* 8 HASTINGS CTR. RPT. (Oct. 1978), at 5.

[346] *E.g.*, Head v. Colloton, 331 N.W.2d 870 (Iowa 1983).

[347] Bosze v. Curran, No. 87 M1 4599 (Ill. Cir. Ct. Cook County July 18, 1990), *as discussed in* 23 J. HEALTH & HOSP. L. 282 (1990).

[348] Curran v. Bosze, No. 70501 (Ill. Aug. 10, 1990), *as discussed in* 23 J. HEALTH & HOSP. L. 282 (1990).

[349] Curran v. Bosze, 141 Ill. 2d 473, 566 N.E.2d 1319 (1990); P. Hughes & R. Wood, *Comment: Curran v. Bosze; Disposing of an incompetent donor consent case: The role of parental autonomy and bodily integrity*, 24 J. HEALTH & HOSP. L. 88 (1991).

DEPENDENTS. Some states assert an interest in protecting dependents, especially minor children, from the emotional and financial damage of the patient's death. This interest has been discussed in cases in which Jehovah's Witnesses refuse transfusions. For example, in 1964, a federal appellate court in the District of Columbia authorized transfusions for a woman in part because she was the mother of a seven-month-old child.[350] In 1972, another District of Columbia court refused to authorize a transfusion for a father of two minor children because adequate arrangements had been made for their future well-being.[351]

In 1989, the Florida Supreme Court ruled that a lower court had erred in ordering transfusions for a competent adult with minor children when there were other arrangements to care for the child, such as a surviving parent.[352]

In 1992, the Florida Supreme Court reversed a transfusion order directed at a mother where no arrangements had been made for her four other children. The court noted that the children had two living parents and, even though they were separated, the law presumed that as natural guardian the father would assume the responsibilities for the children.[353]

These cases involved patients who could probably be restored to normal functioning by appropriate therapy. It is doubtful whether dependents will be a determinative issue in cases involving the terminally ill or irreversibly comatose because emotional and financial damage will seldom be increased by discontinuing treatment.

7-7.4 When Does Criminal Law Enforcement Justify Involuntary Treatment?

Sometimes the state's interest in gathering evidence for criminal law enforcement justifies involuntary medical procedures. Law enforcement officers frequently call on medical personnel to perform such procedures, including examining suspects, taking blood samples, pumping stomachs, removing bullets, and performing

---

[350] Application of President & Directors of Georgetown College, Inc., 118 U.S. App. D.C. 80, 331 F.2d 1000, *reh'g denied*, 118 U.S. App. D.C. 90, 331 F.2d 1010, *cert. denied*, 377 U.S. 978 (1964).
[351] *In re* Osborne, 294 A.2d 372 (D.C. 1972).
[352] Public Health Trust v. Wons, 541 So. 2d 96 (Fla. 1989).
[353] *In re* Dubreuil, 629 So. 2d 819 (Fla. 1993).

other interventions. Courts have addressed these procedures primarily in two contexts: admissibility of the resulting evidence[354] and liability for performing the procedures.

STOMACH PUMPING. In 1951, the United States Supreme Court ruled that police-ordered pumping of a suspect's stomach "shocks the conscience;" so the stomach contents were not admissible.[355]

DRAWING BLOOD. In 1957, the United States Supreme Court ruled that blood drawn from an unconscious person after a traffic accident was admissible if the blood was drawn after a proper arrest with probable cause to believe the person was intoxicated while driving.[356] In 1966, the United States Supreme Court ruled that blood drawn from an objecting defendant without a search warrant is admissible if five conditions are satisfied:

1. the defendant is arrested,
2. the blood is likely to produce evidence for the criminal prosecution,
3. delay would lead to destruction of evidence,
4. the test is reasonable and not medically contraindicated, and
5. the test is performed in a reasonable manner.[357]

If these conditions are present and properly documented, hospital personnel can safely cooperate in drawing blood for law enforcement officers to the extent authorized by state law. Any additional state requirements concerning by whom, how, and when blood may be withdrawn should be observed. In most states, hospitals and health professionals have no legal duty to perform tests requested by law enforcement officers. When providers who perform the tests frequently must testify at criminal trials, some health professionals refuse to perform tests to avoid the disruption of their clinical schedules. When subjects physically resist tests,

---

[354] *See* Annotation, *Admissibility, in criminal case, of physical evidence obtained without consent by surgical removal from person's body,* 41 A.L.R. 4TH 60.

[355] Rochin v. California, 342 U.S. 165 (1951).

[356] Breithaupt v. Adams, 352 U.S. 432 (1957).

[357] Schmerber v. California, 384 U.S. 757 (1966); Graham v. Connor, 490 U.S. 386 (1989) [force seizing person must meet "objectively reasonable" standard]; *see also* Hammer v. Gross, 932 F.2d 842 (9th Cir.), *cert. denied,* 502 U.S. 980 (1991) [forcible blood sample from suspect in DUI case not objectively reasonable; city liable but individuals escaped liability because standard not clear at time]; Nelson v. City of Irvine, 143 F.3d 1196 (9th Cir. 1998) [compelled blood test of suspected drunken driver after consent to breath or urine test violates Fourth Amendment].

most professionals refuse to perform the tests to avoid injury to the subject and themselves.

URINE TESTS. In 2001, the United States Supreme Court decided that it was a violation of the Fourth Amendment prohibition of unreasonable searches and seizures when a hospital had an arrangement with the local police to routinely perform nonconsensual testing of the urine of pregnant women for cocaine when they were suspected of illegal drug use and to refer them to the police when cocaine use was discovered.[358]

BULLET REMOVAL. Several cases have involved requests for authorization to remove bullets from suspects. In 1985, the United States Supreme Court ruled that the reasonableness and, thus, the constitutionality of court-ordered surgery to remove bullets for evidence is to be decided on a case-by-case basis, weighing the individual's interest in privacy and security against the societal interest in gathering evidence.[359] The Court indicated that the privacy interest was very strong when general anesthesia would be required or other dangers to life and health were present. The Court also indicated that state interests could prevail in few situations. However, when other evidence demonstrates the surgery is likely to produce helpful evidence, that evidence is likely to be sufficient without consideration of the bullet.

WITNESSES. In one case, the state sought involuntary treatment to preserve the life of a witness. In 1985, the Mississippi Supreme Court ruled that the state's interest in prosecuting crimes, even murder, was not sufficient to outweigh the right of an adult Jehovah's Witness to refuse lifesaving transfusions even though she was the only eyewitness to a murder.[360]

SMUGGLING DRUGS IN THE BODY. Courts have addressed the steps that can be taken to assure that drugs being smuggled internally are detected and recovered. While suspected carriers intercepted by immigration officials at the borders and other points of entry can be detained, even in a hospital, to be observed until drugs can be expelled, there is disagreement among the courts concerning (1) how soon a court must be involved to authorize continued detention and (2) whether a court order is required before a person can

---

[358] Ferguson v. City of Charleston, 532 U.S. 67 (2001).
[359] Winston v. Lee, 470 U.S. 753 (1985); *see also* People v. Richard, 145 Misc. 2d 755, 548 N.Y.S.2d 369 (1989) [denial of order to surgically remove bullet].
[360] *In re* Brown, 478 So. 2d 1033 (Miss. 1985).

be x-rayed.[361] In 1992, a federal appellate court ruled that medical treatment to save the life of a drug carrier was not subject to Fourth Amendment constraints.[362] In 2005, a Wisconsin appellate court ruled that a suspected drug carrier could not be forced to take laxatives to recover plastic bags of heroin that had been swallowed.[363]

7-7.5 When Does Civil Law Discovery Justify Involuntary Treatment?

There are many situations where parties to civil litigation seek medical examination and testing of persons as part of the discovery process. Usually, examination and testing cannot be forced,[364] but a party who refuses to comply with a proper order may have to waive claims or other benefits and may even lose the lawsuit. Thus, most cases focus on what tests can reasonably be demanded as a condition of preserving rights in the suit.

In 1992, an Illinois court ruled that the lower court should not have ordered a minor to undergo magnetic resonance imaging (MRI) where the child would require sedation and it was not shown that this was minimal risk.[365]

However, in civil cases where the purpose of the case is to gain medical information, courts will order mandatory tests in some

---

361 United States v. Montoya de Hernandez, 473 U.S. 531 (1985) [particularized, objective basis for suspecting alimentary canal smuggling justifies detention at border for observation]; United States v. Vega-Bravo, 729 F.2d 1341 (11th Cir.), *cert. denied*, 469 U.S. 1088 (1984) [search warrant not required for X-ray]; United States v. Esieke, 940 F.2d 31 (2d Cir.), *cert. denied*, 502 U.S. 992 (1991) [in Second Circuit must notify U.S. Attorney within 24 hours of detention, who must notify court]; United States v. Adekunle, 980 F.2d 985 (5th Cir. 1992), *cert. denied*, 113 S. Ct. 2380 & 2455 (U.S. 1993) [X-rays performed pursuant of federal magistrate order; forcible laxatives justified under circumstances], *other parts of opinion vacated & superceded*, 2 F.3d 559 (5th Cir. 1993) [judicial determination must be sought within reasonable time, usually within 48 hours of detention]; United States v. Ibekwe, 760 F. Supp. 1546 (M.D. Fla. 1991), *aff'd without op.*, 990 F.2d 1267 (11th Cir. 1993) [insufficient justification for forced X-rays]; Velez v. United States, 693 F. Supp. 51 (S.D. N.Y. 1988) [X-rays justified, but false imprisonment to delay review by qualified radiologist who would have determined not smuggling].

362 United States v. Chukwubike, 956 F.2d 209 (9th Cir. 1992) [X-rays, endoscopy, digital & surgical by physician acting to save life of drug courier carrying balloons of heroin in stomach not subject to Fourth Amendment, balloons could be used as evidence].

363 State v. Payano-Roman, 2005 Wisc. App. LEXIS 413.

364 *E.g.*, C.S. v. Manning, 713 So. 2d 1026 (Fla. 3d DCA 1998) [taking woman into custody to assure appearance at psychology examination unjustified].

365 Stasiak v. Illinois Valley Comm. Hosp., 226 Ill. App. 3d 1075, 590 N.E.2d 974 (3d Dist. 1992); *accord* State *ex rel.* Letts v. Zakaib, 189 W.Va. 616, 433 S.E.2d 554 (1993) [denial of order for MRI examination of minor]; *see also* Lefkowitz v. Nassau County Med. Ctr., 94 A.D.2d 18, 462 N.Y.S.2d 903 (2d Dept. 1983) [deny order of test involving radiated material where no proof without danger].

cases. The Wisconsin Supreme Court ruled in 1993 that a trial court could order involuntary HIV testing of a person who bit a social worker and shouted she had AIDS after the biting. The court determined that the victim's need for the information for medical planning could not be satisfied in any other way.[366]

7-7.6 When Do the Needs of the Management of Governmental Institutions Justify Involuntary Treatment?

In unusual individual cases, the state's interest in management of its institutions can justify involuntary treatment. In 1979, the highest court of Massachusetts authorized dialysis for a prisoner because he attempted to manipulate his placement by refusing dialysis until he was moved.[367] Although prisoners ordinarily have the same rights as others to decline treatment, the state's interest in orderly prison administration was found to outweigh those rights.[368] In 1995, a federal appellate court upheld involuntary catheterization of a prisoner to obtain a urine sample for a blood test.[369]

Similarly, in some situations courts have ordered forced feeding of prisoners engaged in hunger strikes but have denied orders in other cases.[370]

Note that generally military requirements have not been considered sufficient to authorize involuntary treatment, but in some circumstances, military personnel can be punished for refusal to submit.[371]

However, it has long been the position of the U.S military that surgery generally cannot be forced. On December 15, 1917, the U.S. Judge Advocate General of the Army published an official ruling

---

[366] Syring v. Tucker, 174 Wis. 2d 787, 498 N.W.2d 370 (1993).

[367] Commissioner of Corrections v. Myers, 379 Mass. 255, 399 N.E.2d 452 (1979).

[368] *E.g.*, Walker v. Shansky, 28 F.3d 666 (7th Cir. 1994) [cruel, unusual punishment claim stated against officials for forced injections of tranquilizing drugs in prisoners]; *but see* Doe v. Dyett, 1993 U.S. Dist. LEXIS 13,450 (S.D. N.Y.) [not constitutional violation to give involuntary antipsychotic drugs to prisoner in emergency situation where safety of inmate or others threatened].

[369] Sparks v. Stutler, 71 F.3d 259 (7th Cir. 1995).

[370] *E.g.*, Commonwealth, Dep't of Public Welfare v. Kallinger, 134 Pa. Commw. 415, 580 A.2d 887 (1990) [forced feeding ordered]; Von Holden v. Chapman, 87 A.D.2d 66, 450 N.Y.S.2d 623 (4th Dept. 1982) [forced feeding ordered]; *Florida: New feeding tube battle*, N.Y. TIMES, Apr. 16, 2005, A9 [court cleared force feeding of hunger striking prisoner]; *contra*, Thor v. Superior Ct., 5 Cal. 4th 725, 21 Cal. Rptr. 2d 357, 855 P.2d 375 (1993) [inmate can refuse life-sustaining treatment; deny application by prison physician to force feed irreversible quadriplegic inmate where no showing it would undermine prison security]; Zant v. Prevatte, 248 Ga. 832, 286 S.E.2d 715 (1982); *Ethiopian imprisoned in Arizona dies following a hunger strike*, N.Y. TIMES, Jan. 5, 1998, A11 [court had denied order to force feed].

[371] *E.g.*, *Marine pilot dismissed, jailed for refusing anthrax vaccination*, AP, July 8, 2003.

that enlisted men have the right to refuse to undergo a surgical operation unless the attending surgeon certifies that there is no danger to the life of the patient. This was a follow-up to the release of Private Brady E. Cross. Private Cross had been convicted by a court martial and sentenced to two months in prison for refusing to obey orders to undergo surgery necessary to remove a disability that prevented him from performing his duties. The proceedings were declared null and void because there was no certificate of the absence of danger of fatal consequences.[372]

7-7.7 When Do the Other Traditional State Interests Justify Involuntary Treatment?

Several other state and family interests have been asserted, but they generally have not been found to outweigh the right of an adult with decision-making capacity to refuse treatment.

PRESERVATION OF LIFE. The state asserts an interest in the preservation of life. Nearly all courts have ruled that this interest does not outweigh the right of terminally ill patients to refuse treatment. For example, the *Quinlan* decision[373] ruled that the state's interest in preserving life decreases as the prognosis dims and the degree of bodily invasion of the proposed procedure increases. In the *Saikewicz* decision,[374] which authorized withholding chemotherapy from a patient with leukemia, the court concluded: "The value of life as so perceived is lessened not by a decision to refuse treatment, but by the failure to allow a competent human being the right of choice." Even when the patient is not terminally ill, courts have generally declined to order lifesaving transfusions,[375] amputations of gangrenous limbs,[376] and other procedures.[377] Thus, it is not clear when the state's interest in preser-

---

[372] *Can't compel operation*, N.Y. TIMES, Dec. 16, 1917, 8.

[373] *In re* Quinlan, 70 N.J. 10, 355 A.2d 647 (1976).

[374] Superintendent of Belchertown State School v. Saikewicz, 373 Mass. 728, 370 N.E.2d 417, 426 (1977).

[375] *E.g.*, Public Health Trust v. Wons, 541 So. 2d 96 (1989); *In re* Brooks Estate, 32 Ill. 2d 361, 205 N.E.2d 435 (1965).

[376] *E.g.*, Lane v. Candura, 6 Mass. App. Ct. 377, 376 N.E.2d 1232 (1978).

[377] *E.g.*, *In re* Farrell, 108 N.J. 335, 529 A.2d 404 (1987) [respirator]; Bouvia v. Superior Court, 179 Cal. App. 3d 1127, 225 Cal. Rptr. 297 (2d Dist. 1986) [tube feeding]; *In re* Milton, 29 Ohio St. 2d 20, 505 N.E.2d 255, *cert. denied*, 484 U.S. 820 (1987) [cancer treatment]; *In re* Lydia E. Hall Hosp., 116 Misc. 2d 477, 455 N.Y.S.2d 706 (Sup. Ct. 1982) [dialysis]; *see also* Commonwealth v. Konz, 498 Pa. 639, 450 A.2d 638 (1982) [no duty to intervene when competent diabetic husband discontinued insulin].

vation of life alone could justify involuntary treatment of an adult with decision-making capacity. At least one court has adopted a minority position that this state interest can justify involuntary treatment,[378] but no reported appellate decisions have upheld court-ordered involuntary treatment of an adult with decision-making capacity based on the interest in preservation of life without other state interests being present.

PREVENTION OF IRRATIONAL SELF-DESTRUCTION. The prevention of irrational self-destruction (suicide) is another interest asserted by the state. In 1975, a Pennsylvania trial court authorized transfusions for a bleeding ulcer to prevent self-destruction of a twenty-five-year-old Jehovah's Witness.[379] Other courts have refused to consider refusal of transfusions by adult Jehovah's Witnesses to be irrational self-destruction. Courts have generally recognized that there can be a competent, rational decision to refuse treatment.

Courts generally do not view refusals as suicidal if the patient is not seeking death but is seeking to live without the particular medical treatment. One California appellate court found that the state interest was not sufficient to overcome the refusal of tube feeding by a competent quadriplegic patient who stated that she wanted to die.[380]

Some courts have declined to intervene when terminal patients have taken active steps to hasten death. In 1984, a Florida court addressed the situation of a fifty-five-year-old patient, terminally ill with cancer and in intense pain. After attempting suicide by stabbing herself, she refused surgery for her stab wounds. Even though the wounds were due to a suicide attempt, the court refused to order the surgery.[381]

PROTECTION OF THE ETHICAL INTEGRITY OF HEALTH CARE PROVIDERS. Several courts have discussed whether they should recognize a state interest in maintaining the ethical integrity of the medical profession and allowing hospitals the opportunity to care for patients who have been admitted. The courts have concluded that it is not a countervailing interest. Some courts have found that the right of privacy is superior to these professional and

---

[378] *E.g.*, Cruzan v. Harmon, 760 S.W.2d 408 (Mo. 1988) (en banc), *aff'd on other grounds*, 497 U.S. 261 (1990).

[379] *In re* Dell, 1 D. & C. 3d 655 (Pa. Cm. Pl. Ct. Allegheny County 1975).

[380] Bouvia v. Superior Court, 179 Cal. App. 3d 1127, 225 Cal. Rptr. 297 (2d Dist. 1986).

[381] N. Laughlin & L. Benet, *Dying woman can refuse help, court says,* MIAMI [FL] HERALD, Oct. 23, 1984, 1A; *Judge rules for woman who attempted suicide,* N.Y. TIMES, Oct. 24, 1984, A16.

institutional considerations. Other courts have concluded that honoring directives of patients or their representatives is consistent with medical ethics; so there is no conflict. The state interest in preserving the ethical integrity of the medical profession should not be interpreted to permit individual professionals to impose their own standards on patients.[382]

This state interest still affects one aspect of court decisions. Some courts have used this interest as a rationale for not forcing the objecting provider to carry out the directive of the patient or representative, so that the patient must be transferred to another institution or professional.[383] Other courts have refused to require transfers, ordering objecting providers to withhold or withdraw refused treatment,[384] especially when no other institution will accept the transfer[385] or the institution gave no notice of its policies prior to admission.[386]

7-8 What Are the Consequences of Stopping Treatment or Providing Unauthorized Treatment?

There are potential licensing, liability, and criminal consequences for (a) providing treatment without appropriate authorization, (b) withholding or withdrawing life-sustaining treatment in circumstances where this is not permitted, or (c) taking steps other than withholding or withdrawing treatment that cause death.

This section addresses the following questions:

7-8.1. What is the civil liability for providing services without consent or other authorization?

7-8.2. What is the civil liability for providing services with consent that is not informed consent?

---

[382] *E.g.*, Warthen v. Toms River Comm. Mem. Hosp., 199 N.J. Super. 18, 488 A.2d 229 (App. Div. 1985) [upholding termination of nurse who refused to dialyze a seriously ill patient due to moral objections].

[383] *E.g.*, Gray v. Romeo, 697 F. Supp. 580 (D. R.I. 1988); *see also* Miles et al., *Conflicts between patients' wishes to forgo treatment and the policies of health care facilities*, 321 N. ENG. J. MED. 48 (1989).

[384] *E.g.*, Bouvia v. Superior Court, 179 Cal. App. 3d 1127, 225 Cal. Rptr. 297 (2d Dist. 1986).

[385] *E.g.*, *In re* Rodas, No. 86PR139 (Colo. Dist. Ct. Mesa County Jan. 22, 1987), *damages denied*, Ross v. Hilltop Rehabilitation Hosp., 676 F. Supp. 1528 (D. Colo. 1987).

[386] *E.g.*, *In re* Requena, 213 N.J. Super. 443, 517 A.2d 869 (App. Div. 1986).

7-8.3. What is the civil liability for withholding or withdrawing services?

7-8.4. What are the licensing consequences for decisions concerning the treatment of individuals?

7-8.5. What are the criminal law consequences of decisions concerning the treatment of individuals?

7-8.1 What Is the Civil Liability for Providing Services Without Consent or Other Authorization?

BATTERY. The common law has long recognized the right of persons to be free from harmful or offensive touching. The intentional harmful or offensive touching of another person without authorization is called *battery* (see the discussion in Chapter 11). When there is no consent or other authorization for a procedure, the physician or other practitioner doing the medical procedure can be liable for battery even if the procedure is properly performed, is beneficial, and has no negative effects. The touching alone leads to liability.

Medical procedures without express or implied consent constitute a battery unless one of the exceptions to the consent requirement applies. Those exceptions to the consent requirement, in which the law authorizes treatment without consent or despite refusal, are discussed early in this chapter. When express consent is given for one procedure and a different procedure is performed, the procedure performed can be a case of battery.[387] When conditions or restrictions are placed on consent, violations can lead to liability. In 1997, the Louisiana Supreme Court decided that a surgeon was liable for failing to use mesh to close a hernia repair when patient had expressly requested mesh and had specified it on the consent form.[388] One court has found that violations of express restrictions can be a breach of contract.[389]

UNWANTED LIFESAVING PROCEDURES. Courts have struggled with what to do when unwanted lifesaving procedures are provided.

---

[387] *E.g.*, Szkorla v. Vecchione, 231 Cal. App. 3d 1541, 283 Cal. Rptr. 219 (4th Dist. 1991), *rev. dismissed*, 13 Cal. Rptr. 2d 53, 838 P.2d 781 (Cal. 1992) [subcutaneous mastectomy performed instead of breast reduction].

[388] Lugenbuhl v. Dowling, 701 So. 2d 447 (La. 1997).

[389] Dauven v. St. Vincent Hosp. & Med. Center, 130 Or. App. 584, 883 P.2d 241 (1994).

No Liability. In most cases, courts have clearly been troubled with punishing providers for prolonging life and have not imposed liability.[390]

When the husband of a terminally ill woman requested that she be taken off a respirator, an Ohio hospital refused to permit removal until a court order was obtained. After the court order was obtained,[391] the husband filed suit against the physician and the hospital, claiming that his wife's constitutional right of privacy was violated and seeking payment for her pain, suffering, and medical expenses during the time the order was sought. An Ohio court refused to dismiss the suit, ruling that the providers could be sued for battery for continuing treatment for too long a period after authorization was withdrawn.[392] The hospital settled, and the trial judge ruled in favor of the physician.[393]

In another Ohio case, a patient sued a hospital for resuscitation after a no-code order had been written. The court ruled that providers could be sued for battery and negligence, but prolonged life was not a compensable injury as "wrongful living."[394] In the same case, in 1996, the Ohio Supreme Court agreed but ruled that damages could be awarded only for complications that were caused by the unwanted therapy other than by simply prolonging life. Since the patient had suffered no such damages, the court ruled that the patient could recover no more than nominal damages.[395]

In 1996, the North Carolina Supreme Court found that there should be no liability for alleged delay in removing a feeding tube

---

[390] *E.g.*, Ross v. Hilltop Rehabilitation Hosp., 676 F. Supp. 1528 (D. Colo. 1987); Westhart v. Mule, 213 Cal. App. 3d 542, 261 Cal. Rptr. 640 (4th Dist. 1989), *rev. denied & op. withdrawn*, 1989 Cal. LEXIS 4990 (Nov. 22, 1989) [not citable in Cal.] [dismissal of suit arising from insertion of feeding tube contrary to directions of wife's directions; she never asked to have tube removed]; Bartling v. Glendale Adventist Med. Ctr., 184 Cal. App. 3d 961, 229 Cal. Rptr. 360 (2d Dist. 1986) [refusal to find intentional infliction of emotional injuries]; *see also* Benoy v. Simons, 66 Wash. App. 56, 831 P.2d 167, *rev. denied*, 120 Wash. 2d 1014, 844 P.2d 435 (1992) [family challenged putting child on respirator without consent, but did not claim refusal; refusal to recognize wrongful prolongation of life as cause of action; refusal to find intentional infliction of emotional injuries]; Spring v. Geriatric Auth., 394 Mass. 274, 475 N.E.2d 727 (1985) [after court authorized ending dialysis—*In re* Spring, 380 Mass. 629, 405 N.E.2d 115 (1980)—wife sued institution that had forced the matter to be taken to court, second jury awarded $1 million based solely on a letter opposing the court order, sent to newspaper by institutional employees with administration approval, award was reversed on appeal].

[391] Leach v. Akron Gen. Med. Ctr., 68 Ohio Misc. 1, 22 Ohio Op. 3d 49, 426 N.E.2d 809 (C.P. Ct. Summit County 1980).

[392] Estate of Leach v. Shapiro, 13 Ohio App. 3d 393, 469 N.E.2d 1047 (1984).

[393] *Doctor is cleared in death plea case,* N.Y. TIMES, Sept. 19, 1985, 16.

[394] Anderson v. Saint Francis-Saint George Hosp., 83 Ohio App. 3d 221, 614 N.E.2d 841 (1992), *rev. denied*, 66 Ohio St. 3d 1459, 610 N.E.2d 423.

[395] Anderson v. Saint Francis-Saint George Hosp., 77 Ohio St. 3d 82, 671 N.E.2d 225 (1996), *rev'g*, 1995 Ohio App. LEXIS 911.

until a court order was obtained, notwithstanding an advance directive.[396]

In 1998, a Texas appellate court ruled that there should be no liability for the unwanted lifesaving treatment in the case due either to statutory immunity or to failure to meet the conditions of the directive.[397]

In 1998, a Texas jury awarded $42.9 million for resuscitating a severely brain-damaged premature baby against the parents' wishes.[398] The Texas Supreme Court reversed the jury award finding that the parents did not have right to refuse treatment for the infant.[399]

In 1999, the highest court of Maryland decided that there should be no liability for unwanted lifesaving treatment when the technical steps necessary to trigger the application of the advance directive had not occurred.[400]

In 1999, a California appellate court decided that providers had statutory immunity from liability for failure to follow family directions to end life support.[401]

Liability. Some courts have vindicated the right to refuse treatment and have found providers liable, but have often limited the scope of the liability. In one of the first such cases, in 1935, a Canadian appellate court affirmed the liability of a physician for battery for providing lifesaving emergency treatment to a competent adult who had refused the treatment.[402]

In 1990, a federal appellate court affirmed provider tort liability for providing refused care. The physicians involved in implanting a Hickman catheter in a minor pursuant to an ex parte court order could be sued for the death of the minor two weeks later from a massive pulmonary embolus.[403] The implantation was a battery because the court order was not valid because it was not properly obtained. The hospital had been dismissed from the case by agreement of the parties without explanation. At trial, the father, who had opposed the implantation, was awarded nearly two million dollars, which the appellate court

---

[396] First HealthCare Corp. v. Rettinger, 342 N.C. 886, 467 S.E.2d 243 (1996), *rev'g,* 118 N.C. App. 600, 456 S.E.2d 347 (1995).

[397] Stolle v. Baylor College of Med., 981 S.W.2d 709 (Tex. Ct. App. 1998).

[398] Miller v. Woman's Hosp. of Tex., No. 92-07830 (Tex. Dist. Ct. Jan. 14, 1998), *as discussed in* 7 H.L.R. 183 (1998).

[399] Miller v. HCA. Inc., 118 S.W.3d 758 (Tex. 2003).

[400] Wright v. Johns Hopkins Health Sys. Corp., 353 Md. 568, 728 A.2d 166 (1999).

[401] Duarte v. Chino Comm. Hosp., 72 Cal. App. 4th 849, 85 Cal. Rptr. 2d 521 (4th Dist. 1999).

[402] Mulloy v. Hop Sang, [1935] 1 W.W.R. 714 (Alta. C.A.).

[403] Bendiburg v. Dempsey, 909 F.2d 463 (11th Cir. 1990), *cert. denied,* 500 U.S. 932 (1991).

affirmed.[404] It is important to insist that proper procedures be followed when court orders are obtained.

In 1996, a Michigan jury awarded a verdict against a hospital for providing treatment contrary to the patient or family directions. Forgoing appeal, the parties entered a confidential settlement.[405]

In 1998, an Illinois appellate court addressed a case in which the hospital and physicians had refused to follow the patient's daughter's direction to discontinue life support pursuant to the patient's advance directive.[406] The court ruled that a medical battery claim was allowed. In addition, a claim of intentional infliction of emotional distress was stated based on the repeated accusations that the wife and daughter were trying to kill the patient.

In 1999, the highest court of Massachusetts decided that providers could be liable for forcible emergency room care over the patient's objections.[407] The court ruled that the emergency exception to the requirement of consent did not apply when a competent patient refuses. A new trial was ordered because the jury in the first trial had not been properly instructed.

Billing. Even when no liability is imposed, there is a question whether providers can bill for refused treatment. Courts have disagreed. In 1993, the highest court of New York permitted a nursing home to charge for refused services, due to the uncertain state of the law during the period the services were provided.[408] In 2003, a Connecticut court ruled that a hospital could not collect the extra cost of a stay in the intensive care unit from a patient who had refused ICU care.[409]

7-8.2 What Is the Civil Liability for Providing Services with Consent That Is Not Informed Consent?

When consent is given but the person consenting does not have sufficient information for an informed decision, the provider can

---

[404] Bendiburg v. Dempsey, 19 F.3d 557 (11th Cir. 1994).

[405] Osgood v. Genesys Reg. Med. Ctr. (Mich. Cir. Ct. Genesee County jury verdict Feb. 1996); discussion at http://www.afs.com/ethics/osgood.htm (accessed Mar. 15, 1999).

[406] Gragg v. Calandra, 297 Ill. App. 3d 639, 696 N.E.2d 1282 (2d Dist. 1998), *app. denied*, 181 Ill. 2d 570, 706 N.E.2d 496 (1998).

[407] Shine v. Vega, 429 Mass. 456, 709 N.E.2d 58 (1999).

[408] Grace Plaza v. Elbaum, 82 N.Y.2d 10, 603 N.Y.S.2d 386, 623 N.E.2d 513 (1993); G.J. Annas, *Adding injustice to injury: Compulsory payment for unwanted treatment*, 327 N. Eng. J. Med. 1885 (1992).

[409] Rockville Gen. Hosp. v. Wirzulis, 2003 Conn. Super. LEXIS 567.

be liable for violating the duty to disclose such information. In some early cases, courts ruled that providing incorrect or insufficient information invalidated the consent, making the physician liable for battery. Today, in most jurisdictions, failure to disclose necessary information does not invalidate consent; so the procedure is not a battery.[410] There is still a minority position that a medical procedure without informed consent is a battery.[411] The majority rule is that failure to disclose is a separate wrong for which there can be liability based on principles applicable to negligent torts discussed in Chapter 11. Uninformed consent protects from liability for battery, but informed consent is necessary to protect from liability for negligence.

CAUSATION. After it is shown that required information has not been disclosed, causation is the most difficult element to prove in an informed consent case. Since informed consent suits are based on negligence principles, the plaintiff must prove that the deviation from the standard caused the injury. Thus, the plaintiff must prove that consent would not have been given if the risk that occurred had been disclosed.

The two standards of causation are the objective standard and the subjective standard. Some states apply an "objective" standard of what a prudent person in the patient's position would have decided if informed of the risk or alternative.[412] Other courts apply a "subjective" standard, so that it must be proved that the patient would have refused to consent if informed of the risk or alternative.[413]

Either standard provides substantial protection for the conscientious health care professional who discloses major risks and then has a more remote risk occur. A patient who consents to a procedure knowing of the risk of death and paralysis will find it difficult to convince a court that knowledge of a minor risk would have led

---

[410] *E.g.*, Batzell v. Buskirk, 752 S.W.2d 902 (Mo. Ct. App. 1988); Kohoutek v. Hafner, 383 N.W.2d 295 (Minn. 1986); Moser v. Stallings, 387 N.W.2d 599 (Iowa 1986).

[411] *E.g.*, Fox v. Smith, 594 So. 2d 596 (Miss. 1992); Marino v. Ballestas, 749 F.2d 162 (3d Cir. 1984) [battery action permitted]; Hales v. Pittman, 118 Ariz. 305, 576 P.2d 493 (1978) [battery action permitted]; ARIZ. REV. STAT. ANN. § 12-562(B) (1982) [battery action eliminated by statute]; Rubino v. DeFretias, 638 F. Supp. 182 (D. Ariz. 1986) [Arizona statute unconstitutional].

[412] *E.g.*, Caputa v. Antiles, 686 A.2d 356 (N.J. Ct. App. 1996); Boyd v. Louisiana Med. Mut. Ins. Co., 593 So. 2d 427 (La. Ct. App. 1991); McKinley v. Stripling, 763 S.W.2d 407 (Tex. 1989); Latham v. Hayes, 495 So. 2d 453 (Miss. 1986); Pardy v. United States, 783 F.2d 710 (7th Cir. 1986); Canterbury v. Spence, 150 U.S. App. D.C. 263, 464 F.2d 772, *cert. denied*, 409 U.S. 1064 (1972).

[413] *E.g.*, Arena v. Gingrich, 305 Or. 1, 748 P.2d 547 (1988); Wilkinson v. Vesey, 110 R.I. 606, 295 A.2d 676 (1972).

to refusal. However, courts may be more easily convinced when there are undisclosed alternatives.[414]

A few jurisdictions do not require proof of causation. The Vermont Supreme Court ruled that even though the vasectomy patient could not prove he would have refused if informed of the risk of recanalization, he could still sue for failure to provide accurate information.[415] In 1992, the Pennsylvania Supreme Court ruled that it was not necessary to prove causation in any informed consent case.[416] In Pennsylvania informed consent is required only for operations and surgery.[417] In effect, Pennsylvania considers operations and surgeries without informed consent to be batteries.

FRAUD. Attempts have been made to claim that failure to obtain informed consent is fraud. In 2000, the Georgia Supreme Court rejected an attempt to establish liability for fraud based on a physician's nondisclosure of his personal drug use. Nondisclosure could not be the basis for a fraud claim.[418]

7-8.3 What Is the Civil Liability for Withholding or Withdrawing Services?

Because they fear liability, physicians and hospitals have sometimes been reluctant to follow the directives of patients and their families. While liability is theoretically possible, it is no more likely that physicians and other health care providers will be held liable for following treatment refusals than for their many other decisions and actions.

Civil liability for withholding or withdrawing medical treatment would have to be based on negligent or deliberate failure to act in accordance with some duty to the patient. The duty to the patient is shaped by the patient's directions and condition. There is no duty to provide properly refused treatment or to treat terminally ill or irre-

---

[414] *E.g.*, Caputa v. Antiles, 296 N.J. Super. 123, 686 A.2d 356 (App. Div. 1996).

[415] Begin v. Richmond, 555 A.2d 363 (Vt. 1988).

[416] Gouse v. Cassel, 532 Pa. 197, 615 A.2d 331 (1992).

[417] *See* Wu v. Spence, 413 Pa. Super. 352, 605 A.2d 395 (1992) [informed consent not required for drug administration]; *accord* Boyer v. Smith, 345 Pa. Super. 66, 497 A.2d 646 (1985); *but see* Jones v. Philadelphia College of Osteopathic Med., 813 F. Supp. 1125 (E.D. Pa. 1993) [transfusion part of surgery, informed consent must be obtained].

[418] Albany Urology Clinic, P.C. v. Cleveland, 272 Ga. 296, 528 S.E.2d 777 (2000); *see also* Saylor v. Providence Hosp., 680 N.E.2d 193 (Ohio App. 1996) [failure to state fraud claim against hospital concerning surgical implantation of plate, screws, where no specific allegations of misrepresentations]; *but see* Luciano v. Levine, 232 A.D.2d 378, 648 N.Y.S.2d 149 (2d Dept. 1996) [only negligence action allowed; no fraud claim allowed for surgeon's assurances of safety of liquid silicone injection where injuries were the same as injuries from alleged malpractice].

versibly unconscious patients as if they are curable. Explicit refusal by an informed patient with decision-making capacity relieves the physician and hospital of further duty to provide the refused treatment unless it is a situation in which involuntary treatment is authorized. If refused treatment is given without legal authorization, liability for battery is possible. The same principles generally apply to proper refusals by an incapacitated patient's representative.

A medical decision can be questioned in subsequent litigation and be found to have been negligent. The risk for decisions regarding the treatment of terminally ill and irreversibly unconscious patients is no greater than is the risk for the treatment of other patients. Liability is even possible when physicians act pursuant to a court order if they are negligent in implementing the order. Limited statutory immunity has been granted in some circumstances by living will laws, but those laws have broad exceptions that preserve accountability.

One indication of the limited exposure to civil liability is the small number of civil lawsuits brought against physicians and hospitals for withholding or withdrawing medical treatment from terminally ill patients.[419] One case arose after the physician and the patient's husband decided to discontinue the patient's dialysis at a Minnesota hospital.[420] Six months after the wife's death, the husband died. Three years later, the patient's children sued the physician for her death, but a jury found in favor of the physician. Other courts have found no liability when family members have sued because they had no right to participate in a competent patient's decision.[421]

Liability exposure is possible in cases of misdiagnosis of terminal illness or unjustifiable failure to obtain the concurrence of the patient or, in the case of incapacitated patients, the family.[422]

---

[419] *E.g*, Payne v. Marion Gen. Hosp., 549 N.E.2d 1043 (Ind. Ct. App. 1990) [patient died after no resuscitation pursuant to DNR order entered at sister's request; in suit by estate, sufficient evidence patient still awake, alert, capable of communicating to require remand to determine whether incapacitated]; Evans v. Salem Hosp., 83 Or. App. 23, 730 P.2d 562 (1986), *rev. denied*, 303 Or. 331, 736 P.2d 565 (1987) [dismissal on procedural grounds of intentional infliction of emotional distress claim for not resuscitating patient where no patient or family approval not to resuscitate].

[420] *See* S. Neu and C.M. Kjellstrand, *Stopping long-term dialysis*, 314 N. Eng. J. Med. 14, 17 (1986).

[421] *E.g.*, Brooks v. United States, 837 F.2d 958 (11th Cir. 1988).

[422] *E.g.*, Hartsell v. Fort Sanders Reg. Med. Ctr., 905 S.W.2d 944 (Tenn. Ct. App. 1995) [dismissal of outrageous conduct suit by child's representative against obstetrician, hospital for disconnecting newborn's life support after premature birth in 1983; doctor determined child not viable, but child still breathing one hour after disconnection; child eventually survived with no evidence of mental injury].

There is some exposure to civil liability from refusing to honor the directives of the patient and the family.[423] Several suits have been brought against providers who continued treatment for a prolonged period after refusal. Although the exposure to liability still varies between states, liability has been found in some cases. This is discussed in Section 7-8.2.

Several decisions have required providers to pay the attorney's fees of the patient and the family in seeking court orders.[424]

7-8.4 What Are the Licensing Consequences for Decisions Concerning the Treatment of Individuals?

Decisions concerning the treatment of individuals can result in discipline by licensing agencies. Cases involving consent, refusal, and care of persons at the end of life continue to be unusual, but they have occurred.

In one reported case, failure to obtain required consent was the basis for discipline.[425]

Treatment at the end of life has resulted in discipline in a few cases. In some cases, health professionals have surrendered their licenses during criminal investigations as part of defense strategies or bargains with prosecutors.

Licensing boards have imposed discipline that does not appear to be part of a bargain. Here are some examples that have either been reported in newspapers or have resulted in court decisions.

In 2003, the Texas medical licensing board revoked the license of an emergency room physician accused of suffocating a patient who was near death by blocking the breathing tube. The two administrative judges who had conducted the hearing for the board had found that the physician's actions had not harmed the patient and recommended that she not be disciplined. The board overruled them.[426]

---

[423] Annotation, *Tortious maintenance or removal of life supports*, 58 A.L.R. 4TH 222.

[424] *E.g.*, Hoffmeister v. Coler, 544 So. 2d 1067 (Fla. 4th DCA 1989); Gray v. Romeo, 709 F. Supp. 325 (D. R.I. 1989); McMahon v. Lopez, 199 Cal. App. 3d 829, 245 Cal. Rptr. 172 (2d Dist. 1988); Bartling v. Glendale Adventist Med. Ctr., 184 Cal. App. 3d 97, 228 Cal. Rptr. 847 (2d Dist. 1986); *see also* Ross v. Hilltop Rehabilitation Hosp., 124 F.R.D. 660 (D. Colo. 1988) [after unsuccessfully seeking damages for continuation of unwanted treatment, plaintiff required to pay costs of hospital, physician].

[425] *E.g.*, Colorado State Bd. of Dental Exam'rs v. Micheli, 928 P.2d 839 (Colo. App. 1996).

[426] *Doctor loses license over suffocation*, AP, Oct. 11, 2003.

In 2003, Vermont reprimanded a physician for giving a dying patient a paralyzing drug.[427]

In 2003, an Iowa nursing home was fined $103,600 by the state because a respiratory therapist allegedly removed two residents from ventilators without a physician's order and one died. The nursing home announced that it was appealing the fine.[428]

In 1998, Illinois suspended the license of a physician who was accused of injecting a dying kidney patient with a lethal dose of potassium chloride. Even though the Cook County Medical Examiner ruled the case a homicide, prosecutors decided that they could not prove homicide; so no charges were filed. In 2002, a local court ordered that his license be reinstated but stayed its action while the state appealed. In 2003, an Illinois appellate court ordered the licensing board to hold a new hearing.[429] As of September 2004, the license was still revoked.

A Nevada physician ordered a morphine drip to control the pain of a dying patient. When the nurse found the bag empty six hours later, she contacted her supervisor who instructed her to fill out a variance report. The patient's son, who was a physician at the hospital, requested another bag, but the nurse would not accept his verbal order. Another staff physician ordered the morphine. The nurse was accused of back-timing the order. The hospital fired the nurse and reported her to the licensing board, which suspended her license. In 1997, the Nevada Supreme Court ordered the state nurse licensing agency to reconsider the suspension of a nurse's license.[430]

In 1996, an Oregon physician allegedly ordered a lethal injection for a patient. In 1997, the state licensing board reprimanded him, suspended his license for sixty days, and imposed a fine. In 1999, a state appellate court upheld the sanctions. In 1997, the local prosecutor announced that no criminal charges would be filed.[431]

---

[427] *Case of disciplined doctor sparks life and death debate*, AP, July 4, 2003.

[428] *Nursing home fined after patient dies*, AP, April 4, 2003.

[429] *Doctor has license suspended in euthanasia investigation*, AP, Oct. 9. 1998; J. Carpenter, *No charge for doc in homicide*, Chicago Sun-Times, Sept. 29, 1999, 1; A. Sweeney, *Doctor accused of killing patient wins appeal*, Chicago Sun-Times, April 11, 2002, 16; Wilson v. Dep't of Prof. Reg., 344 Ill. App. 3d 897, 801 N.E.2d 36 (1st Dist. 2003).

[430] Nevada State Bd. of Nursing v. Merkley, 113 Nev. 659, 940 P.2d 144 (1997); L.J. Gold, *End of life care: Nurse discipline case highlights problem issues in palliative care*, 6 H.L.R. 971 (1997).

[431] Gallant v. Bd. of Med. Examiners, 159 Ore. App. 175, 974 P.2d 814 (1999); *Ore. Board sanctions physician for 'active euthanasia,'* Am. Med News, Aug. 11, 1997, 26.

These cases illustrate that there are potential consequences from these actions. It is prudent to stay within the parameters of accepted practice.

7-8.5 What Are the Criminal Law Consequences of Decisions Concerning the Treatment of Individuals?

In some decisions involving terminally ill patients, courts have discussed the potential criminal liability for withholding or withdrawing medical treatment. In the *Quinlan* decision, after observing that termination of treatment would accelerate death, the court concluded that "there would be no criminal homicide but rather expiration from existing natural causes." It added as a second reason, "even if it were to be regarded as homicide, it would not be unlawful. . . . The termination of treatment pursuant to the right of privacy is, within the limits of this case, ipso facto lawful." The court discussed the constitutional dimensions:

> Furthermore, the exercise of a constitutional right such as we have here found is protected from criminal prosecution. [Citation omitted.] We do not question the State's undoubted power to punish the taking of human life, but that power does not encompass individuals terminating medical treatment pursuant to their right of privacy. [Citation omitted.] The constitutional protection extends to third parties whose action is necessary to effectuate the exercise of that right where the individuals themselves would not be subject to prosecution or the third parties are charged as accessories to an act which could not be a crime.[432]

Thus, there is little risk of criminal liability for these actions.[433] The criminal trials of physicians in the United States for the deaths of unrelated terminally ill patients generally have involved alleged injections of substances to hasten death. In most cases, either the jury has acquitted the physician or an appellate court has reversed the jury conviction. There are few isolated exceptions. The results of these cases illustrate the difficulty in obtaining convictions when the patient is terminally ill, even in cases alleging active euthanasia.

---

[432] *In re* Quinlan, 70 N.J. 10, 355 A.2d 647, 669-670 (1976).
[433] *See* Annotation, *Homicide: physician's withdrawal of life supports from comatose patient*, 47 A.L.R. 4TH 18.

This is one reason prosecutors seldom pursue cases that involve withholding or withdrawing treatment from the terminally ill. The other reason is that it would be difficult to establish a duty to provide the withheld or withdrawn treatment.

There are cases where physicians, nurses, or others have murdered patients. Some of these cases are included in this section to illustrate the range of potential cases. Sometimes law enforcement personnel have had a difficult time distinguishing appropriate medical actions from inappropriate actions. Prudent providers properly document their consultations, decision-making, and orders and stay within accepted practice.

This section focuses on deaths of patients. Other criminal cases against providers are discussed in the criminal law chapter. Some of the other consequences of these cases are mentioned, such as loss of license or time in jail or length of time the case was open, to illustrate the impact on the lives of those involved even when no criminal conviction resulted.

PHYSICIANS. Several cases have involved physicians. Some of these cases do not involve consent issues. They are discussed together to facilitate comparisons.

No Charges. Several criminal investigations of physicians for the deaths of their patients have resulted in no charges.[434]

In 1981, the head of cardiovascular surgery at George Washington University Hospital removed the bullet from President Reagan's heart after the assassination attempt. Five years later, in 1986, he was placed on administrative leave while a hospital and criminal investigation were conducted of the death of a patient. The patient had been declared dead and removed from life support systems with her family's permission, when the physician injected potassium chloride which stops the heart. At the conclusion of the investigation about one month later, he was reinstated with full privileges.[435]

In 1991, a physician published an article in the *New England Journal of Medicine* reporting that he had assisted in a suicide. Later that year, a New York grand jury refused to indict him.[436]

---

[434] *E.g., Doctors reportedly won't be prosecuted in mercy killings*, UPI, Mar. 28, 1990 [five Minnesota physicians allegedly induced the deaths of two terminally patients with morphine].

[435] *D.C. heart surgeon suspended*, MIAMI HERALD [FL], May 10, 1986, 3A; *Doctor reinstated*, N.Y. TIMES, May 6, 1986, 10.

[436] W. Kates, *Grand jury: No charges against doctor in suicide case*, AP, July 26, 1991.

Charges Dismissed. In several cases, charges were dismissed before trial.[437] For example, in 1981, the parents and physician of newborn conjoined twins were charged with attempted murder for denying the twins food, water, and treatment at the request of the parents. An Illinois judge dismissed the charges finding lack of probable cause. The state's attorney sought an indictment from the grand jury, but it refused to indict the parents or physician. The case was then dropped.[438]

In 1983, two California physicians were charged with murder for terminating all life support, including intravenous feeding, of an irreversibly comatose patient upon the written request of the family. A California appellate court ordered the charges dismissed because the physicians had no legal duty to continue futile treatment and, thus, they did not unlawfully fail to fulfill a legal duty that could be the basis for a murder charge.[439]

Jury Did Not Convict. Juries have acquitted physicians in several cases.[440] In one of the first such cases, in 1915, a Chicago physician was indicted for murder for allowing microcephalic infants to die. A jury acquitted him, but his medical career was ended.[441]

In 1949, a New Hampshire physician was charged with murder for an allegedly lethal injection into a terminal cancer patient. In a widely publicized trial, he was acquitted by the jury in 1950. The physician lost his medical license, but it was reinstated several months later.[442]

In 1972, a New York chief surgical resident was charged with murder for injecting potassium chloride into a patient with terminal throat cancer. In 1974, the jury acquitted. The defense argued that

[437] *E.g.*, C. McInnerney, *Charge dropped in Wash. baby death*, AP, Feb. 2, 1999 [pediatrician charged with second-degree murder for allegedly blocking a three-day-old boy's breathing]; *Prosecutor decides against charging doctor*, AP, Nov. 5, 2001 [eighteen-year-old patient died two days after liposuction].

[438] R.L. Zimmer, *Judge dismisses charges against doctor, parents of deformed twins*, AP, July 17, 1981; *State's attorney won't pursue Siamese twins case*, AP, Apr. 16, 1982.

[439] Barber v. Superior Court, 147 Cal. App. 3d 1006, 195 Cal. Rptr. 484 (2d Dist. 1983).

[440] D.M. Gianelli, *Test case? Physician acquitted after taking infant son off respirator*, AM. MED. NEWS Feb. 20, 1995, 3 [Mich. physician charged with disconnecting his own premature child from respirator].

[441] *Jury clears, yet condemns Dr. Haiselden*, CHICAGO DAILY TRIB., Nov. 20, 1915.

[442] *Physician is charged with murder in 'mercy killing' of cancer patient*, N.Y. TIMES, Dec. 30, 1949, 1; R. Porter, *Sander acquitted in an hour; crowd outside court cheers*, N.Y. TIMES, Mar. 10, 1950, 1; *Sander is stripped of medical license*, N.Y. TIMES, Apr. 20, 1950, 1; *Sander's medical license restored and he gets a patient in 10 minutes*, N.Y. TIMES, June 29, 1950, 31.

the state had not proven the patient was alive before receiving the injection.[443]

In 1976, a New Jersey physician was indicted for five murders in the deaths of patients after a *New York Times* reporter wrote about the deaths. The case received a great deal of publicity because the reporter was jailed for not revealing his sources. The trial judge dismissed two of the indictments. The physician voluntarily surrendered his medical license. In 1978, a jury acquitted the physician for the remaining three murders. In 1982, a court upheld the revocation of his medical license.[444]

In 1983, a Texas jury acquitted a physician who was charged with hastening the death of terminally ill man by injecting air into a vein.[445]

In 1994, a Georgia jury deadlocked seven to five in favor of acquitting a neonatologist accused of killing a premature, terminally ill infant. In 1995, the prosecutor decided to drop the charges. In 1996, the state medical licensing board decided not to impose discipline.[446]

In 1995, a Michigan jury acquitted a physician of manslaughter when he was charged with disconnecting the respirator that was keeping his premature son alive.[447]

In 1997, a jury acquitted a physician charged with the death of a terminally ill cancer patient by the administration of morphine and potassium chloride. The jury is reported to have believed the physician administered the drugs to relieve pain and reduce the patient's rapid heart rate.[448]

Convictions Overturned. Convictions of physicians have been overturned in some cases.[449] In 1995, a Kansas physician who was

---

[443] R.R. Silver, *Physician acquitted in patient's death*, N.Y. TIMES, Feb. 6, 1974, 1; L.K. Altman, *L.I. physician's trial raises problem of doctor's relationship with a dying patient*, N.Y. TIMES, Feb. 4, 1974, 15.

[444] C. Feldman, AP, Oct. 24, 1978; *Jersey examiner's board revokes medical license of Dr. Jascalevich*, N.Y. TIMES, Oct. 9, 1980, B6; *In re* Jascalevich License Revocation, 182 N.J. Super. 455, 442 A.2d 635 (App. Div. 1982) [upholding license revocation]; *see also* Shaw v. Riverdell Hosp., 150 N.J. Super. 585, 376 A.2d 228 (1977) [denying stay of civil case during criminal trial].

[445] R. Hackley, *Jury acquits popular small-town doctor*, AP, Feb. 18, 1983.

[446] R. Ellis, *Infanticide case ends in mistrial 'Impossible' deadlock bound jury, foreman says*, ATLANTA JOURNAL & CONST., Nov. 5, 1994, A1; R. Ellis, *Carrizales won't face second trial*, ATLANTA JOURNAL & CONST., Apr. 15, 1995, 1B; R. Ellis, *No sanctions against physician tried for death of newborn*, ATLANTA JOURNAL & CONST., Feb. 8, 1996, 1C.

[447] *Appeals court reverses ruling on documents in infant death case*, AP, Nov. 18, 1999.

[448] Florida v. Pinzon-Reyes, No. CF-96-00666A-XX (Fla. Cir. Ct. Highlands County verdict June 26, 1997), *as discussed in* 6 H.L.R. 1050 (1997).

[449] *E.g.*, United States v. Wood, 207 F.3d 1222 (10th Cir. 2000); *No retrial planned for former VA physician*, AP, July 28, 2000.

charged with trying to kill an elderly patient surrendered his license. In one case, he had given painkillers to a dying patient at the request of relatives. He was convicted of murder, but an appellate court overturned the conviction, finding no medical consensus that the actions were homicidal. The criminal intent necessary for a conviction could not be established. His license was reinstated several months later. The state medical society supported the physician, maintaining that the prosecution was deterring physicians from providing needed pain relief to patients.[450]

In 2000, a Utah jury convicted a physician of manslaughter and negligent homicide. The psychiatrist was accused of prescribing fatal amounts of morphine for five elderly patients. The jury verdict was overturned because the prosecutor withheld evidence from the defense. A second jury acquitted the physician.[451]

Convictions Not Overturned. One conviction of a physician that was not overturned on appeal was the conviction for assisted suicide mentioned in Section 7-6.1.

A Texas physician was charged with criminally negligent homicide for allegedly blocking a patient's breathing tube with her finger in 2000. She said that she did it to stop agonal breathing after the patient had died. In 2003, the physician lost her medical license. In 2004, a jury convicted the physician. The appeal by the physician was still pending in the fall of 2005.[452]

There are several cases not involving terminally patients where physicians have been convicted of manslaughter for the deaths of patients after they were prescribed large amounts of drugs.[453]

In 1994, a New York appellate court upheld the conviction of a physician for reckless endangerment for his failure to promptly transfer a patient from a nursing home to a hospital after he mistakenly fed her through a peritoneal dialysis catheter. In 1997, a federal appellate court affirmed a lower federal court's denial of a

---

[450] J. Hanna, *Court of Appeals panel acquits former osteopath accused of murder*, AP, July 24, 1998; *Naramore's medical license reinstated*, AP, Oct. 19, 1998; *Medical Society head says many reluctant to treat pain of terminally ill*, AP, Nov. 16, 1998.

[451] C.G. Wallace, *Doctor convicted in drug deaths*, AP ONLINE, July 11, 2000; P. Heintz, *Prosecutor's actions against doctors have landmark results*, AP, Jan. 24, 2003.

[452] *Jury convicts doctor in patient death*, AP, Aug. 31, 2004; R. Casey, *Indict a doc?* HOUSTON CHRONICLE, Feb. 11, 2005, B1.

[453] *E.g.*, T. Albert, *Florida physician guilty of manslaughter in OxyContin case*, AM. MED. NEWS, Mar. 11, 2002; Commonwealth v. Youngkin, 285 Pa. Super. 417, 427 A.2d 1356 (1981); People v. Schade, 30 Cal. App. 4th 1515; 32 Cal. Rptr. 2d 59 (6th Dist. 1994).

petition for federal habeas corpus relief. In 1997, the state commuted his sentence to community service.[454]

Guilty Pleas. In 1986, a New Jersey physician pled guilty to killing his aged mother by injecting Demerol into her feeding tube in a nursing home. She had Alzheimer's disease and had lost control of her bodily functions. He was sentenced to two years probation, a fine, and 400 hours of community service.[455]

In 1989, a Michigan physician pled guilty after being charged with injecting a terminally ill and comatose inpatient with potassium chloride in the presence of other medical staff. He was sentenced to five years of probation and community service.[456]

OTHER HEALTH CARE PROFESSIONALS. Other health care professionals have been investigated, charged, tried, and convicted for patient deaths. Some investigations have been dropped.[457]

Charges Dismissed. In 1980, a Nevada nurse was indicted for the death of terminally ill patient. A judge dismissed the murder charge concluding that there was insufficient evidence. She was reinstated to her job in the ICU.[458]

Jury or Judge Did Not Convict. In 1978, a Maryland nurse was accused of disconnecting three patients' respirators and turning down the oxygen flow to a fourth. Tried for one of the disconnection cases, she surrendered her license before the trial. In 1979, the jury deadlocked, and she was not convicted. All charges were then dropped.[459]

In 1980, a Massachusetts grand jury indicted three nurses for murder for the death of a cancer patient to whom they allegedly gave an overdose of morphine as a pain medication. The trials were

---

[454] People v. Einaugler, 208 A.D.2d 946, 618 N.Y.S.2d 414 (2d Dept. 1994); Einaugler v. Supreme Court of State of N.Y., 109 F.3d 836 (2d Cir. 1997); E.B. Fein, *Doctor in negligence case gets his sentence eased*, N.Y. TIMES, June 28, 1997, 25; *see* M.B. Kapp, *Treating medical charts near the end of life: how legal anxieties inhibit good patient deaths*, 28 U. TOL. L. REV. 521 (1997).

[455] A.A. Narvaez, *Jersey physician is spared prison sentence for mercy killing*, N.Y. TIMES, Dec. 20, 1986, 10.

[456] *Juries kind to doctors who assist*, CAP. TIMES (Madison WI), Mar. 17, 1992, 1D.

[457] *E.g.*, J.B. Frazier, *Grand jury refuses to indict nurse in care center morphine deaths*, AP, Sept. 14, 2000 [Oregon]; *North Memorial nurse won't be charged with felonies*, AP, Dec. 19, 2003 [MN nurse investigated for amount of morphine given to patients].

[458] P. Arnold, *Indictment dismissed, nurse reinstated*, AP, May 31, 1980; P.A. Kalisch, B.J. Kalisch & E. Livesay, *The "angel of death,"* 19 NURSING FORUM (No.3) (1980), 212.

[459] Wiley, *Liability for death: nine nurses' legal ordeals*, 11 NURSING 81 (Sept. 1981), at 37 [hereinafter cited as WILEY]; C. Hanson, *Jury deadlocked, mistrial ruled in nurse's murder case*, WASHINGTON STAR, Mar. 21, 1979, A-1; *Nurse admits plug-pulling but is acquitted of murder*, MED. WORLD NEWS, Apr. 30, 1979, 48; AP, July 2, 1979 [licensing board revoked nursing license after rejecting surrender of license].

separated. In 1981, in the first trial, a licensed practical nurse was acquitted. One of the issues in dispute was whether the physician had given verbal orders for the drug. Charges were then dropped against the other two.[460]

In 1984, a Massachusetts nurse was charged with attempting to murder a patient with Lou Gehrig's disease by pulling the plug on his respirator. She surrendered her license after she was indicted. He survived and provided videotaped testimony against her at the trial. She was acquitted by the jury.[461]

In 1986, a Georgia nurse was accused of injecting six ICU patients with a heart-stopping drug and was found innocent by a jury. She was found guilty but mentally ill of one count of aggravated assault. She was sentenced to seventeen years.[462]

In 1985, a Maryland nurse was charged with giving a lethal drug to an elderly patient in an apparent mercy killing. A judge dismissed the charges, and the case was suspended. She was again charged with three deaths. In January 1988, a court suppressed her confession finding it had been improperly obtained. The federal center for the Centers for Disease Control (CDC) did a statistical analysis of the deaths in the hospital where the nurse worked and found that cardiac arrests in the ICU occurred at a higher rate when she was on duty. In 1988, a judge acquitted her of all charges, finding that the statistic analysis was not sufficient to tie her to the deaths.[463]

In 2001, a New Hampshire nurse was charged with assault for giving morphine to an elderly nursing home resident who died the next day. In 2003, a jury acquitted him of the charges.[464]

Convictions Overturned. Two nurses were accused of poisoning eleven patients at the Ann Arbor Veterans Administration Hospital by injecting a muscle relaxant into their intravenous tubes. The nurses were convicted on several of the counts in 1977, but when the court ordered a new trial, their indictments were dismissed.[465]

---

[460] F. Bayles, *Grand jury probing mercy killing returns indictments*, AP, Aug. 13, 1980; *Nurse acquitted of killing cancer patient*, UPI, Oct. 24, 1981; AP, Nov. 13, 1981.

[461] *Patient testifies against his nurse*, N.Y. TIMES, Oct. 7, 1984, 16; *Nurse is acquitted in respirator case*, N.Y. TIMES, Oct. 17, 1984, 10.

[462] *Find nurse innocent in patients' death*, AP, Sept. 25, 1986; *Sentence nurse in patient injection*, AP, Oct. 1, 1986; *State releases former nurse tried for killing patients*, AP, Apr. 2, 2003.

[463] *Embattled nurse*, N.Y. TIMES, Nov. 11, 1985, 30Y; M. Miller, *Murder, by the numbers*, NEWSWEEK, May 30, 1988, 58; *Judge acquits a nurse accused in deaths of 3*, N.Y. TIMES, June 23, 1988, 9.

[464] H.R. Weber, *Nurse charged in morphine death; two other deaths investigated*, AP, Sept. 14, 2001; S. Macomber, *Jurors find self-described 'Angel of Death' innocent in nursing home deaths*, AP, Feb. 10, 2003.

[465] United States v. Narciso, 446 F. Supp. 252 (E.D. Mich. 1976); WILEY *supra* note 59, at 34.

Convictions Not Overturned. In 1981, a California nurse was charged with killing twelve elderly patients by injecting them with overdoses of lidocaine while working as a temporary overnight nurse in a hospital ICU. In 1984, he was convicted by a judge and sentenced to death. In 1992, the California Supreme Court upheld the murder conviction.[466]

In 1983, a Texas grand jury investigated a number of suspicious deaths. The CDC conducted an analysis for the grand jury. In 1983, a judge found the University of Texas medical school dean in contempt for withholding documents from the grand jury investigating the case. In 1984, a Texas vocational nurse was convicted of murdering an infant and was sentenced to ninety-nine years. Later the same year, she was convicted of injuring a child and was sentenced to sixty years. During the period between the two trials, the hospital where the death occurred was accused of shredding documents and was enjoined from further document shredding. In 1986, the first conviction was affirmed by the appellate court.[467]

In 1987, a New York nurse was charged with assault for injecting a patient with a potentially lethal drug. It was reported that he had done this to several patients so that he could play the hero and revive the patients. The hospital where the events occurred was cited by the state for poor record-keeping and inadequate patient monitoring. In 1989, the nurse was convicted of killing four patients. She was sentenced to fifty years to life in prison. In 1996, the highest court of New York affirmed the conviction.[468]

In 1999, an Indiana nurse was found guilty of murdering six patients. The nurse was accused of injecting lethal doses of potassium chloride. He was sentenced to 360 years in prison. In

---

[466] *Nurse convicted of murdering 12*, N.Y. TIMES, Mar. 30, 1984, 9; *Nurse sentenced to death for 12 hospital murders*, AP, June 15, 1984; People v. Diaz, 3 Cal. 4th 495 & 757, 11 Cal. Rptr. 2d 353, 834 P.2d 1171 (1992), *cert. denied*, 508 U.S. 916 (1993), *related proceeding*, Diaz v. Lukash, 82 N.Y.2d 211, 604 N.Y.S.2d 28, 624 N.E.2d 156 (1993) [convicted nurse permitted to inspect autopsy reports to develop theory that no murder occurred].

[467] *Nurse gets 99 years in Texas injection death*, N.Y. TIMES, Feb. 17, 1984, 8; *Nurse gets 60 years for injuring Texas child*, N.Y. TIMES, Oct. 25, 1984, 10; P. Elkind, *Death shift*, TEXAS MONTHLY (Aug. 1983), 106; *CDC investigator finishes gathering infant death data*, AP, Apr. 20, 1983; K. Gazlay, *Dean held in contempt for failing to turn over documents*, AP, Dec. 12, 1983; K. Gazlay, *Judge issues injunction barring record shredding*, AP, Mar. 19, 1984; Jones v. State, 716 S.W.2d 142 (Tex. App. 1986).

[468] P. Milton, *DA: Nurse admits administering fatal drugs*, AP, Nov. 16, 1987; M. Humbert, *State cites hospital in 'angel of death' case*, AP, Dec. 17, 1987; P. Milton, *Nurse sentenced to 50 years to life*, AP, Jan. 24, 1990; People v. Angelo, 88 N.Y.2d 217, 666 N.E.2d 1333, 644 N.Y.S.2d 460 (1996).

2002, the Indiana Supreme Court rejected a challenge to the conviction.[469]

In 2001, a Veterans Administration nurse in Massachusetts was convicted of killing four patients and sentenced to life in prison. The civil suits by the four families against the VA were dismissed in 2002 because they were filed too late; one case was allowed to proceed.[470]

Guilty or No Contest Pleas. In 1984, a Wisconsin nurse pled no contest to practicing medicine without license after an elderly comatose patient died when the nurse unhooked the life support system allegedly at the request of the family. The nurse was sentenced to twenty months probation. In 1985, the nursing license was revoked for one year.[471]

In 1987, an Ohio nurse's aide pled guilty to killing twenty-four people. He had fed poisons to chronically ill hospital patients. It was reported that the CEO and three other employees of the hospital where the deaths occurred were fired as a result of the aide's confessions. The aide was sentenced to multiple life terms. In 1988, the former hospital administrator was sentenced to thirty days in jail after he pled no contest to falsifying the personnel file of the aide in a plea arrangement that resulted in dropping other charges of tampering with evidence.[472]

In 1988, a California nurse pled guilty to attempted murder and forgery. He had posed as a physician and had called in a verbal order for insulin for an AIDS patient. The patient went into a coma, was revived, and survived four days. It was determined that the insulin did not cause the death. The nurse then used the patient's credit cards and forged his signature to access his money. He was sentenced to nine years.[473]

---

[469] L. Renze-Rhodes, *Judge closes book on Majors case,* INDIANA LAWYER, Nov. 24, 1999, 3; Majors v. State, 773 N.E.2d 231 (Ind. 2002).

[470] *Judge dismisses five families' suits against VA hospital,* AP, June 13, 2002; Skwira v. United States, 344 F.3d 64 (1st Cir. 2003) [affirming dismissal]; *Appeals court clears way for widow to sue VA hospital,* AP, May 27, 2004.

[471] A.H. Malcolm, *Medical workers face ethical dilemmas in new technology,* N.Y. TIMES, Dec. 17, 1984, 12; *Wisconsin board revokes license of nurse in mercy killing of man,* N.Y. TIMES, Mar. 20, 1985, 10.

[472] J. Nolan, *Former nurse's aide sentenced for mass killings,* AP, Aug. 18, 1987; *Personnel changes planned in wake of Harvey disclosures,* AP, Aug. 25, 1987; M. Embry, *Judge doesn't buy 'mercy' killing explanation,* AP. Nov. 3, 1987; J. Kay, *Former hospital administrator sentenced to 30 days,* AP, May 13, 1988.

[473] *Nurse sentenced to 9 years for murder attempt, forgery,* MOD. HEALTHCARE, Aug. 12, 1988, 67.

In 2000, a Virginia nurse pled guilty to one count of administering a controlled substance after being investigated for allegedly administering a large dose of morphine to a comatose terminally ill patient. Her two-year sentence was suspended conditioned on her surrender of her nursing license.[474]

In 2002, a former Florida nurse pled guilty to involuntary manslaughter for the death of a patient in a Veterans Affairs hospital. He had been charged with injecting the patient with Propofol, a sedative, which had not been ordered.[475]

In 2002, a California respiratory therapist pled guilty to murdering six elderly patients in a plea agreement to avoid the death penalty. He was accused of injecting the patients with paralyzing drugs. He was sentenced to life without parole. A confession to more than one hundred murders was unsealed at the time of sentencing. In 2003, he settled civil claims with four of the families.[476]

In 2003, a Missouri nurse pled guilty to voluntary manslaughter and was placed on five years probation during which she could not work in health care. She was accused of administering more morphine than had been ordered and Propofol that had not been ordered to an elderly inpatient on life support who died ten minutes later.[477]

In 2004, a Missouri nurse pled guilty to second-degree murder. She was accused of suffocating an elderly nursing home resident by cutting off her oxygen.[478]

In 2004, a New Jersey nurse pled guilty to sixteen deaths. In 2003, he had been arrested after disclosing that forty terminally ill patients under his care had died after he had administered fatal drugs. He surrendered his license. Numerous private lawsuits were filed against the institutions where the deaths occurred and where he had worked. Some of these suits were dismissed. New Jersey fined one hospital for violating state standards for handling suspicious deaths.

---

[474] *V.J. Vollmar, Virginia nurse pleads guilty to administering morphine to patient,* posted at: http://www.willamette.edu/wucl/pas/2000-reports/062000.htm [accessed Nov. 3, 2005].

[475] *Former VA nurse pleads guilty to manslaughter in patient death,* AP, Oct. 31, 2002.

[476] E. Werner, *Angel of death pleads guilty,* AP ONLINE, Mar. 12, 2002; P. Lieberman, *Hospital 'angel of death' gets life without parole,* L.A. TIMES, Apr. 18, 2002, A1; *'Angel of death' settles claims with 4 families,* L.A. TIMES, Dec. 20, 2003.

[477] *Nurse gets probation for killing dying woman,* AP, Dec. 1, 2003.

[478] *Nurse pleads guilty to killing 91-year-old patient,* AP, Jan. 22, 2004.

Pennsylvania officials announced that institutions in their state had complied with its laws.[479]

These cases demonstrate the importance of proper documentation of the circumstances under which medical treatment can be withheld or withdrawn so that authorized actions can be distinguished from unauthorized actions. It is prudent for nurses and other hospital personnel to appropriately document the decision-making by the physicians and decisionmakers for the patient before withholding or withdrawing medical treatment in order to minimize the risk of investigation or prosecution in the absence of documented authorization of the actions.

Discussion Points

1. When do adults have decision-making capacity? What is usual presumption?
2. What is the effect of an advance directive?
3. Who makes decisions for adults who cannot decide for themselves? How do emergencies differ from other situations?
4. What is the difference between a guardian and a health care agent?
5. When can minors make their own decisions? What is an emancipated minor? What is a mature minor? What are necessaries?
6. Who makes decisions for minors who cannot decide for themselves? When can persons other than a parent or guardian decide?
7. When is an informed consent required? What information must be provided for an informed consent?
8. What are some of the barriers to communication?
9. When may information be withheld?
10. Who is responsible for providing the information?

---

[479] T. Bell, *Charges filed against nurse who says he killed dozens of patients*, AP, Dec. 16, 2003; T. Bell, *Nurse who claims to have killed 40 voluntarily surrenders license*, AP, Dec. 17, 2003; D. Caruso, *Lawsuits fly over nurse charged with overdosing patients*, AP, Jan. 15, 2004; *New Jersey fines last hospital of nurse accused of killings*, N.Y. TIMES, Feb. 21, 2004, B5; D.B. Caruso, *Officials say medical centers complied with law in case of nurse accused of killing patients*, AP, Feb. 21, 2004 [PA]; G. Mulvihill, *Former nurse pleads guilty in 13 patient deaths*, AP, Apr. 29, 2004 [NJ cases]; J. Fisher, *Former nurse pleads guilty in killings of another 3*, N.Y. TIMES, May 20, 2004, B5; W. Parry, *Judge dismisses 2 lawsuits in killer nurse cases*, AP, Sept. 14, 2004 [institutions not obligated to contact prospective future employers regarding suspicions]; *Nurse who pleaded guilty to killing 24 patients meets with New Jersey attorney general*, AP, May 20, 2005 [part of plea bargain to avoid death penalty required tips on catching other serial killers].

11. What is the difference between express and implied consent? When is implied consent sufficient?
12. When should consent be documented by a signed consent form?
13. When is express consent ineffective?
14. What are the limits on the decisions that adults can make for themselves?
15. What are the limits on the decisions that others can make for adults?
16. What are the limits on the decisions that can be made for minors?
17. When may the law authorize involuntary treatment?
18. What happens when treatment is provided without proper authorization?
19. What are the consequences for unwanted lifesaving procedures?
20. What happens when health care providers are investigated or charged with murder of patients?

CHAPTER EIGHT

Health Care Information

Objectives

The objective of this chapter is to provide an overview of the legal issues related to the collection, use, and disclosure of health care information. The reader will learn some of the underlying issues concerning health care information, ownership of the information, requirements about content, privacy requirements, and uses and disclosure of health care information. Audio and video transmissions and recordings and computerized records issues are also discussed.

The collection, use, and disclosure of health care information have become some of the most heavily regulated areas of health care. Health care providers must record, generate, and handle a large amount of information. This includes sensitive information about patients that is necessary to provide treatment. It also includes a wide range of information that is required for business and other internal operations, payment, and regulatory purposes.

Providers and others who obtain health care information need to be aware of the applicable requirements when collecting, using, and disclosing health care information. The details of the requirements are beyond the scope of this book.

This chapter addresses the following questions:

8-1. What are the underlying issues addressed through the laws concerning health care information?
8-2. Who owns medical records?
8-3. What records must be created, and how must they be maintained?

8-4. What are the laws concerning privacy of health care information?

8-5. What are the laws concerning use of health care information?

8-6. What are the laws concerning disclosure of health care information?

8-7. What legal issues flow from the use of audio and video transmissions and recordings?

8-8. What legal issues flow from the use of computers and the Internet?

8-1 What Are the Underlying Issues Addressed Through the Laws Concerning Health Care Information?

Some of the underlying problems of health care law in this area are (1) balancing patient concerns for confidentiality with the need for access to health care information and the cost of implementing confidentiality protections, (2) balancing accountability for health care services with the cost to satisfy documentation requirements, and (3) addressing government and business desires to access information for a wide variety of purposes ranging from law enforcement to budgeting to marketing. The following are some of the underlying interests and issues.

PROVIDING HEALTH CARE SERVICES. Health care providers must collect and access accurate health care information to provide health care services. This is the primary reason that health care information is collected. The complex level of care that is frequently required to treat a patient can only be provided by a team of practitioners who are able to use medical records as a communication tool. Continuity of care frequently requires care in multiple settings, again requiring exchange of information. Care of individuals often requires access to records of prior care because the patient does not know or cannot communicate needed information. Requirements that curtail provider access to information can jeopardize patient care.

CONFIDENTIALITY. Individuals have at least two legitimate concerns with confidentiality. First, there is a desire for privacy; they want limits on who can know their health information. Second, there is a concern that information will be misused, for example, to discriminate against the individual in the workplace or by insurers or to harass the individual through focused marketing.

ACCOUNTABILITY. Individuals, payers, society, and others desire to maintain accountability for the services provided. Documentation is the primary proof of services. Review of the documentation is one mechanism for this accountability. Documentation is used in quality review, liability suits, and regulatory/accreditation requirements.

COST OF IMPLEMENTING REQUIREMENTS. Each requirement for documentation content or for special review to implement confidentiality/disclosure requirements consumes health care resources and diverts clinical time and attention from providing services.

USES OF INFORMATION FOR OTHER PURPOSES. There is a great desire by a wide variety of entities to access and use identifiable health care information. Some of these uses include:

1. Performance improvement (finding ways to improve services);
2. Clinical research (advancing medical knowledge and practice);
3. Public health and safety (e.g., protecting from contagious diseases);
4. Billing and collections (justifying payment);
5. Planning and marketing by health care providers;
6. Documenting individuals' conditions (e.g., to be excused from specific duties[1] and to make benefits and other legal claims);
7. Law enforcement (e.g., to investigate and prove crimes);
8. Government planning;
8. Media reporting; and
9. Other business uses (e.g., building databases for marketing and planning).[2]

8-2 Who Owns Medical Records?

The hospital or other health care institution owns the medical record, which is its business record. Institutional ownership is explicitly stated in the statutes and regulations of some states, and courts have recognized this ownership.[3] If a physician has separate records, they are the physician's property, but the physician is still responsible for maintaining complete institutional records.

---

[1] *Inside trader avoids prison*, N.Y. TIMES, Jan. 16, 1999, A16 [convicted lawyer given no prison sentence because his cerebral palsy made him vulnerable to prison hardships].

[2] *See Massachusetts board probes shared Rx information*, AM. MED. NEWS, May 25, 1998, 13 [sharing prescription drug information with marketing company]; Legal Economic Evaluations v. Metropolitan Life Ins. Co., 39 F.3d 951 (9th Cir. 1994), *cert. denied*, 514 U.S. 1044 (1995) [summary judgment for defendants in suit by consultants who provided services to tort claimants on costs of structured settlements, not antitrust violation for life insurance companies to refuse to provide information other than for defense].

[3] *E.g.*, Pyramid Life Ins. Co. v. Masonic Hosp. Ass'n, 191 F. Supp. 51 (W.D. Okla. 1961); *see also* Archive America, Inc. v. Variety Children's Hosp., 873 So. 2d 359 (Fla. 3d Dist. 2004) [warehouseman's lien transferred from stored hospital records to bond].

The medical record is an unusual type of property because, physically, it belongs to the institution and the institution must exercise considerable control over access, but the patient and others have an interest in the information in the record. The institution owns the paper or other material on which the information is recorded,[4] but it has responsibilities concerning access to and use and disclosure of the information. The patient and others have a right of access to the information in many circumstances, but they do not have a right to possession of original records.[5] Courts have also ruled that patients do not have a right to pathological slides[6] or X-ray negatives.[7] The patient does not purchase a picture; the patient purchases the professional service of interpreting the X-ray. Thus, the patient could not use the physician's retention of the X-ray as a defense to a suit to collect professional fees.

The institutional medical record belongs to the institution. While associated with the institution, physicians and other individual providers have access to the records for patient care, administrative uses, and some legal purposes.[8] After physicians or other providers no longer have association with the institution, they have more limited access but generally can obtain access for legal purposes, for example, defending lawsuits and administrative proceedings or collecting bills. However, individual providers generally are not custodians of the records. Subpoenas and other efforts to discover institutional records should be directed to the institutional custodian, not the individual provider.

Ownership issues sometimes arise between providers, especially when physicians are terminated from employment. The outcomes vary depending on state law and what the employment agreement says.[9]

---

4 *But see* University of Tex. Med. Branch v. York, 871 S.W.2d 175 (Tex. 1994) [medical record not tangible personal property; information intangible, fact of recordation does not render information tangible].

5 *E.g.,* Cannell v. Medical & Surg. Clinic, 21 Ill. App. 3d 383, 315 N.E.2d 278 (3d Dist. 1974).

6 Cornelio v. Stamford Hosp., 246 Conn. 45, 717 A.2d 140 (1998); Lucarello v. North Shore Univ. Hosp., 184 A.D.2d 623, 584 N.Y.S.2d 906 (2d Dept. 1992).

7 *E.g.,* McGarry v. J. A. Mercier Co., 272 Mich. 501, 262 N.W. 296 (1935); Gerson v. New York Women's Medical, 249 A.D.2d 265, 671 N.Y.S.2d 104 (2d Dept. 1998) [provider owns mammogram films].

8 *E.g.,* Caldwell v. Shalala, 114 F.3d 216 (D.C. Cir.), *cert. denied,* 522 U.S. 916 (1997) [physician with conditionally reinstated privileges at Army hospital entitled to access medical records].

9 *E.g.,* Simmons v. Southwest Florida Reg. Med. Ctr., No. 98-2046 CA RWP (Fla. Cir. Ct. Lee County Apr. 24, 1998), *as discussed in* 26 HEALTH L. DIG. (July 1998), 57 [office-generated patient medical records developed by physicians while employed by hospital belong to physicians not hospital that terminated them]; State *ex rel.* O'Donnell v. Clifford, 948 S.W.2d 451 (Mo. Ct. App. 1997) [per written employment agreement, terminated physician entitled to copy medical records of patients he had treated only on request by patient].

8-3 What Records Must Be Created, and How Must They Be Maintained?

Health care providers are required by both governmental and non-governmental agencies (NGOs) to have accurate and complete medical records. The licensing laws and regulations of many states include specific requirements with which hospitals and other providers must comply. In addition, nongovernmental agencies, such as the Joint Commission on Accreditation of Healthcare Organizations (JCAHO), establish medical records standards.

The primary purpose of medical records is to facilitate diagnosis, treatment, and patient care. Records provide a communications link among the team members caring for the patient. Records also document what was found and what was done so that patient care can be evaluated, billing and collections can be performed, and other administrative and legal matters can be addressed. Medical records are also valuable in hospital educational and research programs.

This section addresses:

8-3.1. What elements must health care records contain?
8-3.2. Why must medical records be accurate, timely, and legible?
8-3.3. How should corrections and alterations in records be handled?
8-3.4. How long should records be retained, and how should they be destroyed?

8-3.1 What Elements Must Health Care Records Contain?

Many statutes and regulations require health care providers to maintain medical records. Health care providers that participate in Medicare must comply with minimum content requirements.[10] Some local governments require additional information to be kept. Billing requirements of other payers also add requirements.

To be accredited, hospitals must meet JCAHO medical records standards, including a long list of items that must be in the medical record to assure identification of the patient, support for the diagnosis, justification for the treatment, and accurate documentation of results.[11] While some items apply only to inpatients, the general standards apply to all patients.

---

[10] 42 C.F.R. § 482.24(c).
[11] Joint Commission on Accreditation of Healthcare Organizations, 2005 COMPREHENSIVE ACCREDITATION MANUAL FOR HOSPITALS, Elements of Performance for IM.6.10–6.40 [hereinafter 2005 JCAHO CAMH].

Individual health care providers can lose their licenses for failure to maintain required records.[12]

The medical record consists of three types of data: (1) personal, (2) financial, and (3) medical.

Personal information, usually obtained upon admission, includes name, date of birth, sex, marital status, occupation, other items of identification, and the next of kin or other contact person. The accuracy of this information often depends on the knowledge and honesty of the person providing the information. Providers can generally rely on the information provided unless there is significant reason to doubt it. In 1998, a New York court ruled that a hospital could rely on information provided on a patient's behalf; so it was proper to serve a collection action at the address given by an adult patient's father when she was admitted.[13]

Financial data usually include the patient's employer, health insurance identification, and other information to assist billing.

Medical data forms the clinical record, a continuously maintained history of patient condition and treatment, including physical examinations, medical history, treatment administered, progress reports, physician orders, clinical laboratory reports, radiological reports, consultation reports, anesthesia records, operation records, signed consent forms, nursing notes, and discharge summaries. The medical record should be a complete, current record of the history, condition, and treatment of the patient.

Incomplete hospital record-keeping can sometimes be used to infer negligence in treatment.[14] One federal court found a hospital negligent for permitting its nurse to chart by exception in postoperative monitoring.[15] An infection was missed. However, minor variations from hospital standards concerning charting do not automatically prove that an examination or treatment did not meet legal standards. A federal court found that an emergency screening satisfied EMTALA even though the full hospital screening procedure was not followed.[16]

---

[12] *E.g.*, J. Olson, *Pediatrician loses license for failure to keep up records*, OMAHA WORLD HERALD, Mar. 18, 2002, 5B.

[13] Nassau County Med. Ctr. v. Zinman (N.Y. Dist. Ct. Aug. 1998), *as discussed in* N.Y. L.J, Aug. 3, 1998, 25.

[14] *E.g.*, Valendon Martinez v. Hospital Presbiteriano de la Communidad, Inc., 806 F.2d 1128 (1st Cir. 1986).

[15] Lama v. Borras, 16 F.3d 473 (1st Cir. 1994).

[16] Repp v. Anadarko Municipal Hosp., 43 F.3d 519 (10th Cir. 1994).

Governmental and private third-party payers and managed care organizations are demanding that an increased amount of information be documented to justify treatment, referral, or payment.[17] This is changing the nature of medical practice and diverting clinical time and institutional resources to comply with these requirements.

CODING. Medicare and most managed care companies require providers to code their services, which means that a number must be assigned to each service from a complex coding system. Generally, provider records must include documentation of the diagnosis and treatment to support the coding.

Due to the complexity and changing nature of the coding systems and the liability for coding errors, most institutional providers have had to hire professional coders to assign the codes on each bill.

8-3.2 Why Must Medical Records Be Accurate, Timely, and Legible?

Accurate and timely completion of medical records is essential to maximize availability of information for treatment; expedite payment; comply with governmental and accreditation requirements; and minimize liability exposure.

State licensing statutes and regulations and JCAHO standards require accurate records.[18] An inaccurate record can increase the hospital's exposure to liability by destroying the entire record's credibility. In a 1974 Kansas case, the court found that one discrepancy between the medical record and what actually happened to the patient could justify a jury finding that the record could also be erroneous in other parts and be considered generally invalid.[19]

Complete records include observations that the patient's condition has not changed, as well as observations of change. If there is no notation of an observation, many courts permit juries to infer that no observation was made. In 1974, the Illinois Supreme Court decided a case involving a patient admitted with a broken leg.[20] The leg suffered irreversible ischemia while in traction and required amputation. The physician had ordered the nurse to observe the patient's toes, and the medical record indicated hourly observations

---

[17] *E.g.,* M. Greenberg, *Writer's cramp has reached epidemic levels*, AM. MED. NEWS, Aug. 3, 1998, 18 [documentation requirements for referrals]; *Budget-killer progress notes tamed*, AM. MED. NEWS, Feb.1, 1999, 18.

[18] 2005 JCAHO CAMH, IM.6.10.

[19] Hiatt v. Groce, 215 Kan. 14, 523 P.2d 320 (1974).

[20] Collins v. Westlake Commun. Hosp., 57 Ill. 2d 388, 312 N.E.2d 614 (1974).

during the first day of hospitalization. No observations were documented during the seven hours prior to finding the foot cold and without sensation. Though the nurse might have observed the foot during that period, the jury was permitted to infer from the lack of documentation that no observations were made, indicating a breach of the nurse's duty. The hospital, as the nurse's employer, could be liable for resulting injuries.

Failure to document is often also used as an additional offense when providers are charged with other offenses. In 1997, a New York court upheld revocation of a physician's license for a sexual relationship, improper prescribing, and failure to maintain records.[21]

In 1997, a New Jersey court ruled that when errors in records as to time and cause of injury resulted in a low settlement with the person responsible for the injuries, the physician group responsible for the record errors could be sued.[22]

Complete records can often protect hospital and staff. A Kentucky hospital was found not liable for a patient death approximately thirteen hours after surgery because the medical record included documentation of proper periodic nursing observation, contacts with the physician concerning patient management, and compliance with physician directions.[23] Compliance with physician directions does not provide protection when the directions are clearly improper. When the directions are within the range of acceptable professional practice, properly documented compliance provides substantial liability protection.

Medical record entries should usually be made when treatment is given or observations are made. Entries made several days or weeks later have less credibility than those made during or immediately after the patient's hospitalization. Medicare conditions of participation require completion of hospital records within thirty days following patient discharge.[24] JCAHO accreditation standards require medical staff regulations to specify a time limit for completion of the record that cannot exceed thirty days after discharge.[25]

---

21 Sunnen v. Administrative Review Bd., 244 A.D.2d 790, 666 N.Y.S.2d 239 (3d Dept. 1997).
22 Illiano v. Seaview Orthopedics, 299 N.J. Super. 99, 690 A.2d 662 (App. Div. 1997).
23 Engle v. Clarke, 346 S.W.2d 13 (Ky. 1961); *contra* Thome v. Palmer, 141 Ill. App. 3d 92, 489 N.E.2d 1163 (3d Dist. 1986); Hurlock v. Park Lane Med. Ctr., 709 S.W.2d 872 (Mo. Ct. App. 1985).
24 42 C.F.R. § 482.24(c)(2)(viii).
25 2005 JCAHO CAMH at Elements of Performance 9 for IM.6.10 (completion within 30 days of discharge; *see also* Elements of Performance 2 & 3 for PC.2.120 [medical admission history & physical (H&P), nursing assessment within 24 hours of admission]; Elements of Performance 1 & 2 for IM.6.30 [H&P before surgery, operative progress note immediately after surgery].

Persistent failure to conform to this medical staff rule is a basis for suspension of the staff member.[26]

A West Virginia court ruled in favor of a hospital in a case in which a director of social services ordered social workers to review patient charts and complete missing information in master treatment plans for an upcoming accreditation survey. One social worker refused claiming that it was illegal and then resigned under pressure. The court ruled that completing the plans based on information in the charts was not unethical altering of records.[27]

Medical records should be legible. This does not mean that the patient or another nonhealth care professional must be able to read the records, but it does mean that other health care professionals should be able to read the entries. Otherwise, there is a risk of communication errors that defeat the purpose of the record. Medicare/Medicaid and JCAHO have long required legible records.[28] In addition, illegible records will not satisfy the other uses of medical records. In 1996, a federal appellate court remanded a disability case because "nontrivial" parts of the medical record were illegible.[29] In 1997, another federal appellate court reversed a judgment in favor of a life insurance company because the only evidence that might support the company was an illegible page of the medical record.[30] In 1999, a physician and pharmacist were found liable for the death of a patient when an illegible prescription was misread.[31] There has been increased public and regulatory attention on legibility.[32] Florida mandated legibility of prescriptions effective July 1, 2003, without specifying penalties, leaving it to the medical licensing board to enforce.[33] In 2003, an Alabama physician lost his license in part for the inability of others to read his prescriptions.[34]

---

[26] *E.g.,* Board of Trustees v. Pratt, 72 Wyo. 120, 262 P.2d 682 (1953). Some hospitals use financial incentives, *E.g., Incentives spur physicians to complete record-keeping,* MOD. HEALTH-CARE, Dec. 6, 1985, 64; L. Perry, *Emphasis on coordination hastens submission of bills,* MOD. HEALTHCARE, July 14, 1989, 39.

[27] Birthisel v. Tri-Cities Health Services Corp., 188 W.Va. 371, 424 S.E.2d 606 (1992).

[28] 42 C.F.R. § 482.24(c)(1); 2005 JCAHO CAMH at Elements of Performance 13 for IM.6.10 [readability]; Elements of Performance 3 for MS.3.20 [legibility].

[29] Manso-Pizarro v. Secretary of Health & Human Servs., 76 F.3d 15 (1st Cir. 1996).

[30] Eldridge v. Metropolitan Life Ins. Co., 123 F.3d 456 (7th Cir. 1997).

[31] *Misread prescription brings $450K award,* NATIONAL L. J., Nov. 8, 1999, A4.

[32] R.A. Friedman, *Do spelling and penmanship count? In medicine, you bet,* N.Y. TIMES, Mar. 11, 2003, D5.

[33] § 456.42, Fla. Stat.; D. Adams, *Florida tells doctors: Print clearly or else,* AM. MED. NEWS, Aug. 4, 2003, 1; *see also* REV. CODE WASH. § 69.41.120 [requiring legible prescriptions].

[34] *Doctor blames poor penmanship for losing license,* AP, Feb. 8, 2003.

In some circumstances, it is appropriate to use aliases in the place of the names of patients for security or special privacy reasons. This is generally not considered to make the record inaccurate.[35] For example, hospitals that care for high-profile prisoners sometimes give them other names so that persons who seek to help them escape cannot locate them. This is also sometimes done for patients who are celebrities or are under threat from spouses or others. However, there is generally no right to have an alias used.

8-3.3 How Should Corrections and Alterations in Records Be Handled?

Medical record corrections should be made only by proper methods. Improper alterations reduce record credibility, exposing the hospital to increased liability risk.

Medical record errors can be (1) minor errors in transcription, spelling, and the like or (2) more significant errors involving test data, orders, omitted progress notes, and similar substantive entries. Persons authorized to make record entries may correct minor errors in their own entries soon after the original entry. Hospital policies generally limit who may correct substantive errors and errors discovered at a later date. Those who might have been misled by the error should be notified of changes.

Corrections should be made by placing a single line through the incorrect entry, entering the correct information, initialing or signing the correction, and entering the time and date of the correction. Erasing or obliterating errors can lead jurors to suspect the original entry.

After a claim has been made, changes should not be made without first consulting defense counsel. After some New York physicians won a malpractice suit, it was discovered that a page of the medical record had been replaced before the suit; so the court ordered a new trial.[36] A Maryland court ruled that a malpractice insurer could cancel a physician's coverage for alteration of patient records.[37]

---

[35] *E.g.,* Humphreys v. Drug Enforcement Admin., 105 F.3d 112 (3d Cir. 1996) [DEA should not have revoked physician's registration to distribute controlled substances for prescribed drugs for famous patient in another's name to protect patient's privacy].

[36] Kaplan v. Central Med. Group, 71 A.D.2d 912, 419 N.Y.S.2d 750 (2d Dept. 1979).

[37] Murkin v. Medical Mut. Liability Ins. Society, 82 Md. App. 540, 572 A.2d 1126 (1990).

Altering or falsifying a medical record to obtain reimbursement wrongfully is a crime.[38] In some states, a practitioner who improperly alters a medical record is subject to license revocation or other discipline for unprofessional conduct.[39] In some states, improper alteration of a medical record is a crime regardless of the purpose. In 1998, a Virginia appellate court affirmed the conviction of a physician for forging a cardiac stress test record by altering the date. The forgery was used to obtain authorization for coverage of a liver transplant. The physician could be convicted even though the insurer was never billed for the transplant. His medical license was automatically suspended for the conviction, but later reinstated.[40]

Some patients request modification of medical records. Because records are evidence of what occurred and were relied on in making patient care decisions, hospitals should usually not modify records except to update patient name changes. If a patient disagrees with an entry, some hospitals permit amendments in the same manner as corrections of substantive errors if the physician concurs in the amendment. Such an amendment should note the patient's request as a means of explaining the change if it is questioned later. Instead of changing original entries, some hospitals permit patients to add letters to the record. Staff concurrence, if any, can be noted on the letter. Occasionally, courts will order record modifications, especially for records of involuntary evaluation or treatment for mental illness.[41]

---

[38] *E.g.,* Vest v. United States, 116 F.3d 1179 (7th Cir. 1997), *cert. denied,* 522 U.S. 1119 (1998) [affirming physician mail fraud conviction for falsifying medical records, ordering unnecessary procedures]; *Dentist pays for altering records,* AP, Jan. 7, 2003 [Idaho MD sentenced to 10 months home confinement for altering records to obstruct Medicaid fraud investigation]; *Waterbury Hospital fined in audit scandal,* AP, Mar. 4, 2003 [Conn. hosp. staff added treatment plans and signatures to records selected by federal auditors].

[39] *E.g.,* Tang v. De Buono, 235 A.D.2d 745, 652 N.Y.S.2d 408 (3d Dept. 1997) [upholding revoking medical license for falsifying CT scan report for insurance fraud]; Jimenez v. Department of Professional Reg., 556 So. 2d 1219 (Fla. 4th DCA 1990) [one-year suspension of physician's license, $5,000 fine, and two years probation after suspension for adding false information to records after death of patient]; *Doctor fined in teen's death to keep license,* PALM BEACH (FLA.) POST, Aug. 6, 1995, 23A [violated state law by ordering partner to falsify medical records; fine, probation, community service].

[40] Stevenson v. Comm., 27 Va. Ct. App. 453, 499 S.E.2d 580 (1998), *aff'd without op.* en banc *by equally divided court,* 28 Va. Ct. App. 562, 507 S.E.2d 625 (1998).

[41] *E.g., In re* Morris, 482 A.2d 369 (D.C. 1984); *see also* Caraballo v. Secretary of HHS, 670 F. Supp. 1106 (D. P.R. 1987) [judicially altered birth certificate not conclusive evidence of age].

8-3.4 *How Long Should Records Be Retained, and How Should They Be Destroyed?*

RECORD RETENTION. Because health care records are maintained primarily for patient care purposes, decisions concerning record retention periods should be based on sound institutional and medical practice, as well as on applicable regulations. Some states specify minimum retention periods for some or all records. Medicare requires records to be kept for at least five years.[42] Medicare providers must include in contracts with subcontractors a provision requiring the subcontractor to retain records for at least four years after services are provided and to permit the Department of Health and Human Services (HHS) to inspect them.[43] Several state regulations provide that records be kept permanently, but some require retention for the period in which suits may be filed. Some states provide that records cannot be destroyed without state agency approval.

Where there are no controlling regulations, any retention beyond the time needed for medical and administrative purposes should be determined by institutional administration with advice of legal counsel. In institutions where extensive medical research is conducted, a longer retention period may be appropriate to facilitate retrospective studies.

The importance of retaining records until the time has passed for lawsuits is illustrated by a 1984 Florida appellate court decision.[44] The anesthesia records concerning a patient were lost; so the proof necessary to sue the physician was not available. The court ruled that the hospital could be sued for negligently maintaining its records and that the hospital could avoid liability only by showing that the treatment recorded in the missing records was performed nonnegligently, which would be difficult to do without the records.

An independent tort of *spoliation* of evidence has been recognized by some jurisdictions.[45] Some jurisdictions have limited

---

[42] 42 C.F.R. § 482.24(b)(1).

[43] 42 U.S.C. § 1395x(v)(1)(I).

[44] Bondu v. Gurvich, 473 So. 2d 1307 (Fla. 3d DCA 1984); DeLaughter v. Lawrence County Hosp., 601 So. 2d 818 (Miss. 1992) [missing records create rebuttable adverse presumption]; Phillips v. Covenant Clinic, 625 N.W.2d 714 (Iowa 2001) [can create inference but not in this case]; Annotation, *Medical malpractice: presumption or inference from failure of hospital or doctor to produce relevant medical records*, 69 A.L.R. 4TH 906.

[45] *E.g.,* Ortega v. Trevino, 938 S.W.2d 219 (Tex. Ct. App. 1997); Holmes v. Amerex Rent-A-Car, 710 A.2d 846 (D.C. App. 1998).

its applicability.[46] Other jurisdictions have rejected the independent tort.[47]

Sometimes records are lost due to catastrophe such as fire. One federal court permitted the use in a trial of noncontemporaneous medical records created long after the contemporaneous Veterans Administration (VA) hospital records were destroyed in a fire.[48]

RECORD DESTRUCTION. The issue of record destruction arises when the retention period has passed or when a patient requests destruction.

Some state hospital licensing regulations specify the methods for destroying records. The method should protect confidentiality by complete destruction. When required, certificates of destruction should be retained permanently as evidence of record disposal. Some states require creation of a permanent abstract prior to destruction.

Some patients request premature destruction. Some states forbid destruction on an individual basis.[49] In states without specific statutes, it is still prudent not to destroy individual records unless ordered to do so by a court. Courts have generally refused to order destruction. For example, in 1978, the highest court of New York ruled that records could be ordered sealed, but not destroyed.[50] One exception is a 1978 case in which the Pennsylvania Supreme Court ordered destruction of records of the illegal hospitalization of a mental patient.[51]

8-4 What Are the Laws Concerning Privacy of Health Care Information?

On April 14, 2003, the laws concerning privacy of health care information in the United States were fundamentally changed when the federal privacy regulations under the Health Insurance Portability and Accountability Act (HIPAA) took effect. Any state laws that

---

[46] *E.g.,* Miller v. Gupta, 174 Ill. 2d 120, 672 N.E.2d 1229 (1996) [lost X-ray; duty to preserve evidence can only arise from agreement, contract, statute, or special circumstance].

[47] *E.g.,* Fletcher v. Dorchester Mut. Ins. Co., 437 Mass. 544, 773 N.E.2d 420 (2002);Temple Comm. Hosp. v. Superior Court, 20 Cal. 4th 464, 976 P.2d 223, 84 Cal. Rptr. 2d 852 (1999); Goff v. Harold Ives Trucking Co. Inc., 27 S.W.3d 387 (Ark. 2000); Meyn v. State, 594 N.W.2d 31 (Iowa 1999); *see also* Keene v. Brigham & Women's Hosp., 439 Mass. 223, 786 N.E.2d 824 (2003) [trial court cannot bypass rejection of separate spoliation action by imposing a default against hospital].

[48] Elmer v. Tenneco Resins, Inc., 698 F. Supp. 535 (D. Del. 1988).

[49] *E.g.,* Tenn. Code Ann. § 68-11-305(c).

[50] Palmer v. New York State Dep't of Mental Hygiene, 44 N.Y.2d 958, 408 N.Y.S.2d 322, 380 N.E.2d 154 (1978).

[51] Wolfe v. Beal, 477 Pa. 447, 384 A.2d 1187 (1978).

provide less protection are superseded. State laws that provided more protection remain in effect.

This section addresses the following:

8-4.1. What are the fundamentals of the HIPAA privacy regulations?

8-4.2. What state privacy-related laws remain in effect?

8-4.3. What other federal privacy laws are still applicable?

8-4.1 What Are the Fundamentals of the HIPAA Privacy Regulations?

The Health Insurance Portability and Accountability Act mandated that the United States Department of Health and Human Services (HHS) issue regulations for the privacy of individually identifiable health information.[52] The privacy rules were initially published in December 2000[53] and then substantially amended in August 2002.[54] The privacy rules took effect April 14, 2003. Courts have rejected challenges to the initial rules and the amended rules.[55]

The HHS Office of Civil Rights (OCR) enforces the privacy rules. Unlike many other HHS enforcement efforts, OCR has kept a low profile in its enforcement, focusing its efforts on promoting compliance rather than punishment. As of July 2004, there were no publicized impositions of penalties, although there were reports that unidentified cases had been referred to the Department of Justice for possible prosecution.[56] In August 2004, the first conviction was announced. A Washington health care worker pled guilty to having used information from a patient's medical records to obtain credit cards in the patient's name.[57] The facility cooperated in the investigation and was not charged. In June 2005, the United States Department of Justice announced that the criminal penalties of HIPAA

---

[52] PUB. L. 104-191, §§ 264(b), (c)(1) (1996).

[53] 65 FED. REG. 82,461 (Dec. 28, 2000).

[54] 67 FED. REG. 53,181 (Aug. 14, 2002), codified as 45 C.F.R. Parts 160, 164, Subparts A, E.

[55] South Carolina Med. Ass'n v. Thompson, 327 F.3d 346 (4th Cir. 2003), *cert. denied*, 540 U.S. 981 (2003) [initial rule]; Association of Am. Physicians & Surgeons v. U.S. D.H.H.S., 224 F. Supp .2d 1115 (S.D. Tex. 2002) [initial rule]; Citizens for Health v. Thompson, 2004 U.S. Dist. LEXIS 5745 (E.D. Pa.) [amended rule] *app'd*, 2005 U.S. App. LEXIS 23516 (3d Cir).

[56] *Privacy complaints filed with HHS show confusion over rule's scope, requirements*, HEALTH LAW RPTR. [BNA], Feb. 26, 2004, 282 [4266 complaints—41% closed]; *No prosecutions yet under privacy rule, intent to sell, profit key factors in decision*, HEALTH LAW RPTR. [BNA], Mar. 11, 2004, 356.

[57] P. Shukovsky, *Hospitalized man catches identity thief, ex-lab tech pleads guilty to using private health files, credit cards*, SEATTLE POST-INTELLIGENCER, Aug. 20, 2004, B1; *First sentence for violating privacy act*, N.Y. TIMES, Nov. 7, 2004, 22 [16-month sentence].

generally do not apply to individual employees of providers; instead, they apply to insurers, physicians, hospitals, and other providers.[58]

There is no private cause of action for enforcement of the HIPAA privacy rules.[59] This means that patients and their representatives cannot sue providers seeking payment for violation of HIPAA privacy rules. Patients and their representatives must rely on remedies under other laws. Enforcement of the HIPAA privacy rules is left to OCR.

COVERED ENTITIES. The HIPAA privacy rules apply to *covered entities*.[60] Most health care providers, health plans, and health care clearinghouses are considered covered entities. Health care providers for whom no health information is transmitted electronically are excluded, but this exception is illusory because it is virtually impossible to provide treatment or bill without electronic transmission of health information, especially because Medicare requires electronic submission of bills.

PROTECTED HEALTH INFORMATION. The HIPAA privacy rules apply to confidential patient information, which is called *protected health information* or *PHI* in the rules.[61] PHI includes virtually all *individually identifiable health information*, which is defined to include any health information, including demographic information collected from the individual, that:

(1) Is created or received by a health care provider, health plan, employer, or health care clearinghouse; and
(2) Relates to the past, present, or future physical or mental health or condition of an individual; the provision of health care to an individual; or the past, present, or future payment for the provision of health care to an individual; and
   (i) That identifies the individual; or
   (ii) With respect to which there is a reasonable basis to believe the information can be used to identify the individual.

When there is no reasonable basis to believe the information can be used to identify the individual, the PHI and the HIPAA rules do

---

[58] R. Pear, *Ruling limits prosecutions of people who violate law on privacy of medical records*, N.Y. TIMES, June 7, 2005, 16. The DOJ memo appears at http://www.worldprivacy forum.org/pdf/hipaa-opinion-06-01-2005.pdf [accessed June 8, 2005].

[59] *E.g*, Univ. of Colo. Hosp. Auth. v. Denver Publ. Co., 340 F. Supp. 2d 1142 (D. Colo. 2004).

[60] 45 C.F.R. §§ 160.102, 160.103.

[61] 45 C.F.R. §§ 164.500(a), 160.103 ["health information"], 164.501 ["individually identifiable health information," "protected health information"].

not apply. The HIPAA privacy rules apply to PHI in all formats — written, spoken, or electronic.

NOTICE OF PRIVACY PRACTICES. Upon initial presentation to a health care provider, all patients must be given a notice of privacy practices.[62] A record must be kept of giving this notice. Generally, the patient or patient's representative will be asked to sign an acknowledgment.

SAFEGUARDS. HIPAA requires covered entities to take steps to safeguard PHI.[63] They must train their workforce to take common sense steps so that unauthorized persons do not come into contact with PHI. This ranges from not leaving medical records where they can be seen by the public to not talking about patients in cafeterias and elevators.

PATIENT AUTHORIZATION. HIPAA permits many internal uses and external disclosures of PHI without patient authorization. In general, uses and disclosures for treatment, payment, or health care operations are permitted without authorization.[64] Many disclosures that are required to benefit the public, such as child abuse reporting, are also permitted.[65] These and other permitted uses and disclosures are discussed in Sections 8-5 and 8-6.

Other uses and disclosures generally require authorization from the patient or the patient's representative. There are a few uses, such as listing in a facility directory, where all that is required is that the patient be given an opportunity to object.[66]

It is important for staff members to understand which activities can be conducted without patient authorization and which activities require patient authorization.

MINIMUM NECESSARY. Most of the permitted uses and disclosures of PHI are subject to the *minimum necessary* rule which requires that uses or disclosures be the minimum necessary for the permitted purpose.[67]

ALTERNATIVE COMMUNICATIONS. Patients may request that health care providers contact them in a certain way, such as to leave a message on voice mail. Reasonable requests should usually be accommodated.[68]

---

[62] 45 C.F.R. § 164.520.

[63] 45 C.F.R. § 164.530.

[64] 45 C.F.R. § 164.506.

[65] 45 C.F.R. § 164.512.

[66] 45 C.F.R. § 164.510(a).

[67] 45 C.F.R. § 164.502(b).

[68] 45 C.F.R. § 164.522(b).

ACCESS TO RECORDS. Patients generally may look at their medical and billing records and make copies.[69]

CHANGES TO RECORDS. Patients may ask for their medical or billing records to be changed but do not have a right to compel changes.[70]

TRACKING OF DISCLOSURES. Covered entities must maintain a record of some types of disclosures. With a few exceptions, patients have the right to see this list and get a copy of it.[71]

RESTRICTIONS ON USE. Patients may request restrictions on the use of their patient information, but covered entities are not required to agree to such restrictions.[72] When they do agree, they must comply with their agreements. Due to the complexity of health care institutions, few institutions will be able to implement such agreements; so it is anticipated that they will be rare.

BUSINESS ASSOCIATES. Outsiders who provide services to covered entities and need to use or disclose PHI to provide those services must also follow the HIPAA rules. The covered entity must have a business associate (BA) agreement with a business associate.[73] Examples of business associates include attorneys, accountants, collection agencies, and transcription agencies.

ADMINISTRATIVE STEPS. Covered entities are required to have a designated privacy officer, create policies and procedures, train workers, accept privacy complaints, and take corrective steps when there are violations.[74]

MARKETING AND FUND-RAISING. The HIPAA privacy rules generally prohibit using PHI for marketing of health care services or fund-raising, unless authorization is obtained from the patient or patient's representative.[75]

8-4.2 What State Privacy-related Laws Remain in Effect?

HIPAA preempts any state laws that provide less protection, but any state law that provides as great or greater protections than

---

[69] 45 C.F.R. § 164.524.
[70] 45 C.F.R. § 164.526.
[71] 45 C.F.R. § 164.528.
[72] 45 C.F.R. § 164.522.
[73] 45 C.F.R. §§ 164.502(e), 164,504(e).
[74] 45 C.F.R. § 164.530.
[75] 45 C.F.R. § 164.514(e),(f).

HIPAA remains in effect.[76] Thus, state laws that restrict access to certain information at least as strictly as HIPAA remain in effect.

The general state laws concerning confidentiality of health care information also remain important. Because there is no private cause of action under the HIPAA privacy rules, state laws remain as the basis for some private causes of action. States can still enforce individual and institutional licensing rules and criminal laws[77] that generally require confidentiality.

The HIPAA privacy rules permit attorneys to issue subpoenas of PHI without a court order when certain procedural steps are followed. Some states, such as Wisconsin, do not permit this practice, requiring a court order when discovery of PHI is sought without a written authorization of the patient.

In addition, HIPAA looks to state law to determine some aspects of privacy. Thus, most issues regarding the rights of minors to privacy in relation to their parents are left to state law.

Examples of laws that provide greater protection than HIPAA are state laws concerning mental health and HIV/AIDS test results.

In some states, there is a common law duty to maintain confidentiality that may apply in some situations.

The HIPAA privacy rules also recognize the broad authority of courts to order release of PHI. Most states have placed significantly more limitations on the scope of courts to order release of PHI than has the federal government. These state laws continue to be constraints on the judiciary, at least in the cases where state law must be followed. The physician-patient privilege is one of the most important constraints on judicial disclosure of PHI.

MENTAL HEALTH. Many states have statutes that limit access to and disclosure of mental health information. In 1998, an Illinois appellate court ruled that it was a violation of the state confidentiality statute to voluntarily disclosure mental health records to a physician appointed by a court to examine a patient for involuntary commitment.[78] In 1996, a federal appellate court applied the state mental health records law to issue a writ of mandamus commanding a lower court not to require a hospital to produce the records of two male patients who had allegedly raped the plaintiff.[79]

---

[76] 45 C.F.R. §§ 160.201–160.205.

[77] *E.g., Former Houston hospital worker arrested for stealing, selling patient records,* AP, Aug. 28, 2003 [patient care assistant sold records to investigator].

[78] Sassali v. Rockford Mem. Hosp., 296 Ill. App. 3d 80, 693 N.E.2d 1287 (2d Dist 1998).

[79] Hahnemann Univ. Hosp. v. Edgar, 74 F.3d 456 (3d Cir. 1996).

HIV/AIDS. Many states have statutes that specify when an HIV test result or a diagnosis of AIDS can be disclosed.[80] These statutes are often strictly interpreted.

A California physician was sued for writing a patient's HIV status in a medical record without the written consent required by state law even though the patient had given oral consent. The physician settled the suit.[81] A New York physician was found to have violated the law by disclosing a positive HIV test to an out-of-state workers' compensation board, where the authorization from the patient did not satisfy the statutory requirements.[82] Placing a red sticker on the possessions of a HIV-positive inmate and segregating her improperly disclosed her HIV status to persons who were not authorized to know.[83] In 2004, a District of Columbia court ruled that the law did not prohibit a physician from discussing the case with another physician in the same office.[84]

However, a Pennsylvania court permitted a hospital to make limited disclosure of a resident physician's HIV-positive status, including disclosure to patients without naming the resident.[85]

A North Carolina court upheld revocation of the clinical privileges of a physician for not complying with a hospital policy that required disclosure to the hospital of any inpatient who was HIV-positive.[86]

A federal court in Pennsylvania found that a plaintiff had waived the confidential status of his HIV status by seeking damages that required a determination of life expectancy.[87]

In some states, these laws have been revised to require reporting of HIV/AIDS and disclosure to partners and others.[88]

---

[80] *E.g.,* FLA. STAT. § 381.609(2)(f) [AIDS], § 455.2416 [permitting disclosure of AIDS to sexual partner, needle-sharing partner]; Woods v. White, 689 F. Supp. 874 (W.D. Wis. 1988), *aff'd without op.,* 899 F.2d 17 (7th Cir. 1990) [prisoner could sue staff for disclosing AIDS test to other prisoners]; Annotation, *Validity, construction, and effect of state statutes or regulations expressly governing disclosure of fact that person has tested positive for acquired immunodeficiency syndrome (AIDS),* 12 A.L.R. 5TH 149.

[81] F.W. Hafferty, *A new MD "nightmare": HIV status disclosure can mean lawsuits for breach of confidentiality,* AM. MED. NEWS, Nov. 4, 1988, 27.

[82] Doe v. Roe, 155 Misc. 2d 392, 588 N.Y.S.2d 236 (Sup. Ct. 1992), *modified & aff'd,* 190 A.D.2d 463, 599 N.Y.S.2d 350 (4th Dept. 1993).

[83] Nolley v. County of Erie, 776 F. Supp. 715 (W.D. N.Y. 1991).

[84] Suesbury v. Caceres, 840 A.2d 1285 (D.C. App. 2004).

[85] *In re* Milton S. Hershey Med. Ctr., 535 Pa. 9, 634 A.2d 159 (1993).

[86] Weston v. Carolina Medicorp, Inc., 102 N.C. App. 370, 402 S.E.2d 653 (1991).

[87] Agosto v. Trusswal Sys. Corp., 142 F.R.D. 118 (E.D. Pa. 1992).

[88] *E.g.,* D. Shelton, *Naming names,* AM. MED. NEWS, Apr. 6, 1998, 11 [Illinois becomes 32nd state to require reporting names of HIV-positive persons]; L. Richardson, *New York state sets regulations on H.I.V. reporting and partner notification,* N.Y. TIMES, Mar. 13, 1999, A13; *H.I.V. secrecy is proving deadly,* N.Y. TIMES, Nov. 25, 2003, F6 [failure to disclose to partners is factor in spreading HIV].

COMMON LAW. The common law usually does not provide any protection from disclosure in testimonial contexts (e.g., trials, court hearings, subpoenas). Courts generally refuse to impose liability for testimonial disclosures.[89] Physicians and hospitals are usually not obligated to risk contempt of court to protect confidences (except for substance abuse records), although they might choose to do so.

In nontestimonial contexts courts have found limitations on permissible disclosure based on the implied promise of confidentiality in the physician-patient relationship, violation of the right of privacy, and violation of professional licensing standards.[90] For example, a New York court permanently enjoined a psychoanalyst from circulating a book that included detailed information concerning a patient.[91] The patient was identifiable to close friends despite the psychoanalyst's efforts to disguise her identity. The court ruled that the book violated the implied covenant of confidentiality and the right of privacy. The Oregon Supreme Court held that a physician could be liable for revealing his patient's identity to the patient's natural child, who had been adopted.[92] The court ruled that while it was not a violation of the patient's right of privacy that it was a breach of the professional duty to maintain secrets.

Courts have ruled in favor of health care providers in cases where disclosure was intended to prevent the spread of contagious disease.[93] As discussed in the section on the common law duty to disclose information, there could be liability in some circumstances for failing to disclose a contagious disease. Disclosures to the patient's employer or insurance company have resulted in several suits.[94] The Alabama Supreme Court ruled that disclosures to an employer without authorization violated the implied promise of confidentiality and could result in liability.[95] The employer who induces the disclosure can also be liable.[96] However, a New York court ruled that when a patient authorized incomplete disclosure to his employer that the

---

[89] *E.g.,* Boyd v. Wynn, 286 Ky. 173, 150 S.W.2d 648 (1941).

[90] Annotation, *Physician's tort liability for unauthorized disclosure of confidential information about patient,* 48 A.L.R. 4TH 668.

[91] Doe v. Roe, 93 Misc. 2d 201, 400 N.Y.S.2d 668 (Sup. Ct. 1977).

[92] Humphers v. First Interstate Bank, 298 Or. 706, 696 P.2d 527 (1985).

[93] *E.g.,* Simonsen v. Swenson, 104 Neb. 224, 177 N.W. 831 (1920) [physician]; Knecht v. Vandalia Med. Ctr., Inc., 14 Ohio App. 3d 129, 470 N.E.2d 230 (1984) [receptionist].

[94] *E.g.,* Crippen v. Charter Southland Hosp., 534 So. 2d 286 (Ala 1988) [disclosure to employer's psychiatrist]; Tower v. Hirshhorn, 397 Mass. 581, 492 N.E.2d 728 (1986) [disclosure to insurer's physician].

[95] Horne v. Patton, 291 Ala. 701, 287 So. 2d 824 (1973).

[96] *E.g.,* Alberts v. Devine, 395 Mass. 59, 479 N.E.2d 113, *cert. denied,* 474 U.S. 1013 (1985).

physician was not liable for giving a complete disclosure.[97] It is questionable whether other courts would rule this way; so the prudent practice is to refuse to release any information when only a misleading partial release is authorized.

Suits for disclosures of confidential information have also been based on defamation. In most cases involving physicians, courts have found a qualified privilege to make the specific disclosures.[98] The few cases of liability have involved disclosure of a misdiagnosed embarrassing condition (such as venereal disease) that the patient did not actually have in a manner that demonstrated malice, defeating the qualified privilege.[99]

Misuse of confidential information without disclosure can also lead to sanctions. In 1991, a New York psychiatrist pled guilty to securities fraud for trading in stocks based on inside information received from a patient.[100]

Courts have disagreed on whether claims concerning release of information are subject to state medical malpractice claims procedures.[101]

PHYSICIAN-PATIENT PRIVILEGE. The physician-patient privilege is the rule that a physician is not permitted to testify as a witness concerning certain information gained in the physician-patient relationship. There was no physician-patient privilege from testimonial disclosure under the English common law. Nearly all U.S. courts also have adopted this position; so with few exceptions, the privilege exists only in states that have enacted privilege statutes. One exception is Alaska, which established a common law psychotherapist-patient privilege for criminal cases.[102] Federal courts must apply state privileges in suits concerning state law, but state privileges do not apply in most federal suits concerning federal law.[103]

---

[97] Clark v. Geraci, 29 Misc. 2d 791, 208 N.Y.S.2d 564 (Sup. Ct. 1960).

[98] *E.g.,* Thomas v. Hillson, 184 Ga. App. 302, 361 S.E.2d 278 (1987); *see* Annotation, *Libel and slander: privilege of statements by physician, surgeon, or nurse concerning patient,* 73 A.L.R. 2D 325.

[99] *E.g.,* Beatty v. Baston, 130 Ohio L. Abs. 481 (Ct. App. 1932).

[100] United States v. Willis, 778 F. Supp. 205 (S.D. N.Y. 1991), 737 F. Supp. 269 (1990); *Psychiatrist is sentenced,* N.Y. TIMES, Jan. 8, 1992, C12.

[101] *E.g.,* Brand v. Seider, 697 A.2d 846 (Me. 1997) [claim against psychiatrist alleging breach of confidentiality subject to state malpractice act]; *contra* Champion v. Cox, 689 So. 2d 365 (Fla. 1st DCA 1997) [defamation action based upon medical disclosure to patient's employer not subject to state malpractice act].

[102] Allred v. State, 554 P.2d 411 (Alaska 1976).

[103] Fed. R. Evid. 501; United States v. Bercier, 848 F.2d 917 (8th Cir. 1988) [criminal]; United States v. Moore, 970 F.2d 48 (5th Cir. 1992) [IRS summons]; *see* Annotation, *Situations in which federal courts are governed by state law of privilege under Rule 501 of Federal Rules of Evidence,* 48 A.L.R. FED. 259.

Approximately two thirds of the states have enacted a statutory physician-patient privilege. Privilege statutes address only situations in which the physician is being compelled to testify, such as in a deposition, administrative hearing, or trial or to release subpoenaed records. There is a widespread misperception that privilege statutes apply to other disclosures, but in most states, this is not true.[104] The duty to maintain confidentiality outside of testimonial contexts is grounded on other statutes and legal principles. Thus, privilege statutes are usually of concern only when providers are responding to legal compulsion.

The privilege applies only when a bona fide physician-patient relationship exists. The privilege usually does not apply to court-ordered examinations or other examinations solely for the benefit of third parties, such as insurance companies.

The scope of the privilege varies. Pennsylvania limits the privilege to communications that tend to blacken the character of the patient,[105] while Kansas extends the privilege to all communications and observations.[106] Michigan limits the privilege to physicians,[107] while New York extends the privilege to dentists and nurses.[108] When a nurse is present during a confidential communication between physician and patient, some states extend the privilege to the nurse, while other states rule that the communication is no longer privileged for the physician. Generally, the privilege extends to otherwise privileged information recorded in the hospital record.[109] However, information that is required to be reported to public authorities has generally been held not to be privileged unless the public authorities are also privileged not to disclose it.

Even when privileges otherwise apply, most states statutes include numerous exemptions from the privilege.[110] They vary between states.

Psychotherapist-Patient Privilege. In many states, a separate statute establishes a psychotherapist-patient privilege. The

---

[104] *E.g.,* Roosevelt Hotel Ltd. Partnership v. Sweeney, 394 N.W.2d 353 (Iowa 1986).
[105] Pa. Stat. Ann. title. 42, § 5929; *In re* June 1979 Allegheny County Investigating Grand Jury, 490 Pa. 143, 415 A.2d 73 (1980).
[106] Kan. Stat. Ann. § 60-427.
[107] Mich. Comp. Laws § 600.2157.
[108] N.Y. Civil Practice L. & R. § 4504.
[109] *E.g., In re* New York City Council v. Goldwater, 284 N.Y. 296, 31 N.E.2d 31 (1940).
[110] *E.g.,* Edelstein v. Department of Public Health, 240 Conn. 658, 692 A.2d 803 (1997) [physician-patient privilege not applicable to subpoena by state public health department investigating billing practices].

definition of a psychotherapist varies. The Georgia Supreme Court ruled that the state psychiatrist-patient privilege applied to non-psychiatrists who devoted a substantial part of their time to mental diseases.[111]

In 1996, the United States Supreme Court recognized a federal psychotherapist-patient privilege.[112] The Supreme Court left open the possibility that a dangerous patient exception might develop, but federal appellate courts have refused to create such an exception.[113] In 2000, a federal appellate court ruled that parties waive the privilege when they place their medical condition in issue.[114]

Because most third-party payers require waiver of the privilege before providing payment, some psychotherapists make other arrangements with patients for payment to protect confidentiality.[115]

Waiver. The patient may waive the privilege, permitting the physician to testify. The privilege can be waived by contract. Insurance applications and policies often include waivers. Other actions can constitute implied waiver. Introducing evidence of medical details or failing to object to physician testimony generally waives the privilege.[116] Authorization of disclosure outside the testimonial context usually does not waive the privilege.[117] Thus, the patient generally may authorize other persons to have access to medical records outside of court and still successfully object to having them introduced into evidence unless other actions have waived the privilege. In a few states, authorization of any disclosure to opposing

---

111 Wiles v. Wiles, 264 Ga. 594, 448 S.E.2d 681 (1994).

112 Jaffee v. Redmund, 518 U.S. 1 (1996); Newton v. Kemna, 354 F.3d 776 (8th Cir. 2004) [denied access to challenge competency of witness); Oleszko v. State Comp. Ins. Fund, 243 F.3d 1154 (9th Cir. 2001) [Employee Assistance Program information protected]; Henry v. Kernan, 197 F.3d 1021 (9th Cir. 1999) [must have reasonable belief doctor is psychotherapist for privilege to apply]; United States v. Schwensow, 151 F.3d 650 (7th Cir. 1998) [communications with the Alcoholics Anonymous telephone hotline volunteers not protected, since not psychotherapists].

113 *E.g.,* United States v. Chase, 340 F.3d 978 (9th Cir. 2003) (en banc), *cert. denied,* 540 U.S. 1220 (2004); United States v. Hayes, 227 F.3d 578 (6th Cir 2000); United States v. Glass, 133 F.3d 1356 (10th Cir.1998) [refuse to apply dangerous patient exception to facts of case]; *but see also In re* Grand Jury Proceedings (Violette), 183 F.3d 71 (1st Cir. 1999) [crime-fraud exception recognized].

114 Schoffstall v. Henderson, 223 F.3d 818 (8th Cir. 2000); *contra,* Vanderbilt v. Town of Chilmark, 174 F.R.D. 225, 225-30 (D. Mass. 1997) (declining to find waiver where plaintiff sought emotional distress damages).

115 See *Medical records increasingly open,* WIS. ST. J., May 26, 1997, 3B.

116 *E.g.,* Inabnit v. Berkson, 199 Cal. App. 3d 1230, 245 Cal. Rptr. 525 (5th Dist. 1988) [patient's failure to challenge subpoena waived privilege].

117 *E.g.,* Cartwright v. Maccabees Mut. Life Ins. Co., 65 Mich. App. 670, 238 N.W.2d 368 (1975), *rev'd on other grounds,* 398 Mich. 238, 247 N.W.2d 298 (1976) [when misrepresentations in insurance application, life insurer entitled to verdict when widow invoked privilege].

parties waives the privilege.[118] One federal appellate court has ruled that any disclosure to a third party waives the federal psychotherapist-patient privilege.[119]

Making a claim based on emotional distress or other mental condition usually waives the psychotherapist-patient privilege.[120] In some states, if the mental claim is dropped from the suit, the privilege is restored.[121]

Waiver of the privilege usually permits only formal discovery and testimony, not informal interviews. Express patient consent is generally required before informal interviews are permitted.[122] Other courts have permitted informal interviews based on waiver of the privilege.[123] However, in some states, it may be breach of the physician's duty to the patient to engage in informal interviews.[124] Most providers limit disclosures to formal channels unless express patient consent is obtained. One federal trial court has ruled that the HIPAA privacy rules impose this requirement of express consent to informal interviews.[125]

8-4.3 *What Other Federal Privacy Laws Are Still Applicable?*

The HIPAA privacy rules are not the only federal privacy laws applicable to health care information. For example, the federal substance abuse confidentiality rules remain in effect.

SUBSTANCE ABUSE. Special federal rules deal with confidentiality of information concerning patients treated or referred for treatment for alcoholism or drug abuse.[126] The rules apply to any

---

[118] *E.g.,* Willis v. Order of R.R. Telegraphers, 139 Neb. 46, 296 N.W. 443 (1941).

[119] United States v. Bishop, 1998 U.S. App. LEXIS 15147 (6th Cir.) [conviction for murdering fellow VA patient upheld; disclosure to police permitted therapists to testify].

[120] *E.g.,* Maynard v. City of San Jose, 37 F.3d 1396 (9th Cir. 1994); Premack v. J.C.J. Ogar, Inc., 148 F.R.D. 140 (E.D. Pa. 1993).

[121] *E.g.,* Sykes v. St. Andrews School, 619 So. 2d 467 (Fla. 4th DCA 1993).

[122] *E.g.,* State *ex rel.* Kitzmiller v. Henning, 190 W.Va. 142, 437 S.W.2d 452 (1993); McClelland v. Ozenberger, 841 S.W.2d 227 (Mo. Ct. App. 1992); Loudon v. Mhyre, 110 Wash. 2d 675, 756 P.2d 138 (1988); Nelson v. Lewis, 130 N.H. 106, 534 A.2d 720 (1987).

[123] *E.g.,* Huzjak v. United States, 118 F.R.D. 61 (N.D. Ohio 1987) [treating physician may voluntarily engage in ex parte contacts, but cannot be compelled to do so]; Trans-World Invs. v. Drobny, 554 P.2d 1148 (Alaska 1976); Gobuty v. Kavanagh, 795 F. Supp. 281 (D. Minn. 1992) [state law permitted defending physician to informally communicate with plaintiff's treating physician with 15 days notice].

[124] *E.g.,* Requena v. Franciscan Sisters Health Care Corp., 212 Ill. App. 3d 328, 570 N.E.2d 1214 (3d Dist. 1991).

[125] Law v. Zuckerman, 307 F. Supp. 2d 705 (D. Md. 2004) [HIPAA precludes ex parte contacts with treating MD].

[126] 42 C.F.R. pt. 2, implementing 42 U.S.C § 290dd-2.

specialized program for substance abuse in any facility receiving federal funds for any purpose, including Medicare or Medicaid reimbursement. Since 1994, the rules have not applied to treatment outside of specialized programs; so they do not apply to most emergency room treatments.[127]

The regulations preempt any state law that purports to authorize disclosures contrary to the regulations, but states are permitted to impose tighter confidentiality requirements. The rules apply to any disclosure, even acknowledgment of the patient's presence in the facility. Information may be released with the patient's consent if the consent is in writing and contains all the elements required by the federal rules.

A court order, including a subpoena, does not permit release of information unless the requirements of the regulations have all been met.[128] The regulations require a court hearing and a court finding that the purpose for which the order is sought is more important than the purpose for which Congress mandated confidentiality. The regulations have been interpreted to permit hospitals to tell the court why they cannot comply with the order until after a hearing. After a hearing, courts have ordered disclosures to assist probation revocation and child abuse proceedings,[129] to assist an Internal Revenue Service investigation of a surgeon,[130] and other situations.[131] Courts have declined to order disclosure when the information was sought to challenge the credibility of witnesses, assist in determining the rehabilitation potential of a convicted person for purposes of sentencing, or assist in a drug possession investigation.[132]

---

[127] Center for Legal Advocacy v. Earnest, 320 F.3d 1107 (10th Cir. 2003); 59 FED. REG. 42,561 (Aug. 18, 1994).

[128] *E.g.*, United States *ex rel.* Chandler v. Cook County, 277 F.3d 969 (7th Cir. 2002) [mandamus striking down discovery order contrary to regulations].

[129] *E.g.*, United States v. Hopper, 440 F. Supp. 1208 (N.D. Ill. 1977) [probation revocation]; *In re* Baby X, 97 Mich. App. 111, 293 N.W.2d 736 (1980) [child neglect]; *see also* United States v. Corona, 849 F.2d 562 (11th Cir. 1988), *cert. denied*, 489 U.S. 1084 (1989) [trial court did not err in permitting use of records of defendant when court could have found criteria for disclosure met].

[130] United States v. Providence Hosp., 507 F. Supp. 519 (E.D. Mich. 1981).

[131] *E.g.*, *In re* August, 1993 Regular Grand Jury, 854 F. Supp. 1380 (S.D. Ind. 1994) [grand jury investigation of possible criminal conduct by psychotherapist]; State Bd. of Medical Examiners v. Fenwick Hall, Inc., 308 S.C. 477, 419 S.E.2d 222 (1992) [disclosure to licensing board]; O'Boyle v. Jensen, 150 F.R.D. 519 (M.D. Pa. 1993) [civil rights suit for death in police custody].

[132] *E.g.*, United States v. Cresta, 825 F.2d 538 (1st Cir. 1987), *cert. denied*, 486 U.S. 1042 (1988) [credibility]; United States v. Smith, 789 F.2d 196 (3d Cir. 1986) [credibility]; D. Canedy, *Judge upholds privacy for Jeb Bush's daughter,* N.Y. Times, Oct. 1, 2002, A22 [drug possession investigation].

Child abuse reports may be made under state law without patient consent or a court order, but release of records to child abuse agencies requires consent or an order.

Federal courts have ruled that the federal substance abuse rules do not create a private cause of action for violations, so that only the federal government can sue for violations.[133]

FAMILY EDUCATIONAL RIGHTS AND PRIVACY ACT (FERPA). Strict federal rules preclude universities from sharing information about students with their parents or others without the students consent.[134] This has created controversial situations where schools have not been able to involve parents in dealing with suicidal behaviors.[135] The HIPAA privacy rules do not apply to records that are subject to FERPA.[136]

FAIR AND ACCURATE CREDIT TRANSACTIONS ACT. There are federal restrictions on the use of medical information in credit reports.[137]

PRIVACY ACT. The Privacy Act[138] prohibits disclosures of records contained in a system of records maintained by a federal agency (or its contractors) without the written request or consent of the individual to whom the record pertains, subject to various statutory exceptions.

In some cases, the Privacy Act may prohibit some disclosures permitted by the HIPAA privacy rules. The preamble to the December 2000 HIPAA privacy rules indicates that the HIPAA privacy rules may prohibit some disclosures permitted by the Privacy Act and in those cases the HIPAA privacy rules must be followed.

8-5 What Are the Laws Concerning Use of Health Care Information?

The HIPAA privacy rules permit broad uses of PHI for treatment, payment, and health care operations without patient authorization. This is subject to the requirement that the covered entity has privacy poli-

---

[133] *E.g.,* Ellison v. Cocke County, Tenn., 63 F.3d 467 (6th Cir. 1995); Chapa v. Adams, 168 F.3d 1036 (7th Cir. 1999); Doe v. Broderick, 225 F.3d 2000 (4th Cir. 2000).

[134] 20 U.S.C. § 1232g(d).

[135] *See* S. Tavernise, *In college and in despair, with parents in the dark,* N.Y. TIMES, Oct. 26, 2003, 1.

[136] 45 C.F.R. 164.501 ["protected health information"].

[137] 15 U.S.C. 1681b(g); D. Paletta, *Medical data rules: exceptions proposed,* AM. BANKER, Apr. 7, 2004, 4; 69 FED. REG. 23,380 (Apr. 28, 2004) [proposed rules].

[138] 5 U.S.C. § 552a.

cies, workforce members be trained on the requirements, and contractors who have access to the information have a business associate agreement with the covered entity addressing the requirements.

These uses are generally subject to the minimum necessary standards mentioned in Section 8-4.1.

The December 2000 HIPAA privacy rules would have required a signed consent from the patient or a patient representative. However, this was deleted in the August 2003 amendments when it was realized that the consent requirement would have been a tremendous administrative expense and a barrier to access to care without presenting patient with any real choice. No provider could function without being able to use the information in this manner; so patients who would not or could not sign the consent would have had to forgo care. The consent requirement would have been a barrier to timely access for children, mentally disabled persons, and others who could not sign and had no representative readily available.

State law has long recognized that providers must be able to use PHI; so the HIPAA privacy rules are consistent with the law of most states.

TREATMENT. Those who are involved in patient care must have timely access to records to fulfill the patient care functions of the records. Records must be readily accessible for present and future patient care. There will always be some risk of occasional unauthorized access by others. Tremendous steps have been taken to find ways to reduce the opportunities for others to gain access while maintaining the necessary access for patient care, but each innovation must be carefully examined to be sure that the new zeal for privacy does not compromise patient care.

In the past, some courts have tried to draw a distinction between diagnosis and treatment. HIPAA expressly rejects this distinction; *treatment* is defined to include "the provision, coordination, or management of health care and related services by one or more health care providers" and *health care* is defined to include diagnosis.[139]

HIPAA includes within the definition of permitted treatment uses the exchange of information among providers for consultation, referrals, and other treatment purposes. It is not unusual for a provider to need to know about the prior or concurrent treatment from other providers.

---

[139] 45 C.F.R. §§ 160.103 ["health care"], 164.501 ["treatment"].

PAYMENT. Providers must be able to use health care information to process claims for payment. Payers have a legitimate need for data to justify their payments, and providers must be able to provide that data. State laws also recognize this.[140] HIPAA broadly defines what is in the scope of payment.[141]

HEALTH CARE OPERATIONS. Medical records are also business records. Many staff members must have access to them to operate the health care organization. The organization has authority to permit internal access by professional, technical, and administrative personnel who need access. Examples of uses requiring access include auditing, filing, replying to inquiries, quality improvement, risk management, and defending potential litigation. HIPAA broadly defines the scope of health care operations.[142]

Under prior law, these administrative uses were so widely understood that they were seldom addressed in reported court decisions. The few cases were decided in favor of administrative access. In 1965, the highest court of New York authorized a trustee to examine medical records of patients involved in a controversial research project.[143] In 1975, a Missouri court upheld the authority of hospitals to review records for quality assurance purposes.[144] In 1979, a Canadian court ruled that the hospital's insurers and lawyers may have access to prepare to deal with patient claims.[145] However, in 1999, the Ohio Supreme Court ruled that a hospital could not share its records with a law firm that was hired to screen medical records to locate patients who could seek government payments.[146] Other courts have not placed this limit on the ability of hospitals to use agents. Some plaintiffs' attorneys have attempted to bar hospital attorneys from communicating with physicians and hospital employees involved in the case with-

---

[140] *E.g.*, Wilkinson v. Methodist, Richard Young Hosp., 259 Neb. 745, 612 N.W.2d 213 (2000) [hospital staff may access, use computer information for billing purposes].

[141] 45 C.F.R. § 164.501 ["payment"].

[142] 45 C.F.R. § 164.501 ["health care operations"].

[143] Hyman v. Jewish Chronic Disease Hosp., 15 N.Y.2d 317, 258 N.Y.S.2d 397, 399, 206 N.E.2d 338 (1965).

[144] Klinge v. Lutheran Med. Ctr., 518 S.W.2d 157 (Mo. Ct. App. 1974).

[145] *In re* General Accident Assurance Co. of Canada & Sunnybrook Hosp., 23 O.R.(2d) 513 (Ont. High Ct. of Justice 1979); *accord* Rea v. Pardo, 132 A.D.2d 442, 522 N.Y.S.2d 393 (4th Dept. 1987) [patient request to send record to attorney justified physician sending copy to his insurer]; Archambault v. Roller, 254 Va. 210, 491 S.E.2d 729 (1997) [nonparty physician being deposed in malpractice action may disclose patient information to attorney].

[146] Biddle v. Warren Gen. Hosp., 86 Ohio St. 3d 395, 715 N.E.2d 518 (1999).

out the presence of the plaintiffs' attorneys. Courts have generally rejected these attempts.[147]

RESEARCH. Prior to the HIPAA privacy rules, health care providers generally could use their own records to conduct medical research without patient consent. Federal human subject regulations and many state laws expressly authorized this practice. Federal human subject regulations exempted some research involving only records from review processes or made the research eligible for expedited review.[148] Important medical discoveries have been made through researching medical records.[149]

The HIPAA privacy rules essentially eliminated the exemption from review. An Institutional Review Board or Privacy Board must review all records research, and patient authorization must be obtained unless an Institutional Review Board or Privacy Board grants a waiver of authorization.[150]

8-6 What Are the Laws Concerning Disclosure of Health Care Information?

This section discusses the circumstances in which health care information can or must be disclosed outside of the covered entity and those working for the covered entity. The following questions are addressed:

8-6.1. When can the patient or representative authorize disclosure of PHI?

8-6.2. When and how can disclosure be compelled in legal proceedings?

---

[147] *E.g.*, Lancaster v. Loyola Univ. Med. Ctr., 1992 U.S. Dist. LEXIS 15207 (N.D. Ill.) [hospital employees]; Morgan v. Cook County, 252 Ill. App. 3d 947, 625 N.E.2d 136 (1st Dist. 1993) [treating physician, when suit seeks to make hospital vicariously liable]; Alachua Gen. Hosp. v. Stewart, 649 So. 2d 357 (Fla. 1st DCA 1995) [physician, when suit seeks to make hospital vicariously liable]; *but see* Ritter v. Rush-Presbyterian-St. Luke's Med. Ctr., 177 Ill. App. 3d 313, 532 N.E.2d 327 (1st Dist. 1988) [hospital not even permitted to interview its codefendant employee treating physicians].

[148] 45 C.F.R. § 46.101(b)(5); 46 FED. REG. 8,392 (1981); *see also* 56 FED. REG. 67,078 (1991) [HCFA allowed release of patient identifiable information from Uniform Clinical Data Set for research purposes].

[149] See, *E.g.*, T. Meyer, *Chest radiation linked to breast cancer*, WIS. ST. J., Feb. 13, 1998, 6A [discovery from review of medical records of 3,436 patients]; D. McKenzie, *Harvesting data: A little less privacy leads to better care*, AM. MED. NEWS, Jan. 26, 1998, 14; *Scientists use medical-record data bases to detect adverse side effects of drugs*, WALL ST. J., Mar. 24, 1988, 33; L. Gordis & E. Gold, *Privacy, confidentiality, and the use of medical records in research*, 207 SCIENCE 153 (1980).

[150] 45 C.F.R. § 164.512(i).

8-6.3. When are providers required or authorized to report PHI to legal authorities and others?

8-6.4. When may providers disclose PHI in response to inquiries from legal authorities?

8-6.5. When may providers disclose PHI in response to inquiries from others?

8-6.1 When Can the Patient or Representative Authorize Disclosure of PHI?

With rare exceptions, the patient (or representative of an incapacitated patient) may authorize release of PHI to themselves or others.

AUTHORIZATION BY PATIENT. Competent patients can generally authorize access to themselves and others. The HIPAA privacy regulations recognize this right, while permitting withholding of information in limited circumstances if specified procedures are followed.[151]

The right of access by the patient has been widely recognized prior to HIPAA either through statutes or court decisions.[152] In 1986, a Pennsylvania court found that denial of access could be intentional infliction of emotional distress.[153] In 1990, the Maryland high court ruled that a hospital could be assessed punitive damages for failing to provide requested medical records within a reasonable time.[154]

In 1994, a Florida appellate court ruled that a health care provider could require that the patient's signature on a release form be notarized.[155] This case should not be interpreted to suggest that notarization is necessary. However, it is clear that courts will accept identity checks that are appropriate to the situation.

Providers generally cannot condition release of records on prior arrangements for payment for the documented care. In 1997, a California appellate court ruled that a provider could not require the patient to sign a lien before releasing records.[156]

The right to authorize others to have access has also been widely recognized prior to HIPAA.[157]

---

[151] 45 C.F.R. §§ 164.524 [self], 164.508 [others].

[152] *E.g.,* FLA STAT. § 395.017 [hospitals]; § 455.241 [individual professionals]; ILL. REV. STAT. ch. 110 §§ 8-2001-8-2004; Annotation, *Patient's right to disclosure of his or her own medical records under state freedom of information act,* 26 A.L.R. 4TH 701; Wallace v. University Hosps. of Cleveland, 84 Ohio L. Abs. 224, 170 N.E.2d 261 (Ct. App. 1960).

[153] Pierce v. Penman, 357 Pa. Super. 225, 515 A.2d 948 (1986).

[154] Franklin Square Hosp. v. Laubach, 318 Md. 615, 569 A.2d 693 (1990).

[155] Lee County v. State Farm Mutual Auto. Ins. Co., 634 So. 2d 250 (Fla. 2d DCA 1994).

[156] Person v. Farmers Ins. Group, 52 Cal. App. 4th 813, 61 Cal. Rptr. 2d 30 (2d Dist. 1997).

[157] *E.g.,* Pyramid Life Ins. Co. v. Masonic Hosp. Ass'n, 191 F. Supp. 51 (W.D. Okla. 1961).

HIPAA generally permits disclosures to family members, relatives, and close friends who are involved in the patient's care, unless the patient objects.[158] In essence, there is implied authorization to keep those involved in the patient's care informed, unless the patient objects or other law prohibits the disclosure. The federal substance abuse confidentiality rules discussed in Section 8-4.3 restrict disclosures related to substance abuse treatment.

Release of psychiatric information is subject to special restrictions in some states. In 1982, a New York court stated that a spouse should not be given psychiatric information, even when there is no estrangement, unless (1) the patient authorizes disclosure or (2) a danger to the patient, spouse, or another person can be reduced by disclosure.[159] Some states authorize disclosure of psychiatric information to spouses and others in additional circumstances.[160]

Providers can refuse to release records until presented with a release form that complies with their reasonable policies. A Missouri court upheld a hospital's refusal to release records to an attorney who presented a form with an altered date.[161]

When providers agree to release information, they may be liable for failing to do so. In 1999, a federal appellate court ruled that a former patient could sue a psychiatric facility, when a staff member failed to fulfill a promise to inform the patient's employer that the employee was unable to come to work.[162]

Exceptions. The HIPAA privacy rules recognize that there are some circumstances where release of the information to the patient can endanger the life or physical safety of the patient and permit withholding information in such cases subject to a right to have the decision reviewed.[163] Courts had previously recognized some exceptions to the general rule in favor of access. Courts have generally insisted that medically contraindicated information be made available to the patient's representative, who is frequently an outside professional acting on behalf of the patient. For example, in 1979, a federal appellate court addressed the withholding of information from patients preparing for hearings challenging their transfer to a lower level of care.[164]

---

[158] 45 C.F.R. § 164.510(b).

[159] MacDonald v. Clinger, 84 A.D.2d 482, 446 N.Y.S.2d 801 (4th Dept. 1982).

[160] *E.g.,* IOWA CODE ANN. § 229.25.

[161] Thurman v. Crawford, 652 S.W.2d 240 (Mo. Ct. App. 1983).

[162] Byers v. Toyota Motor Manufacturing Ky., Inc., 1998 U.S. App. LEXIS 33155 (6th Cir.) (unpub).

[163] 45 C.F.R. § 164.524(a)(3).

[164] Yaretsky v. Blum, 592 F.2d 65 (2d Cir. 1979), *appeal after remand*, 629 F.2d 817 (2d Cir. 1980), *rev'd*, 457 U.S. 991 (1982) [no right to hearing before transfer].

The court ruled that it was not enough for the state to offer to release information to a representative when the patient did not have a representative. The state was permitted to withhold medically contraindicated information from patients only when they had representatives, provided by the state if necessary.

Mental health information is treated differently in some circumstances. In 1995, the Utah Supreme Court ruled that a mental health clinic could assert a privilege not to disclose its records even after the patient executed a release document.[165] In a 1983 case, a New York mental hospital attempted to enforce its policy of releasing records only to physicians.[166] The court ruled that the records could be protected from disclosure only if the hospital proved release would cause detriment (1) to the patient, (2) to involved third parties, or (3) to an important hospital program. Because none of these was proved, the court ordered disclosure to the persons authorized by the patient. In 1997, a federal court ruled that a Florida statute denying persons with mental conditions access to obtain their medical records after discharge discriminated against persons with mental disabilities, violating the Americans with Disabilities Act.[167]

AUTHORIZATION BY THE PATIENT'S REPRESENTATIVE. When authorization is required and the patient is unable to authorize access because of incapacity, minority, or death, someone other than the patient must authorize access. The HIPAA privacy rules state that a personal representative of the patient has the same rights as the patient and specifies how to determine who may be a personal representative.[168]

Mentally Incapacitated Patients. The HIPAA privacy rules generally look to state law to identify the personal representative. Anyone that state law permits to make medical decisions is a personal representative. Some courts have suppressed family confidences and information that could upset the patient severely.[169] Similarly, the HIPAA privacy rules permit withholding information that is reasonably likely to cause substantial harm.[170]

---

[165] Salt Lake Child & Family Therapy Clinic, Inc. v. Frederick, 890 P.2d 1017 (Utah 1995).

[166] Cynthia B. v. New Rochelle Hosp. Med. Ctr., 60 N.Y.2d 452, 470 N.Y.S.2d 1221, 458 N.E.2d 363 (1983).

[167] Doe v. Stincer, 990 F. Supp. 1427 (S.D. Fla. 1997).

[168] 45 C.F.R. § 164.502(g).

[169] *E.g.,* Gaertner v. State, 385 Mich. 49, 187 N.W.2d 429 (1971).

[170] 45 C.F.R. § 164.524(a)(3)(iii).

In 2004, a New York court ruled that under the HIPAA privacy rules an agent under an activated health care proxy was entitled to access.[171]

When the mental incapacity is temporary and the release of the information can reasonably wait, it usually is appropriate to wait for the patient's authorization.

Minors. The HIPAA privacy rules generally look to state law to determine when a parent or other person *in loco parentis* is the personal representative and may authorize disclosure of PHI.[172] For most minors, state laws provide for the decision whether to release records to be made by a custodial parent. Access rights of noncustodial parents vary from state to state and can depend on the specific wording of the applicable court order assigning custodial rights.[173]

States vary greatly in the extent to which older minors are allowed to control access of parents and guardians to records.[174] Some state statutes specify that information regarding certain types of treatment, such as treatment for venereal disease and substance abuse, cannot be disclosed without the minor's consent. Some statutes specify that parents must be informed before a minor obtains certain kinds of services.[175]

In some states, when minors may legally consent to their own care, parents do not have a right to information concerning the care. If the minor fails to make other arrangements to pay for the care and relies on the parents to pay, the parents can be entitled to more information.

Providers generally can release information concerning immature minors to custodial parents without substantial risk of liability unless state statutes expressly prohibit release. When a mature minor wishes information withheld from parents, the provider must

---

[171] Mougiannis v. North Shore-Long Island Jewish Health System (N.Y. Sup Ct. May 2004), *as reported in* N.Y.L.J., May 19, 2004, 19.

[172] 45 C.F.R. § 164.502(g)(2),(3).

[173] *E.g.,* Leaf v. Iowa Methodist Med. Ctr., 460 N.W.2d 892 (Iowa Ct. App. 1990) [noncustodial parent's access right to minor's medical records].

[174] *E.g.* In the Matter of Marriage of Jones, 983 S.W.2d 377 (Tex. App. 1999) [psychologist must disclose records of treatment of minor to parent]; Attorney ad litem for D.K. v. Parents of D.K., 780 So. 2d 301 (Fla. 4th DCA 2001) [minor may block parent access to mental health records]; S.C. v. Guardian ad litem, 845 So. 2d 953 (Fla. 4th DCA 2003) [guardian ad litem cannot have unlimited access to minor's mental health records]; *see also* T.L. Cheng et al., *Confidentiality in health care*, 269 J.A.M.A. 1404 (1993) [survey of adolescent attitudes indicated they would not seek health services to avoid disclosure of certain information]; Council on Scientific Affairs, American Med. Ass'n, *Confidential health services for adolescents*, 269 J.A.M.A. 1420 (1993) [encouraging increased confidentiality].

[175] *E.g.,* H.L. v. Matheson, 450 U.S. 398 (1981) [Utah parental consent requirement for abortions].

make a professional judgment concerning information release to the parents except in the few circumstances where the law is settled, such as when a constitutional statute requires or forbids notification. Disclosure is generally permitted when there is likelihood of harm (such as contagious disease) to the minor or others and avoidance of that harm requires parental involvement.

State statutes should be followed. A Georgia court ruled that a father could sue a psychiatrist for releasing his minor daughter's mental health records to his former wife's attorney for use in custody litigation.[176] The daughter had requested the release and had ratified it after becoming an adult, but the release did not comply with the state statute.

Deceased Patients. The HIPAA privacy rules apply after the death of the patient.[177] The executor, administrator, or other person authorized to act on behalf of the deceased individual or estate may act as the personal representative.[178] Disclosures can be made without authorization for some law enforcement purposes, disposal of the body, or cadaveric organ donation.[179]

If there is an executor or administrator of the estate, required authorizations should usually be sought from that person.[180] If there is no executor or administrator, in most states authorization should be obtained from the next of kin, such as a surviving spouse[181] or a child.[182] Authorizations signed by the patient before death may still apply. In 1992, the Canadian Supreme Court ruled that a hospital must release records to a life insurance company pursuant to the release signed by the patient in the insurance application.[183]

The Wisconsin Supreme Court ruled that a hospital could insist that the person signing an authorization for release of the records of a deceased person state the authority of the person signing.[184]

---

[176] Mrozinski v. Pogue, 205 Ga. App. 731, 423 S.E.2d 405 (1992).

[177] 45 C.F.R. § 146.502(f).

[178] 45 C.F.R. § 146.502(g)(4).

[179] 45 C.F.R. § 146.512 (f)(4), (g), (h).

[180] *E.g.,* Scott v. Henry Ford Hosp., 199 Mich. App. 241, 501 N.W.2d 259 (1993) [only executor may authorize release; wife does not have authority]; In Interest of Roy, 423 Pa. Super. 183, 620 A.2d 1172 (1992) [only executor can authorize release of mental health records]; Annotation, *Who may waive privilege of confidential communication to physician by person since deceased,* 97 A.L.R. 2D 393.

[181] *E.g.,* Gerkin v. Werner, 106 Misc. 2d 643, 434 N.Y.S.2d 607 (Sup. Ct. 1980).

[182] *E.g.,* Emmett v. Eastern Dispensary and Casualty Hosp., 130 U.S. App. D.C. 50, 396 F.2d 931 (1967).

[183] Metropolitan Life Ins. Co. v. Frenette, [1992] 1 S.C.R. 647.

[184] Fanshaw v. Medical Protective Ass'n, 52 Wis. 2d 234, 190 N.W.2d 155 (1971).

8-6.2 When and How Can Disclosure Be Compelled in Legal Proceedings?

Even if the patient or representative opposes information release, health care providers can be compelled by law to disclose information in legal proceedings through the subpoenas and other procedures to discover evidence.

In lawsuits and administrative proceedings, the parties are authorized by law to demand relevant unprivileged information in the control of others. Lawyers call this the *discovery* process.

SUBPOENAS AND OTHER DISCOVERY ORDERS. The most frequent discovery demand is called a subpoena. A subpoena is a demand for a person to appear at a certain place at a certain time, and it frequently requires the person to bring certain documents. In federal courts and in most states, demands to parties are generally called notices of deposition or notices to produce, while actual subpoenas are used only for persons who are not parties to the suit. Notices and subpoenas have essentially the same effect; so what is said about subpoenas in the rest of this chapter also applies to notices. When the demands are ignored, a court can order compliance, and further noncompliance can be punished as contempt of court.

Other discovery orders can require a person to submit to a physical or mental examination or to permit inspection of land, buildings, or other property.

In some jurisdictions, a subpoena is issued by the court and constitutes a court order. A court order is generally sufficient authorization to release a medical record, unless special protections apply. For example, federal rules require a court order before substance abuse records may be released.

In some jurisdictions where individual attorneys are permitted to issue subpoenas without involvement of a court, noncourt subpoenas are not sufficient authorization to release medical records in some circumstances.[185] In those circumstances, the provider should assert the confidentiality of the records and demand a court order or authorization from the patient or an appropriate representative.

---

[185] *E.g., In re* Grand Jury Subpoena for Medical Records of Curtis Payne, 150 N.H. 436, 839 A.2d 837 (2004); Rost v. State Bd. of Psychology, 659 A.2d 626 (Pa. Commw. 1995) [affirming reprimand of psychologist for complying with subpoena by releasing patient records without consent]; Simms v. Bradach, No. MON-L-393-01 (N.J. Super Ct. Monmouth County Sept. 13, 2002), *as discussed in* H. Gottlieb, *Judge bars use of subpoenas for medical records patient's authorization is required*, N.J.L.J. Nov. 4, 2002.

When the subpoena is sufficient, it is important to submit the documents to the right person. In 1997, the Rhode Island Supreme Court ruled that subpoenaed records should be delivered to the court, not to the requesting attorney.[186]

Some states have sought to simplify the discovery process by mandating exchange of records. In 1997, the Illinois Supreme Court declared such a law to be an unconstitutional violation of the separation of powers and of privacy rights.[187]

HIPAA REQUIREMENTS. The HIPAA privacy rules permit subpoenas and other court-ordered releases of PHI, but there is a change from the prior practice in most states. When a subpoena is issued without a court order, the covered entity must be provided with assurances that there have been reasonable efforts to notify the patient or obtain a protective order.[188]

MEDICAL INFORMATION. A subpoena can require that medical records (or copies) be provided to the court or to the other side in the suit. A subpoena can require a person to submit to formal questioning under oath prior to the trial. This question-and-answer session is called a *deposition* and often is used as testimony in the trial if the person questioned cannot be at the trial. If the person questioned is at the trial and gives different testimony, the deposition can be used for *impeachment*, which means to cast doubt on what is said at the trial.

Parties. Under the current liberal discovery practices, medical records of parties can nearly always be subpoenaed if the mental or physical condition of the party is relevant. When records can be subpoenaed, those who provided the health care usually can be ordered also to give depositions.

Nonparties. In most circumstances, courts will not permit discovery of information concerning health care of persons who are not parties.[189] Some attorneys have sought such information to establish what happened when similar treatment was given to other patients. Providers have resisted these attempts on the basis that they invade patient privacy, violate the physician-patient privilege

---

186 Washburn v. Rite Aid Corp., 695 A.2d 495 (R.I. 1997).
187 Kunkel v. Walton, 179 Ill. 2d 519, 689 N.E.2d 1047 (1997).
188 45 C.F.R. § 164.512(e)(1)(ii); *E.g.*, Hutton v. City of Martinez, 219 F.R.D. 164 (N.D. Cal. 2003).
189 *E.g.*, Bristol-Meyers Squibb Co. v. Hancock, 921 S.W.2d 917 (Tex. Ct. App. 1996) [when surgeon sued breast implant manufacturer for injury to his reputation, income, company denied discovery of medical records of his patients]; Parkson v. Central Du Page Hosp., 105 Ill. App. 3d 850, 435 N.E.2d 140 (1st Dist. 1982).

discussed later in this chapter, and are not relevant because of the uniqueness of the condition and reaction of each patient.

The only widely accepted exceptions in which discovery of nonparty records has been permitted have been cases of billing fraud or professional discipline.[190] Some courts have permitted access to medical records of nonparties in malpractice suits but have required all "identifiers" to be deleted.[191] However, other courts have reaffirmed the traditional rule and declined to order access even with identifiers deleted.[192]

A series of cases in 2004 illustrate the strengths and weaknesses of the privacy protections from subpoenas of nonparty records in federal courts. The constitutionality of a new federal law banning certain abortion procedures was challenged in a series of cases. The United States Department of Justice (DOJ) subpoenaed the records of patients at the institutions where the expert physicians who were testifying in support of the challenge practiced.[193] Thus, DOJ sought the abortion records of nonparty patients ostensibly to cross-examine the plaintiff's experts.[194] The Seventh Circuit Court of Appeals in Chicago did not permit the records to be released.[195] However, it reached this conclusion on a basis that provides little assurance of how future cases will be handled. The court applied the established law to conclude that state privileges did not apply because the issue presented was a federal issue. It also decided that HIPAA created no privilege in federal cases; so it provided no protection from court orders. The court grounded its refusal to permit the release of the records on the basis that the burden of compliance with the subpoena would exceed the benefit of production of

---

[190] *E.g.,* St. Lukes Reg. Med. Ctr. v. United States, 717 F. Supp. 665 (N.D. Iowa 1989) [government entitled to disclosure of physician's medical records by administrative subpoena to investigate Medicaid civil violations]; Goldberg v. Davis, 151 Ill. 2d 267, 602 N.E.2d 812 (1992) [professional discipline]; Dr. K v. State Bd. of Physician Quality Assurance, 98 Md. App. 103, 632 A.2d 453, *cert. denied,* 513 U.S. 817 (1994) [professional discipline].

[191] *E.g.,* Amente v. Newman, 653 So. 2d 1030 (Fla. 1995); Todd v. South Jersey Hosp. Sys., 152 F.R.D. 676 (D. N.J. 1993); Terre Haute Reg. Hosp. v. Trueblood, 600 N.E.2d 1358 (Ind. 1992); Community Hosp. Ass'n v. District Court, 194 Colo. 98, 570 P.2d 243 (1977); State *ex rel.* Lester E. Cox Med. Ctr. v. Keet, 678 S.W.2d 813 (Mo. 1984) (en banc).

[192] *E.g.,* Buford v. Howe, 10 F.3d 1184 (5th Cir. 1994); Glassman v. St. Joseph Hosp., 259 Ill. App. 3d 730, 631 N.E.2d 1186 (1st Dist. 1994); Ekstrom v. Temple, 197 Ill. App. 3d 120, 553 N.E.2d 424 (2d Dist. 1990).

[193] E. Lichtbau, *Defending '03 law, Justice Dept. seeks abortion records,* N.Y. TIMES, Feb. 12, 2004, A1; R. Pear & E. Lichtbau, *Administration sets forth a limited view on privacy,* N.Y. TIMES, Mar. 6, 2004, A8.

[194] C. Anderson, *Justice Dept. wants doctors barred from testifying without abortion records,* AP, Mar. 1, 2004.

[195] Northwestern Mem. Hosp. v. Ashcroft, 362 F.3d 923 (7th Cir. 2004).

the material sought, since DOJ had articulated any benefit from the release. The court expressed concerns about the privacy of the records and expressed skepticism that removal (called *redaction*) of the patients' names and other identifiers would actually protect the patients from being identified. In the end, these privacy concerns could only be used as one factor in determining that the burden outweighed the benefit.

In the parallel New York case, the District Court ordered that the records be produced. The Second Circuit Court of Appeals in New York refused to hear the case until the hospital had been found in contempt. The hospital was found in contempt, but before the Second Circuit could hear the appeal, DOJ dropped its efforts to obtain the records.[196] Similarly, a District Court in Michigan ordered release of redacted records because the HIPAA procedure had been followed. The subpoenaed Michigan hospital had no records within the scope of the subpoena; so the decision was not appealed.[197]

PATIENT NAMES. Some attorneys have attempted to bypass the rule against disclosure of nonparty medical records by seeking nonparty patients' names and obtaining their permission to get the records. Providers have resisted these attempts for reasons similar to those for resisting discovery of records. Most courts have not permitted discovery of nonparty patient names. For example, the Michigan Supreme Court ruled that patients' names are protected by the physician-patient privilege.[198] Similarly, in 1987, the Florida Supreme Court denied discovery of blood donor names in an AIDS case.[199] In 1976, the Arizona Supreme Court ruled that the physician-patient privilege does not protect patient names in Arizona but

---

[196] E. Lichtbau, *Hospital is ordered to release abortion records*, N.Y. TIMES, Mar. 20, 2004, A1; M. Hamblett, *U.S. ends effort to gain abortion patient files, trial phase concludes*, N.Y.L.J., Apr. 27, 2004, 1.

[197] National Abortion Fed. v. Ashcroft, 2004 U.S. Dist. LEXIS 4491 (E.D. Mich.); S. Karush, *University of Michigan finds no abortion records to hand over in battle over ban*, AP, Mar. 25, 2004; *see also Federal judge blocks Justice Department abortion records request in Philadelphia*, AP, Mar. 27, 2004; D. Kravets, *Judge denies request for abortion records*, AP, Mar. 5, 2004 [CA case]; E. Lichtbau, *Justice Dept. backs off its demand for abortion records*, N.Y. TIMES, Mar. 10, 2004 [CA case].

[198] Schechet v. Kesten, 372 Mich. 346, 126 N.W.2d 718 (1964); Dorris v. Detroit Osteopathic Hosp. Corp., 559 N.W.2d 76 (Mich. Ct. App. 1996) [affirming denial of disclosure of name of nonparty patient who may have witnessed patient's refusal of drug]; *accord* Gunn v. Sound Shore Med. Ctr., 5 A.D.3d 435, 772 N.Y.S.2d 714 (2d Dept. 2004) [reject release of log of patients in rehab center when accident happened].

[199] Rasmussen v. South Fla. Blood Serv., 500 So. 2d 533 (Fla. 1987); *see* Annotation, *Discovery of identity of blood donor*, 56 A.L.R. 4TH 755.

still refused to order release of other names because it did not consider them relevant.[200]

In 1987, a Texas court allowed discovery of donor names in an AIDS case but prohibited contact with the donors.[201] In 1988, the Colorado Supreme Court ordered disclosure to the court clerk of the name of a donor with AIDS so that the plaintiff could submit written questions to the donor through the clerk.[202] In 1995, a federal court allowed the deposition of a donor with AIDS under a protective order to protect the donor's identity.[203] One attorney violated a court order restricting use of donor specific information. In 1994, a federal court ruled that, while the attorney could be punished, the case could not be dismissed as punishment.[204] There is a risk that records obtained without identifiers could be linked later to patient names through another exception.

COMMITTEE REPORTS. Many states have enacted statutes protecting quality improvement and peer review activities and committee reports from discovery or admission into evidence. These laws are designed to permit the candor necessary for effective peer review to improve quality and reduce morbidity and mortality. Courts have found these laws constitutional.[205]

Some courts have strictly interpreted statutory protections, reducing their effectiveness. For example, a New Jersey court refused to apply the statutory protection for "utilization review committees" to related committees, such as the medical records committee and infection control committee.[206] The Louisiana Supreme Court ruled that its statute did not protect nosocomial infection studies.[207] Nosocomial infections are the infections that are acquired in a hospital. The hostility of some courts to such privileges is illustrated by a West Virginia case that ruled that courts should not rely on a hospital's assertion of the privilege, but instead

---

[200] Banta v. Superior Court, 112 Ariz. 544, 544 P.2d 653 (1976); *accord* Mason v. Regional Med. Ctr., 121 F.R.D. 300 (W.D. Ky. 1988).
[201] Tarrant County Hosp. Dist. v. Hughes, 734 S.W.2d 675 (Tex. Ct. App.), *cert. denied*, 484 U.S. 1065 (1987).
[202] Belle Bonfils Mem. Blood Ctr. v. District Court, 763 P.2d 1003 (Colo. 1988).
[203] Marcella v. Brandywine Hosp., 47 F.3d 618 (3d Cir. 1995); *accord,* Watson v. Lowcountry Red Cross, 974 F.2d 482 (4th Cir. 1992).
[204] Coleman v. American Red Cross, 23 F.3d 1091 (6th Cir. 1994).
[205] *E.g.,* City of Edmund v. Parr, 587 P.2d 56 (Okla. 1978); Jenkins v. Wu, 102 Ill. 2d 468, 468 N.E.2d 1162 (1984); *but see* Southwest Commun. Health Servs. v. Smith, 107 N.M. 196, 755 P.2d 40 (1988) [law upheld, but court may ignore law when records sufficiently needed in litigation].
[206] Young v. King, 136 N.J. Super. 127, 344 A.2d 792 (Law Div. 1975).
[207] Smith v. Lincoln Gen. Hosp., 605 So. 2d 1347 (La. 1992).

should inspect all documents for which a privilege was claimed and require the hospital to prove that each document was protected by the privilege.[208]

Some courts have interpreted statutory protections broadly.[209] In 1997, the Iowa Supreme Court ruled that peer review law permitted state hospital to refuse to disclose nosocomial infection reports requested under open records law.[210] The Minnesota Supreme Court found that a complications conference report was protected under a statute that protected "the proceedings and records of a review organization."[211] Under some states' laws, the identities of persons involved in peer review are also protected.[212] In 2005, an Ohio appellate court ruled that a hospital did not have to produce a list of peer reviewed documents in order to assert the privilege for them.[213]

Some state laws only protect peer review records from discovery; if they are obtained through other channels they can be used in court.[214] Other laws protect the records from being introduced in lawsuits even if they are obtained outside discovery channels.[215]

Even when the privilege does apply, many state laws permit state licensing agencies to gain access.[216] This can become a significant loophole in the protection of this information. In 1998, the Kansas Supreme Court permitted private plaintiffs to access and use most of the records the state licensing agency had obtained.[217]

State law protections for peer review records do not apply in suits in federal court that involve federal law.[218] A few federal courts

---

[208] State *ex rel.* Shroades v. Henry, 187 W.Va. 723, 421 S.E.2d 264 (1992).

[209] *E.g.,* Carr v. Howard, 426 Mass. 514, 689 N.E.2d 1304 (1998) [reports for peer review committee confidential, cannot be provided to trial judge for in camera review]; Application to Quash a Grand Jury Subpoena, 239 A.D.2d 412, 657 N.Y.S.2d 747 (2d Dept. 1997) [quashing grand jury subpoena of hospital's quality assurance records].

[210] Burton v. University of Iowa Hosps. & Clinics, 566 N.W.2d 182 (Iowa 1997).

[211] Warrick v. Giron, 290 N.W.2d 166 (Minn. 1980).

[212] *E.g.,* Cedars-Sinai Med. Ctr. v. Superior Court, 12 Cal. App. 4th 579, 16 Cal. Rptr. 2d 253 (2d Dist. 1993).

[213] Huntsman v. Aultman Hosp., 160 Ohio App. 3d 196, 2005 Ohio 1482, 826 N.E.2d 384.

[214] *E.g.,* Ashokan v. Department of Ins., 109 Nev. 662, 856 P.2d 244 (1993).

[215] *E.g.,* FLA. STAT. §§ 395.0191–395.0193, 766.101; Young v. Saldanha, 189 W.Va. 330, 431 S.E.2d 669 (1993) [physician's use of peer review materials in suit against hospital concerning clinical privileges did not waive evidentiary privilege, so patient could not use materials in malpractice suit against physician].

[216] *E.g.,* St. Elizabeth's Hosp. v. State Bd. of Prof. Med. Conduct, 174 A.D.2d 225, 579 N.Y.S.2d 457 (3d Dept. 1992).

[217] Adams v. St. Francis Reg. Med. Ctr., 264 Kan. 144, 955 P.2d 1169 (1998).

[218] Fed. R. Evid. 501; *In re* Subpoena Duces Tecum, 2004 U.S. Dist. LEXIS 6494 (N.D. Ill.); Memorial Hosp. for McHenry County v. Shadur, 664 F.2d 1058 (7th Cir. 1981); Pagano v. Oroville Hosp., 145 F.R.D. 683 (E.D. Cal. 1993) [patient and physician identifiers deleted; HCQIA does not create privilege].

have recognized a common law qualified privilege based on the public interest in peer review activities. A District of Columbia court refused to order release of information concerning a peer review committee's activities.[219] In 1998, a federal court in Maryland limited discovery of peer review information in a federal antitrust suit.[220] However, other courts have refused to limit such discovery.[221] In 1997, the Missouri Supreme Court found a federal privilege for certain nursing home committee records.[222]

Because the status of committee reports is still an open question in many states, these reports should be carefully written so that, if they must be released, they will not inappropriately increase liability exposure.

RESPONSES TO SUBPOENAS AND OTHER DISCOVERY ORDERS. In most situations, the proper response to a valid subpoena or discovery order is compliance. However, prompt legal assistance should be sought because some subpoenas or orders are not valid and others should be resisted.[223] A discovery order should never be ignored.

Subpoenas from state courts in other states are usually not valid unless they are given to the person being subpoenaed while that person is in the state of the issuing court. For example, in 1993, a New York appellate court ruled that a New York physician could be sued for releasing information pursuant to a Pennsylvania state subpoena.[224] Courts in some states have authority to issue subpoenas to persons only in a limited area. Most states have a procedure for obtaining a valid subpoena from a local court to require the release of information for a trial in a distant court that does not have the

---

[219] Bredice v. Doctors Hosp., Inc., 50 F.R.D. 249 (D. D.C. 1970), *aff'd without op.*, 156 U.S. App. D.C. 199, 479 F.2d 920 (1973); *accord*, Laws v. Georgetown Univ. Hosp., 656 F. Supp. 824 (D. D.C. 1987).

[220] Price v. Howard County Gen. Hosp., No. Y-95-3355 (D. Md. June 6, 1997), *as discussed in* 7 H.L.R. 675 (1998).

[221] *E.g.*, Pagano v. Oroville Hosp., 145 F.R.D. 683 (E.D. Cal. 1993); Davison v. St. Paul Fire & Marine Ins. Co., 75 Wis. 2d 190, 248 N.W.2d 433 (1977).

[222] State *ex rel.* Boone Retirement Ctr. v. Hamilton, 946 S.W.2d 740 (Mo.1997) [records of nursing home QA committee privileged under federal law; writ of prohibition against criminal subpoena by state grand jury; privileged under 42 U.S.C. §§ 1395i-3(b)(1)(B), 1396r(b)(1)(B)].

[223] *E.g.*, Thomas v. Benedictine Hosp., 296 A.D.2d 781, 745 N.Y.S.2d 606 (3d Dept. 2002) [affirming order rejecting plaintiff's effort to depose hospital officials in malpractice lawsuit concerning physician treatment for leg fracture]; Allen v. Smith, 179 W.Va. 360, 368 S.E.2d 924 (1988) [if not protected by statute of limitations, psychiatrist could have been sued for complying with insufficient subpoena].

[224] Doe v. Roe, 190 A.D.2d 463, 599 N.Y.S.2d 350 (4th Dept. 1993).

authority to issue a valid subpoena. Some state courts will order a party to sign a document requesting and authorizing release of records, especially out-of-state records, instead of going through the process of obtaining an order where the records are located.[225]

Subpoenas from federal courts in other states are usually valid.

Sometimes challenges to subpoenas are successful. A New Jersey court refused to order a woman or her psychiatrist to answer questions concerning nonfinancial matters in a marriage separation case because the husband had failed to demonstrate relevance or good cause for the order.[226] When judges are not certain whether to order a release, they sometimes will order that the information be presented for court review before ruling. An Illinois court ruled that this review should be by a judge, not an administrative hearing officer.[227]

In some situations, the only way to obtain prompt appellate review of an apparently inappropriate discovery order is to risk being found in contempt of court. In one case a physician challenged a grand jury subpoena of records of sixty-three patients.[228] The trial court found him to be in contempt for failing to comply. The Illinois Supreme Court held that he must release the records of the one patient who had waived her physician-patient privilege but reversed the contempt finding on the other sixty-two records. They were protected by the physician-patient privilege in Illinois until a showing of a criminal action relating to the treatment documented in the records was made. In another Illinois case, the appellate court ruled that the trial court had erred in jailing a physician and his attorney for contempt of court concerning a deposition. The applicable statute did not permit more discovery than had been given, and the trial court failed to show any accommodation for the patients scheduled for the physician's care.[229]

Valid subpoenas should never be ignored and should never be challenged except on advice of an attorney. In 1978, an Illinois court affirmed a $1,000 fine assessed against an orthopedic surgeon for ignoring a subpoena and refusing to appear at a trial involving his patient.[230] In a Kansas case, a treating physician was jailed for refus-

---

[225] *E.g.,* Rojas v. Ryder Truck Rental, Inc., 641 So. 2d 855 (Fla. 1994); Doelfel v. Trevisani, 644 So. 2d 1359 (Fla. 1994).

[226] Ritt v. Ritt, 52 N.J. 177, 244 A.2d 497 (1968).

[227] Laurent v. Brelji, 74 Ill. App. 3d 214, 392 N.E.2d 929 (4th Dist. 1979).

[228] People v. Bickham, 89 Ill. 2d 1, 431 N.E.2d 365 (1982).

[229] Roth v. Saint Elizabeth's Hosp., 241 Ill. App. 3d 407, 607 N.E.2d 1356 (5th Dist. *appeal denied*), 151 Ill. 2d 577, 616 N.E.2d 347 (1993).

[230] Schmoll v. Bray, 61 Ill. App. 3d 64, 377 N.E.2d 1172 (4th Dist. 1978).

ing to testify until he was paid an expert witness fee.[231] In 2003, a Nebraska physician was arrested for failing to testify at a competency hearing. Due to confusion in communications over the schedule, charges were dropped after the physician apologized.[232]

Attorneys need to be cautious in giving such advice. A federal court found an attorney to be in contempt and fined the attorney for advising the client to resist a subpoena in a Medicare investigation.[233]

8-6.3 When Are Providers Required or Authorized to Report PHI to Legal Authorities and Others?

The law compels disclosure of medical information in many contexts other than discovery or testimony. Reporting laws have been enacted that require medical information to be reported to governmental agencies. The most common examples are vital statistics, communicable diseases, child abuse, and wound reporting laws. Familiarity with these and other reporting laws is important to assure compliance and to avoid reporting to the wrong agency. Reports to the wrong agency may not be legally protected, resulting in potential liability for breach of confidentiality.[234]

HIPAA. The HIPAA privacy rules generally permit covered entities to comply with state laws that require reports or other disclosures.[235]

VITAL STATISTICS. All states require the reporting of births and deaths.[236] These laws are a valid exercise of the state police power.[237]

PUBLIC HEALTH. Most states require reports of venereal disease and other communicable diseases.[238] A California court observed that in addition to criminal penalties for not reporting, civil liability is possible in a suit by persons who contract diseases that might have been avoided by proper reports.[239] Some states require reports of cancer and other selected noncontagious diseases.

---

[231] Swope v. State, 145 Kan. 928, 67 P.2d 416 (1937).
[232] *Regional center doctor arrested for failing to testify*, AP, Aug. 5, 2003; *Action ends against doctor who missed court date*, AP, Aug. 15, 2003.
[233] United States v. Fesman, 781 F. Supp. 511 (S.D. Ohio 1991).
[234] *E.g.*, Hope v. Landau, 398 Mass. 738, 500 N.E.2d 809 (1986) [immunity lost if child abuse report made to wrong agency]; *see also* Searcy v. Auerbach, 980 F.2d 609 (9th Cir. 1992) [psychologist who failed to follow statutory procedure for reporting child abuse not immune from civil liability].
[235] 45 C.F.R. §§ 164.512(a), 164.501 ["required by law"].
[236] *E.g.*, FLA. STAT. §§ 382.16, 382.081.
[237] *E.g.*, Robinson v. Hamilton, 60 Iowa 134, 14 N.W. 202 (1882).
[238] *E.g.*, FLA. STAT. § 381.231 [communicable diseases], § 384.25 [venereal diseases].
[239] Derrick v. Ontario Comm. Hosp., 47 Cal. App. 3d 145, 120 Cal. Rptr. 566 (4th Dist. 1975).

In 1998, the Alabama Supreme Court ruled that it was constitutional to require physicians to report the names of persons with AIDS.[240]

In 1994, a Missouri appellate court barred enforcement of a local court rule requiring correction facilities to disclose the infectious disease reports of inmates before court appearances.[241]

CHILD ABUSE. Most states require reports of suspected cases of child abuse or neglect.[242] The HIPAA privacy rules and the federal substance abuse confidentiality rules expressly permit child abuse reports.[243]

Some professionals, such as physicians and nurses, are mandatory reporters and thus are required to make reports. Anyone who is not a mandatory reporter may make a report as a permissive reporter. In some states, any report arising out of diagnosis or treatment in an institution must be made through the institutional administration. In some states, a professional is a mandatory reporter only when the child has been examined or treated but is a permissive reporter when the abuse is learned from the abuser or another person.[244] In some states, providers are required to report abuse that they learn from others but only if the abuse occurred in the state.[245]

Most child abuse reporting laws extend some degree of immunity from liability for reports made through proper channels.[246] A mandatory reporter who fails to report child abuse is subject to both criminal penalties[247] and civil liability for future injuries to the child that

---

[240] Mark Middlebrooks, M.D., P.A. v. Alabama Bd. of Health, 710 So. 2d 891 (Ala. 1998).

[241] State *ex rel.* Callahan v. Kinder, 879 S.W.2d 677 (Mo. Ct. App. 1994).

[242] *E.g.,* FLA. STAT. § 415.504; L.S. Wissow, *Current concepts: Child abuse and neglect,* 332 N. ENG. J. MED. 1425 (1995).

[243] 45 C.F.R. § 164.512(b)(1)(ii); 42 C.F.R. § 2.12(c)(6).

[244] *E.g.,* WIS. STAT. § 48.981(2)(a).

[245] *See* A. Goldstein, *Hospital for priests not required to report all abuse,* WASH. POST, June 30, 2002, C5 [Maryland AG opinion, provider not required to report abuse outside of state].

[246] *E.g.,* O'Heron v. Blaney, 276 Ga. 871, 583 S.E.2d 834 (2003); Meyer v. Lashley, 44 P.2d 553 (Okla. 2002); Casbohm v. Metrohealth Med. Ctr., 746 N.E.2d 661 (Ohio. App. 2000); Martinez v. Mafchir, 35 F.3d 1486 (10th Cir. 1994) [social worker protected]; *see also* People v. Wood, 447 Mich. 80, 523 N.W.2d 477 (1994) [social worker could contact police to obtain assistance in investigating possible neglect]; Bryant-Bruce v. Vanderbilt Univ. Inc., 974 F. Supp. 1127. (M.D. Tenn. 1997) [immunity only for report within scope of state duty to report; deny dismissal for other aspects of report]; Bol v. Cole, 561 N.W.2d 143 (Minn. 1997) [no immunity for copy of report given to patient's mother; only qualified privilege to release to mother to protect child who cannot otherwise protect self].

[247] *E.g.,* Gladson v. State, 258 Ga. 885, 376 S.E.2d 362 (1989); *Doctor faces penalty for failing to report child abuse,* AP, Nov. 8, 2002 [Iowa MD fined $5,000 in settlement with licensing board]; *Prosecutors drop charges against doctors accused of failing to report child abuse,* AP, Feb. 11, 2004 [Mich.].

could have been avoided if a report had been made.[248] In 2003, in a prosecution of an emergency nurse, a Missouri trail court decided that the criminal penalties for not reporting were unconstitutional.[249]

There have been disputes in some states over when some activities, such as sexual activity of younger minors, must be reported as child abuse.[250]

ADULT ABUSE/DOMESTIC VIOLENCE. Some states have enacted adult abuse reporting laws that are similar to the child abuse reporting laws.[251] Unlike child abuse laws, these laws are usually more permissive, with no required reporting.[252] The HIPAA privacy rules permit required reports; permissive reports are required in some limited circumstances.[253] These laws are controversial.[254]

WOUNDS. Many states require the reporting of certain wounds.[255] Some states specify that all wounds of certain types must be reported. For example, New York requires the reporting of wounds inflicted by sharp instruments that may result in death and

---

[248] *E.g.,* IOWA CODE ANN. § 232.75(2); Stecker v. First Commercial Trust Co., 962 S.W.2d 792 (Ark. 1998); Landeros v. Flood, 17 Cal. 3d 399, 131 Cal. Rptr. 69, 551 P.2d 389 (1976); *contra,* Vance v. T.R.C., 229 Ga. App. 608. 494 S.E.2d 714 (1997) [statute requiring child abuse report did not create private cause of action against physician for failure to report]; Annotation, *Validity, construction, and application of state statute requiring doctor or other person to report child abuse,* 73 A.L.R. 4TH 782; *Jury reaches $2 million verdict in injuries to abused infant,* AP, Apr. 29, 2002 [Missouri physician, day care center liable]; *but see* Cuyler v. United States, 362 F.3d 949 (7th Cir. 2004) [no implied duty of rescue in Ill. child abuse statute, so no civil liability].

[249] *Missouri reporting law for health care workers is unconstitutional,* AP, Sept. 11, 2003; *Missouri Supreme Court to hear arguments in nurse appeal,* AP, Apr. 30, 2004.

[250] *E.g.,* People v. Stockton Pregnancy Control Med. Clinic, 203 Cal. App. 3d 225, 249 Cal. Rptr. 762 (3d Dist. 1988) [must report sexual conduct of minors under age 14 if with person of disparate age]; Planned Parenthood Affiliates v. Van de Camp, 181 Cal. App. 3d 245, 226 Cal. Rptr. 361 (1st Dist. 1986) [not required to report all sexual activity of minors under age 14]; *Doctor seeks special probation,* AP, Dec. 12, 2002 [two-year probation for Conn. MD accused of failing to report pregnancy of 10-year-old]; J. Hanna, *Kline: Doctors must report youngsters' pregnancies,* AP, June 18, 2002 [Kansas AG opinion]; R. Hegeman, *Kansas judge says doctors cannot be forced to report underage sex,* AP, July 26, 2004; *see also* WIS. STAT. § 48.981(2m) [providers not required to report some sexual activities of minors].

[251] *E.g.,* FLA STAT. § 415.103; M.S. Lachs & K. Pillemer, *Current concepts: Abuse and neglect of elderly persons,* 332 N. ENG. J. MED. 437 (1995) [42 states required reporting in 1991].

[252] *E.g.,* WIS. STAT. § 46.90 [elder abuse].

[253] 45 C.F.R. § 164.512(c).

[254] S. Stapleton, *Confidentiality is key in protecting patients,* AM. MED. NEWS, July 14, 1997, 3 [Am. Med. Ass'n opposes reporting domestic violence]; A. Hyman et al., *Laws mandating reporting of domestic violence: Do they promote patient well-being?* 273 J.A.M.A. 1781 (1995) [questioning helpfulness where there are inadequate responses to reports]; *see also* S. Stapleton, *Plans ask doctors to address domestic violence,* AM. MED. NEWS, Dec. 21, 1998, 28 [internal reporting within managed care].

[255] *See* D. Hancock, *Hospital's inaction delayed arrest,* MIAMI (FL) HERALD, Jan. 24, 1996, 6B [no notice to authorities of gunshot victim as required, gave clothing (potential evidence) to family].

all gunshot wounds.[256] Other states limit the reporting requirement to wounds caused under certain circumstances. For example, Iowa requires the reporting of wounds that apparently resulted from criminal acts.[257] Thus, wounds that are clearly accidental or self-inflicted do not have to be reported in Iowa.

In 2002, a New York district attorney sought to compel New York City hospitals to produce all records pertaining to male Caucasian emergency room patients between the ages of 30 and 45 who sought treatment for knife wounds on two dates. The highest court of New York ruled that the subpoena could not be enforced. The state law that mandated reporting knife wounds was limited to life-threatening stab wounds. Treatment for other stab wounds was privileged.[258]

DRIVERS. A few states require reports to be submitted to state driver licensing agencies of conditions such as seizures that could lead to loss of license. Most states permit such reports but do not require them.[259]

OTHER REPORTING LAWS. Some states require reports of other information, such as industrial accidents and radiation incidents.[260] National reporting laws apply to hospitals that are involved in manufacturing, testing, or using certain substances and devices. For example, fatalities due to blood transfusions must be reported to the Food and Drug Administration (FDA).[261] A sponsor of an investigational medical device must report to the FDA any unanticipated adverse effects from use of the device.[262] There is a duty to report deaths or serious injuries in connection with devices.[263]

---

[256] N.Y. PENAL LAW § 265.25.

[257] IOWA CODE ANN. § 147.111.

[258] In the Matter of Grand Jury Investigation in New York County, 98 N.Y.2d 525, 779 N.E.2d 173, 749 N.Y.S.2d 462 (2002); *but see* State v. Baptist Mem. Hosp., 726 So. 2d 554 (Miss. 1998) [state can subpoena records of all patients treated for lacerations during a specified time period as part of a homicide investigation, where the law requires reporting knifings which the court broadly interpreted to include the cases sought by the subpoena].

[259] See *American Medical Association wants doctors more involved with older drivers*, AP Sept. 10, 2003; J.E. Allen, *Medicine: Drivers not telling doctors of seizures: Some report concealing episodes because they don't want to lose their licenses, a survey finds*, L.A. TIMES, Apr. 7, 2003, 3 [6 states require reports of seizures]; WIS. STAT. § 146.82(3)(a) [permissive]; *see also Edina hospital cited for allowing drugged patient drive*, AP Aug. 5, 2003 [MN hospital given three citations]; M. Raffaele, *Six-pack-a-day drinker loses license*, AP, July 13, 2004 [challenge to loss after MD report].

[260] *E.g.*, FLA. ADMIN. CODE §§ 10D-91.425, 10D-91.426, 10D-91.428 [radiation incidents].

[261] 21 C.F.R. § 606.170(b).

[262] 21 C.F.R. § 812.150(b).

[263] 63 FED. REG. 26,069 (May 12, 1998).

Some states require that major adverse incidents be reported to a state agency.[264] The director of nursing at a nursing home was personally fined in New York for failing to make such a report.[265]

In 1977, the United States Supreme Court upheld a state law that required reports to a central state registry of all prescriptions of Schedule II controlled substances.[266]

At least one state requires reports to private individuals. Florida requires hospitals to notify emergency transport personnel and other individuals who bring emergency patients to the hospital if the patient is diagnosed as having a contagious disease.[267]

COMMON LAW DUTY TO DISCLOSE. In addition to these statutory requirements, the common law has recognized a duty to disclose medical information in several circumstances. Persons who could have avoided injury if information had been disclosed have won civil suits against providers who failed to disclose such information.

Contagious Diseases. When a contagious disease is diagnosed, there is a duty to warn some persons at risk of exposure unless forbidden by statute.[268] Hospital staff, family members, and others caring for the patient should be warned. In a 1928 case, an Ohio court ruled that a physician could be liable for the death of a neighbor who contracted smallpox while assisting in the care of the physician's patient with smallpox because the physician failed to warn the neighbor of the contagious nature of the disease.[269] In 1998, the Alaska Supreme Court found that a residential care facility owed a duty to employees' spouses to take reasonable measures to control infections and warn employees of dangers of infections.[270] However, in most states there is no duty to warn all members of the general public. In a California case, the court observed that liability to the general public might result from failure to make a required report

---

[264] *E.g.,* Beth Israel Hosp. Ass'n v. Board of Registration in Med., 401 Mass. 172, 515 N.E.2d 574 (1987).

[265] Choe v. Axelrod, 141 A.D.2d 235, 534 N.Y.S.2d 739 (3d Dept. 1988).

[266] Whalen v. Roe, 429 U.S. 589 (1977).

[267] *E.g.,* FLA. STAT. § 395.0147.

[268] *See* Annotation, *Liability of doctor or other health practitioner to third party contracting contagious disease from doctor's patient,* 3 A.L.R. 5TH 370.

[269] Jones v. Stanko, 118 Ohio St. 147, 160 N.E. 456 (1928); *but see* D'Amico v. Delliquadri, 114 Ohio App. 3d 579, 683 N.E.2d 814 (1996) [physician owes no duty to girlfriend of patient to warn her of his genital warts; refusal to extend existing duty to warn those in dangerous proximity to deadly incurable disease]; *see also* S.A.V. v. K.G.V., 708 S.W.2d 651 (Mo. 1986) (en banc) [wife permitted to sue husband for failing to disclose herpes].

[270] Bolieu v. Sisters of Providence, 953 P.2d 1233 (Alaska 1998).

to public health authorities.[271] In at least one state, there is a duty to warn a broader range of individuals. In 1986, the South Carolina Supreme Court ruled that a hospital could be sued by the parents of a girl who had died of meningitis. Her friend had been diagnosed and treated at the hospital for meningitis, and the hospital had not notified persons who had prior contact with its patient during the likely period of contagiousness.[272] In 1997, the Tennessee Supreme Court ruled that hospitals could place HIV-positive patients in semi-private rooms without advising or obtaining consent from the other patient in the room. The placement was in accordance with current health care standards; as a matter of law, the placement did not constitute outrageous conduct.[273]

In 1991, the West Virginia Supreme Court ruled that a hospital security guard should have been warned that a patient had AIDS before being asked to help restrain the patient.[274] In 1994, a federal appellate court ruled that a man who got HIV infection from his brother while transporting him between hospitals could sue the first hospital for failure to disclose the brother's condition.[275] When a statute forbids disclosure of certain diseases, such as AIDS, there is generally no duty to disclose.[276]

Threats to Others. Some courts have ruled that there is a duty to warn identified persons that a patient has made a credible threat to kill them. Other courts have expanded the duty. The first decision to impose this duty was *Tarasoff v. Regents of University of California.*[277] When the Tarasoffs sued for the death of their daughter, the California Supreme Court found the employer of a psychiatrist liable for the psychiatrist's failure to warn the daughter that one of his patients had threatened to kill her. The court ruled that he should have either warned the victim or advised others likely to apprise the victim of the danger. In a 1980 case, the same court clarified the scope of this duty by ruling that only threats to readily identified individuals create a duty to warn; so there is no duty to warn a threatened group.[278] In 1989, the Arizona Supreme Court ruled that foreseeable victims had to be warned

271 Derrick v. Ontario Commun. Hosp., 47 Cal. App. 3d 154, 120 Cal. Rptr. 566 (4th Dist. 1975).
272 Phillips v. Oconee Mem. Hosp., 290 S.C. 192, 348 S.E.2d 836 (1986).
273 Bain v. Wells, 936 S.W.2d 618 (Tenn. 1997).
274 Johnson v. West Va. Univ. Hosps., Inc., 186 W.Va. 648, 413 S.E.2d 889 (1991).
275 J. B. v. Sacred Heart Hosp., 27 F.3d 506 (11th Cir. 1994).
276 *E.g.,* N.O.L.v. District of Columbia, 674 A.2d 498 (D.C. App. 1995).
277 Tarasoff v. Regents of Univ. of Cal., 17 Cal. 3d 425, 131 Cal. Rptr. 14, 551 P.2d 334 (1976).
278 Thompson v. County of Alameda, 27 Cal. 3d 741, 167 Cal. Rptr. 70, 614 P.2d 728 (1980).

even without specific threats.[279] In 1983, the Washington Supreme Court ruled that the duty to warn extended to unidentifiable victims.[280] In 1985, the Vermont Supreme Court extended the duty to warn to include property damage, imposing liability on a counseling service when a patient burned his parents' barn.[281] Some courts have declined to establish a duty to warn even readily identified individuals.[282] In states that have not addressed the issue, it is prudent to follow the California rule and warn identified individuals of credible threats when the patient is not detained.

The HIPAA privacy rules generally permit Tarasoff-type reports.[283]

There is no general duty to inform others of the release of a psychiatric patient absent such threats.[284]

OTHER DUTIES. Courts have recognized other situations that lead to a duty to disclose. One example is the duty of referral specialists to communicate their findings to the referring physician.[285] A competent patient can waive this duty by directing the referral specialist not to communicate with the referring physician.[286]

In 1988, the Oklahoma Supreme Court held that a physician could not be sued by a patient who was convicted of rape after the physician informed police that he suspected the patient was the rapist the police were seeking. The disclosure was protected by public policy.[287] However, there is no general right of law enforcement

---

[279] Hamman v. County of Maricopa, 161 Ariz. 58, 775 P.2d 1122 (1989); *see also* Morgan Estates v. Fairfield Family Counseling Ctr.*, 77 Ohio St. 3d 284, 673 N.E.2d 1311 (1997) [psychotherapist duty to protect society from violent acts by outpatient if knew or should have known and in position to control]; O'Keefe v. Orea, 731 So. 2d 680 (Fla. 1st DCA 1998) [psychiatrist duty to warn parents of minor patient of dangerous propensity].

[280] Peterson v. State, 100 Wash. 2d 421, 671 P.2d 230 (1983).

[281] Peck v. Counseling Serv., 146 Vt. 61, 499 A.2d 422 (1985).

[282] *E.g.,* Thapar v. Zezulka, 994 S.W.2d 635 (Tex. 1999); Shaw v. Glickman, 45 Md. App. 718, 415 A.2d 625 (1980).

[283] 45 C.F.R. § 164.512(j).

[284] *E.g.,* Nasser v. Parker, 455 S.E.2d 502 (Va. 1995) [no duty of psychiatrist, hospital to warn woman of release of mentally ill former boyfriend]; Limon v. Gonzaba, 940 S.W.2d 236 (Tex. Ct. App. 1997); Rousey v. United States, 115 F.3d 394 (6th Cir. 1997).

[285] *E.g.,* Thornburg v. Long, 178 N.C. 589, 101 S.E. 99 (1919); *see also* Gross v. Allen, 22 Cal. App. 4th 354, 27 Cal. Rptr. 2d 429 (2d Dist. 1994) [original psychiatrists had duty to tell subsequent attending psychiatrist of patient's prior suicide attempts; subsequent psychiatrist called to obtain history].

[286] *E.g.,* Watts v. Cumberland County Hosp. Sys., 75 N.C. App. 1, 330 S.E.2d 242 (1985), *rev'd on other grounds*, 317 N.C. 321, 345 S.E.2d 201 (1986).

[287] Bryson v. Tillinghast, 749 P.2d 110 (Okla. 1988); *see also* State v. Beatty, 770 S.W.2d 387 (Mo. Ct. App. 1989) [anonymous tip by physician linking patient to robbery did not violate privilege]; Porter v. Michigan Osteopathic Hosp. Ass'n, 170 Mich. App. 619, 428 N.W.2d 719 (1988) [hospital required to disclose to court information concerning patient suspects in rape]; Ohio Att'y Gen. Op. No. 88-027 (Apr. 21, 1988) [psychologists may but do not have to report felonies].

officials to access patient records. In 1998, a federal court found a county prosecutor liable for illegally obtaining a defendant's psychiatric records.[288]

8-6.4 When May Providers Disclose PHI in Response to Inquiries from Legal Authorities?

The HIPAA privacy rules authorize disclosures without patient authorization for some public health activities,[289] health oversight activities,[290] administrative proceedings,[291] law enforcement purposes,[292] cadaveric organ, eye, or tissue donation purposes,[293] research purposes,[294] to avert a serious threat to health or safety,[295] and various specialized governmental functions.[296] The rules define in detail when disclosures can be made for each of these purposes without consent. This section discusses law enforcement disclosures.

While it is true that HIPAA privacy rules have reduced the access of law enforcement to PHI, there are still many circumstances where information can be disclosed to law enforcement officers. There is still disagreement about the scope of permitted disclosures. The following is one analysis.

PRESENCE IN FACILITY. Providers may confirm the presence in the facility of a named patient or a patient with a physical description (e.g., height, weight, hair and eye color, race, gender, scars, presence or absence of facial hair, scars, and tattoos), except for patients subject to the substance abuse treatment confidentiality rules.[297]

However, generally providers cannot respond to individual law enforcement requests to report when a patient arrives with a particular medical condition. There are at least three exceptions. First, when the law requires or permits reports about the medical condition (such as certain wounds) to law enforcement, a report can be made. Second, if the law enforcement officer is trying to locate a sus-

---

[288] Schwenk v. Kavanaugh, 4 F. Supp. 2d 116 (N.D. N.Y. 1998) [$1 in punitive damages awarded].
[289] 45 C.F.R. § 164.512(b).
[290] 45 C.F.R. § 164.512(d).
[291] 45 C.F.R. § 164.512(e).
[292] 45 C.F.R. § 164.512(f).
[293] 45 C.F.R. § 164.512(h).
[294] 45 C.F.R. § 164.512(i).
[295] 45 C.F.R. § 164.512(j).
[296] 45 C.F.R. § 164.512(k).
[297] 45 C.F.R. §§ 164.512(a)(1) [named patient], 164.512(f)(2) [suspect, fugitive, material witness, missing person]; 164.512(f)(3) [victim].

pect, victim, or material witness to a crime, in most states providers may disclose type of injury and date and time of treatment or death. Third, when a law enforcement officer calls to ask for information and discloses that a person who could become a patient is dangerous, providers can take appropriate steps to protect themselves and others from dangerous persons, which in some cases can involve notifying law enforcement officials to assist in protection.

EFFORTS TO USE MEDICAL RECORDS TO IDENTIFY CRIMINALS. Courts generally will not permit law enforcement to rummage through the files of large numbers of patients in an effort to identify a criminal suspect.[298] However, the temptation to use this shortcut is great; so there unfortunately are several examples of unsuccessful attempts. One example is the attempt in New York described in the discussion on wound reporting in Section 8-6.3. Here are two other examples.

Law enforcement officers in Pennsylvania were investigating larceny of a jewelry store in which the suspect escaped in a car stolen from a parking lot near a methadone clinic. The law enforcement officers obtained a search warrant and searched confidential medical records in the methadone clinic. One patient sued the policeman who conducted the search. In 2000, a federal appellate court ruled that there was no probable cause to justify seeking the search warrant because the search violated the patient's Fourth Amendment right against unreasonable searches.[299]

In 2002, an Iowa county attorney was investigating the death of an unidentified newborn. He issued a subpoena for the names of all women tested for pregnancy at a Planned Parenthood clinic for the period of the pregnancy that resulted in the newborn. The trial court rejected a challenge to the subpoena but stayed the effect of the subpoena during appeal. After several months, the trial court vacated the order at the request of the county attorney and the appeal was dismissed as moot.[300]

---

[298] *E.g.*, People v. Doe, 211 Ill. App. 3d 962, 570 N.E.2d 733 (1st Dist. 1991) [in homicide investigation, quashing grand jury subpoena of identities of all residents of facility for alternative housing and treatment for chronically mentally ill persons during a 54-week period].

[299] Doe v. Broderick, 225 F.3d 440 (4th Cir. 2000); B.A. Masters, *Fairfax police concede seizure was wrong*, WASH. POST, Sept. 1, 1998, D1.

[300] *Search for baby's mother turns to courts*, AP, July 2, 2002; M.S. Welte, *Iowa Planned Parenthood granted stay*, AP, Aug. 6, 2002; *Court guards results of pregnancy tests*, N.Y. TIMES, Oct. 24, 2002, A18; *Iowa Supreme Court dismisses Planned Parenthood case*, AP, Nov. 1, 2002.

DISCHARGE OF PRISONERS. When persons in law enforcement custody are discharged from the provider back to a jail or prison, generally medical authorities at the jail or prison can be told the information that is necessary for the ongoing care of the prisoner. Guards who are transporting the prisoner generally cannot be told medical information. However, information that is necessary for a safe transport is permitted, for example, a propensity for violence that is not known by the guards.[301]

POLICE REPORTS. In most circumstances, providers are not permitted to provide PHI to law enforcement officers for the purposes of investigating a crime or completing a police report, unless there is written authorization from the patient or court action (search warrant or court order). This includes requests for the extent of injury, diagnoses, treatment plans, personal impressions (e.g., "Did you smell alcohol on his breath?"), and medications. Law enforcement should generally obtain a search warrant, court order, or patient authorization before accessing PHI. Failure to do so can bar the admissibility of any information obtained.[302] Generally, if a patient has provided false identification to obtain a prescription or other services, information necessary to investigate this crime on the provider's premises can be disclosed to law enforcement.

INCIDENTAL EXPOSURE. Law enforcement officers often incidentally overhear PHI when they bring suspects or victims of a crime to a health care facility or accompany an arrested or detained person. Law enforcement is permitted and even required to accompany arrested or detained individuals in order to secure the environment. Some incidental disclosure is unavoidable and permissible, but to the extent possible, consistent with good patient care and security concerns, attention should be given to limiting what is discussed in the presence of a law enforcement officer.

COLLECTION AND TESTING OF SAMPLES. It is permissible for providers to draw blood and other forensic samples at the request of law enforcement officers to the extent permitted by state law. The most common example of this is the drawing of a blood sample of someone who is suspected of driving while under the

---

[301] *See* 45 C.F.R. § 512(k)(5); Johnson v. West Va. Univ. Hosps., Inc., 186 W.Va. 648, 413 S.E.2d 889 (1991) [liability for failure to warn hospital security guard of HIV status of patient before asking him to assist in restraint of patient].

[302] *E.g.,* M. Stolz, *Politician's drug records protected; Judge says police lacked warrant to get evidence from pharmacy*, PLAIN DEALER, Mar. 15, 2002, B3 [Ohio trial court threw out records in prosecution for allegedly lying to obtain pain drugs].

influence of alcohol or drugs. Drawing the sample and delivering it to the law enforcement officer for testing by a forensic laboratory is not a disclosure of PHI.

However, providers generally should not let law enforcement officers influence their decisions whether to draw blood or collect other samples for clinical purposes and testing by the provider. Clinical sample collection at the direction of law enforcement officers can be a constitutional violation, and the results are generally not admissible in court.[303]

When law enforcement officers seek a sample collected for clinical purposes or the results of hospital testing on the sample, they should obtain a court order or search warrant. Providers should not voluntarily release the samples or results. In most states, voluntarily released samples or results generally are not admissible in court.[304]

The inadmissibility of improperly obtained samples and results is generally not a concern of health care providers, but it can be useful information when trying to deal with law enforcement officers who are demanding the samples or results. Most law enforcement officers do not want to jeopardize their cases.

PATIENT PROPERTY. Providers generally should not release personal property of the patient to a law enforcement officer, unless there is a search warrant, court order, or patient consent.[305] However, when a patient is in law enforcement custody, law enforcement officers may generally assist in searching the patient (unless the physician determines such involvement is medically contraindicated) and may retain

---

[303] *E.g.,* Ferguson v. City of Charleston, 532 U.S. 67 (2001) [performing urine tests at request of law enforcement to obtain evidence of cocaine use by maternity patients for law enforcement purposes was unreasonable search violating Fourth Amendment].

[304] *E.g.,* Comm. v. Shaw, 564 Pa. 617, 770 A.2d 295 (2001) [clinical blood test results obtained by police without warrant not admissible]; State v. Dyal, 97 N.J. 229, 478 A.2d 390 (1984) [court-issued subpoena required when police seek to obtain hospital blood test]; *contra,* People v. Ernst, 311 Ill. App. 3d 672, 725 N.E.2d 59 (2d Dist. 2000) [hospital may disclose blood alcohol results to police without court order]; Hannoy v. State, 793 N.E.2d 1109 (Ind. App. 2003) [clinical blood alcohol results may be released to police without court order]; *but see* State v. Schreiber, 122 N.J. 579, 585 A.2d 945 (1991) [doctor initiated disclosure of blood test result admissible]; Tapp v. State, 108 S.W.3d 459 (Tex. App. 2003) [upholding obtaining clinical blood test results with a grand jury subpoena].

[305] *E.g.,* People v. Maltbia, 273 Ill.App. 3d 622, 653 N.E.2d 402 (3d Dist. 1995) [physician gave drugs found in medical exam; inadmissible]; Jones v. State, 648 So. 2d 669 (1994) [warrantless seizure of clothing not justified, but admission harmless error]; People v. Watt, 118 Misc. 2d 930, 462 N.Y.S.2d 389 (Sup. Ct. 1983) [seized clothes inadmissible where no warrant, consent or exigent circumstances]; Morris v. Comm., 208 Va. 331, 157 S.E.2d 191 (1967) [clothes given to police on request when patient incapacitated; inadmissible]; *but see* State v. Smith, 88 Wn. 2d 127, 559 P.2d 970 (1977) [warrantless seizure of clothes justified as exigent circumstances].

what law enforcement finds. Weapons, explosives, or other items that present a danger to others in the hospital may be turned over to law enforcement officers to achieve institutional safety.

Patient property is generally not covered by the HIPAA privacy rule. It is subject to applicable state laws concerning property ownership and to federal constitutional restrictions on search and seizure.

REMOVAL OF BULLETS AND OTHER FOREIGN OBJECTS. The law concerning removal of bullets or other foreign objects from patients varies somewhat from state to state. There are constitutional limits on compelling such removal (see Section 7-7.4). Assuming the removal is appropriately authorized, there are three approaches to delivering the object to law enforcement. In some circumstances, providers may authorize law enforcement officers to be present during the removal and directly deliver the objects to the witnessing officer without a court order.[306] The circumstances vary from state to state. Wisconsin permits law enforcement officers to be present in the operating room during surgical removal of bags of cocaine if the patient is in law enforcement custody.[307] When law enforcement is not permitted to assume direct custody, the more conservative position is to require a search warrant, court order, or patient consent before releasing objects to law enforcement, but most of the courts that have addressed the question have permitted bullets to be admitted into evidence even when police obtain them without a warrant, order, or consent.[308]

CRIMES ON THE PREMISES. Providers may report apparent crimes that occur on their premises. Usually, disclosure of PHI is not required to make these reports. When PHI is related to the apparent crime, PHI may be disclosed to the extent necessary to provide evidence of the crime. For example, when drugs are stolen, the name and amount of drug may be disclosed, but the diagnosis should generally not be disclosed

FEDERAL LAW ENFORCEMENT. The HIPAA privacy rules permit disclosures for some national security activities and for protective services for the President and others.[309] Disclosures must also be

---

[306] *E.g.,* People v. Gomez, 147 Misc. 2d 704, 556 N.Y.S.2d 961 (Sup. Ct. 1990) [police witness surgical removal of bags from stomach].

[307] State v. Thompson, 585 N.W.2d 905 (Wis. App. 1998).

[308] *E.g.,* Comm. v. Johnson, 556 Pa. 216, 727 A.2d 1089 (1999) [no reasonable expectation of privacy in bullet removed for medical reasons, so no violation to give to police without warrant]; State v. Cowan, 46 S.W.2d 227 (Tenn. Crim. App. 2000) [no reasonable expectation of privacy in removed bullet, so admissible even though obtained from hospital without warrant].

[309] 45 C.F.R. § 146.512(k)(2),(3).

made when necessary for enforcement of the HIPAA privacy rules,[310] Medicare, Medicaid, and other governmental payment programs.[311]

8-6.5 When May Providers Disclose PHI in Response to Inquiries from Others?

Some statutes do not mandate reporting but authorize access to medical records, without the patient's permission, on request of certain individuals or organizations or the general public.

WORKERS' COMPENSATION. Some state statutes grant all parties to a workers' compensation claim access to all relevant medical information after a claim has been made.[312] In some states, courts have ruled that filing a workers' compensation claim is a waiver of confidentiality of relevant medical information.[313] However, in at least one state the physician-patient privilege applies in workers' compensation cases.[314] States that consider filing a claim to be a waiver vary on whether this includes information about HIV status.[315]

The HIPAA privacy rules permit compliance with these workers' compensation laws.[316]

FEDERAL FREEDOM OF INFORMATION ACT. The federal Freedom of Information Act (FOIA) applies only to federal agencies.[317] A provider does not become a federal agency by receiving federal funds; so the FOIA applies to few hospitals outside of the VA and Defense Department hospital systems. When the FOIA applies, medical information is exempted from disclosure under Exemption 6 when the disclosure would "constitute a clearly unwarranted invasion of personal privacy." Thus, the Act provides only limited protection of confidentiality of medical information in the possession of federal agencies. However, the federal Privacy Act may provide some additional protection to such information.[318]

---

[310] 45 C.F.R. §§ 146.310(c), 164.502(a)(2)(ii).

[311] 45 C.F.R. § 146.512(d).

[312] *E.g.,* IOWA CODE ANN. § 85.27.

[313] *E.g.,* Acosta v. Cary, 365 So. 2d 4 (La. Ct. App. 1978).

[314] Morris v. Consolidation Coal Co., 191 W.Va. 426, 446 S.E.2d 648 (1994).

[315] *Compare* Melo v. Barnett, 157 S.W.3d 596 (Ky. 2005) [disclosure of HIV status permitted] *with* Francies v. Kapla, 127 Cal. App. 4th 1381, 26 Cal. Rptr. 3d 501 (1st Dist. 2005) [disclosure of HIV status not permitted].

[316] 45 C.F.R. § 146.512(l).

[317] 5 U.S.C. § 552.

[318] 5 U.S.C. § 552a; Doe v. Stephens, 271 U.S. App. D.C. 230, 851 F.2d 1457 (1988) [effect of Privacy Act on grand jury subpoena of VA medical records]; Williams v. Department of Veterans Affairs, 879 F. Supp. 578 (E.D. Va. 1995) [Privacy Act is exclusive remedy for wrongful disclosure of medical information by VA].

Although the HIPAA privacy rules permit compliance with disclosures required by other laws, including FOIA, the preamble to the December 2000 HIPAA privacy rules states that in most cases requests for PHI under FOIA should be denied under Exemption 6.

STATE PUBLIC RECORDS LAWS. Many states have public records laws that apply to public hospitals. Some state statutes explicitly exempt hospital and medical records from disclosure.[319] In a 1974 case, Colorado's law was interpreted not to permit a publisher to obtain all birth and death reports routinely.[320] In 1983, the Iowa Supreme Court addressed the effort of a leukemia patient to force the disclosure of an unrelated potential bone marrow donor whose name was in the records of a public hospital.[321] The court ruled that names of patients could be withheld from disclosure and that although the potential donor had never sought treatment at the hospital, the potential donor was a patient for purposes of the exemption because the medical procedure of tissue typing had been performed. However, in a 1978 Ohio case, the state law was interpreted to require access to the names and the dates of admission and discharge of all persons admitted to a public hospital.[322] In states that follow the Ohio rule, it is especially important to resist discovery of nonparty records because removal of "identifiers" does not offer much protection when dates in the records may make it possible to identify the patient from the admission list.

OTHER ACCESS LAWS. Some federal and state statutes give governmental agencies access to medical records on request or through administrative subpoena.[323] For example, Peer Review Organizations (PROs) have access to all medical records pertinent to their federal review functions on request. A federal district court has ruled that Medicare surveyors have a right of access to records of non-Medicare patients, as well as to those of Medicare patients.[324] Hospital licensing laws often grant inspectors access without subpoena for audit and inspection purposes.

---

[319] *E.g.,* Iowa Code Ann. § 22.7; Head v. Colloton, 331 N.W.2d 870 (Iowa 1983).

[320] Eugene Cervi & Co. v. Russell, 184 Colo. 282, 519 P.2d 1189 (1974).

[321] Head v. Colloton, 331 N.W.2d 870 (Iowa 1983).

[322] Wooster Republican Printing Co. v. City of Wooster, 56 Ohio St. 2d 126, 383 N.E.2d 124 (1978).

[323] *E.g.,* Oklahoma Disability Law Ctr. v. Dillon Family & Youth Servs., 879 F. Supp. 1110 (D. Okla. 1995) [plaintiff entitled to discovery of treatment records of its clients, state law authorizing facility to require court order superceded by federal Protection and Advocacy of Mentally Ill Individuals Act].

[324] O'Hare v. Harris, Medicare & Medicaid Guide (CCH) ¶31,054 (D. N.H. Mar. 12, 1981), *see also* F.E.R. v. Valdez, 58 F.3d 1530 (10th Cir. 1995) [not violation of non-Medicaid patients' rights for state investigators to seize records in investigation of psychiatrist for Medicaid fraud].

8-7   What Legal Issues Flow from the Use of Audio and Video Transmissions and Recordings?

AUDIO RECORDINGS. Federal law and the law of many states permit recording of conversations by any party to the conversation.[325] In most circumstances, the other states require the consent of all parties to the conversation. In some jurisdictions, these laws apply primarily to recording of telephone and other transmitted conversations; in other jurisdictions, they apply to all conversations but generally do not apply where there is no reasonable expectation of privacy.

Persons in states that require consent of all parties need to be careful about recordings. In 1998, the highest court of Massachusetts found a hospital liable for recording meetings with a physician without his permission.[326] Persons receiving calls from these states should obtain permission from the caller before recording calls. In 1998, a Florida court found that it had jurisdiction over an out-of-state person who had recorded a telephone conversation with a person in Florida. The court has jurisdiction over torts that occur in Florida, and it concluded the tort occurred where the communication originated, not where it was recorded. Thus, it could apply Florida law to the recording.[327]

In 1989, a California appellate court ruled that to the extent a video recorder also records audio, it is subject to laws against recording conversations.[328]

In 2004, a federal court ruled that a hospital could be sued for an audio recording of an allegedly confidential meeting with a labor management consultant.[329]

Even in states that require all parties to consent, there are exceptions for law enforcement purposes and for recordings in situations where there is no reasonable expectation of privacy.[330]

JCAHO requires consent before audio or video recording of patients for any purpose other than identification, diagnosis, or treatment.[331]

---

[325] 18 U.S.C. § 2511(d).
[326] Birbiglia v. Saint Vincent Hosp., 427 Mass. 80, 692 N.E.2d 9 (1998).
[327] Koch v. Kimball, 710 So. 2d 5 (Fla. 2nd DCA 1998).
[328] People v. Gibbons, 215 Cal. App. 3d 1204, 263 Cal. Rptr. 905 (4th Dist. 1989) [video recorder subject to Calif. Penal Code § 632 restrictions on recording communications].
[329] Care v. Reading Hosp., 2004 U.S. Dist. LEXIS 5485 (E.D. Pa.).
[330] *E.g., Prosecutors say tapes implicate Scrushy*, AP, Feb. 14, 2004 [HealthSouth CFO wore FBI recording device].
[331] 2005 JCAHO CAMH, RI.2.50.

VISUAL RECORDINGS. Physicians usually may take and use photographs of patients for the medical record or for professional educational purposes unless the patient expressly forbids photographs. The highest court of Massachusetts enjoined public showing of a film of inmates of an institution for insane persons charged with crimes or delinquency but permitted continued showings to audiences of a specialized or professional character with a serious interest in rehabilitation.[332] The court observed that the public interest in having these people informed outweighs the rights of the inmates to privacy. The Maine Supreme Court ruled that when a patient had expressly objected to being photographed, there could be liability for photographing the patient even if the photograph was solely for the medical record.[333] It is best to obtain express consent for taking and using photographs,[334] but liability for photographs taken without express consent is not likely if the patient does not object and uses are appropriately restricted. A New York appellate court ruled that a physician and nurse could not be sued for allowing a newspaper photographer to photograph a patient in the waiting areas of an infectious disease unit because the individual's presence did not indicate the individual was a patient and the individual was never identified as a patient.[335] Public or commercial showing without consent can lead to liability.[336]

Visual recordings have lead to a wide variety of situations that courts have addressed. One group of cases deals with the right to make recordings. In 1985, a New York appellate court ruled that

---

[332] Commonwealth v. Wiseman, 356 Mass. 251, 249 N.E.2d 610 (1969), *cert. denied*, 398 U.S. 960 (1970); *Film on hospital provocative after 20 years,* N.Y. TIMES, May 17, 1987, 14; *see also* Adams v. St. Elizabeth Hosp., 1989 Ohio App. LEXIS 913 [written consent not required to show patient to teaching conference in teaching hospital], *as discussed in* 22 J. HEALTH & HOSP. L. 291 (1989).

[333] Estate of Berthiaume v. Pratt, 365 A.2d 792 (Me. 1976); *see* Annotation, *Taking unauthorized photographs as invasion of privacy,* 86 A.L.R. 3D 374.

[334] *E.g., In re* Karlin, 112 Bankr. 319 (Bankr. 9th Cir. 1989), *aff'd without op.,* 940 F.2d 1534 (9th Cir. 1989) [plastic surgeon's use of pictures in article was for instructional or educational purpose within meaning of authorization].

[335] Anderson v. Strong Mem. Hosp., 140 Misc. 2d 770, 531 N.Y.S.2d 735 (Sup. Ct. 1988), *aff'd,* 151 A.D.2d 1033, 542 N.Y.S.2d 96 (4th Dept. 1989).

[336] *E.g.,* Stubbs v. North Mem. Med. Ctr., 448 N.W.2d 78 (Minn. Ct. App. 1989) [publication in promotional, educational materials of before, after photographs of facial cosmetic surgery without patient consent may constitute breach of express warranty of silence arising from physician-patient relationship]; Feeney v. Young, 191 A.D. 501, 181 N.Y.S. 481 (1st Dept.920) [public showing of a film of a caesarean section delivery]; Vassiliades v. Garfinkels, 492 A.2d 580 (D.C. 1985) [public use of before, after photos of cosmetic surgery in department store, on television]; *see* Annotation, *Invasion of privacy by use of plaintiff's name or likeness in advertising,* 23 A.L.R. 3D 865.

representatives of an incompetent patient do not have a right to photograph the patient in the hospital.[337] The petitioners failed to show a sufficient need to justify a court order that they be permitted to film an eight-hour videotape of their comatose daughter in an intensive care unit for use in a suit. In 1986, a New York court ruled that a patient had no right, before filing a malpractice suit, to a videotape of the patient's operation. It was found not to be a part of the medical record because the physician had taken it for his personal use.[338] In an unreported New Jersey appellate court case in 2000, a hospital was ordered to permit videotaping in an intensive care unit.[339]

Other suits have dealt with liability for media recordings.[340] In 1998, the California Supreme Court ruled that an accident victim could sue two television production companies for invasion of privacy for taping the victim's medical helicopter flight to the hospital. The court ruled that some of the recording at the scene of the accident may also have constituted an invasion of privacy.[341]

Other suits have involved the use of recordings.[342] In 2002, a Florida trial court permitted the parents of a comatose woman to televise a videotape of her condition since it had been shown in court.[343] In 2002, a woman used the surgeon's videotape of her surgery to support her suit claiming that he had branded her during the surgery.[344]

In 2003, a federal appellate court ruled that an employer had to negotiate with the union over use of hidden surveillance cameras.[345]

JCAHO requires consent before audio or video recording of patients for any purpose other than identification, diagnosis, or

---

[337] *In re* Simmons, 112 A.D.2d 806, 492 N.Y.S.2d 308 (4th Dept. 1985); *but see* North Broward Hosp. Dist. v. ABC, No. 86-026514 (Fla. Cir. Ct. Broward County Oct. 20, 1986) [hospital cannot prohibit media access to comatose patient when guardian consents].

[338] Hill v. Springer, 132 Misc. 2d 1012, 506 N.Y.S.2d 255 (1986).

[339] R.J. Peach, *Court overrides hospital's ban on photographs in intensive care unit*, LEGAL INTELLIGENCER, Dec. 27, 2000, 6.

[340] *E.g., Jury acquits reporter of trespassing charge*, AP Dec. 23, 2003 [N.C. reporter entered assisted living center with assistance of former staff member and videotaped sleeping residents].

[341] Shulman v. Group W Productions, 18 Cal. 4th 200, 74 Cal. Rptr. 2d 843, 955 P.2d 469 (1998).

[342] *E.g., Nurse accused of torturing brain-damaged child*, AP Oct. 3, 2003 [use of film from surveillance cameras in WA home installed by grandmother]; *Mother accused of contaminating infant daughter's IV*, AP, Jan. 15, 2004 [Ind. woman videotaped injecting fecal matter into daughter's IV tube]; Kinsella v. Welch, 2003 N.J. Super. LEXIS 253 (App. Div.) [under newsperson privilege media not required to produce video of treatment in hospital, but must produce any portions that will be used at trial].

[343] *Judge: Media permitted to broadcast video of woman in coma*, AP, Oct. 2, 2002.

[344] *Lawsuit: Woman claims doctor branded her during surgery*, AP, Jan. 24, 2003.

[345] National Steel Corp. v. National Labor Relations Board, 324 F.3d 928 (7th Cir. 2003).

treatment.[346] This means that JCAHO-accredited hospitals should obtain consent for recordings that are for educational purposes.

8-8   What Legal Issues Flow from the Use of Computers and the Internet?

FEDERAL POLICY. There is an increasing push for use of computerized medical records. In 2004, the President announced an effort to achieve electronic medical records by 2014.[347] The Veterans Administration has adopted a computerized medical record.[348] The federal Consolidated Health Informatics Initiative is seeking to establish the framework for sharing health information among federal agencies and is pursuing interoperability standards.[349] An Executive Order in 2004 established a federal Office of Health Information Technology.[350]

COMPUTERIZED RECORD-KEEPING. Computerized records are generally more accessible than paper records for their many functions. Multiple uses can occur concurrently, reducing the need for waiting for others to complete their uses of the paper record. They permit more standardization of data-keeping. They remove some of the problems with legibility of some paper records and assist in reducing some preventable errors. Computer programs can assist physicians in making diagnostic and treatment decisions through clinical decision support. There is an opportunity to build in checking procedures that can call attention to and even bar potentially problematic orders. Computerized records provide an opportunity for more automatic analysis of data.

There are potential disadvantages to computerized systems.[351] Computerized systems are costly.[352] In addition, they can divert professional time from patient care. Data still must be entered by

---

[346] 2005 JCAHO CAMH, RI.2.50.

[347] *Bush promotes technology*, UPI, Apr. 26, 2004.

[348] *See* Schmidt v. U.S. Dep't Of Veterans Affairs, 218 F.R.D. 619 (E.D. Wis. 2003).

[349] Described in http://www.whitehouse.gov/omb/egov/gtob/health_informatics.htm (accessed Aug. 25, 2004).

[350] The office website is http://www.hhs.gov/onchit/ (accessed Aug. 25, 2004).

[351] M. Freudenheim, *Many hospitals resist computerized patient care*, N.Y. TIMES, Apr. 6, 2004, C1; R. Koppel et al., *Role of computerized physician order entry systems in facilitating medication errors*, J.A.M.A., Mar. 9, 2005, 1197.

[352] *See* S. Lohr, *Health care technology is a promise unfinanced*, N.Y. TIMES, Dec. 3, 2004, C5; J. Morrissey, *It's more than just the purchase; make clear the commitments that it will trigger*, MOD. HEALTHCARE, July 12, 2004, 30.

someone. Many approaches require data entry by physicians and other professionals that can divert their time from other functions, reducing the quantity of patient care that can be provided. They create a temptation to require the collection of more data that further diverts resources from patient care. These are not necessarily arguments against computerization. Rather they need to be kept in mind by those structuring the systems.

Another potential disadvantage is the security risk. Unauthorized users can sometimes gain access. Authorized users can access records for unauthorized purposes. However, this is a strong argument against computerized records. Similar risks exist with paper records. In addition, computerized systems are more effective in tracking uses of records than are paper records. Steps are being taken to provide more security for computerized records.

HIPAA privacy and security rules apply to access to and use of computerized records. HIPAA privacy rules are in effect. HIPAA security rules require that computerized records and communications meet basic security standards, effective April 21, 2005.

It is cumbersome to structure computerized records so that authorized persons cannot access records beyond those they need for their job because it is usually not possible to determine in advance which records they will need to access. Thus, training, professional standards, and monitoring of lookups are used to deter and detect inappropriate lookups. There have been few legal cases involving inappropriate lookups.[353]

For several years, some health care providers have been developing computerized methods for handling some health care information. For a time, one legal barrier was the requirement of authentication of physician entries and orders by a physician signature that could only be performed on a hard copy. Electronic signatures are now generally accepted; so this barrier has largely been

---

[353] *E.g.*, Doe v. Medlantic Health Care Group, 814 A.2d 939 (D.C. App. 2003) [hospital liable under D.C. law for staff member's dissemination of HIV status after unauthorized lookup]; Doe v. Dartmouth-Hitchcock Med. Ctr., 2001 U.S. Dist. LEXIS 10704 (D.N.H.) [hospital not liable under federal law for MD lookup]; J. Mandak, *Researcher sentenced in Wynette case,* AP Online, Dec. 1, 2000 [using former physician's password, former research assistant accessed computerized hospital records of late country singer Tammy Wynette and sold them to tabloids; sentenced to six months, fined amount received from tabloids]; Arbster v. Unemployment Comp. Bd. of Rev., 690 A.2d 805 (Pa. Commw. 1997) [nurse fired for lookup of computer records of her family denied unemployment compensation]; *see also* Schmidt v. U.S. Dep't of Veterans Affairs, 218 F.R.D. 619 (E.D. Wis. 2003) [challenge to access to employee social security numbers in VA hospital computerized medical record; description of steps VA had taken to restrict, trace lookups].

removed. In 2000, the federal government adopted a law recognizing electronic signatures for most purposes.[354] However, care must still be exercised in the structuring and use of electronic signatures.[355] Some states have had centralized computer records of some health care information. In 1977, the United States Supreme Court upheld New York's mandatory reporting of prescriptions, discussing how the information was placed into a centralized state computer system.[356]

Another legal barrier was that some jurisdictions would not accept computerized records as official records. Computerized records are now generally accepted as official records for regulatory and evidentiary purposes if they meet basic standards of reliability.[357]

One barrier to the standardization of documentation has been the difficulty in establishing standard terminology. Progress is being made in addressing this issue. On May 6, 2004, the United States Department of Health and Human Services (HHS) announced that it had licensed the College of American Pathologists Systematized Nomenclature of Medicine Clinical Terms® (SNOMED-CT®) for laboratory result contents, nonlaboratory interventions and procedures, anatomy, diagnosis and problems, and nursing and announced that it was making SNOMED-CT® available for use in the United States at no charge to users.[358]

E-MAIL. Many providers use e-mail to communicate with patients and other providers.[359] With appropriate attention to confidentiality and the different nature of interaction, this practice appears to offer advantages. In 1998, a Wisconsin appellate court recognized the validity of e-mail prescriptions.[360] One of the impediments to broader

---

[354] Electronic Signatures in Global and National Consumer Act, Pub. No. L. 106-229, 114 Stat, 464 (2000), *codified in part at* 15 U.S. §§ 7001 et seq.

[355] *E.g., Second doctor sues hospital over Pap smear tests*, AP, Jan. 23, 2004 [accusation of misuse of electronic signatures]; *Feds find no significant problems with Magee Pap smears*, AP, Apr. 13, 2004.

[356] Whalen v. Roe, 429 U.S. 589 (1977); *see also Letcher woman convicted on drug fraud charges*, AP, Apr. 4, 2001 [use of KY computerized prescription tracking system to achieve conviction].

[357] *E.g.,* 15 U.S.C. § 7001; United States v. Fujii, 301 F.3d 535 (7th Cir. 2002) [admissibility of printouts in federal court].

[358] *See* http://www.whitehouse.gov/omb/egov/gtob/health_informatics.htm (accessed Aug. 25, 2004).

[359] *See* L. Stevens, *Virtually there,* AM. MED. NEWS, Dec. 21, 1998, 24; B. Kane & D.Z. Sands, *Guidelines for the clinical use of electronic mail with patients,* 5 J. AM. MED. INFORMATICS ASS'N 104 (1998) [http://www.jamia.org/cgi/reprint/5/1/104 [accessed Nov. 17, 2005]; S.M. Borowitz & J.C. Wyatt, *The origin, content, and workload of e-mail consultations,* J.A.M.A., Oct. 21, 1998, 1321; A.R. Spielberg, *On call and online: Sociohistorical, legal, and ethical implications of e-mail for the patient physician relationship,* J.A.M.A., Oct. 21, 1998, 1353; G. Baldwin, *Doctor benefits from e-mail efficiency with patients,* AM. MED. NEWS, Dec. 21, 1998, 24.

[360] Walgreen Co. v. Wisconsin Pharmacy Examining Bd., 217 Wis. 2d 290, 577 N.W.2d 387, 1998 Wisc. App. LEXIS 201 (Unpub).

adoption of e-mail communications with patients has been the lack of payment for the time spent in this function.[361] Some payers have experimented with payments.[362]

E-mail communications should be treated with the same degree of care and formality as other written communications. They can be discovered and used in criminal investigations and civil lawsuits.[363] Federal courts have generally determined that they are not subject to the same degree of protection as telephone calls; so it may not be a violation of federal wiretap laws to intercept e-mail at several stages in their transmission.[364] Some employers have increased the monitoring of e-mail and other computer use.[365]

E-mail is also sometimes used for threats and harassment.[366]

Care must be taken when sending e-mail in a health care environment. There have been a few incidents where medical information was accidentally distributed to the wrong recipients.[367] The HIPAA security rules apply to e-mail and will require encryption and other steps to improve the security of e-mail.

INTERNET. Computerized records have been stolen through the Internet.[368] It is important for those responsible for computers to monitor and implement security precautions.[369]

Computerized records have been accidentally posted on the Internet.[370] It is important to train staff on how to minimize these accidents.

---

[361] *See Online consultations slow to take off*, AM MED. NEWS, Apr. 12, 2004, 21 [consumers say they want e-mail, but unwilling to pay more than $10].

[362] *E.g.*, L. Kowalczyk, *The doctor will e-you now: Insurers to pay doctors to answer questions over Web*, BOSTON GLOBE, May 24, 2004, A1.

[363] *E.g.*, A. Michaels & D. Wells, *HealthSouth investigators reveal damning new e-mail*, FINANCIAL TIMES (London), July 11, 2003, 13; J. Sarche, *Beware of e-mail, text messages*, WIS. ST. J., June 7, 2004, A3.

[364] *E.g.*, United States v. Councilman, 2004 U.S. App. LEXIS 13352 (1st Cir.).

[365] *E.g.*, M.A. Nusbaum, *New kind of snooping arrives at the office*, N.Y. TIMES, July 13, 2003, 12BU.

[366] *E.g.*, *Georgia man accused of sending Internet threat to hospital*, AP, Mar. 6, 2003.

[367] *E.g.*, J. Wells, *Wrong MDs got patient records; psychiatric privacy violated*, SAN FRANCISCO CHRONICLE, Dec. 30, 2000, A13; M.W. Salganik, *Health data on 858 patients mistakenly e-mailed to others; medical information was among messages sent out by Kaiser Health Care*, BALTIMORE SUN, Aug. 10, 2000, 1C.

[368] *E.g.*, *Hacker steals files on patients from UW*, SEATTLE TIMES, Dec. 9, 2000, B1 [hacker stole files on 4,700 patients].

[369] *See* S. Bakerand & M. Shenk, *A patch in time saves nine: Liability risks for unpatched software*, CORP. COUNSELLOR, Apr. 5, 2004. 3.

[370] *E.g.*, M. Lerner & J. Marcotty, *Web posting has health and university officials scrambling; mental health records of children from 20 families were mistakenly put onto the Internet*, STAR TRIBUNE (Minneapolis, MN), Nov. 8, 2001, 1B; C. Pillar, *Web mishap: Kids' psychological files posted*, L.A. TIMES, Nov. 7, 2001, A1.

There have been challenges to postings on the Internet. In 1999, a jury awarded $107 million verdict against an antiabortion group who had produced wanted posters of abortion providers and had supplied then to a Web site. The trial court enjoined production of the posters and the supplying of them to the Web site. A federal appellate court upheld the injunction and the verdict against the group but required that the lower court review the amount of the judgment. The appellate court found that there was a sufficient threat of force on the posters to overcome the First Amendment protection for the posters. In 2004, the lower court affirmed the amount of the judgment.[371] In 2001, another antiabortion group created a Web site that includes photographs and medical records of women who had obtained abortions. A Missouri state lower court enjoined removal of the photographs and records.[372]

In 2002, a Massachusetts court required a patient to remove misleading photos and defamatory statements from a Web site about a physician.[373] In 2003, a Pennsylvania judge ordered attorneys to close a Web site for recruiting patients for a class action lawsuit, but it was reopened later after a settlement with the hospital that involved deleting the hospital's name from the Web site name.[374]

The law related to computers, e-mail, and the Internet is still developing. It can be anticipated that new legal issues will continue to flow from this changing area.

---

371 Planned Parenthood v. American Coalition of Life Activists, 41 F. Supp. 2d 1130 (D. Or. 1999), *rev'd*, 244 F.3d 1007 (9th Cir. 2001), *rev'd*, 290 F.3d 1058 (9th Cir. 2002) (en banc) [reinstating district court injunction and verdict against defendants], *cert. denied*, 123 S. Ct. 2637 (U.S. 2003), *on remand*, 300 F. Supp. 2d 1055 (D. Ore. 2004) [jury award of punitive damages affirmed].

372 T. Hillig & J. Mannies, *Woman sues over posting of abortion details; her records from Granite City hospital were put on Web site; hospital, protesters are defendants*, St. Louis Post-Dispatch, July 3, 2001, A1; J. Mannies, *Abortion foes are ordered to take woman's records, photo off Web; patient had complications at clinic in Granite City*, St. Louis Post-Dispatch, July 11, 2001, B1; *Judge keeps woman's records off net*, AP Online, Aug. 23, 2001.

373 A. Barnard, *Facing criticism cosmetic surgeon sues over postings by a former patient*, Boston Globe, Sept. 24, 2002, B1; *see also* M. Ko, *Judge limits police data online; Web site operators must remove officers' Social Security numbers*, Seattle Times, May 11, 2001, B; A. Liptak, *Dispute simmers over Web site posting personal data on police*, N.Y. Times, July 12, 2003, A1.

374 J. Mandak, *Judge orders attorneys to shut down hospital lawsuit Web site*, AP, Dec. 23, 2003 [E.D. Pa. judge ordered closing site recruiting for class action suit against hospital]; *Law firms, hospital agree on Web site*, AP, Jan. 21, 2004.

Discussion Points

1. What are some of the underlying issues that must be balanced in developing laws and policies concerning health care information?
2. Who owns the medical record?
3. What information must be collected in a record?
4. How should a provider determine how long to keep records?
5. What are the basic HIPAA requirements concerning privacy of protected health care information?
6. Which state laws are still in effect? What other federal privacy laws remain in effect?
7. When may patients and their representatives authorize disclosure?
8. When may the law compel disclosure?
9. When are reports to legal authorities still required?
10. When may providers release information in response to requests from others?
11. Has HIPAA struck the proper balance between privacy and uses of health care information?
12. What restrictions are there on audio and visual recordings in health care settings?
13. What are some of the legal issues related to the use of computers and the Internet in health care?
14. What are some of the advantages and disadvantages of computerized medical records?

CHAPTER NINE

Paying for Health Care Resources and Services

Objectives

The objective of this chapter is to provide an overview of the ways that health care services are financed. Issues related to managed care and eligibility for third-party coverage are discussed in Chapter 10. This chapter focuses primarily on payment mechanisms. The reader will learn about regulation of provider budgets and charges; Medicare, Medicaid, and other major government payer programs; employee-sponsored payment programs and other private payment programs; collection of out-of-pocket amounts; sources of financing; and tax issues.

Payment for the creation and maintenance of health care resources and the delivery of health care services is one of the most difficult problems of health care law and public policy. The United States Department of Health and Human Services (HHS) estimates that $1.7 trillion was spent in the United States on health care services in 2003 and that this will increase to $3.6 trillion by 2014. In 2003, the federal government spent $507.5 billion on health care, and state governments spent $214.2 billion. Of the federal expenditures, $283.1 billion was for Medicare, and $157.5 billion was for Medicaid. Of the state and local expenditures, $109.5

billion was on Medicaid.[1] In 2005, it was estimated that the average annual family medical costs were $12,200.[2]

The issue of payment is inextricably intertwined with the problem of what facilities and services should be available and how they should be accessed.

There is no one decisionmaker that addresses these concerns. The existing delivery system and payment system is the result of the complex interaction among decisions by governments, payers, providers, and individuals, all of which are beyond the scope of this book. Instead this chapter focuses on the current legal structure.

Payment can occur at least at four levels.

First, those paying for health care obtain their revenues from some payment source. For example, employers sell their products or services, governments collect taxes or borrow money, and philanthropists receive donations. There are political, market, and other constraints on the amount of revenue that can be obtained from each source. This aspect of payment is beyond the scope of this book.

Second, in many cases, the payers do not pay directly for health services but instead purchase insurance or contribute to health plans; the second level of payment is the premium for insurance or other prepaid health care coverage. The insurer or other plan that accepts the premium agrees to provide or pay for a set of services for covered individuals. Unless there is a subsidy from some other source, the aggregate of the premiums and the investment income from the premiums must cover the services promised or the plan fails.

Third, in most cases, the insurers or other prepaid health care plan do not directly provide health care, but instead they purchase health care from providers. The next level of payment is to the institutional or individual provider. Those without insurance buy their services directly from the provider.

---

[1] *Overall health care cost growth projections slow from 2003 Medicare drug coverage expected to lower prices*, HHS Press Release, Feb. 23, 2005, https://www.cms.hhs.gov/media/press/release.asp?Counter=1356 [accessed Oct. 1, 2005]; HHS, Table 3: National Health Expenditures, by Source of Funds and Type of Expenditure: Selected Calendar Years 1997–2003, http://www.cms.hhs.gov/statistics/nhe/historical/t3.asp (accessed Oct. 1, 2005); HHS, Table 10: Expenditures for Health Services and Supplies Under Public Programs, by Type of Expenditure and Program: Calendar Year 2003, http://www.cms.hhs.gov/statistics/nhe/historical/t10.asp (accessed Oct. 1, 2005).

[2] K. Whitehouse, *Average family medical costs will exceed $12,200 this year*, WIS. ST. J, May 26, 2005, D2.

Fourth, providers must pay their workers; construct and maintain facilities and other infrastructures; and pay for the equipment, supplies, and services that are necessary to deliver health care services. Businesses that supply equipment, supplies, and services to the primary provider face similar payment issues in their own businesses; they will not be addressed separately.

This brief sketch is just the skeleton of the system. At each level there are multiple participants with a variety of competing views and demands. No one participant and no one level can control the system. The existing system is the result of the complex interaction of the decisions and actions of all the participants.

Each of these levels sees the issues somewhat differently, but there is an underlying reality. There are ultimate costs to provide a certain amount of health care in a certain manner. Either those costs are paid, or the health care is not provided in the amount or the manner desired. There are ultimate limits to what can be paid, and there are limits to the amount and manner of care. There are few examples of explicit rationing of care. These limits generally appear in other ways. Managed care is discussed in the following chapter.

This chapter addresses the following questions:

9-1. What attempts have been made to directly address provider charges and budgets?

9-2. How are Medicare, Medicaid, and other major government payment programs structured?

9-3. How are employer-sponsored and other payment programs structured?

9-4. What are the laws governing collection of copayments, deductibles, and uninsured amounts?

9-5. How can capital financing be arranged?

9-6. What are the other sources of financing for providers?

9-7. What is the impact of the tax structure on the health care system?

9-1 What Attempts Have Been Made to Directly Address Provider Charges and Budgets?

There have been governmental attempts to try to directly control the third level of payment by controlling provider charges or budgets as a mechanism for controlling the overall costs of health care.

These attempts have been abandoned in most states. The market for health care is so complex that direct control of budgets or charges lead to unacceptable dislocation in available services. Most jurisdictions rely on market forces and government payer policies to address payments to providers.

FINANCIAL REQUIREMENTS. Any effort to control budgets or charges of providers needs to be examined in the context of the financial requirements for viable providers.

One duty of the governing body of a health care provider is to maintain the financial integrity of the institution. Most actions necessary to accomplish this goal are the responsibility of the CEO, who must conceptualize and recommend actions to the governing body, and then implement its decisions.

The institution's mission and resulting scope of activities must be within its attainable financial means. The resulting financial requirements must be met, or the institution cannot continue to operate. This is accomplished through realistically establishing the scope of activities within available resources; entering appropriate contracts and other arrangements with insurers, providers, and others to assure the planned role in health care delivery with appropriate payment; developing a realistic budget to allocate resources to carry out those activities; setting appropriate charges and pricing practices; obtaining payment from third parties and individuals; initiating appropriate cost containment and restructuring measures; arranging for appropriate capital financing; protecting the hospital's assets; and minimizing the impact of taxes, including preserving appropriate tax exemptions.

A hospital's financial requirements include its current operating needs plus an operating margin. In addition to caring for paying patients, many hospitals also provide charity care, education, and research, and these activities also contribute to current operating needs. An operating margin is necessary to provide working capital and meet other capital requirements. For-profit hospitals also seek profit so that they can pay dividends to their investors. Working capital is needed to assure immediate stability and the ability to make timely payment of current obligations without costly short-term borrowing. Other capital requirements include renovations and major repairs, replacement of buildings and equipment, expansion, and acquisition of new technology. These capital requirements are frequently financed through bonding and other long-term debt; hospitals must have an adequate operating margin to qualify for this borrowing, unless some other entity is guarantying the debt.

SETTING CHARGES. Even though an increasing portion of hospital payments are determined by contracts with managed care entities and insurers, hospitals still must set charges for those not covered by contracts. These charges are often limited by law either for specific groups of patients, such as those covered by workers' compensation or Medicare, or for all patients. In some states, they are still limited through rate regulation. This section focuses on some legal considerations in setting charges.

When hospitals borrow money through bonds or other mechanisms, they usually pledge certain property or revenues to guarantee repayment. One pledge is usually a promise to set rates sufficiently high to repay the loan and maintain hospital operations until the loan is repaid. These pledges must be respected to the extent permitted by law.

RATE REGULATION. In the past, several states had an agency that monitored, reviewed, or established charges or revenue limits for hospitals. The role of this agency varied greatly among the states. Legal challenges against these programs were generally unsuccessful.[3] As market forces developed, state rate regulation was increasingly recognized as obsolete. As early as 1989, Washington repealed its rate-setting law.[4] By 2004, only one state, Maryland,

---

[3] *E.g., In re* William B. Kessler Mem. Hosp., 78 N.J. 564, 397 A.2d 656 (1979); Rebaldo v. Cuomo, 749 F.2d 133 (2d Cir. 1984), *cert. denied*, 472 U.S. 1008 (1985) [New York system preventing self-insured employee benefit plans from negotiating rates lower than those set by system not violation of ERISA]; United Hosp. Ctr., Inc. v. Richardson, 757 F.2d 1445 (4th Cir. 1985) [West Virginia law freezing all hospital rate schedules upheld]; Panama City Med. Diagnostic Ltd. v. Williams, 13 F.3d 1541 (11th Cir. 1994), *cert. denied*, 513 U.S. 826 (1994) [not violation of equal protection for Florida to exempt hospitals, group practices from fee cap on diagnostic imaging services]; *see* Massachusetts Nurses Ass'n v. Dukakis, 726 F.2d 41 (1st Cir. 1984) [state rate regulation does not violate nurses' collective bargaining rights, affected labor-management relations only indirectly]; for other rate regulation issues, *see* Bath Mem. Hosp. v. Maine Health Care Fin. Comm'n, 853 F.2d 1007 (1st Cir. 1988); Matter of 1983 Final Reconciliation Adjustments for Greenville Hosp., 214 N.J. Super. 607, 520 A.2d 809 (App. Div. 1987); Griffin Hosp. v. Commission on Hosps. & Health Care, 200 Conn. 489, 512 A.2d 199 (1986), *cert. denied*, 479 U.S. 810 (1986); Prince George's Doctor's Hosp., Inc. v. Health Servs. Cost Review Comm'n, 302 Md. 193, 486 A.2d 744 (1985); Baltimore & Ohio R.R. v. United States, 345 U.S. 146 (1953) [broad power of states to regulate rates without regulation being "taking" of private property that requires compensation under Fifth Amendment]; F.C. Dreyer, Jr., *Health care rate regulations: The need for a reinvigorated "takings" analysis*, 26 J. HEALTH & HOSP. L. 161 (1993) [hereinafter J. HEALTH & HOSP. L. will be cited as J.H.H.L.].

[4] *Washington forms health agency, will end rate-setting policy*, MOD. HEALTHCARE, June 16, 1989, 12

still had hospital rate-setting, and only a few states maintained some rate review.[5] At least one state, Vermont, has maintained hospital budget review.[6]

CHARGES TO THE UNINSURED. Some uninsured patients have challenged having to pay full charges.[7] The challenges have been based on the fact that the implied contract for hospital services is to pay "reasonable" charges. Some cases focus on the fact that higher charges are designed to help cover the cost of those who cannot pay, so called "cost-shifting." Courts have generally recognized that this is necessary and reasonable. The law cannot mandate care to those who cannot pay for that care and then block the other avenues to cover the associated costs. The other focus of the challenges is on the markup on individual items, for example, the $10 aspirin. Most courts place the burden on the challenger to show that the charges were not reasonable. In those jurisdictions, these cases seldom reach appellate courts. Some courts place more of the burden on the provider. In those jurisdictions, occasionally uninsured patients have succeeded in their challenges when the hospital has provided insufficient evidence of reasonableness.[8]

In 2004, another organized attack on charges to the uninsured was launched. Lawsuits were filed against hundreds of hospitals in many states.[9] The suits made various claims including that hospitals should be required to lower their charges to the uninsured as a condition of their federal tax exemption. In 2004, a federal court refused to consolidate the cases into a single case.[10] Federal courts

---

5   MD. HEALTH-GENERAL CODE ANN. §§ 19-201 et seq.; L. Page, *Florida ends hospital rate review; Maryland now alone*, AM. MED. NEWS, July 20, 1998, 16; L. Page, *Maryland rate-setting faces overhaul or extinction*, AM. MED. NEWS, Nov. 16, 1998, 18 [only Maryland sets rates, few other states review hospital charges].

6   18 V.S.A. §§ 9451 et seq.; *see* G. D'Ambrosio, *Vermont approves embattled Fletcher Allen Health's $579 million budget*, BOND BUYER, Sept. 8, 2003, 29.

7   *E.g.*, Johnson v. Plantation Gen. Hosp., 641 So. 2d 58 (Fla. 1994) [claims of patients in class action challenge for overcharging could be aggregated to meet amount in controversy]; Galloway v. Methodist Hosps., Inc., 658 N.E.2d 611 (Ind. Ct. App.1995) [in collection action, hospital controller testimony as to reasonableness of charges sufficient; not unreasonable to base charges on hospital's budgetary needs]; Hall v. Humana Hosp. Daytona Beach, 686 So. 2d 653 (Fla. 5th DCA) [payment ratified agreement to pay charges, so could not sue for refund].

8   *E.g.*, St. Francis Med. Ctr. v. Hargrove, 956 S.W.2d 949 (Mo. Ct. App. 1997) [charges not reasonable]; *contra*, St. Luke's Episcopal-Presbyterian Hosp. v. Underwood, 957 S.W.2d 496 (Mo. Ct. App. 1997) [charges reasonable].

9   *See* R. Abelson & J. Glater, *Suits contend that hospitals bilked the poor*, N.Y. TIMES, June 17, 2004, C1; L.W. Clark, K.M. Kelton & D. Flynn, *What may arrive in tomorrow's mail? An analysis of class action lawsuits concerning hospital billing of uninsured patients*, HEALTH L. RPTR [BNA], July 29, 2004, 1134 [hereinafter Health L. Rptr. cited as H.L.R.]; *Mississippi nonprofit hospital system agrees to settle uninsured patients' claims*, H.L.R., Aug. 12, 2004, 1204.

10   *In re* Not-For-Profit Hospitals/Uninsured Patients Litigation, 341 F. Supp. 2d 1354 (J.P.M.L. 2004).

have consistently dismissed these suits.[11] At least one state court has allowed the suits to proceed on state law theories.[12] One hospital entered a preliminary settlement of the suit that was brought against it, but later withdrew from the settlement.[13] One positive outcome of the suits is that the Center for Medicare and Medicaid Services (CMS) announced that providers could grant discounts to all of the uninsured, not just the needy, without adversely affecting certain Medicare payments.[14] Some states have pursued efforts to promote discounts for the uninsured. For example, the Minnesota Attorney General has actively pursued a program that has resulted in new discount practices by many hospitals in that state.[15] It is not yet clear what other impact these suits will have beyond diverting health care dollars to legal defense.

9-2 How Are Medicare, Medicaid, and Other Major Government Payment Programs Structured?

There are several federal government programs that provide payment for health care, including Medicare; Civilian Health and Medical Program for the Uniformed Services (CHAMPUS);[16] Federal Employee Health Benefits Program (FEHBP);[17] and the Veterans Administration. There are federal-state programs, especially Medicaid. There are also various state programs. Participation in some government programs is limited to those who have a contract with the appropriate government agency. However, because of the latitude of government to unilaterally change most of the programs, the right to payment is often determined not by contract, but more

---

[11] *E.g.,* Sabeta v. Baptist. Hosp., 2005 U.S. Dist. LEXIS 6132 (S.D. Fla.); Peterson v. Allina Health Sys., 2005 U.S. Dist. LEXIS 1962 (D. Minn) & cases cited therein; *See generally* L.T. Crowley, *Hospitals prevailing in charity care cases,* N. Y. LAW J., Dec. 28, 2004, 3.

[12] *E.g.,* Servedio v. Our Lady of the Resurrection Med. Ctr., No. 04 L 3381 (Ill. Cir. Ct. Jan. 7, 2005) [dismissal denied], *as reported in* H.L.R., Feb. 3, 2005, 165.

[13] *Mississippi nonprofit hospital system shuns proposed charity care settlement,* H.L.R., Apr. 14, 2005, 513 [decision not to finalize tentative settlement due to overwhelming demand for charity care services].

[14] CMS guidance (Dec. 27, 2004) [www.cms.hhs.gov/providers/FAQ_Uninsured_Additional.pdf]; *HCA says it will provide discounts to uninsured, cites new CMS guidance,* H.L.R., Jan. 13, 2005, 68.

[15] *Four Minnesota health systems agree to drop prices for uninsured patients,* H.L.R., May 12, 2005, 652; *but see* A. Dembner, *Romney aide targets debt at hospitals: aggressive collecting from patients urged,* BOSTON GLOBE, May 18,2005, A1 [MA urging more aggressive collection of copayments, deductibles].

[16] 10 U.S.C. §§ 1079–1086, 1095; 32 C.F.R. pt. 199.

[17] 5 U.S.C. §§ 8901–8914; 5 C.F.R. pt. 890; 48 C.F.R. chaps.1, 16.

by the current statute and regulations and the practices of those who have been assigned administrative responsibility to make payments. This section focuses on Medicare (9-2.1) and Medicaid (9-2.2) and then discusses state programs (9-2.3).

9-2.1 Medicare

The 1965 Amendments to the Social Security Act[18] added Title XVIII to the Act. Title XVIII established a two-part program of health insurance for the aged known as Medicare. In 2002, $267.1 billion was spent on the Medicare program.

Persons are eligible to participate in Part A, the hospital insurance program, if they (1) are 65 or older and are receiving retirement benefits under Title II of the Social Security Act or the Railroad Retirement Act, (2) qualify under a special program for persons with end-stage renal (kidney) disease, or (3) qualify under the special transitional program. Persons not qualifying otherwise who are 65 or older may still participate in Part A by paying premiums. Anyone age 65 or older who is a U.S. citizen or has been a permanent resident alien for five years may elect to enroll in Part B, a program of supplementary medical insurance. Medicare applies to all qualified people without regard to financial need. It is administered federally; so it is intended to have nationally uniform benefits. Provider relations and payments are federally administered on a regional basis, and some regional variations exist.[19]

In 1998, the President proposed expanding Medicare eligibility to persons from age 55 to 64, but this was not enacted.[20]

Congress passed the Balanced Budget Act of 1997 making a number of significant cuts in Medicare expecting to slow the growth of Medicare spending. However, Medicare spending was actually reduced, with less being spent in the first half of fiscal year 1999 than in the first half of the prior fiscal year.[21] This created serious problems for providers. Many home health care providers went out

---

[18] Pub. L. No. 89-97, 79 Stat. 290 (1965).

[19] C. Culhane, *Medicare denial rates vary widely: Carriers inconsistent in judging medical necessity*, AM. MED. NEWS, Apr. 18, 1994, 3; *HCFA defends program appeal process, announces national coverage procedures*, 8 H.L.R. 695 (1999) [response to criticism of inconsistency in local determinations].

[20] J. Broder, *Clinton proposes opening Medicare to those 55 to 65*, N.Y. TIMES, Jan. 7, 1998, A1; R. Pear, *Clinton revives proposal to expand Medicare*, N.Y. TIMES, Jan. 10, 1999, 17.

[21] R. Pear, *With budget cutting, Medicare spending fell unexpectedly*, N.Y. TIMES, May 4, 1999, A20 [$103.9 billion compared to $106.5 billion].

of business.[22] Nursing homes were also threatened.[23] In late 1999, legislation was passed increasing payments.[24]

One significant area of health care that was not addressed by Medicare for many years is outpatient drug costs. Drugs were covered only when they are administered to inpatients, with a few limited exceptions, such as for some transplant drugs. There was increasing political attention to the portion of the income of many Medicare recipients that is spent on outpatient drugs. In 2003, the law was amended to create a new Part D outpatient drug benefit program, effective in 2006.[25] In the interim, a controversial, complex program of drug discount cards was offered to Medicare participants. Initially, enrollment was slow.

Due to the many out-of-pocket costs associated with Medicare, there is a substantial market for Medi-Gap insurance to cover the costs not covered by Medicare.

Between the pressures to expand the program and the pressures to keep the program fiscally sound, it is likely that Medicare coverage and payments will continue to significantly change. The Hospital Insurance Trust Fund Board of Trustees reported in 2004 that the fund is expected to be exhausted in 2019.[26]

PARTS A, B, C, AND D. The Medicare program is divided into four parts, lettered A through D.

Part A. Part A is a program of hospital insurance benefits for the aged and selected others. Part A is financed by a special tax on employers, employees, and the self-employed. The coverage includes a specified number of days of care in hospitals and extended care facilities for each benefit period plus posthospital home care. The Medicare Catastrophic Coverage Act of 1988[27] removed the limits on the number of hospital days and increased the limits for other coverages. There was strong opposition by the elderly to the surtax which funded the 1988 benefit expansion, and

---

[22] *IPS has caused 763 home health agencies to close, home care association reports,* 7 H.L.R. 1607 (1998); *Reductions in Medicare payments three times worse than CBO first thought,* 8 H.L.R. 451 (1999) [original projection $16.1 billion in cuts over five years, now projecting $47 billion over same period; state licensing agencies report 1,067 home health agency closures since Oct. 1997].

[23] *Domenici, at hearing, says changes in Medicare may shut nursing homes,* WALL ST. J., Apr. 23, 1999, B2; *Vencor misses debt payment, raising question of its survival,* N.Y. TIMES, May 4, 1999, C2.

[24] *Provider relief becomes law,* MOD. HEALTHCARE, Dec. 6, 1999, 2.

[25] Pub. No. L. 108-173, Title I, 117 Stat. 2071, *codified* as 42 U.S.C. § 1395w-101 et seq.

[26] A. Goldstein, *A dire report on Medicare finances,* WASH. POST, Mar. 24, 2004, A1.

[27] Pub. L. No. 100-360, 102 Stat. 683 (1988).

Congress repealed the Act in 1989, restoring the coverage limits and eliminating the surtax.[28]

Claims must be presented to trigger reimbursement. Until 1983, reimbursement under Part A was based on the allowable costs of the facility providing the care but was subject to several reimbursement limits. This was changed by the Social Security Amendments of 1983,[29] so that payment to hospitals for inpatient care is based on a prospectively determined amount per discharge according to the patient's diagnosis and the facility's location. In 2000, home health care and many hospital outpatient procedures were converted to prospective payment systems.[30]

Beneficiaries have to pay certain deductible and coinsurance payments. A deductible is the amount of health care charges that the patient must incur and owe before Medicare pays for any of the remainder. Medicare will pay only a percentage of some of the remaining allowable payments for some services; the percentage not paid by Medicare is called a coinsurance payment and is owed by the patient. In some circumstances, hospitals and physicians waive deductibles and copayments.[31] At least one state forbids routine waivers.[32] There is concern that some waivers may be viewed as violations of Medicare antifraud and abuse laws. Some waivers by hospitals are within the safe harbors permitted by regulation.[33]

Part B. Part B is a program of supplementary medical insurance covering a substantial part of physician and other practitioner services, medical supplies, and X-rays and laboratory tests incident to physician services, as well as other services not covered under Part A, such as ambulance services and prosthetic devices. The program is funded from contributions by beneficiaries and the federal government. Beneficiaries must pay a deductible and usually a twenty per-

---

[28] Pub. L. No. 101-234 (1989); M. Tolchin. *Lawmakers tell the elderly: "Next year" on health-care,* N.Y. TIMES, Nov. 23, 1989, A20.

[29] Pub. L. No. 98-21, 97 Stat. 65 (1983), *as amended by* Pub. L. No. 98-369, 98 Stat. 1073 (1984); 42 C.F.R. §§ 405.470–405.477; J. Tieman, *It was 20 years ago today...; some say it's complex and vulnerable to political whims, but Medicare's PPS has helped impose order on hospital finances,* MOD. HEALTHCARE, Sept. 29, 2003, 6.

[30] V. Galloro, *Embracing PPS; Home-care providers see opportunity under new system,* MOD. HEALTHCARE, Sept. 25, 2000, 2; V. Galloro, *Flipped out over outpatient PPS,* MOD. HEALTHCARE, Nov. 20, 2000, 30.

[31] *See* M. Freudenheim, *Some doctors letting patients skip co-payments,* N.Y. TIMES, Dec. 27, 2003, B1.

[32] Parrish v. Lamm, 758 P.2d 1356 (Colo. 1988); Annotation, *Validity of statute prohibiting health providers from the practice of waiving patients' obligation to pay health insurance deductibles or copayments, or advertising such practice,* 8 A.L.R. 5TH 855.

[33] 42 C.F.R. § 1001.952(k).

cent coinsurance amount. Enrollment is voluntary; persons are responsible for their own decisions whether to enroll in Part B. In 1998, a federal appellate court refused to order retroactive enrollment when the plaintiff claimed a federal employee gave misinformation.[34]

Some categories of providers are paid under Part B on the basis of "reasonable charges," which are subject to numerous arbitrary limits.[35] Since 1992, most payments to physicians have been paid based on a resource-based relative value scale (RBRVS).[36] Effective January 1, 1999, the resource-based, relative value payment system for paying physicians was expanded to include practice expenses.[37] Prior to the change, the practice expense component of payments had continued to be derived from historical charges. Effective January 1, 2000, the system was expanded to include malpractice expenses.[38]

Medicare payments can be made only to the provider who provides the services and certain entities permitted to bill for the provider; other reassignments of payments are prohibited.[39] Thus, some billing arrangements are not permitted. Each physician has a unique physician identification number (UPIN) that must be put on each bill.[40] Another billing issue is that physicians may bill for services, such as X-rays, provided by others, such as technicians, usually only when the services are provided in a way that meets the technical requirements to be "incident to" the physicians' services.[41]

Part C. The Balanced Budget Act of 1997 reorganized Part C of Medicare Part C, establishing the Medicare+Choice program that permitted eligible individuals to elect to receive their Medicare benefits through enrollment in a variety of private health plans.[42] Each plan must meet detailed requirements to be qualified to participate.

The payments associated with the plans led many HMOs either to withdraw from participation or to reduce their scope of benefits.[43]

---

[34] McGowan v. Shalala, 135 F.3d 531 (7th Cir. 1998).

[35] *E.g.*, 42 U.S.C. § 1395u(b).

[36] 42 U.S.C. § 1395w-4.

[37] 63 FED. REG. 58,813 (Nov. 2, 1998), *codified in* 42 C.F.R. § 414.22.

[38] 64 FED. REG. 59,380 (Nov. 2, 1999), *codified in* 42 C.F.R. § 414.22.

[39] 42 U.S.C. §§ 1395g, 1395u(b)(6); 42 C.F.R. §§ 424.73, 424.66; *Physician staffing companies may not receive Medicare payment, HCFA says*, 6 H.L.R. 608 (1997); CMS Transmittal No. 111 (Feb. 27, 2004) [relaxing assignment rules].

[40] 42 U.S.C. § 1395l(q).

[41] 42 U.S.C. § 1395x(s)(2)(A).

[42] 42 U.S.C. §§ 1395w-21 et seq., as added by the Balanced Budget Act of 1997, Pub. L. No. 105-33, § 4001; 42 C.F.R. pt. 422, added by 63 FED. REG. 34,967 (June 26, 1998), amended by 64 FED. REG. 7,967 (Feb. 17, 1999).

[43] *See* L.B. Benko, *Hopping mad; Medicare HMOs' restrictions on drug coverage prompt high enrollee turnover*, MOD. HEALTHCARE, Apr. 9, 2001, 35.

Effective in 2004, the program was renamed Medicare Advantage and payments were increased.[44]

One state attempted to require Medicare HMOs to provide unlimited drug coverage. A federal appellate court declared the law to be preempted by federal law.[45] In 2001, a federal appellate court rejected challenge to the geographic differences in payment rates.[46]

Part D. The 2003 amendments to the Social Security Act added a prescription drug benefit, effective in 2006. This provides federal payment for part of the costs of outpatient prescription drugs. Rules have been promulgated establishing geographic regions and establishing rules for creating the drug formularies that will determine which drugs are covered.[47]

ADMINISTRATION. The Secretary of HHS has the overall responsibility for Medicare. The operation of the program has been assigned to CMS. Congress authorized the delegation of much of the day-to-day administration to state agencies and public and private organizations operating under agreements with the Secretary of HHS.

Most payment claims are processed by private agencies that have entered agreements to serve as "intermediaries" for Part A or "carriers" for Part B. They make initial determinations whether services provided to beneficiaries are payable by the program and how much payment is due. Hospitals must be cautious in acting on information provided by intermediaries and carriers. The United States Supreme Court ruled in 1984 that HCFA could recover Medicare overpayments from a provider despite the fact that the overpayments were due to erroneous information from the intermediary.[48] The Court stated that providers are expected to know the law and cannot rely on information provided by governmental agents. In areas that have not been addressed nationally, local intermediaries have the power to adopt local coverage rules; so there is regional variation in what services are covered by Medicare.[49] In 2004, a fed-

---

[44] *See* J. Tieman, *Pay increase; increased HMO funding excites many*, MOD. HEALTHCARE, Feb. 9, 2004, 17; 70 FED. REG. 4,587 (Jan. 28, 2005).

[45] Massachusetts Ass'n of HMOs v. Ruthardt, 194 F.3d 176 (1st Cir. 1999).

[46] Minnesota Senior Fed. v. United States, 273 F.3d 805 (8th Cir. 2001).

[47] Pub. L. No. 108-173, Title I, 117 Stat. 2071, *codified as* 42 U.S.C. § 1395w-101 et seq.; R. Pear, *U.S. settles on regions for dispensing Medicare drug benefits*, N.Y. TIMES, Dec. 17, 2004, A16; R. Pear, *New Medicare rules on drugs balance access against costs*, N.Y. TIMES, Jan. 22, 2005, A1 [formularies]; 70 FED. REG. 4193 (Jan. 28, 2005) [formularies]; R. Pear, *Defying experts, insurers join Medicare drug plan*, N.Y. TIMES, Mar. 6, 2005, 1.

[48] Heckler v. Community Health Servs., 467 U.S. 51 (1984).

[49] *See* L. McGinley, *Behind Medicare's decisions, an invisible web of gatekeepers*, WALL ST. J., Sept. 16, 2003, A1.

eral appellate court ruled that local coverage determinations by intermediaries are merely interpretive rules that are not subject to the formal federal rulemaking requirements.[50]

Some intermediaries have been charged with defrauding the government while acting in that capacity.[51] Federal courts have ruled that since intermediaries and carriers are administering a federal program that they are immune when providers sue.[52]

PARTICIPATING PROVIDERS. To be a participating provider of services and receive payments from Medicare, a hospital must sign an agreement with HHS and meet the conditions of participation.[53] The only exception is that Medicare will pay for some emergency services in nonparticipating hospitals. The participating provider agreement specifies that the hospital will not bill Medicare patients for services except for (1) deductible and coinsurance payments required by law and (2) charges for services that Medicare does not cover. Charges can be made for noncovered services only if the patient has been given adequate notice that they are not covered. A hospital is deemed to meet the conditions of participation if it is accredited by JCAHO or the American Osteopathic Association unless a Medicare inspection indicates noncompliance.[54]

Physicians who become participating providers are paid directly by Medicare and may charge patients only allowed copayments and deductibles. When patients are treated by nonparticipating physicians, Medicare pays the patient directly. The physician then bills the patient. The amount the nonparticipating physician may bill the patient is limited to a maximum allowable actual charge (MAAC).[55] Physicians who bill more than the MAAC can be assessed substantial civil money penalties and barred from Medicare payments for

---

[50] Erringer v. Thompson, 371 F.3d 625 (9th Cir. 2004).

[51] *E.g.*, United States v. Blue Cross & Blue Shield of Mich., No. L93-1794 (D. Md. settlement Jan. 10, 1995), *complaint reprinted in* M.M.G. ¶43,019; *Illinois Blues to pay $144 million to settle fraud charges*, AM. MED. NEWS, Aug. 3, 1998, 8.

[52] *E.g.*, Midland Psychiatric Assocs., Inc. v. United States, 145 F.3d 1000 (8th Cir. 1998) [Medicare intermediary immune from tortious interference suit by provider]; Pani v. Empire Blue Cross & Blue Shield, 152 F.3d 67 (2d Cir. 1998), *cert. denied*, 525 U.S. 1103 (1999) [Medicare intermediary immune from tort suits for investigating, reporting possible fraud].

[53] 42 U.S.C. § 1395x(e); 42 C.F.R. pt. 482. There are also conditions of participation for other providers, *E.g.*, 42 C.F.R. §§ 405.1101–405.1137 [skilled nursing facilities].

[54] 42 U.S.C.A. §§ 1395aa, 1395bb; Cospito v. Heckler, 742 F.2d 72 (3d Cir. 1984), *cert. denied*, 471 U.S. 1131 (1985) [not improper delegation to Joint Commission because HHS retains ultimate authority].

[55] *E.g.*, Garelick v. Sullivan, 987 F.2d 913 (2d Cir. 1993), *cert. denied*, 510 U.S. 821 (1993) [fee limits not taking].

up to five years.[56] Some states have required physicians to accept the Medicare payment amount as payment in full.[57]

In 1997, the Medicare law was amended to permit physicians to opt out of Medicare and reach separate payment arrangements with their patients, but those who opt out cannot receive payment from Medicare for any of their patients for two years.[58] Challenges to the limited scope of this exception were unsuccessful.[59]

Health and Human Services frequently threatens to revoke participating provider status, but most hospitals are able to make changes and reach settlements that avoid revocation.[60] Rarely hospitals have had their status revoked.[61] In rare cases, prior to 2000, providers obtained restraining orders to stop termination.[62] However in 2000, the United States Supreme Court ruled that administrative remedies must be exhausted before courts may consider such terminations.[63] Occasionally, administrative remedies do reverse terminations.[64]

PROSPECTIVE PAYMENT. The Social Security Amendments of 1983[65] established a Medicare prospective payment system (PPS) based on diagnosis-related groups (DRGs) to pay hospitals for inpatient care. The system has been modified by numerous amendments.[66] All Medicare acute care inpatients are divided into twenty-five major diagnostic categories that are further divided into

---

[56] 42 U.S.C. §§ 1395u(b)(3)(G), 1395u(j).

[57] *E.g.*, Medical Soc'y of N.Y. State v. Cuomo, 976 F.2d 812 (2d Cir. 1992) [no preemption of state statute forbidding balanced billing of Medicare]; Pennsylvania Med. Soc'y v. Marconis, 942 F.2d 842 (3d Cir. 1991).

[58] Balanced Budget Act of 1997, Pub. L. No. 105-33, § 4507; 63 FED. REG. 58,813 (Nov. 2, 1999); R. Pear, *New flexibility for Medicare, but at a price*, N.Y. TIMES, Aug. 5, 1997, A1.

[59] *E.g.*, United Seniors Ass'n v. Shalala, 2 F. Supp. 2d 39 (D. D.C. 1998).

[60] *E.g, In re* Westchester County Med. Center, Docket No. 91-504-2 (H.H.S. Sept. 29, 1992), *as discussed in* 2 H.L.R. 61 (1993) [revocation of participation of hospital ordered for violation of Rehabilitation Act by restricting HIV-positive worker, but case settled].

[61] *E.g.*, Our Lady of Mt. Carmel Hosp. v. Secretary of HEW, Civ. No. 72 CA 84 (W.D. Tex. Oct. 4, 1973), *reprinted in* M.M.G. ¶26,778 [noncompliance with conditions of participation]; Milo Commun. Hosp. v. Weinberger, 525 F.2d 144 (1st Cir. 1975) [noncompliance with Life Safety Code]; Summit Health, Ltd. v. Inspector Ge., Doc. No. C-108, Dec. 1173 (HHS D.A.B., App. Div. June 29, 1990), *reprinted in* M.M.G. ¶38,653 [exclusion of convalescent hospital after guilty plea to criminal patient neglect]; *see also* Kings View Hosp. v. H.C.F.A., DAB Dec. No. CR442, Docket No. C-96-233 (Nov. 5, 1996) [Medicare participation agreement automatically terminated on day hospital failed to maintain its license].

[62] *E.g.*, Mediplex v. Shalala, 39 F. Supp. 2d 88 (D. Mass. 1999).

[63] Shalala v. Illinois Council on Long Term Care, 529 U.S. 1 (2000).

[64] *E.g.*, CSM Home Health Servs. Inc. v. H.C.F.A., HHS DAB, App. Div., Dec. No. 1622 (July 23, 1997), *as discussed at* 6 H.L.R. 1270 (1997) [provider wrongfully terminated from Medicare, not out of compliance with conditions of participation].

[65] Pub. L. No. 98-21, 97 Stat. 65 (1983).

[66] Pub. L. No. 98-21, 97 Stat. 65 (1983) (codified as amended primarily at 42 U.S.C. § 1395ww); 42 C.F.R. pt. 412.

approximately five hundred DRGs based on their principal diagnoses, complications, comorbidities, and whether certain procedures are performed.[67] The principal diagnosis is the one chiefly responsible for the admission. Medicare will pay for nearly all of the groups. A small number of groups involve unacceptable diagnoses and invalid data. Each year adjustments are made in the groups and in the assignments to the groups. By statute, no administrative or judicial review is permitted for either the DRG groups, assignment to a group, or the weight given to the group.[68] One criticism of the DRG system is that it does not equitably adjust for the cost of treating more severely ill patients in each group. Various severity of illness adjustments have been proposed,[69] but none has been adopted. There is one adjustment to all prospective payments to each hospital based on the average severity of all Medicare patients treated in the hospital.

With a few exceptions, the hospital receives one payment for the entire admission based on the DRG and facility location. The payment also covers some preadmission services.[70] The payment rate varies geographically based on regional wages and other factors. This has lead to periodic controversy as states have sought to reduce or preserve the differences.[71]

There is no extra payment for longer stays or more procedures unless the patient becomes an outlier. An outlier is a patient with a high total cost of care. Medicare makes an extra payment for outliers, some bad debts, and some other items.[72] Another exception is that some educational costs and kidney acquisition costs are paid separately from the prospective payment.[73] Initially capital costs were paid separately on a cost basis, but since 1991, capital costs have been paid prospectively.[74]

---

[67] 69 FED. REG. 48,916 (Aug. 11, 2004).

[68] 42 U.S.C. § 1395ww(d)(7); *E.g.*, Little Co. of Mary Hosp. v. Shalala, 24 F.3d 984 (7th Cir. 1994) [no right to hearing after hospital failed to correct its own DRG assignment within 60 days].

[69] *See* discussion in 59 FED. REG. 45,341 (Sept. 1, 1994).

[70] 42 C.F.R. § 412.2(c)(5), first printed in 59 FED. REG. 1654 (Jan. 12, 1994).

[71] *E.g.*, *State to appeal proposed Medicare rules*, AP, July 4, 2003 [Iowa]; R. Pérez-Peña, *Hospital cash to be shifted across Hudson*, N.Y. TIMES, July 3, 2004, A15 [NY, NJ]; R. Hernandez, *'Big four' governors working together to lobby Congress*, N.Y. TIMES, July 20, 2004, A20 [CA, NY, TX, FL]; M. Santora, *New York hospitals to sue over Medicare rule change*, N.Y. TIMES, Aug. 25, 2004, B2; *but see* Minnesota Senior Fed. v. United States, 273 F.3d 805 (8th Cir. 2001) [rejecting challenge to geographic difference in Part C payment rates].

[72] *E.g.*, 42 U.S.C. § 1395ww(d)(5)(A) [outliers]; 42 C.F.R. §§ 412.80–412.86 [outliers]; 42 C.F.R. §§ 412.115(a), 413.80 [bad debts]; 42 C.F.R. §§ 412.115(c), 466.78 [some copying costs].

[73] 42 U.S.C. § 1395ww(d)(5)(B); 42 C.F.R. § 413.85 [indirect medical education costs]; 42 C.F.R. § 412.100 [kidney acquisition costs].

[74] 42 C.F.R. §§ 412.300–412.352.

An adjustment for indirect medical education costs increases payments to hospitals with medical residency programs.[75] Children's hospitals, long-term care hospitals, psychiatric hospitals, and rehabilitation hospitals were initially exempt from the PPS so they could continue to receive cost-based payment from Medicare.[76] A prospective payment system has been implemented for rehabilitation hospitals,[77] and in 2004, one was being implemented for psychiatric hospitals.[78]

There is an adjustment for some hospitals that serve a disproportionate share of low-income or Medicaid patients,[79] are sole community providers,[80] are referral centers,[81] are essential access community hospitals,[82] or experience other extraordinary circumstances.

PPS is prospective only in the sense that the amount paid is calculated based on circumstances at the time of admission. Payment is made only after services are provided. PPS completely changed provider incentives. Under the previous cost-based system, additional hospital days and services meant additional payment; there was an incentive to give patients all the services that could possibly benefit them. In some situations, unnecessary services were provided, but Medicare refused to pay for them, when discovered.

Under PPS the incentive is to minimize services and shorten stays. Hospitals lose money if services exceed the prospective payment, and they keep the savings when services cost less than the payment.

Interhospital transfers presented a problem when structuring the prospective payment system. Those fashioning PPS wanted to make one payment to be shared by all hospitals that provided care to the patient, but the Act did not authorize shared payment. The hospital from which the patient is finally discharged receives a full prospective payment based on the patient's DRG. The hospital that cares for the patient before transfer is paid a per diem rate equal to the prospective payment for the DRG divided by the average length of stay for that DRG, but the total cannot exceed the full DRG pay-

---

[75] 42 U.S.C. § 1395ww(h); 42 C.F.R. § 412.105.

[76] 42 U.S.C. § 1395ww(d)(1)(B); 42 C.F.R. § 412.23.

[77] 42 C.F.R. Part 412, Subpart P, §§ 412.602 et seq.; 70 FED. REG. 30188 (May 25, 2005).

[78] 42 C.F.R. Part 412, Subpart N, § 412.400 et seq.; 69 FED. REG. 66922 (Nov. 15, 2004).

[79] 42 U.S.C. § 1395ww(d)(5)(F); 42 C.F.R. § 412.106; North Broward Hosp. Dist. v. Shalala, 172 F.3d 90 (D.C. Cir. 1999) [upholding disproportionate share regulations].

[80] 42 U.S.C. § 1395ww(d)(5)(D); 42 C.F.R. § 412.92; *E.g.*, Macon County Samaritan Mem. Hosp. v. Shalala, 7 F.3d 762 (8th Cir. 1993) [affirming sole community provider criteria].

[81] 42 U.S.C. § 1395ww(d)(5)(C); 42 C.F.R. § 412.96.

[82] 42 U.S.C. § 1395ww(d)(5)(D)(v); 42 C.F.R. § 412.109.

ment. The transferring hospital can qualify for additional payment if the patient becomes an outlier due to high costs.[83]

Other institutional providers are now also paid on a prospective payment basis. For example, skilled nursing facilities are paid on the basis of the Resource Utilization Group (RUG) into which the patient fits.[84] In 2005, CMS proposed to expand the number of RUGs from 44 to 55.[85] Hospital outpatient services are paid on the basis of the Ambulatory Payment Classification (APC) system, by which outpatient services and procedures are placed in groups that are comparable clinically and in terms of resource use.[86] Home health agencies are paid on the basis of a national standardized sixty-day episode payment, adjusted for case mix, wage index, and other factors, such as the partial episode payment adjustment (PEP adjustment) and the significant change in condition (SCIC) adjustment. When there are four or fewer visits, payment is on the basis of the national per visit amount for the discipline, called the low utilization payment adjustment (LUPA).[87] Long-term care hospitals (LTCHs) are also paid on a prospective basis.[88]

CODING. One important issue for all providers is proper coding of the services provided. The diagnoses and certain other features of the patient's condition or treatment must be coded on the claim. Hospital claims are coded according to the International Classification of Diseases, Ninth Edition, Clinical Modification (ICD-9-CM). Physician claims are coded according to the CMS Common Procedure Coding System (HCPCS), which includes the Physician's Current Procedural Terminology (CPT).[89] The amount of payment is determined by the codes. In some circumstances, erroneous coding can constitute fraud.

APPEALS. Depending on the amount of money in controversy, hospitals may appeal payment decisions under the old cost reimbursement

---

[83] 42 C.F.R. § 412.4.

[84] 42 C.F.R. Part 413, Subpart J, §§ 413.339 et seq.

[85] 70 FED. REG. 29,070 (May 19, 2005).

[86] 42 C.F.R. Part 419, Subpart C, §§ 419.310 et seq.; 65 FED. REG. 18,434 (Apr. 7, 2000).

[87] 65 FED. REG. 41,128 (July 3, 2000); 69 FED. REG. 62,124 (Oct. 4, 2004).

[88] 42 C.F.R. Part 412, Subpart O; 67 FED. REG. 55,954 (Aug. 30, 2002); 70 FED. REG. 24,168 (May 6, 2005).

[89] United States v. Krizek, 859 F. Supp. 5 (D.D.C. 1994) [although physician barred from participation until he could abide by coding rules, criticism of government for confusing coding requirements]; Practice Management Information Corp. v. American Med. Ass'n, 133 F.3d 1140 (9th Cir. 1998), *cert. denied*, 524 U.S. 952 (1998) [HCFA adoption of CPT code did not cast it into public domain, but terms of AMA exclusive license with agency constituted misuse by specifying agency not to use competitor's products].

systems to the Provider Reimbursement Review Board (PRRB) in the case of larger amounts or to their Medicare intermediary in the case of smaller amounts. When the issues being appealed apply to several hospitals, group appeals are frequently pursued to reduce the cost to individual hospitals. The Secretary of HHS has the authority to modify the decisions of the PRRB or the intermediary. The final decision of HHS concerning a payment issue can sometimes be appealed to the federal courts. Administrative remedies must be exhausted before resort to the courts.[90]

The number of issues that can be appealed is limited.[91] In 1993, the United States Supreme Court decided that HHS is not required to give providers an opportunity to establish entitlement to payment in excess of limits stated in the regulations.[92] In 1999, the Supreme Court decided that there could be no judicial review of denials of reopening of Medicare cost reports.[93]

In 1995, the Supreme Court upheld the HHS guidelines for treatment of bond defeasance losses, finding that HHS did not have to adhere to generally accepted accounting principles (GAPP) in developing its cost determination principles.[94]

Physician challenges to changes in reimbursement policies for individual procedures and specialties have generally been unsuccessful.[95] Product manufacturers have had similar results. In 1994, a federal appellate court ruled that a drug manufacturer does not have standing to challenge the Medicare Part B policy of limiting payments for one of its drugs to the amount paid for a competing product.[96]

Sometimes coverage decisions by CMS are challenged. In most cases, courts defer to CMS and uphold the decisions.[97] However,

---

[90] *E.g.*, National Kidney Patients Ass'n v. Sullivan, 958 F.2d 1127 (D.C. Cir. 1992), *cert. denied*, 506 U.S. 1049 (1993); *see also* T. Albert, *Medicare appeals process too slow, GAO report finds*, AM. MED. NEWS, Nov. 17, 2003, 7 [only 43% of first-level appeals completed with 30 days required by Medicare, Medicaid, & SCHIP Benefits Improvement Act of 2000 (BIPA)]; *see also* 69 FED. REG. 35,716 (June 25, 2004) [proposed changes in provider appeal procedures].

[91] 42 U.S.C. §§ 405(h), 1395ff, 1395ii; Michigan Ass'n of Independent Clinical Labs. v. Shalala, 52 F.3d 1340 (6th Cir. 1994).

[92] Good Samaritan Hosp. v. Shalala, 508 U.S. 402 (1993).

[93] Your Home Visiting Nurse Servs., Inc. v. Shalala, 525 U.S. 449 (1999).

[94] Shalala v. Guernsey Mem. Hosp., 514 U.S. 87 (1995).

[95] *E.g.*, Necketopoulos v. Shalala, 941 F. Supp. 1382 (S.D. N.Y. 1996) [rejecting challenge to abandonment of use of modifier units as basis for Part B payment for anesthesia services]; American Acad. of Dermatology v. H.H.S., 118 F.3d 1495 (11th Cir. 1997) [rejecting challenge to change in payment policy for removal of precancerous skin lesions, failure to exhaust administrative remedies]; Abbott Radiology Assocs. v. Shalala, 160 F.3d 137 (2d Cir. 1998).

[96] TAP Pharmaceuticals v. D.H.H.S., 163 F.3d 199 (4th Cir. 1998).

[97] *E.g.*, Warder v. Shalala, 149 F.3d 73 (1st Cir. 1998), *cert. denied*, 526 U.S. 1064 (1999) [upholding HCFA Ruling 96-1 concerning the scope of coverage for orthotics, reversing a lower court that would have required formal rule-making procedures before the Ruling could take effect].

occasionally challengers succeed. In 1997, HCFA added a requirement that hospitals must be within a certain distance of a skilled nursing facility in order to be paid for providing respiratory services to the facility. A federal court granted injunction against the requirement finding it arbitrary because distance was irrelevant and not authorized by statute or regulation.[98]

Patients must follow the administrative appeal procedures established by CMS.[99] These procedures were adopted after a federal court in Arizona found the prior appeal rights after denials to Medicare HMO members were inadequate and issued an injunction requiring HCFA to monitor and enforce denial of care appeals of Medicare patients. In 1998, a federal appellate court upheld the injunction, but in 1999, the United States Supreme Court vacated the judgment and remanded the case to the appellate court for reconsideration. The appellate court dissolved the injunction.[100] In 2005, CMS substantially limited the access to personal hearings by reducing the number of hearing sites in the nation from 140 to 4.[101]

9-2.2 Medicaid

Medicaid is a joint federal-state program designed to provide medical assistance to individuals unable to afford health care. Although the Medicaid program is authorized by federal law (Title XIX of the Social Security Act[102]), states are not required to have Medicaid programs. Each state must pass its own law to participate. All states now participate. Under Medicaid, the federal government makes grants to states to enable them to furnish (1) medical assistance to families with dependent children and to aged, blind, or disabled individuals whose income and resources are insufficient to pay for necessary health services and (2) rehabilitation and other services to help such families and individuals obtain or retain the capability

---

[98] Vencor, Inc. v. Shalala, 988 F. Supp. 1467 (N.D. Ga. 1997) [permanent injunction]; *see also* Estate of Aitken v. Shalala, 986 F. Supp. 57 (D. Mass. 1997) [preliminary injunction of implementation of national coverage determination denying payment for electrical stimulation therapy treatments to promote healing of open wounds].

[99] 62 Fed. Reg. 25,844 (May 12, 1997); *Medicare beneficiaries' appeal rights codified in HCFA final rule*, 6 H.L.R. 780 (1997).

[100] Grijalva v. Shalala, 152 F.3d 1115 (9th Cir. 1998) [decisions by Medicare HMOs are state action entitled to due process, specific procedural protections mandated], *judgment vacated, case remanded*, 526 U.S. 1096 (1999), *remanded to district court*, 185 F.3d 1075 (9th Cir. 1999) [injunction dissolved].

[101] R. Pear, *Medicare change will limit access to claim hearing*, N.Y. Times, Apr. 24, 2005, 1.

[102] 42 U.S.C. §§ 1396–1396t.

for independence or self-care. The Secretary of HHS is responsible for administration of federal grants-in-aid to states under Medicaid.

Medicaid is different from Medicare in that it provides medical assistance for categories of persons in financial need, while Medicare provides medical assistance primarily to people 65 years of age or older without regard to financial need. Medicaid varies widely among the states, while Medicare is largely uniform. Medicaid is financed by general federal and state revenues, while Medicare is financed by a special tax on employers and employees for hospital insurance and by contributions by beneficiaries and the federal government for supplementary medical services. Medicaid is basically a welfare program, while Medicare is considered a form of social insurance.

BENEFICIARIES AND SCOPE OF BENEFITS. Any state adopting a Medicaid plan must provide certain minimum health benefits to the categorically needy. The categorically needy include individuals receiving financial assistance under the state's approved plan for Supplemental Security Income (Title XVI of the Social Security Act[103]) or for Aid to Families with Dependent Children (Title IV-A of the Social Security Act[104]). Several other groups are included in the categorically needy if they qualify for financial assistance under the state plans except for certain characteristics that Medicaid requires to be ignored. States have the option of including other persons within their plan as medically needy if (1) they would qualify for assistance under one of the preceding programs if their incomes were lower and (2) their incomes would be low enough to qualify for assistance under that program if they were permitted to subtract the health care expenses they have already incurred. This is sometimes called the "spend-down" option because the persons must in effect spend their income down to the threshold level for the other programs to be eligible for Medicaid.

In 1997, Congress authorized expanded Children Health Insurance Programs (CHIP), Title XXI of the Social Security Act. States were given the option of putting their CHIPs in Medicaid or establishing a non-Medicaid program. However, CMS favors Medicaid programs, denying federal vaccines to children in non-Medicaid programs and requiring non-Medicaid CHIPs to screen for Medicaid

---

[103] 42 U.S.C. §§ 1381–1383c.
[104] 42 U.S.C. §§ 601–613.

eligibility and enroll persons who are eligible in Medicaid.[105] Involvement of some states in CHIP was not at the projected level in 2002; so funds were reallocated to other states.[106]

In 2002, HHS allowed states to expand health insurance coverage under CHIP to fetuses by classifying them as unborn children.[107]

Undocumented aliens are ineligible for nonemergency Medicaid.[108]

There have been challenges to the age requirements for certain Medicaid benefits. The United States Supreme Court ruled that Congress can limit coverage in public health institutions to persons under age 21 and over age 65.[109] However, the Arizona Supreme Court ruled that the Medicaid law does not permit states to limit liver transplants to minors.[110] Courts have sometimes enjoined state attempts to drop other categories of persons from eligibility.[111]

Eligible recipients must apply to the designated state agency before Medicaid will pay for the services they receive. State Medicaid plans must meet many conditions before they can be approved, but states are permitted substantial flexibility in the administration of their own programs. States may decide, within federal guidelines, which persons in addition to the categorically needy will be eligible for medical assistance. In determining scope of benefits, states are required to provide some five basic services to the categorically needy but are free to provide additional optional services. Although

---

[105] Pub. L. No. 105-33, § 4901; 62 FED. REG. 48,098 (Sept. 12, 1997) [guidance to help design plans]; *States split evenly between Medicaid, separate programs for kid care effort*, 6 H.L.R. 1753 (1997); *Non-Medicaid CHIP programs not eligible for federal vaccine funds, HCFA says*, 7 H.L.R. 906 (1998); *CHIP reporting requirements released: HCFA reminds states about deadlines*, 7 H.L.R. 1952 (1998) [non-Medicaid CHIPs must screen for Medicaid eligibility, enroll in Medicaid]; R. Pear, *Many states slow to use children's insurance fund*, N.Y. TIMES, May 9, 1999, 1.

[106] *See* C. Ornstein, *States cut back coverage for poor*, L.A. TIMES, Feb. 25, 2002, A1; R. Pear, *States forfeit unspent U.S. money for child health insurance*, N.Y. TIMES, Oct. 14, 2002, A17.

[107] 67 FED. REG. 61,956 (Oct. 2, 2002).

[108] *E.g.*, Greenery Rehab. Group, Inc. v. Hammon, 150 F.3d 226 (2d Cir. 1998) [long-term care for undocumented alien for chronic conditions from accident were not care for emergency medical condition, not covered by Medicaid beyond initial stabilization]; S. Sengupta, *Illegal and with AIDS: New law cuts off help*, N.Y. TIMES, Dec. 29, 1997, A14 [loss of Medicaid benefits in N.Y.]; Norwood Hosp. v. Comm'r of Public Welfare, 417 Mass. 54, 627 N.E.2d 914 (1994); *but see* Lewis v. Grinker, 794 F. Supp. 1193 (C.D. N.Y. 1991) [due to status of fetus as citizen, cannot deny Medicaid coverage for prenatal care to financially eligible undocumented aliens], *aff'd*, 926 F.2d 1206 (2d Cir. 1992); *Lewis* criticized in Douglas v. Babcock, 990 F.2d 875 (6th Cir.), *cert. denied*, 510 U.S. 825 (1993) [pregnant women denied Medicaid for noncooperation in determining paternity of previous children].

[109] Schwieker v. Wilson, 450 U.S. 221 (1981) [strict scrutiny not applied to Medicaid coverage in public health institutions only under 21 and over 64].

[110] Salgado v. Kirschner, 179 Ariz. 301, 878 P.2d 659 (1994), *cert. denied*, 513 U.S. 1151 (1995).

[111] See *Federal court rules in favor of poor in medical insurance lawsuit*, AP, Mar. 26, 2004 [2d Cir. enjoins Conn. from dropping 18,000 from Medicaid].

the states are given wide latitude in the administration of their programs, they are sensitive to federal direction because 50 percent or more of the financial support for Medicaid comes from the federal government. Both federal administrative agencies and courts use the threat of withdrawal of federal funds to coerce changes in the state's program. For example, when a Florida federal court ruled in 1998 that the state Medicaid program must be expanded to provide prompt institutional care to developmentally disabled persons, there was a threat to enjoin all Medicaid funds to the state if the state did not comply.[112]

Enrollment can retroactively cover some services that have been provided.[113] Providers may have to refund monies collected during the period of retroactive coverage.[114] In 2004, the Wisconsin Supreme Court ruled that the refund for the retroactive period is limited to the amount that Medicaid pays; the difference between the Medicaid payment and what was charged may be retained by the provider.[115]

Some participants in Medicare are also eligible for Medicaid. They are called Qualified Medical Beneficiaries (QMB). States are not required to pay providers at more than the Medicaid rate for services to QMBs.[116]

Most Medicaid beneficiaries have a range of choice among participating providers. When services are misutilized, beneficiaries may be limited to specified providers.[117]

Courts have disagreed on whether recipients have a right to sue providers to force compliance with the Medicaid regulations.[118]

---

[112] Doe v. Chiles, No. 92-0589-CIV-Ferguson (S.D. Fla. bench order Nov. 4, 1998), *as discussed in* 7 H.L.R. 1856 (1998), *implementing*, 136 F.3d 709 (11th Cir., 1998).

[113] *See* Seittelman v. Sabol, 91 N.Y.2d 618, 674 N.Y.S.2d 253, 697 N.E.2d 154 (1998) [Medicaid program must not limit coverage of services by Medicaid-enrolled providers during three months prior to application to Medicaid].

[114] See *Nursing facilities must refund money received before Medicaid starts, HCFA says,* 7 H.L.R. 1959 (1998) [refunds after retroactive Medicaid eligibility].

[115] Keup v. Wisconsin Dep't of Health & Fam. Servs., 2004 WI 16, 269 Wis. 2d 59, 675 N.W.2d 755.

[116] Balanced Budget Act of 1997, Pub. L. No. 105-33, 111 Stat. 251, § 4714(a); *see* Paramount Health Systems Inc. v. Wright, 138 F.3d 706 (7th Cir. 1998), *cert. denied,* 525 U.S. 929 (1998).

[117] 42 U.S.C. § 1396n(a)(2); *E.g.,* Gross v. North Dakota Dep't of Human Servs., 673 N.W.2d 910 (2004) [upholding application of lock-in].

[118] *See* Wood v. Tompkins, 33 F.3d 600 (6th Cir. 1994) [private cause of action to enforce 42 U.S.C. § 1396a(a)(10)(B)] *with* Stowell v. Ives, 979 F.2d 65 (1st Cir. 1992) [no private cause of action to enforce 42 U.S.C. § 1396a(c)(1); *compare* Boatman v. Hammons, 164 F.3d 286 (6th Cir. 1998) [when denying transportation assistance to Medicaid recipients, state must send written denial, notice of right to hearing] *with* Harris v. James, 127 F.3d 993 (11th Cir. 1997) [no private cause of action to enforce transportation regulation]; Doe v. Chiles, 136 F.3d 709 (11th Cir. 1998) [private cause of action to enforce reasonable promptness regulation]; R. Pear, *Two federal appeals courts permit the poor to sue states for benefits under Medicaid,* N.Y. TIMES, May 26, 2002, 26.

PROVIDERS AND PAYMENT. Institutional providers of services generally become participants in the Medicaid program by contracting with the state to provide services to Medicaid recipients in exchange for the payment permitted by the state. Payment cannot be collected from the patient except to the extent permitted by federal law.[119] Noninstitutional providers generally are not required to enter into any contract with the state but participate merely by treating Medicaid recipients and then billing the state. States may directly reimburse physicians who provide covered services to the medically needy, or they may pay the individual beneficiaries, leaving them with the obligation to pay the physician. Payment for physician services can be made only if the physician agrees to accept charges determined by the state as the full charges.

States have considerable latitude to determine the services to be covered and the amount of payments.[120] States are generally free to establish their own methods of payment for inpatient hospital services as long as the costs do not exceed the Medicare payment for the same services. For several years, the Boren Amendment required the state to find that the rates are "reasonable and adequate to meet the costs which must be incurred by efficiently and economically operated facilities."[121] In 1990, the United States Supreme Court ruled that the Boren Amendment created a substantive federal right to adequate reimbursement that could be enforced by health care providers.[122] This resulted in many lawsuits challenging the adequacy of Medicaid payment rates.[123] Some decisions required states to reinstate prior payment approaches until proper procedure are followed,[124] while others have upheld the state payment rates.[125] However, the Boren Amendment was repealed.[126] This

---

[119] *See* Public Health Trust v. Jackson Mem. Hosp., 693 So. 2d 562 (Fla. 3d DCA 1996) [Medicaid payment is payment in full, precluding application of third-party recoveries to provider charges in excess of Medicaid rates; contrary state statute preempted].

[120] *E.g.*, Royal Geropsychiatric Servs., Inc. v. Tompkins, 159 F.3d 238 (6th Cir. 1998) [psychiatrists' challenge to reduced payments for nonhospital treatment of mentally ill rejected].

[121] Pub. L. No. 97-35, § 2173 (1981) (codified as amended in 42 U.S.C. § 1395a(a)(13)(A)).

[122] Wilder v. Virginia Hosp. Ass'n, 496 U.S. 498 (1990).

[123] *Suits force U.S. and states to pay more for Medicaid*, N.Y. TIMES, Oct. 29, 1991, A1; R.A. Ringler, *Boren Amendment litigation: An analysis*, 27 J.H.H.L. 65 (1994).

[124] *E.g.*, Abbeville Gen. Hosp. v. Ramsey, 3 F.3d 797 (5th Cir. 1993), *cert. denied*, 511 U.S. 1032 (1994).

[125] *E.g.*, Folden v. Washington State Dep't of Social & Health Serv., 981 F.2d 1054 (9th Cir. 1992); Connecticut Hosp. Ass'n v. O'Neill, 46 F.3d 211 (2d Cir. 1995).

[126] L. Clark, *The demise of the Boren Amendment: What comes next in the struggle over hospital payment standards under the Medicaid Act*, 26 HEALTH L. DIG. (Jan. 1998), at 11; *Impact of Boren repeal to be watched, but warnings of deep cuts lose urgency*, 6 H.L.R. 1276 (1997).

increased the latitude of states in adopting their payment mechanisms. However, the federal Medicaid law still requires state payment rates to be consistent with efficiency, quality of care, and equal
access to services.[127] Some federal appellate courts have held this
requires states to follow certain procedures in adopting payment
rates, but other courts have disagreed.[128] In addition, one state court
found that the state had a contract with the provider that precluded
some changes in payments.[129]

States must require that services are provided at the appropriate level of care. However, in 1999, the highest court of Massachusetts, after upholding the state's right to review inpatient services
for medical necessity, ruled that the state could not deny all payment for medically necessary services that should have been provided in an outpatient setting. The court required payment at the
outpatient rate.[130]

Many states have reduced services. When Tennessee reduced
the covered days of inpatient care from twenty to fourteen, the
reduction was challenged as a violation of the federal laws prohibiting discrimination against the handicapped because they generally
need longer stays. The United States Supreme Court rejected this
challenge, ruling that the handicapped nondiscrimination law does
not guarantee equal results from Medicaid services.[131] The Court
did not rule on whether the limit was consistent with the Medicaid
law. Lower courts have ruled that limits on the number of inpatient
days, such as South Carolina's twelve-day limit, are consistent with
the Medicaid law.[132] However, courts will enjoin reductions that fail
to preserve mandated services.[133]

---

[127] 42 U.S.C. § 1396a(a)(30)(A).

[128] Rite Aid of Pa., Inc. v. Houstoun, 171 F.3d 842 (3d Cir. 1999) [requires certain result, but
does not require particular procedures]; *contra,* Orthopaedic Hosp. v. Belshe, 103 F.3d 1491
(9th Cir. 1997) [courts may review payment rates to determine if they bear a reasonable relationship to provider costs]; *see also* Minnesota Homecare Ass'n v. Gomez, 108 F.3d 917 (8th
Cir. 1997) [consideration of factors required, but not specific analytical procedure; state
methodology met requirements]; *Judge orders state to drop budget measure to cut medical payments,* AP, Dec. 24, 2003 [federal judge enjoins Calif. Medicaid payment cut for violating quality, access requirements].

[129] Physicians Health Care Plans v. Cook, 714 So. 2d 566 (Fla. 1st DCA 1998) [state agency
breached contract by lowering capitation rate for Medicaid services].

[130] Massachusetts Eye & Ear Infirmary v. Division of Med. Assistance, 428 Mass. 805, 705 N.E.2d
592 (1999).

[131] Alexander v. Choate, 469 U.S. 287 (1985).

[132] Charleston Mem. Hosp. v. Conrad, 693 F.2d 324 (4th Cir. 1982).

[133] *E.g.,* Pediatric Specialty Care, Inc. v. Arkansas Dep't of Human Servs., 293 F.3d 472 (8th
Cir. 2002) [injunction of cutback of services required under Medicaid Act even though budget shortfall].

Other states have placed other limits on payment to providers. Several states have adopted prospective payment systems for Medicaid similar to the Medicare payment system.[134] Minnesota went one step further in its nursing home payment system. Minnesota will pay nursing homes through its Medicaid system only when the nursing home agrees not to charge non-Medicaid patients more than Medicaid pays for comparable care. This system has been upheld by both the federal and the state courts.[135] In 1985, a Minnesota court ruled that neither the state nor Medicaid patients could stop a nursing home from phasing out participation in Medicaid.[136]

As late as 1994 almost half of the states continued to use cost-based payment systems.[137] Some calculated allowable costs assuming facility occupancy is at least a certain percentage, such as 85 percent or 90 percent. These formulas were generally upheld by the courts.[138]

Medicaid plans continue to change. In 1994, Medicaid consumed approximately 20 percent of state budgets. Medicaid is one of the fastest growing parts of the budgets of many states. Faced with the unacceptability of tax increases and with other important budgetary needs, especially education and law enforcement, most states continue to seek ways to control that growth.[139] Medicaid is also a major budget element at the federal level. Congress continues to explore ways to change Medicaid. In 2005, the President announced an advisory committee to study Medicaid.[140] Developing changes remains contentious, but further change is likely.

Many states have significantly modified their Medicaid programs, usually by adopting managed care approaches, including contracting with private HMOs. Medicaid includes a freedom-of-choice of

---

[134] *E.g.*, Michigan, M.M.G. ¶15,600; *see also* Presbyterian-Univ. of Pa. Med. Ctr. v. Commonwealth, Dep't of Pub. Welfare, 553 A.2d 1027 (Pa. Commw. Ct. 1989) [Medicaid DRG payment system upheld].

[135] Minnesota Ass'n of Health Care Facilities, Inc. v. Minnesota Dep't of Pub. Welfare, 742 F.2d 442 (8th Cir. 1984), *cert. denied*, 469 U.S. 1215 (1985); Highland Chateau, Inc. v. Minnesota Dep't of Pub. Welfare, 356 N.W.2d 804 (Minn. Ct. App. 1984).

[136] LaZalla v. Minnesota, 366 N.W.2d 395 (Minn. Ct. App. 1985); *accord* Catir v. Commissioner of Dep't of Human Servs., 543 A.2d 356 (Me. 1988).

[137] *NGA report finds 23 states using cost-based reimbursement*, 3 H.L.R. 21 (1994).

[138] *E.g.*, Haven Home, Inc. v. Department of Pub. Welfare, 216 Neb. 731, 346 N.W.2d 225 (1984). These formulas do not require states to take steps to furnish the specified occupancy, Humphrey v. State, Dep't of Mental Health, 14 Ohio App. 3d 15, 469 N.E.2d 981 (1984).

[139] *See* R. Pear, *Rising costs prompt states to reduce Medicaid further*, N.Y. TIMES, Sept. 23, 2003, A1; *State cuts Medicaid*, AM. MED. NEWS, Dec. 22-29, 2003, 6 [Medicaid is on the average 30% of state budgets; 50 states reduced or froze some payments and imposed other changes; 32 states expect shortfalls in 2004 Medicaid budgets].

[140] R. Pear, *New panel will study Medicaid with eyes toward big changes*, N.Y. TIMES, May 12, 2005, A19.

provider requirement under which eligible persons may select any participating provider.[141] Initially the managed care approaches were voluntary.[142] However, the Medicaid law authorizes federal waivers of various requirements, including freedom of choice.[143] Several states have obtained waivers[144] or are requesting waivers. Congress has mandated that some individual waivers be granted.[145] Starting in 1995, waiver requests and decisions were published in the *Federal Register*.[146]

In 2002, Utah obtained a waiver from HHS and reorganized its Medicaid program. It dropped coverage of catastrophic costs and specialty care, relying on charity care from providers. The Utah approach received increasing attention when the Utah governor became Secretary of HHS in January 2005.[147]

Government is confronted with difficult allocation decisions. In ruling that the Medicaid law does not grant an enforceable right to compel expenditure of funds to provide a particular treatment, a federal court in Minnesota stated:

> Unfortunately, funds available for these programs are finite. Ordering the development of the requested facility, at cost far above the currently available funding limits, would rob Peter to pay Paul. Society, through its elected representatives and appointed agency administrators, has made the difficult decisions regarding the amount and allocation of these funds.[148]

However, other federal courts have mandated expensive modifications to state Medicaid programs expressly rejecting that they should consider the cost as a factor in their decision. For example

---

[141] 42 U.S.C. § 1396a(a)(23).

[142] 42 U.S.C. § 1396n(a)(1)(A); *see also* Lackner v. Department of Health Services, 29 Cal. App. 4th 1760, 35 Cal. Rptr. 2d 482 (1st Dist. 1994), *rev. denied*, 1995 Cal. LEXIS 398 (Jan. 25, 1995) [permissible to enroll persons in managed care if they did not choose an alternative within 30 days of joining].

[143] 42 U.S.C. § 1396n [§ 1915 of the Social Security Act], which authorizes waivers for two-year periods; 42 U.S.C. § 1315 [§ 1115], which authorizes broader waivers for longer time periods for demonstration projects.

[144] *E.g.*, Hawaii Health QUEST, Oregon Reform Demonstration, and TennCare Demonstration Project, M.M.G. ¶¶ 41580, 41313, & 41908; *see also* R. Pear, *Report criticizes federal oversight of state Medicaid*, N.Y. TIMES, July 7, 2003, A1 [GAO study of oversight of waivers].

[145] *E.g.*, Pub. L. No. 100-485, § 507 (1988) [Minnesota].

[146] *E.g.*, 60 FED. REG. 4,418 (Jan. 23, 1995), 16,481 (Mar. 30, 1995), 17,791 (April 7, 1995).

[147] K. Johnson & R. Abelson, *Model in Utah may be future for Medicaid*, N.Y. TIMES, Feb. 24, 2005, A1; R. Gehrke, *HHS waiver for Utah provides health care for some, reduces benefits for others*, AP, Feb. 9, 2002.

[148] Jordano v. Steffen, 787 F. Supp. 886, 891 (D. Minn. 1992).

in 1998, a federal appellate court mandated expanded and timely services to the developmentally disabled, quoting an earlier decision that had stated "inadequate state appropriations do not excuse noncompliance."[149] Because the service was an optional service, the plaintiffs and the court took a daring gamble that the state would not abandon all coverage of the services in the face of the tremendous cost increases. They apparently won the gamble because the new governor announced support for making the necessary increases in appropriations for the program.[150]

In 1994, Tennessee began an ambitious program to expand its Medicaid coverage. The history of this program illustrates the difficulties when open-ended entitlement programs such as Medicaid become difficult for governments to finance. The program had financial difficulties from its early days. Attempts to control the costs were challenged by advocacy groups. In 2002, a federal court mandated additional services and took over part of the program. As costs escalated in 2004, the legislature adopted an overhaul plan. A federal court again imposed a costly plan on the state. In 2005, the governor announced major cutbacks in TennCare, but the federal judge again blocked the changes. A federal appellate court twice overturned the federal district court. With federal administrative approval, the disenrollment process of downsizing was scheduled to begin in August 2005.[151]

Actual and proposed changes in Medicaid and other funding can also affect hospital financing in other indirect ways. For example, soon after New Jersey announced plans in early 1994 to reduce Medicaid payments to hospitals, Standard & Poor's Rating Group scheduled meetings with New Jersey hospitals to discuss the impact on their bond ratings.[152]

---

[149] Doe v. Chiles, 136 F.3d 709 (11th Cir. 1998).

[150] Press release by Florida Governor's office, February 8, 1999.

[151] *TennCare timeline: From its start in 1994, to its current crisis*, AP, May 30, 2005; M. Gouras, *Federal government OKs another piece of TennCare reform*, AP, June 8, 2005; T. Sharp, *Judge orders state to follow new plan for TennCare children*, AP, Oct. 26, 2004; 60 FED. REG. 4418 (Jan. 23, 1995); *see* http://www.cms.hhs.gov/medicaid/1115/tn1115tc.asp & http://www.cms.hhs.gov/medicaid/waivers/tnwaiver.asp (accessed June 11, 2005) for information concerning federal waivers for TennCare; Rosen v. Tennessee Comm'r of Finance, 204 F. Supp. 2d 1048 (M.D. Tenn. 2001); 204 F. Supp. 2d 1061 (M.D. Tenn. 2001); 280 F. Supp. 2d 743, (M.D. Tenn., 2002), *aff'd in part & vacated in part*, 288 F.3d 918 (6th Cir. 2002); 2005 U.S. App. LEXIS 6444 (6th Cir.) (unpub); 2005 U.S. App. LEXIS 9743 (6th Cir.).

[152] *New Jersey plans to cut payments for Medicaid 20%*, N.Y. TIMES, Nov. 23, 1994, A1; *S&P, New Jersey hospital to discuss Medicaid cuts*, WALL ST. J., Nov. 25, 1994, A5.

9-2.3 State Programs

Several states have state and local programs that pay for some health care for indigent persons who cannot qualify for Medicaid. These programs vary greatly. Under the statutes of some states, counties or other units of local government are responsible for paying for some health care on behalf of their residents who are unable to pay.[153] Some of these statutes provide that prior notice must be given[154] or authorization must be obtained from appropriate government officials. Other statutes do not require prior approval to create an obligation, especially in emergencies.[155] Some states require that claims for payment be made in a certain way, and courts affirm nonpayment when the proper procedures are not followed.[156] Frequently, these requirements result in disputes between units or levels of government concerning which is responsible to pay for the care of an individual.[157]

In 1999, the United States Supreme Court ruled that state welfare programs could not restrict new residents to the welfare benefits they would have received in the states from which they had moved.[158]

In many states, local governmental units or their police departments are obligated to pay for the care of persons in their custody who are charged with crimes.[159] However, police generally do not assume financial responsibility by bringing to the hospital someone

---

[153] *E.g.*, John C. Lincoln Hosp. & Health Corp. v. Maricopa County, 208 Ariz. 532, 96 P.3d 530 (App. Ct. 2004) [county ordered to pay].

[154] *E.g.*, Washoe Med. Ctr., Inc. v. Churchill County, 108 Nev. 622, 836 P.2d 624 (1992) [hospital not entitled to summary determination of county liability where question whether notice given].

[155] *E.g.*, University of Utah Hosp. v. Bethke, 101 Id. 245, 611 P.2d 1030 (1980) [Idaho county ordered to pay for emergency services to two indigent county residents].

[156] *E.g.*, St. Paul Ramsey County Med. Ctr. v. Pennington County, 875 F.2d 1185 (8th Cir. 1988) [hospital could not collect from county when it had not filed statement of costs]; University of Utah Hosp. v. Minidoka County, 115 Id. 406, 767 P.2d 249 (1989) [claim properly denied because administrative remedies not exhausted]; Middlesex Mem. Hosp. v. Town of North Haven, 206 Conn. 1, 535 A.2d 1303 (1988) [hospital must prove eligibility of recipient; *but see* Sioux Valley Hosp. Ass'n v. Yankton Clinic, 424 N.W.2d 379 (S.D. 1988) [patient's non-cooperation in giving information for application did not justify county denial].

[157] *E.g.*, Temple Univ. v. Philadelphia, 698 A.2d 118 (Pa. Commw. Ct. 1997). [city not responsible for cost of emergency treatment for indigent city residents not eligible for state medical assistance benefits, state's duty to provide medical assistance to poor].

[158] Saenz v. Roe, 526 U.S. 489 (1999).

[159] *E.g.*, Emanuel Hosp. v. Umatilla County, 314 Or. 393, 840 P.2d 56 (1992); Lutheran Med. Ctr. v. City of Omaha, 229 Neb. 802, 429 N.W.2d 347 (1988); *see also* Borgess Hosp. v. County of Berrien, 114 Mich. App. 385, 319 N.W.2d 354 (1982) [no obligation to pay for care of former prisoner after discharge from jail]; *but see* Northeast Indiana Colon & Rectal Surgeons v. Allen County Comm'rs, 674 N.E.2d 590 (Ind. Ct. App. 1996) [sheriff not responsible for medical bills for treatment of inmate's preexisting condition after sheriff gave provider notice to directly bill inmate].

who is not in custody.[160] Some jurisdictions have sought to avoid the cost of caring for prisoners by not charging sick suspects or by releasing sick prisoners.[161] There are frequently disputes over whether an individual was in custody when care was given.[162]

9-3 How Are Employer-Sponsored and Other Private Payment Programs Structured?

Some private payment programs pay the covered person some or all of the charges incurred. The provider collects from the patient and the patient collects from the program, with the patient remaining responsible for the difference between the charges and what the program pays.

Many private payment programs contract directly or indirectly with providers to obtain services at contracted payment rates.

Most private payment programs are designed to manage care in some fashion. One component of this management is often the way that providers are paid. Other components are discussed in Chapter 10.

Private plans that are provided by employers are regulated by the federal Employee Retirement Income Security Act (ERISA) discussed later in this section. Most nonfederal plans are also regulated by state law to the extent that the laws are not preempted by ERISA when it applies.

---

[160] *E.g.*, Dade County v. Hospital Affiliates Int'l, Inc., 378 So. 2d 43 (Fla. 3d DCA 1979); *but see* Susan B. Allen Mem. Hosp. v. Board of County Comm'rs, 12 Kan. App. 2d 680, 753 P.2d 1302 (1988) [county liable for cost of care of intoxicated person taken into protective custody]; Albany Gen. Hosp. v. Dalton, 69 Or. App. 204, 684 P.2d 34 (1984) [county responsible for cost of care of person injured in gunfight with police]; *Hospital accuses City of Macon of not paying bills; sues,* AP, Nov. 27, 2003 [GA suit seeking payment for persons not under arrest].

[161] *E.g., More trouble than he's worth, law says,* N.Y. TIMES, Nov. 26, 1992, A8 [prosecutor says man accused of theft should be cleared because medical care while in custody is costing county too much]; Texas Dep't of Corrections v. Sisters of St. Francis of St. Jude Hosp., 836 S.W.2d 719 (Tex. Ct. App. 1992) [governor's proclamation granting inmate six-month medical reprieve, provided all financial arrangements for care made by inmate or family did not excuse state from responsibility for medical care; inmate did not sign acceptance until after care rendered; hospital did not know of payment condition before rendering services; unconscionable to require waiver of right to medical care as condition of seeking care away from prison; waiver coerced]; Meriter Hosp. v. Dane County, 2004 WI 145, 277 Wis. 2d 1, 689 N.W.2d 627 [county only required to pay while patient was prisoner, even when county changes status after admission].

[162] *E.g.*, Macon-Bibb County Hosp. Auth. v. Reese, 492 S.E.2d 292 (Ga. Ct. App. 1997) [seeking county payment for detainee care, fact question whether detainee in sheriff's physical custody during medical treatment].

MANAGED CARE ORGANIZATIONS. Many health insurance plans are designed either (1) to require the use of a specific provider or a member of a panel of providers or (2) to pay a significantly smaller portion of the costs when a nonpanel provider is selected, creating a strong incentive to use the panel, especially for more expensive treatments, such as hospitalization. Such plans are generally referred to as managed care entities or organizations (MCOs).

The structure of MCOs varies widely. Two types of MCOs are health maintenance organizations (HMOs) and preferred provider organizations (PPOs).

A staff-model HMO generally provides services directly to patients through HMO employees, while an Independent Practice Association (IPA) model HMO provides services through other providers with which the HMO contracts. In exchange the HMO receives a fixed premium payment from or on behalf of the patient. Except for some emergency services and some services provided while the patient is out of the HMO's service area, the HMO pays for services only if they are provided by HMO employees or contractors. While some HMOs own hospitals, most HMOs make arrangements with other hospitals. These arrangements vary widely. In many HMO contracts, the provider agrees not to bill the patient even if the HMO fails to pay. Many hospitals have lost large amounts when HMOs have become bankrupt.[163] Even when the HMO contract does not contain this restriction, federal law prohibits hospitals from billing Medicare patients directly when their HMOs fail to pay the provider.[164] Some states forbid direct provider billing to any HMO patients. One bankruptcy court took the unusual further step of enjoining providers from all direct billing of any of a bankrupt HMO's patients.[165]

A PPO generally does not provide services directly. It contracts with other providers to provide care at an agreed rate. Patients are given a financial incentive to use these preferred providers, such as lower deductibles and copayments. The PPO pays for services provided by other providers, but usually at a lower rate, so that the patient pays higher out-of-pocket expenses. PPOs are often mar-

---

163 *E.g.*, H. Larkin, *Hospitals foot bill for Maxicare Utah's failure*, Hosps., Oct. 5, 1988, 44 [hospitals left with $6 million in unpaid bills]; P.J. Kenkel, *Pa. hospitals denied payment from Maxicare*, Mod. Healthcare, July 7, 1989, 4.

164 42 U.S.C. § 1395cc; 42 C.F.R. §§ 489.20, 489.30; M.E. Klas, *Hospital may lose Medicare over lawsuits*, Palm Beach Post [FL], Nov. 20, 1987, at 7B.

165 *Providers not permitted to bill Maxicare enrollees*, Mod. Healthcare, Sept. 22, 1989, 12.

keted to self-insured employers on a cost-plus-processing-fee basis. Thus, the PPO often does not assume the risk of higher health care costs; the PPO is usually an administrative service, not an insurer. In some cases, there is no PPO entity; the PPO is the result of the direct contracts an insurer enters with providers. Some providers have attempted to convince courts and regulators that PPOs are violations of federal antitrust laws, but these attacks have generally been unsuccessful.[166]

FEDERAL LAW. Numerous federal statutes regulating health care providers and insurers also may apply to MCOs.

HMO Act. The federal HMO Act (Title XIII of the Public Health Service Act, enacted in 1973)[167] established standards in the areas of legal and organizational status, financial viability, marketing, and benefits that had to be met in order for a HMO to be "federally qualified." Federal qualification is entirely voluntary. Initially, federally qualified HMOs had substantial advantages over nonqualified HMOs, including access to federal grants, loans, and loan guarantees. Over time, these advantages have been mostly eliminated, and the restrictive standards required for federal qualification have been eased. Current advantages to federal qualification include (1) increased "credibility" with employers, (2) a shortened Medicare risk-contracting process, and (3) exemption from certain state laws.

ERISA. The Employee Retirement Income Security Act of 1974 (ERISA)[168] established uniform national standards for employee benefit plans and preempts, in many instances, state laws governing employee health plans, including MCOs. Under ERISA, only contract damages (e.g., the cost of improperly denied treatment) are recoverable in the event of a violation of the law. ERISA has been viewed as a shield against malpractice actions (and damage awards for pain and suffering, lost earnings, and costs of future medical care) for those MCOs that provide care as part of employee benefit plans. In recent years, there has been much controversy regarding when state laws can be preempted by ERISA, with inconsistent

---

[166] *E.g.*, Barry v. Blue Cross, 805 F.2d 866 (9th Cir. 1986) [PPO did not violate antitrust laws]; Ball Mem. Hosp., Inc. v. Mutual Hosp. Ins. Co., 603 F. Supp. 1077 (S.D. Ind. 1985) [preliminary injunction of PPO denied]; Associated Foot Surgeons v. National Foot Care Program, Inc., No. 84-271367CZ (Mich. Cir. Ct. Oakland County Feb. 1, 1984) [injunction of PPO denied], *as discussed in* HEALTH L. DIG., June 1984, 4.

[167] 42 U.S.C. §§ 300e – 300e-17.

[168] 42 U.S.C. §§ 1001 et seq.

decisions between jurisdictions. The preemption analysis has three levels. First, all state laws that "relate to" any covered employee benefit plan are preempted.[169] Second, there is an exception so that state laws that "regulate insurance, banking, or securities" are not preempted.[170] Third, most employee benefit plans cannot be deemed to be insurers or banks; so they cannot be subjected to state insurance or banking laws.[171] There has been extensive litigation concerning the scope of this preemption. Many of these decisions have come in legal actions by plan beneficiaries against MCOs for alleged negligence in medical care or other services. These cases are discussed in Chapter 10.

HIPAA. The Health Insurance Portability and Accountability Act of 1996 (HIPAA)[172] contains provisions that affect group health plans, including MCOs. Most significantly, HIPAA limits the ability of group health plans to make coverage decisions based on the health condition of the insured. HIPAA and other federal laws governing coverage and benefits are discussed in more detail in Chapter 10.

STATE LAW. Most states have enabling statutes that define and regulate HMOs, PPOs, and other MCOs. Some provisions of these laws affect the payment arrangements that can be made with providers. The other aspects of these laws that address eligibility and benefits are discussed in Chapter 10.

CONTRACTS BETWEEN HEALTH CARE PROVIDERS AND MANAGED CARE ENTITIES AND OTHER THIRD-PARTY PAYERS. Health care providers and the larger groups of which they are often part, seek contracts with managed care entities and other third-party payers to assure that the health care provider is at least included in the panel of permitted providers for the persons covered by that payer. When possible, they seek exclusive agreements that restrict the extent that competing providers can be on the panel. Some of these restrictions can raise antitrust problems in some circumstances which are discussed in Chapter 7.

Providers need to carefully evaluate what care they are promising to give. One serious problem has been the "silent PPO" where the payer tries to take advantage of the special prices in the contract for patients who are not intended to be covered by

---

[169] 29 U.S.C. § 1144(a).
[170] 29 U.S.C. § 1144(b)(2)(A).
[171] 29 U.S.C. § 1144(b)(2)(B).
[172] Pub. L. No. 104-191.

the contract.[173] Some contracts are worded so broadly that this practice may be authorized by the contract. In other cases, the payer is acting outside the contract.

Another potential problem is that in some cases the patient becomes a third-party beneficiary to the contract so that the patient may sue for breach of contract when the obligation to provide services is not fulfilled.[174] Unless this is required or intended, it can usually be avoided by the wording of the contract.

Structuring of provider contracts/payments. The payer's duty to pay is based on a direct contractual relationship. Generally, the specified payment provided by the contract must be accepted as payment in full. Sometimes part of that payment must be collected directly from the patient as a deductible or coinsurance payment. The remainder is paid by the third-party payer directly to the provider. A discussion of the wide range of contractual arrangements is beyond the scope of this book.

The payment arrangements with managed care plans and other third-party payers can include charges (usually discounted), per diem rates (a fixed payment per day the patient is in the hospital, which may vary depending on whether intensive care or other special services are provided), and per admission rates (which may vary by diagnosis or other factors). These may be adjusted so that the provider shares some of the risk and benefit of overall costs savings from efficient practice.

In some cases, the payment is by capitation, under which the provider agrees to provide to a defined population all the services within the service capacity of the institution for a fixed rate per person per month. Under capitation, the provider receives the same payment whether no services or a large amount of services are provided; the incentive is to promote health, efficient practice, and empty beds, rather than filling the hospital. Capitation was popular in 1990s but has become much less common.[175]

State law needed to be reviewed in structuring capitation arrangements because some arrangements required the hospital to

---

[173] See *AHA, AMA jointly warn members of billing scam by "silent PPO,"* 3 H.L.R. 1779 (1994) ["Special membership alert" distributed in Sept. 1994]; B. McCormick, *Where are your discounts?* AM. MED. NEWS, Feb. 6, 1995, 1.

[174] *E.g.*, St. Charles v. Kender, 38 Mass. App. Ct. 155, 646 N.E.2d 411 (1995).

[175] G. Mays, G. Claxton & J. White, *MarketWatch: Managed care rebound? Recent changes in health plans' cost containment strategies*, HEALTH AFFAIRS, Aug. 11, 2004 [http://content.healthaffairs.org/cgi/content/full/hlthaff.w4.427/DC1 (accessed Sept. 1, 2004)].

qualify as an insurance company. However, under some state laws, as long as the hospital was only accepting capitation to provide its own services and not agreeing to pay other providers that were not part of the hospital, the arrangement did not require the hospital to qualify as an insurer. Under some state laws, the arrangement had to be with a managed care entity, and not directly with an employer, to avoid having to qualify the hospital as an insurer.

Coordination of Benefits. Most plans have a coordination of benefits provision that specifies the priorities when more than one plan or policy potentially applies. These often result in disputes between plans.[176]

Insolvency. With limited exceptions, direct contracts are only as good as the solvency of the payer. Hospitals have lost significant amounts when payers have become unable to pay.[177] Insolvency of payers can be a problem whether or nor there is a direct contract but is particularly significant in the direct contracting situation because the direct contract will usually eliminate or limit the opportunity to pursue collection from the patient and may require acceptance of additional patients for a period of time after the insolvency occurs.

Many contracts specify that the provider cannot bill the patient even if the payer fails to pay. The provider is left with a claim in the bankruptcy or receivership of the payer. Generally, providers are not given a priority in the distribution of assets.[178] Thus, to the extent possible, providers need to structure their arrangements to keep their exposure to loss with sustainable bounds. Attention should be paid to the steps the provider can take to protect itself, including when the contract can be terminated. Generally, a hospital can bill HMO patients for care given after the date the hospital terminates its contract with the HMO.[179]

Insurance companies are not eligible for federal bankruptcy and instead must go through a receivership under state law.[180] When

---

[176] *E.g.*, McGurl v. Trucking Employees of North Jersey Welfare Fund, Inc., 124 F.3d 47 (3d Cir. 1997) [when conflicting, plan of claimant's employer pays]; Principal Health Care v. Lewer Agency, Inc., 38 F.3d 240 (5th Cir. 1994); *see also DHHS OIG advisory opinion holds coordination of benefits provision of provider agreement between nursing home and healthcare plan may violate anti-kickback statute*, 26 HEALTH L. DIG. (May 1998), at 33 [Advisory Opinion 98-5 (Apr. 24, 1998)].

[177] *E.g., Blue Cross collapse in West Virginia puts many in dire straits*, WALL ST. J., Mar. 8, 1991, 1A [first collapse of a Blue Shield plan, leaving $50 million in unpaid medical bills].

[178] *E.g.*, Washington Physicians Serv. v. Marquardt, 867 Wash. App. 650, 38 P.2d 142 (1992).

[179] *E.g.*, St. Elizabeth Hosp. Med. Ctr. v. Moliterno, 1991 Ohio App. LEXIS 6040.

[180] *E.g.*, 11 U.S.C. § 109.

HMOs are treated as insurance companies under state law, they are not eligible for federal bankruptcy.

Due to the adverse effect of payer failures, some states have strengthened the financial qualifications to be a health maintenance organization, insurer, or other payer. Many plans have private reinsurance that will sometimes, but not always, cover some payments.[181] Some plans are required to contribute to state guaranty funds that pay some of the losses when plans become insolvent. However, not all plans are covered.

CONTRACTS BETWEEN MANAGED CARE ENTITIES AND EMPLOYERS AND OTHER ULTIMATE PAYERS. Managed care entities and other third-party payers contract directly with employers and other ultimate payers to provide care through the networks that are created by the agreements discussed in the previous section. In an effort to reduce the number of intermediate layers of administration and control, some hospitals and groups of providers seek to contract directly with employers and other ultimate payers to provide services. These contracts have to be carefully structured to avoid or comply with state insurance and other laws.

9-4 What Are the Laws Governing Collection of Copayments, Deductibles, and Uninsured Amounts?

This section addresses the following questions regarding collection of payment for health care services.

9-4.1. When may a provider pursue collection directly from a health insurance coverage plan?

9-4.2. When may a provider pursue collection directly against the patient, family members, or individual guarantors?

9-4.3. What are some other sources that may be available to pay for services?

9-4.4. What are some of the legal restrictions on the billing and collection process?

9-4.5. What is the scope of responsibility to provide uncompensated care?

---

[181] *E.g.*, *In re* International Med. Ctrs., Inc., 604 So. 2d 505 (Fla. 1st DCA 1992).

9-4.1 When May a Provider Pursue Collection Directly from a Health Insurance Coverage Plan?

When a provider has a direct contract with a payer, the provider generally submits bills and collects payment in accordance with terms of the contract. Similarly, government programs specify how a bill should be submitted and paid and the regulatory requirements that must be followed.

Some third-party payers do not contract with providers. These payers contract with individuals or their employers to reimburse for some or all of the cost of covered services to the individuals. The individuals must make their own arrangements with providers for the services. Some of these payers pay the individual directly, and the provider must collect from the individual. Providers usually seek assignment of these payments so that they can be paid directly.

Generally, a hospital must have an assignment of the beneficiary's claim before the hospital can sue an ERISA plan directly.[182] However, some courts have ruled that a suit against a health plan by a provider with a direct contract with the plan is not affected by ERISA.[183]

Some payers have sought to forbid such assignments.[184] Federal appellate courts have ruled that contractual barriers to assignment in ERISA plans are enforceable.[185] Some states have prohibited non-assignment provisions in plans.[186] Some payers have permitted assignment only when the provider accepts the payment as payment in full. For example, one Michigan insurer required a physician requesting direct payment to sign a form stating the physician would accept the amount as payment in full. One Michigan physician crossed out this statement before signing the form, but a Michigan court ruled that the physician was still bound by the statement.[187]

---

[182] *E.g.*, Hermann Hosp. v. Meba Med. & Benefits Plan, 845 F.2d 1286 (5th Cir. 1988); Kennedy v. Deere & Co., 118 Ill. 2d 69, 514 N.E.2d 171 (1987), *cert. denied*, 484 U.S. 1064 (1987); Misic v. Building Serv. Employees Health & Welfare Trust, 789 F.2d 1374 (9th Cir. 1986).

[183] *E.g.*, Pritt v. Blue Cross, 699 F. Supp. 81 (S.D. W.Va. 1988).

[184] *E.g.*, R. Kazel, *Out of network, out of luck*, AM. MED. NEWS, May 16, 2005, 18; St. Francis Reg. Med. Ctr. v. Blue Cross & Blue Shield, 49 F.3d 1460 (10th Cir. 1995) [upheld ban on assignment of claims to providers that had not signed contracts with Blue Cross]; Obstetricians-Gynecologists, P.C. v. Blue Cross & Blue Shield, 219 Neb.199, 361 N.W.2d 550 (1985) [prohibition of assignment enforceable]; Blue Cross Hosp. Serv. v. Frappier, 681 S.W.2d 925 (Mo. 1984) (en banc) [state law requiring insurers to accept assignment upheld].

[185] *E.g.*, Physicians Multispecialty Group v. Health Care Plan of Horton Homes, Inc., 371 F.3d 1291 (11th Cir. 2004); City of Hope Nat. Med. Ctr. v. Healthplus, Inc., 156 F.3d 223 (1st Cir. 1998).

[186] *E.g.*, 215 ILL. COMP. STAT. 5/370a.

[187] Oakland Neurosurgical Arts, P.C. v. Blue Cross & Blue Shield, 135 Mich. App. 798, 356 N.W.2d 267 (1984).

Physicians have challenged requirements that patients not be billed more than allowed by the insurance company, but these limits have generally been upheld.[188] However, without a contractual agreement or a statutory limit, there is no limit on what the provider may charge, and the patient remains liable for any amount not paid by the payer.

After the provider gives notice to the payer of a valid assignment, the payer is generally obligated to pay amounts due directly to the provider.[189] After assignment, generally only the provider who has received the assignment has the right to sue for unpaid claims.[190]

9-4.2 When May a Provider Pursue Collection Directly Against the Patient, Family Members, or Individual Guarantors?

Adult patients are responsible for paying their own hospital bills, unless the provider is barred by another contract or by law from billing the patient. Some insurers have contracts with providers that bar the provider from billing the patient for amounts covered by the insurance. However, with the growing use of copayment, deductibles, and exclusions from coverage, even persons protected by such insurance contracts may have substantial bills.[191]

This responsibility is based on either an express or implied contract to pay for accepted services.[192] The adult patient is responsible for the reasonable value of services furnished in good faith even if the patient is unconscious, mentally incompetent, or incapacitated at the time the services are provided.[193] The major exceptions occur (1) when the law entitles the patient to free care and (2) when the competent, oriented adult has explicitly refused to accept the services. However, some courts have been reluctant to deny

---

[188] Kartell v. Blue Shield, 749 F.2d 922 (1st Cir. 1984), *cert. denied*, 471 U.S. 2049 (1985).

[189] *E.g.*, Pro Cardiaco Pronto Socorro Cardiologica S.A. v. Trussell, 863 F. Supp. 135 (S.D. N.Y. 1994); *but see* Gray v. State Farm Auto Ins. Co., 491 S.E.2d 272 (S.C. App. Ct. 1997) [language of assignment applied only to patients' insurer, not to third-party insurers, so not violation for third-party insurer to pay patient directly].

[190] *E.g.*, Allianz Life Ins. Co. v. Reidl, 264 Ga. 395, 444 S.E.2d 736 (1994).

[191] *See* J.S. Hacker, *Call it the family risk factor*, N.Y. TIMES, Jan. 11, 2004, 15WK [increasing shift of economic risk from government and corporations to workers and families].

[192] *E.g.*, Galloway v. Methodist Hosps., Inc., 658 N.E.2d 611 (Ind. Ct. App. 1995) [contract implied in law with both spouses for emergency caesarian delivery, care of mother, child].

[193] *E.g.*, Morehead v. Conley, 75 Ohio App. 3d 409, 599 N.E.2d 786 (1991); K.A.L. v. Southern Med. Business Servs., 854 So. 2d 106 (Ala. App. 2003) [prisoner liable for emergency treatment despite no consent].

payment for life-sustaining treatment that allegedly was refused.[194] In some cases, patients negotiate special discounted rates for services directly with providers.[195]

In many states, a husband is responsible for paying for necessary care for his wife. In many states, the wife has a reciprocal duty to pay for necessary care for her husband.[196] A few state courts, when confronted with laws requiring the husband to pay, but not the wife, have found the laws to be unconstitutional so that neither must pay for the other.[197]

Most states make the father responsible for paying for necessary care for minor children. In many states, the mother is also responsible.[198] In some states, minors are not legally responsible for paying for care they receive unless they are emancipated. However, in other states minors are also responsible for paying for their necessary care.[199] When there is doubt under state law concerning parental responsibility, the parents' express promise to pay is frequently obtained. When parents are divorced or separated, special rules concerning parental responsibility apply in

---

[194] *E.g.*, Grace Plaza v. Elbaum, 82 N.Y.2d 10, 603 N.Y.S.2d 386, 623 N.E.2d 513 (1993); G.J. Annas, *Adding injustice to injury: Compulsory payment for unwanted treatment*, 327 N. ENG. J. MED. 1885 (1992).

[195] *E.g.*, L. Lagnado, *Forgoing insurance, Mr. Selby bargains for his health care*, WALL ST. J, Nov. 24, 2004, A1; V. Fuhrmans, *Childbirth for bargain-hunters*, WALL ST. J, Apr. 5, 2005, D1; *see also* S. Rai, *Low costs lure foreigners to India for medical care*, N.Y. TIMES, Apr. 7, 2005, C6.

[196] *E.g.*, IOWA CODE § 597.14 [both spouses liable for necessary care provided to family members]; St. Luke's Episcopal-Presbyterian Hosp. v. Underwood, 957 S.W.2d 496 (Mo. Ct. App. 1997) [wife liable]; St. Francis Reg. Med. Center, Inc. v. Bowles, 251 Kan, 334, 836 P.2d 123 (1992) [both spouses liable]; Richland Mem. Hosp. v. English, 295 S.C. 511, 369 S.E.2d 395 (Ct. App. 1988) [common law wife liable].

[197] *E.g.*, North Ottawa Commun. Hosp. v. Kieft, 457 Mich. 2d 394, 578 N.W.2d 267 (1998) [deny collection from spouse, violation of equal protection]; Schilling v. Bedford County Mem. Hosp., 225 Va. 539, 303 S.E.2d 905 (1983) [unconstitutional to require pay from husband, but not from wife, neither obligated; ruling partially reversed by VA. CODE § 55-37 (1986)].

[198] *E.g.*, Estate of Bonner, 954 S.W.2d 356 (Mo. Ct. App. 1997) [allow claim against mother's estate for medical services to infant son]; Mary Imogene Bassett Hosp. v. Dahlberg, 229 A.D.2d 781, 645 N.Y.S.2d 578 (3d Dept. 1996) [both divorced parents obligated to pay for medical care of unemancipated child under age 21, N.Y. FAMILY COURT ACT § 413]; Ex parte Odem, 537 So. 2d 919 (Ala. 1988) [minor mother may contract for care of her minor child as necessary service, but not bound by attorney fee provision].

[199] *E.g.*, Yale Diagnostic Radiology v. Estate of Fountain, 267 Conn. 351, 838 A.2d 179 (2003) [minor liable for necessary medical services when parent does not pay]; Johns Hopkins Hosp. v. Pepper, 346 Md. 679, 697 A.2d 1358 (1997) [minor medical malpractice victim could make claim for medical expenses in own name when parents unable to meet expenses, minor could ultimately be liable under doctrine of necessaries]; Annotation, *Infant's liability for medical, dental, or hospital services*, 53 A.L.R. 4TH 1249.

some states[200] so that an express promise is frequently required to make the noncustodial parent responsible.[201]

Absent a statute or an express promise, other relatives or friends are not responsible for paying for care. A few state statutes make adult children responsible for their parents' care when their parents are unable to pay.[202] In addition, by expressly promising to pay, a relative or friend or other guarantor may become responsible for paying for care, especially if the promise is written.[203] The promise must be carefully written because some forms have been successfully challenged.[204] In most states merely arranging for care or bringing a person to the hospital does not make a relative, friend, or other person responsible for payment.

Since 1990, when nursing homes participate in Medicare or Medicaid, federal law forbids requiring a third-party guaranty of payment

---

[200] *E.g.*, Sentry Investigations, Inc. v. Davis, 841 P.2d 732 (Utah Ct. App. 1992) [noncustodial parent not responsible for cost of care arranged by custodial parent]; Inter Valley Health Plan v. Blue Cross/Blue Shield, 16 Cal. App. 4th 60, 19 Cal. Rptr. 2d 782 (4th Dist. 1993) [father's plan primarily responsible for cost of bone marrow transplant, chemotherapy because divorce decree required father to maintain child as beneficiary under his employment policy]; *but see* Dean Med. Ctr., S.C. v. Conners, 618 N.W.2d 194 (Wis. App. 2000) [provider may pursue either parent notwithstanding court order assigning responsibility as between parents].

[201] Wagoner v. Joe Mater & Assocs., Inc., 461 N.E.2d 706 (Ind. Ct. App. 1984) [noncustodial parent not required to pay despite support order because he was willing to pay for care at another location, but opposed particular provider]; *but see* Ex parte Davila, 709 S.W.2d 15 (Tex. Ct. App. 1986) [noncustodial father could be imprisoned for contempt for failure to pay hospital for child's treatment].

[202] *E.g.*, Americana Healthcare Ctr. v. Randall, 513 N.W.2d 566 (S.D. 1994) [son liable for nursing home care of elderly mother under S. DAK. C.L. § 25-7-27, reject constitutional challenges to law]; Trinity Med. Ctr., Inc. v. Rubbelke, 389 N.W.2d 805 (N.D. 1986) [secondary liability of adult children, so release of patient, spouse released adult children]; Accounts Management, Inc. v. Nelson, 2003 SD 61 [children not responsible under S. DAK. C.L. § 25-7-27 when patient not unable to provide for himself].

[203] *E.g.*, Sisters of Charity Hosp. of Buffalo v. Riley, 231 A.D.2d 272, 661 N.Y.S.2d 352 (4th Dept. 1997) [son bound by guaranty]; In Matter of Estate of Breen, 171 Misc. 2d 905, 656 N.Y.S.2d 122 (Tr. T. 1997) [guarantor entitled to credit for payments to provider from third-party insurer]; Samaritan Hosp. v. Chodikoff, 97 A.D.2d 937, 471 N.Y.S.2d 20 (3d Dept. 1983) [wife liable based on signed guaranty].

[204] *E.g.*, Service Fin. Corp. v. Hall, 1986 Ark. App. LEXIS 2421 [financial responsibility agreement not valid when signer believed it to be general consent form]; Memorial Hosp. v. Bauman, 100 A.D.2d 701, 474 N.Y.S.2d 636 (3d Dept. 1984) [daughter not bound by signed commitment to pay because no evidence she intended to be personally bound]; Rohrscheib v. Helena Hosp. Ass'n, 12 Ark. App. 6, 670 S.W.2d 812 (1984) [brother-in-law who signed admission form not personally responsible for bill because it did not contain express promise to pay]; McCarthy v. Weaver, 99 A.D.2d 652, 472 N.Y.S.2d 64 (4th Dept. 1984) [form ambiguous because it contained both a promise to pay expenses not covered by insurance and a promise to pay all expenses]; Texas County Mem. Found., Inc. v. Ramsey, 677 P.2d 665 (Okla. Ct. App. 1984) [promise by son to pay for nursing home care for indefinite term could be revoked with 30 days notice]; *see also* Orthopedic & Reconstructive Surgery, S.C. v. Kezelis, 146 Ill. App. 3d 227, 496 N.E.2d 1112 (1st Dist. 1986) [payment contract between hospital and patient did not encompass surgical corporation].

as a condition of admission, expedited admission, or continued stay. DHHS interprets this ban to apply to all residents regardless of the source of their payment.[205] However, solicitation of voluntary guarantees appears to be permitted.[206]

PREPAYMENT. Some providers require prepayment of all or part of the amount due before providing services.[207] This is permissible in many situations, but there are some restrictions. For example, prepayment cannot be required before providing emergency screening and stabilization services required by the federal Emergency Medical Treatment and Active Labor Act (EMTALA), discussed in Chapter 6. Governmental regulations and many managed care contracts bar collection of advance payment of the amounts that are payable under their programs.

9-4.3 What Are Some Other Sources That May Be Available to Pay for Services?

WORKERS' COMPENSATION. State workers' compensation laws often require employers or their insurers to pay for care related to work injuries. These laws frequently specify claims procedures and payment rates. However, in 1999, the United States Supreme Court ruled that workers' compensation payments could be withheld during review of claims.[208]

NO-FAULT AUTOMOBILE INSURANCE. In some states, no-fault automobile insurer payments for health care to persons injured in automobile accidents are governed by statutes that affect claims procedures and the rates that are paid.[209] For example, in 1998,

---

[205] 42 U.S.C. §§ 1395i-3(c)(5)(ii), 1396r(c)(5)(ii); 56 FED. REG. 48,841 (Sept. 26, 1991).

[206] *See* Podolsky v. First Healthcare Corp., 50 Cal. App. 4th 632, 58 Cal. Rptr. 2d 89 (2d Dist. 1996).

[207] *See* R.L. Rundle & P. Davies, *Hospitals start to seek payment upfront*, WALL ST. J., June 2, 2004, D1.

[208] American Manufacturers Mutual Ins. Co. v. Sullivan, 526 U.S. 40 (1999); *see also* Scheffield Med. Group v. Roth, 63 Cal. App. 4th 1465, 74 Cal. Rptr. 2d 752 (2d Dist.1998) [in challenge to alleged plan to avoid, delay payment of workers' compensation medical bills, employees of State Compensation Insurance Fund are immune for their prosecutorial actions].

[209] *E.g.*, Mercy Mt. Clemens Corp. v. Auto Club Ins. Ass'n, 219 Mich. App. 46, 555 N.W.2d 871 (1996) [no fault auto insurers could not base their pay on amounts paid by others, so could not discover those amounts]; Central Gen. Hosp. v. Chubb Group of Ins. Cos., 90 N.Y.2d 195, 659 N.Y.S.2d 246, 681 N.E.2d 413 (1997) [insurer's untimely disclaimer did not preclude no-fault payment denial based on lack of coverage]; Presbyterian Hosp. v. Maryland Cas. Co., 90 N.Y.2d 274, 660 N.Y.S.2d 536, 683 N.E.2d 1 (1997) [no-fault benefits award affirmed, intoxication defense precluded when insurer did not timely deny claim]; New York Hosp. Med. Ctr. v. Country-Wide Ins. Co., 295 A.D.2d 583, 744 N.Y.S.2d 201 (2d Dept. 2002), *see also* Advocacy Organization for Patients & Providers v. Auto Club Ins. Ass'n, 176 F.3d 315 (6th Cir.), *cert. denied*, 528 U.S. 871 (1999) [affirming dismissal of suit claiming no-fault insurers conspired to defraud of reasonable fees].

New Jersey proposed six care paths for treating persons under no-fault automobile coverage.[210] In 1999, a New Jersey appellate court upheld the regulations.[211]

EMTALA. In response to the perceived problem of "dumping" of patients, the Emergency Medical Treatment and Active Labor Act (EMTALA) makes the transferring hospital responsible for the financial loss to the receiving hospital as a result of an impermissible transfer.[212] EMTALA is discussed in Chapter 6.

TRANSFER AGREEMENTS. Some health care entities enter transfer agreements that involve obligations to pay for care. Such commitments generally are not implied; they need to be expressly stated. For example, one Florida hospital sued a nursing home that would not accept the return of a patient. The hospital was trying to collect the cost for care of the patient during the period from when hospitalization was no longer necessary until arrangements could be made for discharge to another nursing home. The court denied the claim because neither state law nor the transfer agreement with the nursing home required such payment.[213]

9-4.4 What Are Some of the Legal Restrictions on the Billing and Collection Process?

CONTENT OF BILL. To ensure that collections can be pursued to the full extent permitted by law, the billings must be accurately prepared and maintained. The correct name and address of the patient and the person responsible for payment must be obtained, the services provided and dates must be clearly described, and any payments or other credits must be promptly reflected on the account. Some states impose additional requirements on the contents of hospital bills.[214] There is increasing consumer scrutiny of bills.[215]

Laws concerning the content, including the amount, of the bill need to be observed. Proper coding is important. Improper billing can result in proceedings under the False Claims Act or the mail fraud law.

---

[210] 30 N.J. REG. 3211 (Sept. 8, 1998) [proposal]; 30 N.J. REG. 4401(a) [modified after hearings, comments].

[211] New Jersey Coalition of Health Care Professionals v. N.J. Dept. of Banking & Ins., 323 N.J. Super. 207, 732 A.2d 1063 (App. Div. 1999).

[212] 42 U.S.C. § 1395dd(d)(2)(B).

[213] In re Senior Care Properties, Inc., 161 Bankr. 294 (Bankr. N.D. Fla. 1993).

[214] E.g., FLA. STAT. § 395.015.

[215] See Decoding your hospital bill, CONSUMER REPORTS, Jan. 2003, 19.

False Claims Act. The False Claims Act[216] imposes criminal penalties on anyone who knowingly presents, or causes to be presented, to the U.S. government a false or fictitious claim for payment. This includes using a false record or statement to get a false or fictitious claim paid. It is not limited to health care; it applies equally to all others who make claims for payment to the government for any item or service. There does not have to be specific intent to defraud the government, recklessness is enough. If the government suffered damages as a result of the false claim, the defendant can be assessed three times those damages. In addition, a penalty of $5,000 to $10,000 per false claim can be assessed. Providers have been found liable under this act.[217]

The Act permits individuals to bring suits, called "qui tam" actions, in the name of the United States as "private attorneys general."[218] The individual must be the "original source" of the information, and the government has to be given an opportunity to pursue the litigation. Regardless, the individual is entitled to keep part of any recovery in the suit. Retaliation against whistleblowers is prohibited. Qui tam actions have been brought against providers and those administering federal health programs.[219]

Mail Fraud. False claims that are sent through the mails can be punished under the mail fraud law.[220] It is not limited to claims to the government. Physicians have been convicted of mail fraud for bills submitted to private insurers.[221]

Fraud by Patients and Others. Patients who submit fraudulent claims can also be prosecuted. A 1993 case addressed friends who had lied about an injured person's identity so that one could use the other's employer-provided health insurance to obtain medical services. They were convicted of wire fraud and conspiracy.[222] In 1995, a federal appellate court upheld the convictions of two physicians for mail fraud. One physician had treated himself, which was not a covered

---

216 31 U.S.C. §§ 3729–3731.

217 *E.g.*, United States v. Lorenzo, 768 F. Supp. 1127 (E.D. Pa. 1991); United States v. Krizek, 859 F. Supp. 5 (D. D.C. 1994).

218 31 U.S.C. § 3730(b).

219 *E.g.*, Cooper v. Blue Cross & Blue Shield of Fla., Inc., 19 F.3d 562 (11th Cir. 1994).

220 18 U.S.C. § 1341; United States v. Woodely, 9 F.3d 74 (9th Cir. 1993) [mail fraud conviction for Medicare claims by nursing home]; United States v. Migliaccio, 34 F.3d 1517 (10th Cir. 1994) [conviction of doctors for mail fraud for sending false CHAMPUS claims reversed and new trial ordered, alleged misrepresentation of surgical procedures performed, inadequate jury instructions].

221 *E.g.*, United States v. Hooshmand, 931 F.2d 725 (11th Cir. 1991).

222 United States v. Milligan, 17 F.3d 177 (6th Cir. 1994), *cert. denied*, 513 U.S. 879 (1994); *Health-care system is issue in jailing of uninsured patient*, N.Y. Times, Jan. 8, 1993, A7.

service under his health insurance; and his medical partner submitted bill as if the partner had provided the service.[223] In 2000, a woman was sentenced to jail for permitting her lover to pose as her husband so that her insurance would pay for his penile implant surgery.[224]

COLLECTION METHODS. When a hospital's internal collection procedures fail to produce payment, hospitals frequently use collection agencies.[225] Both internal billing efforts and collection agency efforts must comply with applicable laws.

A bill is evidence of a contract to pay for services provided and is enforceable by legal action. Although small bills may not be worth the cost of judicial proceedings, legal action may sometimes help educate patients about their obligation to pay medical bills just as they pay other bills. In some states, small claims courts can be used to enforce smaller obligations at lower cost.

After the time period for filing a malpractice suit has passed, providers usually will not want to file a suit to collect the bill because in some states filing a collection suit reopens the opportunity to file the malpractice suit as a counterclaim.[226]

Some health plans impose a much shorter time limit for filing suit to recover benefits. These are valid under some state laws[227] and violate the laws of other states.[228] However, the shorter time limit can be valid for ERISA plans in all states due to preemption of contrary state laws.

When a court judgment is obtained, it can be enforced in several ways, including having a sheriff seize the debtor's property and imposing garnishment of the debtor's wages. Garnishment of a debtor's wages requires a court order to an employer to pay a portion of the debtor's paycheck to the creditor until the debt is paid. The federal Consumer Credit Protection Act[229] and various state laws limit the portion of a paycheck that may be garnished.[230]

---

[223] United States v. Johnson, 71 F.3d 539 (6th Cir. 1995).

[224] S. Maull, *Woman sentenced to weekends in jail for fraud in penis implant case*, AP, June 23, 2000.

[225] *E.g.*, Hauge Assocs. v. McGriff, 666 N.W.2d 151 (Iowa 2003) [collection agency may sue for assigned hospital bill].

[226] *E.g.*, Stein v. Feingold, 629 So. 2d 998 (Fla. 3d DCA 1993); *see also* Harris v. Stein, 207 A.D.2d 382, 615 N.Y.S.2d 703 (2d Dept. 1994) [malpractice suit barred by judgment in prior suit].

[227] *E.g.*, Hale v. Blue Cross & Blue Shield, 862 S.W.2d 905 (Ky. Ct. App. 1993) [one-year limit on lawsuits to recover benefits in group health benefits contract valid].

[228] FLA. STAT. § 95.03; *but see* Burroughs Corp. v. Suntogs of Miami, Inc., 472 So. 2d 1166 (Fla. 1985) [permitting contractual choice of law of state permitting shortening].

[229] 15 U.S.C. §§ 1671–1677.

[230] *E.g.*, St. Ann's Hosp. v. Arnold, 109 Ohio App. 3d 562, 672 N.E.2d 743 (1996) [not violation of equal protection for state to put lower limit on percentage of income that may be garnished for health care debts].

Occasionally, families have alleged that patient suicides were due to collection efforts. In 1987, a New York appellate court ruled that suicide was not a foreseeable risk of aggressive collection efforts; so the hospital was not liable for the death.[231] However, also in 1987, a federal appellate court ruled that a jury properly required a physician to pay $200,000 to the surviving husband when his wife committed suicide after receiving a copy of a Medicare claim that falsely indicated a diagnosis of a brain tumor.[232] The physician had instructed his staff to enter the false diagnosis because payment would have been denied for the test if a negative result had been reported.

Fair Debt Collection Practices Act. The Fair Debt Collection Practices Act (FDCPA)[233] and various state laws[234] regulate techniques that can be used to seek payment of delinquent accounts. Some of these laws apply only to collection activities of collection agencies, while others also apply to internal hospital collection activities. All persons involved in hospital collection activities should be familiar with these laws to assure compliance. In some situations, failure to comply can make the debt unenforceable and even subject the hospital and involved individuals to civil liability and criminal penalties. In 1984, a collection agency attempting to collect a $552.40 bill for the Mayo Clinic was required to pay the debtor $14,400 for his emotional distress, out-of-pocket expenses, and attorney's fees because the agency violated the FDCPA.[235]

Although originally there was an exception for attorneys, the exception was removed; letters and communications from attorneys are also covered by FDCPA.[236]

Fair Credit Reporting Act. The Fair Credit Reporting Act[237] regulates the collection and use of consumer credit information. Obtaining consumer reports for unauthorized uses violates this

---

231 Wells v. St. Luke's Mem. Hosp. Ctr., 129 A.D.2d 952, 515 N.Y.S.2d 335 (3d Dept. 1987).

232 Stafford v. Neurological Med., Inc., 811 F.2d 470 (8th Cir. 1987).

233 15 U.S.C. §§ 1692–1692o; Hamilton v. United Healthcare, 310 F.3d 385 (5th Cir. 2002) [FDCPA applies to subrogation]; Edwards v. Hocking Valley Comm. Hosp., 87 Fed. Appx. 542 (6th Cir. 2004) (unpub) [settlement agreement concerning class action suit over violations of FDCPA].

234 *E.g.*, Forsyth Mem. Hosp. Inc. v. Contreras, 107 N.C. App. 611, 421 S.E.2d 167 (1992) [collection letter by hospital holding company sent on letterhead of attorney did not violate state collection law].

235 Venes v. Professional Serv. Bureau, Inc., 353 N.W.2d 671 (Minn. Ct. App. 1984); *see also* United States v. ACB Sales & Serv., Inc., 683 F. Supp. 734 (D. Ariz. 1987) [each officer fined $25,000, home office fined $150,000 for collection violations after a Federal Trade Commission compliance order]; Bieber v. Associated Collection Servs., 631 F. Supp. 1410 (D. Kan. 1986).

236 *E.g.*, Heintz v. Jenkins, 514 U.S. 291 (1995) [FDCPA applies to lawyer even when engaged in litigation for credit or client].

237 15 U.S.C. §§ 1681–1681t.

Act.[238] In 2000, a federal court in Florida ruled that sending dunning letters extended the time in which complaints could be made under the Act.[239]

Liens. Hospital liens are a special legal collection mechanism. Many states have hospital lien laws to assist hospitals in collecting for services rendered to victims of compensable accidents. If a patient is treated for injuries caused by a person who is insured or otherwise capable of paying damages, the hospital may place a lien on the proceeds of any court judgment or settlement of the patient's personal injury action against the responsible individual.[240] This lien gives the hospital some priority to payment from the proceeds. Some states limit the amount of the lien[241] or require the hospital to be public[242] or located or incorporated[243] in the state to qualify for the lien. In most states, appropriate documents must be filed with the court, negligent party, insurer, and patient's attorney. Some states also have physician's liens.[244]

Some states place limits on when liens can be used. For example, in 2005, the California Supreme Court ruled that a hospital could not file a lien against a personal injury action when the hospital had accepted payment for the treatment from a health plan.[245]

---

[238] *E.g.*, Bakker v. McKinnon, 152 F.3d 1007 (8th Cir. 1998) [violation of Act for plaintiff's attorney to obtain consumer credit report on defendant dentist, his adult daughter]; Duncan v. Handmaker, 149 F.3d 424 (6th Cir. 1998) [violation for attorney to obtain consumer report to defend client]; Ippolito v. W.N.S., Inc., 864 F.2d 440 (7th Cir. 1988), *cert. dismissed*, 490 U.S. 1061 (1989); *but see* Trans Union Corp. v. F.T.C., 317 U.S. App. D.C. 133, 81 F.3d 228 (1996) [certain mailing lists not consumer reports protected by Act].

[239] Kaplan v Assetcare, Inc. 88 F. Supp. 2d 1355 (S.D. Fla. 2000).

[240] *E.g.*, *In re* Estate of Cooper, 125 Ill. 2d 363, 532 N.E.2d 236 (1988) [hospital lien attached to money used to obtain structured settlement annuity]; Wood v. Baptist Med. Ctr., 890 P.2d 1367 (Okla. Ct. App. 1995) [foreclosure of hospital lien]; Amisub (St. Joseph Hosp.), Inc. v. Allied Property & Casualty Ins. Co., 6 Neb. App. 696, 576 N.W.2d 493 (1998) [Neb. hospital lien law applied to services provided in Neb. to Iowans resulting from auto accident in Iowa]; Annotation, *Construction, operation, and effect of statute giving hospital lien against recovery from tortfeasor causing patient's injuries*, 16 A.L.R. 5TH 262.

[241] *E.g.*, Mercy Hosp. & Med. Ctr. v. Farmers Ins. Group, 15 Cal. 4th 213, 61 Cal. Rptr. 2d 638, 932 P.2d 210 (1997) [hospital recovery under statutory lien limited to 50 percent of patient's recovery].

[242] *E.g.*, Schwartz v. Geico Gen. Ins. Co., 712 So. 2d 773 (Fla. 4th DCA 1998) [hospital liens limited to public hospitals].

[243] *E.g.*, Beckett v. Department of Soc. Svcs., Div. of Med. Servs., 948 S.W.2d 250 (Mo. Ct. App. 1997) [hospital must be located or incorporated in state to use state hospital lien].

[244] *E.g.*, Dollieslager v. Hurst, 295 Ill. App. 3d 152, 691 N.E.2d 1181 (3d Dist. 1998) [physicians lien attached only to reasonable charges for services causally connected to underlying event of tort action].

[245] Parnell v. Adventist Health Sys./West, 35 Cal. 4th 595, 109 P.3d 69, 26 Cal. Rptr. 3d 569 (2005); *see also* Dorr v. Sacred Heart Hosp., 228 Wis. 2d 425, 597 N.W.2d 462 (App. 1999) [no hospital lien permitted when patient covered by HMO that has contract with hospital].

There may be other liens against third-party recoveries, such as liens to recover Medicaid payments, and they may have priority in some situations.[246]

Estate Claims. When the patient dies, the patient's estate is responsible for debts of the deceased if the estate is given timely notice of the debt. Many states assign a high priority to payment of expenses for care of the deceased during the last illness. Thus, many of the other debts of the deceased cannot be paid until the hospital bill has been paid.

Bankruptcy. When a hospital receives a notice that a patient has filed for bankruptcy or has obtained discharge of debts in bankruptcy, collection efforts must cease. Federal law forbids most efforts to collect debts during bankruptcy proceedings[247] or after discharge of the debts in bankruptcy.[248] A hospital can be liable for any damage it causes by violating this law. Bankruptcy issues are discussed in Chapter 2.

Ascertaining Indigency and Applying for Benefits. Although hospitals generally help patients identify and qualify for benefits, in most jurisdictions there is no legal duty to do so. However, one California trial court found such a duty and barred a hospital that had not provided such assistance from collecting half of its bill.[249]

Interest. Health care providers also need to be aware of the Truth-in-Lending Act and its implementing regulation[250] called "Regulation Z," which specifies the disclosures that must be made by entities that lend consumers money. These rules are applicable to the credit practices of many providers. Oral agreements involving no finance charges are generally exempt. Some other credit practices might not be affected by the rules.[251]

---

[246] *E.g.*, Moore v. Kaiser Found. Health Plan, 57 Cal. App. 4th 178, 66 Cal. Rptr. 2d 784 (4th Dist. 1997) [affirming Medi-Cal lien against settlement of malpractice suit]; Whelan v. Division of Med. Assistance, 44 Mass. App. Ct. 663, 694 N.E.2d 10 (1998) [affirming state medical assistance lien against medical malpractice judgment]; Estate of Pierce v. State of Missouri Department of Social Services, 969 S.W.2d 814 (Mo. Ct. App.1998) [affirming Medicaid lien].

[247] 11 U.S.C. § 362(a),(h).

[248] 11 U.S.C. § 524(a).

[249] Medico-Dental Adjustment Bureau v. Ruiz, No. MC-44033 (Cal. Mun. Ct. San Luis Obispo County Aug. 31, 1993), *as discussed in* "Year in Review" from 1994 Annual Meeting of American Academy of Hospital Attorneys.

[250] 15 U.S.C. §§ 1601–1667e; 12 C.F.R. pt. 226.

[251] Hahn v. Hank's Ambulance Serv., Inc., 787 F.2d 543 (11th Cir. 1986) [$5 ambulance charge for not paying at time of service was not "credit," not subject to Act].

9-4.5 What Is the Scope of Responsibility to Provide Uncompensated Care?

Many hospitals are required by law to provide uncompensated care to certain patients. State law requires many governmental hospitals to provide uncompensated care, especially to patients who are residents of the area providing tax support to the hospital and who are unable to pay.

HILL-BURTON ACT. The federal Hill-Burton Act[252] provided public and nonprofit community hospitals with funding for construction and modernization. Hospitals that accepted this funding are required to provide a reasonable volume of services to persons unable to pay for twenty years after construction was completed.[253] Most hospitals have fulfilled their Hill-Burton uncompensated obligation. The Hill-Burton program retains significance because of the ongoing community service obligation[254] and because any Hill-Burton funding must be repaid to the U.S. government in certain sales of hospitals.[255]

Some patients have attempted to use a hospital's failure to comply with the Hill-Burton uncompensated care regulations as a defense to collection suits. Courts have disagreed on whether this can be used as a defense.[256]

9-5 How Can Capital Financing Be Arranged?

Hospitals have substantial and growing needs for capital to modernize and expand.

INTERNAL FINANCING. Internal financing from current net operating revenues or funded depreciation is one source of capital, but it has become increasingly difficult to accumulate.

PHILANTHROPY. Private philanthropy is another source of capital and operating funds for nonprofit hospitals. Although funds from philanthropic sources remain important and substantial,[257] the

---

[252] 42 U.S.C. §§ 291a-291o-1.
[253] 42 C.F.R. pt. 124; American Hosp. Ass'n v. Schweicker, 721 F.2d 170 (7th Cir. 1983), *cert. denied*, 466 U.S. 958 (1984); Flagstaff Med. Ctr., Inc. v. Sullivan, 962 F.2d 879 (9th Cir. 1992).
[254] 42 C.F.R. § 124.603.
[255] *E.g.*, United States v. Coweta County Hosp. Auth., 777 F.2d 667 (11th Cir. 1985).
[256] *E.g.*, Falmouth Hosp. v. Lopes, 376 Mass. 580, 382 N.E.2d 1042 (1978) [not defense]; White v. Moses Taylor Hosp., 841 F. Supp. 629 (M.D. Pa. 1992) [not defense]; *contra* Creditors Protective Ass'n, Inc. v. Flack, 93 Or. App. 719, 763 P.2d 756 (1988) [defense permitted]; Yale New Haven Hosp., Inc. v. Wilczynski, 44 Conn. Super. 274, 683 A.2d 1362 (1995) [defense permitted].
[257] S. Strom, *Charitable giving holds steady, report finds*, N.Y. TIMES, June 22, 2004, A10 [$20.9 billion for health in 2003].

percentage of total hospital funds for capital expenditures from these sources has been continually decreasing.

Before a donor of a charitable gift of $250 or more may deduct the gift in calculating federal income taxes, the donor must obtain from the recipient a written acknowledgment confirming the gift and stating whether anything of value was given in return and, if so, what its value was.[258]

Care must be taken to use philanthropic gifts for the purposes intended. The donors and, in most states, the state attorney general can bring actions to compel compliance.[259]

GOVERNMENT GRANTS. Another major source of capital was governmental grants, until the federal government discontinued its programs. Some states still have grant and loan programs to help fund construction and improvement of medical facilities.[260]

This has left bonds, equity, and conventional borrowing as the primary sources of capital.

BONDS. Bonds can be tax-exempt or taxable.

Tax-Exempt Bonds. Sale of tax-exempt bonds is the predominant method by which many nonprofit providers of health care obtain funds for major capital expenditures.[261] A principal advantage of tax-exempt bonds has been a lower interest rate than the rate on loans that pay taxable interest. Tax-exempt bonds are issued by state or local governmental entities. The bonds are usually revenue bonds repayable only from hospital revenues, but bonds for governmental hospitals are sometimes payable from general tax revenues. The exemption of bond interest from federal income taxation is based on Section 103 of the Internal Revenue Code.[262] Bonds for private tax-exempt hospital purposes qualify if certain conditions are met.[263] This law and its implementing regulations must be complied with to assure tax exemption. For example, federal directives place limits on the contracts that may be signed with management companies or with nonemployee physicians.[264]

---

[258] 26 U.S.C. § 170(f)(8).

[259] *E.g.*, Smithers v. St. Lukes-Roosevelt Hosp. Ctr., 281 A.D.2d 127, 723 N.Y.S.2d 426 (1st Dept. 2001).

[260] *E.g.*, *Brandon Regional Hospital gets grant to add beds*, ST. PETERSBURG TIMES [FL], June 14, 2003, 3B [$13 million Fla. state grant].

[261] For an example of trouble selling bonds for a health facility, *see* Ford v. First Mun. Leasing Corp., 838 F.2d 994 (8th Cir. 1988) [prospective bond purchasers' failure to purchase not a breach of contract].

[262] 26 U.S.C. § 103.

[263] 26 U.S.C. §§ 141, 145, 147–149.

[264] Rev. Proc. 97-13, 97-14; *IRS gives more flexibility to issuers in rules on private activity bond use*, 6 H.L.R. 126 (1997).

Some incidental uses outside the scope of otherwise permitted uses are permitted, if they involve a small enough percentage of the proceeds and the space.[265]

The IRS has increased its scrutiny of hospital bonds, with special attention to bonds that are used to finance acquisitions.[266]

Some states place additional limits on hospital use of tax-exempt bonds. One controversial area has been whether these bonds can be used to finance the capital needs of church-owned hospitals, but most courts have upheld such uses.[267]

Most tax-exempt bonds must be in registered form.[268] However, tax-exempt bonds generally do not have to be registered under federal securities laws[269] but are subject to the penalties under those laws if fraudulent or deceptive practices are used. Tax-exempt bonds are not exempt from some state securities laws; they must be registered in some states before they can be sold to residents of the state.

In 1995, the Securities Exchange Commission (SEC) began requiring entities that receive monies from tax-exempt bonds, including hospitals, to make annual and special disclosures.[270]

When a for-profit corporation buys a nonprofit hospital that was financed with tax-exempt bonds, the bonds generally must be redeemed.[271]

Times when bond are being processed can be delicate. A radiologist who lost his contract with a hospital sent allegedly false information to the finance commission that delayed approval of the bonds. A Michigan court ruled that the radiologist could be liable for tortious interference with the bonding.[272]

When selling tax-exempt or exempt bonds, hospitals generally must release a public offering statement. These must be written

---

[265] 26 U.S.C. § 141(b); IRS Notice 87-69, 1987-2 C.B. 378.

[266] 67 FED REG. 17,309 (Apr. 10, 2002) [proposed IRS rules on acquisitions]; S. Duff, *Texas Health settles with no penalty; IRS: Acquisition financing debt OK*, BOND BUYER, Feb. 7, 2003, 1.

[267] *E.g.*, Manning v. Sevier County, 30 Utah 2d 305, 517 P.2d 549 (1973); *contra* Board of County Comm'rs v. Idaho Health Care Facilities Auths., 96 Id. 498, 531 P.2d 588 (1975).

[268] 26 U.S.C. § 149(a).

[269] 15 U.S.C. § 77c(a)(2), (4); Securities & Exch. Comm'n v. Children's Hosp., 214 F. Supp. 883 (D. Ariz. 1963) [exemption does not apply when substantial purpose of hospital is profit for promoters].

[270] S.B. Kite, *SEC mandates secondary market disclosure for 501(c)(3) bonds*, 4 H.L.R. 256 (1995) [effective July 3, 1995, ongoing disclosure requirements by beneficiaries of tax-exempt bonds, including annual information, notices of designated events].

[271] *E.g.*, PLR No. 9427025 (Apr. 11, 1994); *Hospital sale to for-profit firm requires bond redemption in 90 days*, 3 H.L.R. 971 (1994); *but see* PLR No. 9419022 (Feb. 10, 1994); *Hospital's lease to private entity does not change county bonds' status*, 3 H.L.R. 675 (1994).

[272] Trepel v. Pontiac Osteopathic Hosp., 135 Mich. App. 361, 354 N.W.2d 341 (1984).

carefully so that they not only are complete and not misleading, but also so that they cannot be used against the hospital in other contexts. In 2002, a public offering statement by a hospital was used against the hospital in a managed care lawsuit.[273]

When hospitals close or have difficulty meeting their bonding obligations, the resolution can often be complex.[274] It is sometimes difficult to determine who can be involved in the resolution. In 2002, an Illinois appellate court ruled that a township did not have standing to seek to stop the repayment of the bonds for a closed township hospital.[275]

Sometimes localities place conditions on their approval of bonds under programs that they can control. For example in 2003, Oklahoma City supported bonds for a local hospital when it agreed not to relocate out of the city.[276]

Taxable Bonds. For-profit hospitals borrow money using taxable bonds and other taxable debt arrangements. Some nonprofit hospitals have also used taxable bonds.

EQUITY. Hospitals and other health care enterprises owned by investors acquire equity capital by selling stock, partnership interests, or other equity interests to investors. Such sales have been a major source of capital. Enterprises that acquire capital through these means must comply with securities laws. These laws require disclosure of certain information as well as placing some restrictions on the conduct of those involved with the enterprise.

CONVENTIONAL BORROWING. Both for-profit and nonprofit hospitals borrow money through conventional borrowing, often secured by mortgages on the real and personal property of the borrower. This can lead to mortgage foreclosures on buildings that are mortgaged to secure the borrowings.[277]

---

[273] *Chester County Hospital made pitch to investors that contradicts lawsuit against Independence Blue Cross*, PR NEWSWIRE, June 17, 2002.

[274] *E.g.*, *HealthSouth reaches agreement with noteholders*, HEALTH & MED. WEEK, June 28, 2004, 114; G. D'Ambrosio, *Pennsylvania court sets hearing to retire debt of defunct health system*, BOND BUYER, Nov. 3, 2003, 41.

[275] Wood River Township v. Wood River Township Hosp., 331 Ill. App. 3d 599, 772 N.E.2d 308 (5th Dist. 2002), *leave. denied*, 202 Ill. 2d 665; 787 N.E.2d 170 (2002); T.L. Howard, *Wood River seeks back payment for hospital bonds*, ST. LOUIS POST-DISPATCH, Aug. 24, 2000, 1; Y. Shields, *Illinois high court rejects Wood River's appeal on hospital bonds*, BOND BUYER, Dec. 9, 2002, 36.

[276] R. Williamson, *Saving deal: St. Anthony Hospital to stay in Oklahoma City*, BOND BUYER, Oct. 24, 2003, 36 [hospital agreed to maintain location in city with the help of a $250 million bond issue through Oklahoma Industries Auth.].

[277] *E.g.*, Travelers Ins. Co. v. Liljeberg Enters., Inc., 38 F.3d 1404 (5th Cir. 1994) [suit by Travelers seeking seizure, judicial sale of St. Jude Medical Office Building].

Mortgage Guaranties. The Federal Housing Administration (FHA) insures conventional mortgages for constructing, modernizing, and equipping hospitals.[278] Rather than lending funds directly to the hospital, the FHA provides loan insurance. This minimizes the lender's risk, making it easier to borrow money. The FHA also guarantees and insures loans for some capital expenditures of hospitals in rural communities.[279]

LEASING. While purchasing has been the more traditional method within the health care industry for obtaining capital assets, leasing is also used. Although any type of capital asset can be leased, leases are most frequently used to obtain equipment.

Leasing is used as part of capital financing arrangements. Hospitals are sometimes sold to real estate investment trusts or other entities and then leased back on a long-term basis. Leases are also used for off-balance sheet financing of other real estate, such as medical office buildings.

9-6 What Are the Other Sources of Financing for Providers?

BORROWING ON RECEIVABLES. Some hospitals obtain working capital by borrowing against their receivables, the amounts that the hospital is owed by others.[280] In 2002, a prominent lender in receivables trade collapsed, resulting in the bankruptcy of several hospitals that had relied on the lender.[281]

TAX SUPPORT. Many localities support public and nonprofit hospitals through special taxes.[282] Voters generally must approve such taxes and frequently do so.[283] Others provide tax-supported aid from general revenues.[284]

---

[278] 12 U.S.C. § 1715z-7; L. Lagnado, *New York hospitals scramble to keep controversial U.S. loan program alive*, WALL ST. J., Jan. 27, 1997, B6.

[279] 7 U.S.C. §§ 1926, 1932.

[280] *See* J. Spinner, *Health care receivables trade grows; Uncertain payment process expands risk*, WASH. POST, Dec. 25, 2002, E1.

[281] M. O'Neal, *Fallout spreads after collapse of a health services lender*, N.Y. TIMES, Nov. 21, 2002, C1.

[282] *E.g.*, F. Alvarado, *Health trust's properties to get professional treatment*, MIAMI DAILY BUSINESS REV., Nov. 13, 2001, A1 [half cent sales tax in Dade County Fla. supports public hospitals, other health facilities].

[283] *E.g.*, *San Juan County voters approve tax for hospital*, AP, Aug. 6, 2003 [NM], *House race decided; Panhandle hospital receives funding*, AP, Apr. 3, 2002 [two 1-cent sales taxes for Cimarron Memorial Hospital and Nursing Home in Boise City, Okla.]; *but see* T. Bower, *Bexar balks at raising health system tax rate; Commissioners face cutting services for poor*, SAN ANTONIO EXPRESS-NEWS [TX], Aug. 6, 2003, 8B.

[284] *E.g.*, *Michigan: Detroit Medical Center cancels layoffs*, N.Y. TIMES, July 22, 2003, A15 [state and local government aid agreement].

There are usually conditions required to this aid when the institution is not directly controlled by the local government. Sometimes institutions forgo the aid when the conditions are unacceptable.[285]

FEDERAL BAILOUTS. On rare occasions, the federal government has bailed out hospitals, usually in large urban areas that were unable to solve the problem at the state or local level. The Los Angeles County health system was provided $365 million in 1995 and $150 million in 2003.[286]

9-7 What Is the Impact of Tax Structure on the Health Care System?

This section is divided into two parts covering state and local taxes (9-7.1) and federal taxes (9-7.2).

9-7.1 State and Local Taxes

There are a wide variety of state and local taxes. Some examples include income taxes, corporate franchise taxes, revenue taxes, tangible and intangible property taxes, professional and business registration and licensure fees, unemployment taxes, and transactional taxes, such as sales taxes, transfer taxes, and document stamps. In some states, the way a transaction is structured can have a large impact on the amount of taxes that are due.

Governmental and charitable institutions are granted exemption from many taxes at both the state and the local levels for property, sales, and income taxes and at the federal level for income taxes. Classification of a hospital as exempt depends on several factors that vary depending on the type of tax. The state qualifications for exemptions are often different from the qualifications for exemption from federal taxes.

TAXES ON HEALTH SERVICES. Some states levy taxes on health services.[287] Sometimes these are simply revenue generating

---

285 *E.g., Hospital decides it doesn't want property tax funds*, AP, July 21, 2002 [Hardin County, Ohio, voters approved tax].

286 C. Ornstein, *California; Hospitals to Get $150-Million Infusion; U.S. officials approve extra funds for ailing county health system, saving two medical centers from closure*, L.A. TIMES, Feb. 5, 2003, Part 2, 1; J.E. Allen, *Clinton announces $364 million federal bailout for county*, AP, Sept. 22, 1995.

287 *E.g.*, Revenue Cabinet v. Smith, 875 S.W.2d 873 (Ky.1994), *cert. denied*, 513 U.S. 1000 (1994).

measures. Other state taxes on health services are designed to spread the responsibility for financing uncompensated or under-compensated care.[288] Challenges to these taxes are generally unsuccessful. In 2003, a New York court ruled that a state tax on non-Medicaid receipts of nursing homes could be applied to non-profit institutions.[289]

In 1995, the United States Supreme Court addressed a New York tax on third-party payments to hospitals. Different categories of pay-ers had different tax rates, with Blue Cross exempt from the tax. Blue Cross was exempt because it was the only payer who sold indi-vidual health policies on an open enrollment basis. Plans covered by ERISA challenged the tax claiming that it was preempted by ERISA. The Supreme Court ruled that the tax was not preempted by ERISA. The Court concluded that ERISA preemption was focused on per-mitting plans to offer uniform national benefits and claims process-ing. It was not designed to regulate the price of health care.[290]

In 1998, a federal district court ruled that the Federal Employ-ees Health Benefit Act (FEHBA) preempted applying some state taxes for funding uncompensated health care to a FEHBA plan.[291]

Some states tried to generate some of the state share of the cost of Medicaid through special taxes on providers. Most providers accepted this tax because they got the money back with the addition of federal matching funds. In 1991, Congress out-lawed this practice.[292] The tax itself is not illegal;[293] it is the use of the funds to pay for Medicaid that is prohibited. In 1995, the fed-eral government sought repayment of the additional federal matching monies due to continued use of such provider taxes after 1991.[294] Congress included in the Balanced Budget Act of 1997 a special exception permitting certain taxes collected by the state of New York to be used as part of its share of Medicaid fund-ing.[295] The President used the new line item veto to strike down

---

[288] *E.g.,* A. Miller, *Patients pay added costs; New nursing home 'bed tax' affects only some,* Atlanta J. & Constitution, Aug. 17, 2003, 5E [tax on non-Medicaid patients to help pay for Medicaid shortfall].

[289] Charles T. Sitrin Health Care Ctr. Inc. v. State, 195 Misc. 2d 824, 761 N.Y.S.2d 452 (Sup. Ct. 2003).

[290] New York State Conf. of Blue Cross & Blue Shield Plans v. Travelers Ins. Co., 514 U.S. 645 (1995).

[291] Connecticut v. United States, 1 F. Supp. 2d 147 (D. Conn. 1998) [FEHBA preempts some but not all state taxes to finance uncompensated care].

[292] 42 U.S.C. § 1396b(w).

[293] *E.g.,* Revenue Cabinet v. Smith, 875 S.W.2d 873 (Ky. 1994), *cert. denied,* 513 U.S. 1000 (1994).

[294] *U.S. demands repayments from 9 states,* N.Y. Times, Jan. 31, 1995, A9.

[295] Pub. L. No. 105-33, § 4722(c); 42 U.S.C. § 1396b(w).

the exception.[296] However, in 1998, the United States Supreme Court declared the line item veto to be unconstitutional, reinstating the exception.[297] Full enforcement of the restriction on use of provider taxes remains controversial and has not yet been achieved.[298]

PROPERTY TAXES. Each state has the power to tax properties within its boundaries. A hospital must prove eligibility for a specific tax exemption, or its property is taxable. In some states, ownership by a nonprofit or governmental hospital is not sufficient to establish eligibility. In those states, hospitals must also show that the property is used exclusively for hospital or other exempt purposes to qualify.

Federal Hospitals. Federal hospitals are exempt from state and local taxation because the United States has the sovereign right to hold property free of taxation. This right is based in the Supremacy Clause of the Constitution and in the necessity for federal freedom from state interference when dealing with its property. Federal ownership is sufficient to qualify for this exemption.

Other Governmental Hospitals. State, county, district, and municipal hospitals are usually also exempt from property taxation because they fall within state constitutional or statutory exemptions. These exemptions are sometimes based solely on ownership regardless of property use. In some states, exemption from taxation is granted only when governmental property is devoted to a "public use," but hospital purposes are generally considered to be a public use. Questions may arise about whether other uses are valid public uses.

For-profit Hospitals. For-profit hospitals do not qualify for tax exemption even if a profit is not earned. When for-profit hospitals are reorganized as nonprofit hospitals, some states consider the property to be tax-exempt even when hospital net revenue is used to pay off bondholders who are former stockholders in the predecessor for-profit hospital. However, some courts disagree.[299]

Nonprofit Hospitals. Nonprofit hospitals are frequently exempted from state and local property taxation by state constitutions and statutes. Most exemptions require that the institution serve a charitable purpose, but specific wording determines the

---

296 *Clinton uses line-item veto on budget to kill New York provider tax provision*, 6 H.L.R. 1269 (1997).

297 Clinton v. City of New York, 524 U.S. 417 (1998).

298 *See* R. Pear, *U.S. nears clash with governors on Medicaid cost*, N.Y. Times, Feb. 16, 2004, A1.

299 *E.g.*, Benton County v. Allen, 170 Or. 481, 133 P.2d 991 (1943) [reorganized hospital not tax exempt].

qualifications and extent of exemptions. Tax exemption for non-profit hospitals has received renewed scrutiny and challenge.[300] For example, the Utah Supreme Court established tighter criteria for what demonstrates charitable purpose that limited the number of Utah hospitals that could qualify.[301] In 1992, a Pennsylvania hospital lost its tax exemption because it did not donate a substantial portion of its service. The court found that it provided free care only to the extent required by other laws and that it had participated in a lawsuit seeking higher Medicaid reimbursement.[302] The Pennsylvania statute was changed in 1997,[303] but there continued to be mixed results in challenges to exemptions.[304]

In 2002, a religious hospital in Illinois lost its tax exemption when it was found not to be charitable due to the way it treated needy patients. An appeal was pending in 2005.[305]

States and localities apply different tests to determine when tax exemptions apply; familiarity with the tests is important to obtain and retain tax exemptions.

PAYMENTS IN LIEU OF TAXES. In some states, municipal taxing authorities have placed pressure on hospitals and other tax-exempt organizations to make payments in lieu of taxes.[306] Although there is

---

[300] *See* W. Glaberson, *In era of fiscal damage control, cities fight idea of 'tax exempt,'* N.Y. TIMES., Feb. 21, 1996, A1.

[301] Utah County by County Bd. of Equalization v. Intermountain Health Care, Inc., 709 P.2d 265 (Utah 1985); P.S. Rammell & R.J. Parsons, *Utah County v. Intermountain Health Care: Utah's unique method for determining charitable property tax exemptions—A review of its mandate and impact,* 22 J.H.H.L. 73 (1989); Howell v. County Board of Cache County, 881 P.2d 880 (Utah 1994) [upholding Utah State Tax Comm'n standards for charitable property tax exemption].

[302] School Dist. v. Hamot Med. Ctr., 144 Pa. Commw. 668, 602 A.2d 407 (1992), *applying standard adopted in* Hospital Utilization Project v. Commonwealth, 507 Pa. 1, 487 A.2d 1306 (1985); *Challenge to Erie hospital's tax status gains attention of cash-poor U.S. cities,* WALL ST. J., Feb. 16, 1990, B4A.

[303] *Governor signs bill clarifying standards for tax-exempt hospitals,* 6 H.L.R. 1850 (1997) [Pennsylvania HB 55].

[304] *E.g.,* Pinnacle Health Hosps. v. Dauphin County Bd. of Assessment Appeals, 708 A.2d 845 (Pa. Commw. Ct. 1998) [hospital loss of property tax exemption based on affiliated entities' profit motives]; *but see* Lewistown Hosp. v. Mifflin County Bd. of Assessment Appeals, 706 A.2d 1269 (Pa. Commw. Ct. 1998) [hospital was entitled to tax-exempt status where provided care to over 5,100 indigents during three-year period for free or at reduced cost, notwithstanding participation in Hill-Burton Program, Medicare surpluses]; St. Joseph Hosp. v. Berks County Bd. of Assessment Appeals, 709 A.2d 928 (Pa. Commw. Ct. 1998) [distinguishing Pinnacle Health where hospital used surplus to fund profit-oriented activities].

[305] B. Japsen, *Urbana, Ill. hospital faces tax-exemption loss on charity care,* CHICAGO TRIB., Feb. 20, 2004; M. Taylor, *Board tries to revoke status,* MOD. HEALTHCARE, Apr. 25, 2005, 4.

[306] *E.g., Philadelphia nonprofits asked to make voluntary payments in lieu of taxes,* 3 H.L.R. 971 (1994) [for a payment of 40 percent of taxes that would otherwise be owed, city will not challenge exemption of hospitals that sign up]; L. Larkin, *Financial success may invite local tax scrutiny,* 62 HOSPS. (Oct. 5, 1988), at 30.

usually no legal basis for these requests, they have sometimes succeeded in obtaining "voluntary" payments. In fact, some have been made voluntarily. Others have resulted from threats to challenge the hospital's tax-exempt status or to withhold approval of building permits, zoning changes, and other variances, licenses, and approvals. Hospitals may be confronted with the choice of negotiating payments, accepting delays or denials of important approvals, or resisting through the political or legal process.

SALES AND USE TAXES. State and local sales and use taxes vary considerably in their coverage and exemptions. Hospitals sometimes pay taxes on purchases and sometimes collect taxes on sales. Some states exempt qualified charitable organizations from paying sales taxes, while others grant exemptions for specific products or services, rather than for entire institutions.[307] There is usually an exemption for medicines and some medical products.[308] There is sometimes an exemption for items purchased for resale.[309] As state and local governments search for more revenue, exemptions are being more narrowly interpreted, and there is more enforcement activity in some states.

9-7.2 Federal Taxes

Federal income tax laws are an important issue for most hospitals. They either must take the steps to qualify for exemption, as dis-

---

[307] *E.g.*, Fla. Stat. § 212.08; Preston Mem. Hosp. v. Palmer, 578 S.E.2d 383 (W. Va. 2003) [hospital exempt from use tax on payment to reimburse compensation of officers]; *see* Annotation, *Exemption of charitable or educational organization from sales or use tax*, 53 A.L.R. 3d 748.

[308] *E.g.*, Fla. Stat. § 212.08(2); Annotation, *Sales and use tax exemption for medical supplies*, 30 A.L.R. 5th 494; *but see* Feldman v. Huddleston, 912 S.W.2d 161 (Tenn. Ct. App. 1995) [affirming dietary supplements sold by physician in weight loss program not prescribed drugs, so subject to sales tax]; Medcat Leasing Co. v. Whiley, 253 Ill. App. 3d 801, 625 N.E.2d 424 (4th Dist. 1993) [upholding denial of exemption for CT scanner from use tax as not being within medical appliance exemption]; Mississippi State Tax Comm'n v. Medical Devices, 624 So. 2d 987 (Miss. 1993) [sale of enteral feeding systems to Medicare patient not exempt from sales tax]; *see also* Revenue Cabinet v. Humana Inc., 998 S.W.2d (Ky. App. 1998) [error to assess back sales, use taxes for purchases of medications, prosthetic devices, new interpretation, could not be applied due to doctrine of contemporaneous construction].

[309] *E.g.*, Heritage Convalescent Ctr. v. Utah State Tax Comm'n, 953 P.2d 445 (Utah 1997) [sales taxes paid on bulk food used to prepare inpatient meals refunded, no itemized charge required to be considered for resale to patients]; M.S. Osher, M.D. & R.S. Kerstine, M.D., Inc. v. Limbach, 65 Ohio St. 3d 312, 603 N.E.2d 997 (1992) [sale of intraocular lens by manufacturer to ophthalmologist for implantation is not retail sale subject to excise tax; exemption for articles sold for resale in same form received].

cussed later in this section, or they structure their activities to minimize taxes and pay applicable taxes.

A tax-exempt hospital still must pay taxes on unrelated business income.[310] For example, the profit from drug sales to outpatients who are private patients of the medical staff is usually unrelated business income.[311] Another example of unrelated business income is income from the general public's use of a motel operated by the tax-exempt entity.[312] Care needs to be taken in structuring the provision of services to outside entities.[313] If the unrelated business income is too large a portion of total revenues, the entire tax exemption can be lost.

For-profit hospitals must pay taxes on their profits. They can deduct most of its legitimate business expenses in determining its profits. Sometimes corporations try to avoid corporate taxes by paying excessive salaries because salaries are deductible as business expenses while dividends and other distributions of profits are not deductible. The IRS will treat excessive salaries as nondeductible dividends and assess taxes, interest, and penalties.[314]

Insurance companies are taxed differently than other companies. Some for-profit IPA-model HMOs have qualified to be taxed as insurance companies.[315] Staff-model HMOs are generally not taxed as insurance companies.[316]

When reviewing IRS pronouncements, it is important to keep in mind that they have different effects, ranging from rules that are binding on the IRS through Private Letter Rulings (PLRs) that apply only to the entity that obtained the ruling and cannot be cited

---

[310] IRS, TAX ON UNRELATED BUSINESS INCOME OF EXEMPT ORGANIZATIONS (Pub. 598) [available at www.irs.gov].

[311] Carle Found. v. United States, 611 F.2d 1192 (7th Cir. 1979), *cert. denied*, 449 U.S. 824 (1989); Rev. Rul. 85-109, 1985-2 C.B. 165; *but see* PLR 83-49006 [not if physicians are in hospital-based group practice integrally part of hospital operations].

[312] IRS Tech. Adv. Memo 9847002 (Apr. 29, 1998); *IRS advice memo on tax-exempt's income from motel continues existing IRS policy*, 7 H.L.R. 1972 (1998).

[313] *E.g.*, PLR No. 9445024 (Aug. 16, 1994); *Hospital's respiratory care contracts do not generate taxable business income*, 3 H.L.R. 1730 (1994) [contracts with skilled nursing facilities to provide services directly through hospital employees]; *see also* PLR No. 9750056 (Sept. 16, 1997), *as discussed at* 7 H.L.R. 38 (1998) [hospital assumption of home health business of subsidiaries would result in unrelated business income].

[314] *E.g.*, Curtis v. C.I.R., T. C. Memo 1994-15 ["salary" paid to key organizer of psychiatric evaluation practice was corporate earnings distribution because exceeded reasonable compensation]; Klamath Med. Servs. Bureau v. C.I.R., 29 T.C. 339 (1957), *aff'd*, 261 F.2d 842 (9th Cir. 1958), *cert. denied*, 359 U.S. 966 (1959); *but see* Alpha Med., Inc. v. C.I.R., 172 F.3d 942 (6th Cir. 1999) [president compensation of $4,439,180 found to be reasonable under circumstances].

[315] IRS Tech. Adv. Mem. No. 9412002 (Dec. 17, 1993).

[316] Rev. Rul. 68-27, 1968-1 C.B. 315.

by others in any court.[317] Thus, while PLRs are helpful to know what IRS was thinking at the time and, in conjunction with other materials, may suggest ways to structure the hospital's affairs, they cannot be relied on.

FEDERAL EMPLOYMENT TAXES. All hospitals must pay federal employment taxes on employees. Independent contractors pay their own employment taxes. The IRS scrutinizes relationships that are labeled as independent contractor relationships to determine if they should be considered employment relationships under tax law.[318] What the parties call the relationship is not determinative. Retroactive finding of an employer relationship can result in substantial back taxes, interest, and penalties (including the portion of the employee's income that should have been withheld by the employer).[319] Thus, independent contractor relationships need to be structured so that they will not be considered employment relationships under tax law.

Hospitals need to comply with the technical requirements concerning pensions, deferred compensation, and benefits. They have been a focus of some IRS audits.

FEDERAL INCOME TAX EXEMPTION. In 1996, the Internal Revenue Code was amended to authorize intermediate sanctions against tax-exempt organizations and individuals who are considered insiders.[320] In the past, the IRS could only revoke the tax exemption as a sanction. For many offenses this was a disproportionate penalty or the adverse consequences to the community were so great that the sanction could not be applied; and enforcement was difficult. The creation of intermediate sanctions removed

---

[317] *E.g.*, United States v. Wisconsin Power & Light Co., 38 F.3d 329 (7th Cir. 1994) [discussion of weight given to various levels of IRS pronouncements].

[318] *E.g.*, Rev. Rul. 73-417, 1973-2 C.B. 332 [pathologist/hospital laboratory director with guaranteed minimum salary who cannot work for other hospitals is an employee]; Rev. Rul. 70-629, 1970-2 C.B. 228 [full-time associate physician providing services in office furnished by partnership and under their control was employee]; Tech. Adv. Mem. No. 9508004 (Nov. 17, 1994) [mental health worker performing crisis intervention for local government an employee for federal employment tax purposes]; PLR No. 9149001 (TAM) (July 23, 1991) [physician can be employee of hospital for tax purposes even when state law forbids employment of physicians]; *Are you your own boss? Only if the I.R.S. says so*, N.Y. TIMES, Mar. 19, 1995, F13.

[319] 26 U.S.C. § 3403.

[320] Taxpayer Bill of Rights 2, Pub. L. No. 104-68 (1996) [codified as 26 U.S.C. § 4958]; G. Griffith, *IRS intermediate sanctions proposal: Guidance on the eve of enforcement*, 7 H.L.R. 1558 (1998); *Final rules on intermediate sanctions may wait until 2000, IRS officials say*, 7 H.L.R. 1814 (1998).

some of the threat of loss of tax exemption but increased the likelihood that significant sanctions will be applied to violations.

One focus of the intermediate sanctions is on *excess benefit transactions,* which are defined to be transactions in which an economic benefit is provided to one or more of the organization's insiders or other disqualified persons if the fair market value of the benefit exceeds the value of what the organization received in return.[321] Excessive salaries and inadequate payment for asset transfers are the main problem areas. There is a 225 percent tax on such transactions. There are presumptions and safe harbors in the rules. There are self-reporting obligations. Care must be taken in structuring and reviewing transactions with disqualified persons. In one of the few cases to address excess benefit transactions, in 2002, the federal tax court upheld applying the tax but reversed revocation of the exemption of the involved entities.[322]

Section 501(c)(3). Many nonprofit hospitals are eligible for exemption from federal income tax under section 501(c)(3) of the Internal Revenue Code.[323] It exempts organizations created and operated exclusively for certain purposes, including "charitable purposes." The scope of charitable purposes entitled to this exemption is different from the scope used to determine exemption from state and local taxes. Property may be exempt from one and not the other.

All organizations seeking section 501(c)(3) tax exemption must meet six requirements.

1. The organization must be organized and operated exclusively for one or more special purposes (religious, charitable, scientific, literary, or educational purposes; prevention of cruelty to children or animals; testing for public safety; or amateur sports).
2. No part of the net earnings can inure to any private shareholder or individual.
3. No substantial part of its activities can involve passing propaganda or otherwise attempting to influence legislation.
4. The organization cannot participate in or intervene in any political campaign on behalf of any candidate for public office.

---

[321] 29 U.S.C. § 4958.

[322] Caracci v. C.I.R., 118 T.C. 379 (2002) [appeal pending in U.S. 5th Cir. Court of Appeals].

[323] 26 U.S.C. § 501(c)(3); *Qualification of health care entities for federal tax exemption as charitable organization under 26 USCS sec. 501(c)(3)*, 134 A.L.R. FED. 395.

5. The assets of the organization must be dedicated to charity, so that they go to another qualified charity if the organization is dissolved.
6. The organization must apply for classification as a tax-exempt organization on Form 1023 furnished by the IRS.

The second requirement is of particular concern to hospitals. Private inurement can occur when an individual who has a personal and private interest in the activities of the organization receives financial benefit from the organization that exceeds the fair market value of the services provided to the organization.[324] In 1969, the IRS adopted a three-part test for private inurement. (1) Is the compensation arrangement consistent with exempt purposes? (2) Is the compensation arrangement the result of arm's length bargaining? (3) Does the compensation arrangement result in reasonable compensation?[325]

Thus, reasonable pay and benefits can be provided to those who provide services to the organization. When these payments become unreasonable, they can constitute private inurement. In the past, private inurement was found only with respect to person who controlled the organization; so many transactions with noncontrolling physicians received limited scrutiny.[326] In 1986, the IRS stated that it would scrutinize transactions with other "individuals with a close professional working relationship" with the organization; so a broader range of relationships with physicians could constitute private inurement.[327] For example, free or subsidized services or payments to physicians or others in excess of the fair market value of the services they provide to the hospital can constitute private inurement. However, in 1999, a federal appellate court addressed a case in which the IRS had revoked the tax exemption of a cancer charity because of the payments that it had made to a fund-raising company. The IRS considered the fund-raising company to be a "private shareholder or individual" so that payments to the fund-raising company constituted private inurement. The tax court had affirmed the IRS position, but the appellate court reversed, holding that the fund-raiser was not a "private shareholder or other indi-

---

[324] Treas. Reg. § 1.501(a)–1(e).
[325] Rev. Rul. 69-383, 1989-2 CB 113.
[326] *E.g.*, Rev. Rul. 69-383, 1989-2 CB 113 [establishing three-part test for private inurment].
[327] GCM 39498 (April 24, 1986).

vidual" so there was not private inurement.[328] The court did not address the issue of whether there was an excessive payment that would be deemed to be an improper private benefit. The case was subsequently settled with the charity relinquishing its tax-exempt status.[329]

Excessive executive compensation can also constitute private inurement and has received IRS and Congressional attention.[330] In 1998, the tax court upheld the revocation of the tax exemption of a Florida hospital because its sale had allegedly overly benefited its officers and directors. They bought the hospital from the nonprofit entity for $6.3 million and two years later sold it for almost $30 million.[331] In 1999, a federal appellate court rejected a more expansive interpretation of what constitutes private inurement advocated by the IRS and reinstated the tax exemption of an organization that raised money for cancer research.[332] The court rejected the IRS position that a for-profit fund-raising company under long-term contract had become an insider and its compensation had been private inurement.

Not all private benefits are private inurement. The IRS has adopted the position that tax-exempt status is not jeopardized by some private benefits to the organization's control persons, if the private benefit is purely "incidental" to the organization's exempt purposes. A private benefit is considered incidental only if it is incidental in both a qualitative and a quantitative sense. The qualitative test requires that the benefit be a necessary concomitant of the activity which benefits the public at large, that is, the activity can be accomplished only by benefiting certain private individuals. The

---

[328] United Cancer Council v. C.I.R., 165 F.3d 1173 (7th Cir. 1999), *rev'g*, 109 T.C. 326 (1997); D.M. Ford, *COMMENT: Insiders & Inurement: The Seventh Circuit's reversal of the tax court in United Cancer Council v. Commissioner*, 50 CASE W. RES. L. REV. 909 (2000).

[329] R.J. Robes, *United States: Donor-advised funds under attack: IRS business plan unveiled*, MONDAQ BUSINESS BRIEFING, June 1, 2001.

[330] *E.g.*, *IRS launches enforcement effort targeting compensation in tax-exempt organizations*, H.L.R., Aug. 12, 2004, 1183; S. Strom, *I.R.S. broadens an inquiry into salaries at nonprofit groups*, N.Y. TIMES, Aug. 11, 2004, A13; *IRS outlines factors that may cause it to see executive compensation as 'excessive,'* H.L.R., Jan. 8, 2004, 63 [guidance on IRS Web site – www.irs.gov/pub/irs-tege/eotopice04.pdf]; *see also* Lowry Hosp. Ass'n v. C.I.R., 66 T.C. 850 (1976) [retroactive revocation of hospital's tax exemption due to private inurement to benefit of founding physician].

[331] Anclote Psychiatric Ctr. v. C.I.R., T.C. Memo 1998-273 [upholding revocation of tax-exempt status due to inurement]; T. Sullivan et al., *Anclote decision sharpens link between valuation and inurement*, 7 H.L.R. 1379 (1998); *see also* Maynard Hosp. v. C.I.R, 52 T.C. 1006 (1969), *supp. op.*, 54 T.C. 1675 (1970) [retroactive revocation of tax exemption of hospital and liability of stockholder-trustees for distributions they received on sale of hospital and related pharmacy that had been transferred to them several years before].

[332] United Cancer Council, Inc. v. C.I.R., 165 F.3d 1173 (7th Cir. 1999).

quantitative test requires that the benefit not be substantial after considering the overall public benefit conferred by the activity.[333]

The fifth requirement, a charitable purpose, has received considerable attention concerning hospitals. Health care is accepted as a "charitable purpose" by the IRS. Before 1969, the IRS considered free care to the poor to be one of the essential characteristics a hospital must have in order to be "charitable." Then in 1969, the IRS issued a ruling that recognized promotion of health as a purpose of the law of charity; so free or reduced rate services are not required.[334] A federal appellate court upheld this ruling.[335] The United States Supreme Court later vacated the decision on the ground that the organization could not file the suit because it did not have sufficient interest in the outcome.[336] Thus, the 1969 IRS ruling was left in effect. The 1969 ruling found six characteristics to be important in determining whether the hospital was operated for a charitable purpose.

1. The hospital provided care on a nonprofit basis to all persons in the community who were able to pay directly or through third-party reimbursement.
2. The hospital operated an emergency room that was open to all persons.
3. Any surplus of receipts over disbursements was used to improve the quality of patient care, expand facilities, and advance training, education, and research.
4. Control of the hospital rested with a board of trustees composed of independent civic leaders.
5. The hospital maintained an open medical staff, with privileges available to all qualified medical staff.
6. The hospital permitted all members of the active medical staff to lease space in its medical office building, if any.

This ruling was clarified by a 1983 IRS ruling that addressed a hospital that did not have all of the characteristics listed in the 1969 ruling.[337] The hospital did not have an emergency room because the state health planning agency had found it unnecessary. The IRS looked at other factors and concluded that the hospital was oper-

---

[333] GCM 39598 (Jan. 23, 1987).
[334] Rev. Rul. 69-545, 1969-2 C.B. 117.
[335] Eastern Ky. Welfare Rights Org. v. Simon, 165 U.S. App. D.C. 239, 506 F.2d 1278 (1974).
[336] Simon v. Eastern Ky. Welfare Rights Org., 426 U.S. 26 (1976).
[337] Rev. Rul. 83-157, 1983-42 I.R.B. 9.

ated for the exclusive benefit of the community and, thus, was charitable and entitled to tax exemption. Additional flexibility is indicated in other areas, such as the approval of some profit sharing[338] and incentive compensation[339] plans for nonprofit hospitals. It is likely that other flexibility will be recognized. The minimum characteristics necessary to assure tax exemption are not yet clear. Hospitals that desire federal income tax exemption under section 501(c)(3) should seek advice from a tax lawyer before varying from the characteristics listed in the rulings.

In 1983, the United States Supreme Court recognized a new requirement for exemption under section 501(c)(3) by ruling that organizations violating an "established national public policy" are not entitled to exemption.[340] The Court upheld denial of exemptions to a school with a racially discriminatory admission policy and a school with a racially discriminatory code of conduct for students. The IRS has taken the position that the Medicare fraud and abuse and self-referral laws are also such established national policies and that violations can endanger tax exemption.[341]

The IRS has also focused on relationships between hospitals and other entities. For example, there has been attention to the creation of for-profit subsidiaries,[342] joint ventures with for-profit entities,[343] and joint operating agreements and virtual mergers.[344] Hospitals can enter certain Physician-Hospital Organizations (PHOs) without jeopardizing their tax exemption, if the PHOs are not physician controlled and fairly allocate monies.[345] In 1998, the IRS issued a ruling

---

[338] *E.g.*, PLR 84-42-064 (July 18, 1984).

[339] *E.g.*, PLR 88-07-081 (Nov. 30, 1987), *as discussed in* 16 HEALTH L. DIG. (Apr. 1988), at 54.

[340] Bob Jones Univ. v. Simon, 416 U.S. 725 (1983).

[341] *See* K.L. Levine, *IRS application of health care laws: An analysis of IRS enforcement techniques*, 25 J.H.H.L. 334 (1992).

[342] Gen Couns. Mem. 39,326 (Jan. 17, 1985).

[343] Gen Couns. Mem. 39,862 (Nov. 11, 1991) [benefit to hospital not sufficient to justify certain joint ventures that also benefit physicians].

[344] See *'Hospitals' affiliation under JOA does not produce adverse tax effects*, 6 H.L.R. 612 (1997) [PLR No. 9714011 (Dec. 24, 1996)]; *Letter ruling further explains joint operating company powers*, 6 H.L.R. 694 (1997) [PLR No. 9716021 (Jan. 17, 1997)]; *Virtual merger of nonprofit hospitals does not change their tax-exempt status*, 6 H.L.R. 936 (1997) [PLR No. 9722042 (Mar. 7, 1997)]; *IRS approves affiliation agreement involving network of three hospitals*, 6 H.L.R. 1541 (1997) [PLR No. 9738038-54 (June 26, 1997)]; *Some joint operating agreements IRS has approved entail fairly weak control*, 6 H.L.R. 1609 (1997).

[345] PLR # not available (Sept. 29, 1994), 3 H.L.R. 1553 (1994); *Hospital's exempt status not jeopardized by proposed PHO, IRS says*, 3 H.L.R. 1550 (1994) [first PLR on PHOs]; *IRS official clarifies agency view on PHO board representation conditions*, 4 H.L.R. 151 (1995) [for-profit PHOs not subject to 20 percent physician-representation limit; up to 50 percent control probably acceptable if proportional to their investment].

that helped define what was necessary for a whole-hospital joint venture with a for-profit entity.[346] In 2004, a federal jury found that the IRS had wrongly revoked the tax exemption of a hospital for entering a partnership with a for-profit company.[347] Some arrangements are permitted. Care must be taken in structuring relationships with other entities to preserve the federal tax exemption.

When structuring arrangements to satisfy IRS requirements, the arrangements should also be designed to satisfy other legal requirements, such as those to prevent Medicare fraud and abuse. In 1989, the IRS and HHS agreed to share information on potential violations.[348]

Most entities that are tax exempt under section 501(c)(3) must annually file a disclosure form called Form 990. Most government-related organizations are exempt from this reporting requirement. Tax exempt entities are required to disclose their applications for tax exemption and annual Form 990s to anyone who requests them.[349]

Other Organizations. Various new types of health care entities have sought tax exemption with mixed success. One approach has been to seek to qualify as a stand-alone entity. Another way to qualify has been as an "integral part" of an exempt entity.

Geisinger Health Plan, an IPA-model HMO, sought to be recognized as a stand-alone and was denied the exemption based on the finding that it benefited its members and not the community.[350] Geisinger then tried to be recognized as an integral part of the Geisinger system and was denied the exemption again.[351]

There have been other favorable rulings on tax exemption of networks. Friendly Hills Healthcare Network,[352] Facey Medical

---

[346] Rev. Rul. 98-15 [text at 7 H.L.R. 394 (1998)]; *IRS details guidelines for exempt entities involved in whole-hospital joint ventures,* 7 H.L.R. 391 (1998); R.C. Louthian, *IRS provides whole hospital joint venture guidance in Revenue Ruling 98-15,* 7 H.L.R. 477 (1998); T. Sullivan & M. Peregrine, *Revenue ruling 98-15: Is control now the 'name" of the joint venture 'game'?* 26 HEALTH L. DIG., Apr. 1998, 3.

[347] St. David's Health Care System v. United States, 349 F.3d 232 (5th Cir. 2003) [reversing summary judgment for hospital in challenge to revocation of tax exemption due to partnership with for-profit company]; *Federal jury rules for nonprofit Texas system in tax-exempt status case,* H.L.R., Mar. 11, 2004, 343 [jury verdict for St. David's].

[348] *IRS-HHS agreement calls for caution, experts warn,* MOD. HEALTHCARE, June 2, 1989, 10; L.C. Homer, *Feds staging tag-team attack on physician-hospital ties,* MOD. HEALTHCARE, Oct. 6, 1989, 56.

[349] T.D. 8818, 64 FED. REG. 17279 (Apr. 9, 1999), effective June 8, 1999.

[350] Geisinger Health Plan v. C.I.R., 985 F.2d 1210 (3d Cir. 1993).

[351] Geisinger Health Plan v. C.I.R., 30 F.3d 494 (3d Cir. 1994).

[352] 2 H.L.R. 253 (1993) [a foundation-type IDS affiliated with a university medical center].

Foundation,[353] Billings Clinic,[354] and Rockford Memorial Health Services Corporation[355] were granted stand-alone exemptions. Northwestern Healthcare Network was granted tax exemption of the parent and superparent (the parent's parent) in its regional health network as integral parts of an exempt entity.[356]

Some tax exemptions are of short-lived utility. In 1994, after obtaining tax exemption, Friendly Hills was unable to work out various issues with its affiliated medical center; so the foundation was sold to a for-profit corporation.[357]

In 1994, the IRS unofficially outlined several factors that it considered important for exemption of systems, including nondiscriminatory treatment of Medicare and Medicaid patients; open medical staff at the hospital component; community control; no more than twenty percent control of the governing board by physicians; and purchase of assets at fair market value.[358] The 20 percent rule remains controversial with physicians seeking greater representation. One option has been to make the system for profit.[359] Other nonprofit arrangements may be possible. In 1995, one Physician-Hospital Organization in a university context with a board that was over 80 percent physician-controlled received approval where the quorum and voting requirements gave the hospital an effective veto.[360]

Some medical groups have obtained tax exemption as integral parts of hospitals, especially in academic settings.[361]

Some hospitals share services, such as data processing; warehousing; billing and collections; and laboratory and clinical services.

---

[353] 2 H.L.R. 429 (1993) [a foundation-type IDS affiliated with a tax-exempt parent of a multi-hospital system].

[354] *Entity operating physician clinic gets tax exemption in third IDS ruling*, 3 H.L.R. 55 (1994); J. Johnsson, *Montana foundation 1st to test new IRS safe harbor*, AM. MED. NEWS, Feb. 7, 1994, 6 [a direct employment model IDS affiliated with a hospital].

[355] 3 H.L.R. 498 (1994) [a direct employment model IDS affiliated with a hospital].

[356] *IRS issues landmark determinations on creation of regional health network*, 2 H.L.R. 1191 (1993) [Sept. 1, 1993, letter to Northwestern Healthcare Network, Chicago granting tax exemption to superparent as integral part, an unusual example of double derivative exempt status].

[357] J. Somerville, *California foundation calling it quits*, AM. MED. NEWS, Sept. 26, 1994, 3.

[358] *IRS official outlines factors that help determine tax-exempt status of systems*, 3 H.L.R. 1550 (1994); more detailed essays concerning the requirements appear in the IRS EXEMPT ORGANIZATION CONTINUING PROFESSIONAL EDUCATION TECHNICAL INSTRUCTION PROGRAM textbooks for 1994, 1995.

[359] *IRS official clarifies agency view on PHO board representation conditions*, 4 H.L.R. 151 (1995) [for-profit PHOs not subject to 20 percent physician-representation limit, with up to 50 percent control probably acceptable if proportional to their investment].

[360] IRS Determination Letter to University Affiliated Health Care, Inc., Feb. 17, 1995, *as discussed in* 23 HEALTH L. DIG. (May 1995), at 79 [approval of § 501(c)(3) exemption for PHO with 11 directors, two from hospital, four from nonprofit group practice associations, five from employed physicians, where quorum and voting requirements gave hospital an effective veto].

[361] *E.g.*, University of Mass. Med. School Group Practice v. C.I.R., 74 T.C. 1299 (1980), *acq.* 1980-2 C.B. 2; B.H.W. Anesthesia Found., Inc. v. C.I.R. 72 T.C. 681 (1979), *nonacq.*, 1980-2 C.B. 2.

The sharing of some services has been facilitated by section 501(e) of the Internal Revenue Code,[362] which permits the formation of tax-exempt organizations to provide some services to several hospitals. Only the services listed in section 501(e) are entitled to exemption under the section; so it is not helpful for other services, such as shared laundry services, that are not listed.[363]

Government Entities. Some governmental hospitals are tax exempt under Section 115 of the Internal Revenue Code[364] on the basis of being an instrumentality of the state, rather than under section 501(c)(3).

Discussion Points

1. Discuss the efforts to change institutional practices concerning charges to the uninsured.
2. What is the difference between Medicare and Medicaid? What is the difference between the four parts of Medicare (A, B, C, and D)?
3. Discuss the efforts by states to control the growth of Medicaid expenditures.
4. Discuss the scope of preemption by ERISA.
5. Pick a payment plan and discuss the allocation of risk of excessive demand and nonpayment among providers, insurers, and premium payers.
6. When may providers seek to collect outstanding bills directly from health insurance plans?
7. When may providers seek to collect outstanding bills directly from patients, their families, or guarantors?
8. What legal constraints are there on collection efforts?
9. What are legal issues involved in tax-exempt bond financing?
10. Discuss the uses of taxes on health care services.
11. Discuss the challenges to hospital property tax exemption.
12. What must a provider do to qualify for federal tax exemption under § 501(c)(3)?
13. What is an excessive benefit transaction, and what are the consequences?
14. What is private inurement?

---

[362] 26 U.S.C. § 501(e).
[363] HCSC-Laundry v. United States, 450 U.S. 1 (1981) [statutory list is exclusive, laundry not exempt]; *see also* IRS Tech. Adv. Memo 9822004 (Nov. 10, 1997); *IRS revokes long-standing tax exemption to organization that serves rural hospitals*, 7 H.L.R. 920 (1998) [did not provide hospital services, management services not charitable].
[364] 26 U.S.C. § 115.

CHAPTER TEN

Third-party Health Care Coverage

Objectives

The objective of this chapter is to provide an overview of how third-party coverage is structured. The reader will learn some ways plans determine who is covered; manage utilization; handle appeals from adverse utilization determinations; and are held liable for the consequences of plan decisions.

Third-party coverage of health care benefits is structured in a wide variety of ways. Most third-party coverage has some elements of managed care. All third-party coverage places some limits on the scope of coverage. This chapter discusses some of the aspects of the structuring of third-party coverage. The following questions are addressed:

10-1. Who is covered by the plan?
10-2. How is utilization managed?
10-3. What are the appeal rights from adverse utilization determinations?
10-4. When can third-party payers be liable for the consequences of their decisions?

10-1 Who Is Covered by the Plan?

QUALIFICATION FOR COVERAGE. Most plans are open only to certain qualified persons. Government plans are usually open only to persons who are qualified by age, condition, government employment, indigency, or other criteria. Employer plans are generally open only to employees. There are private group plans that are open only to members of the sponsoring organization. Some insurance carriers cover association plans that are open to association members, and usually eligibility for association membership is limited to those in specified professions or other occupations.

In 2004, California mandated that employers with fifty or more workers either provide health care coverage or contribute toward a state plan.[1] However, there was a vote on a challenge to the requirement on the November 2004 ballot, and the plan was defeated by a 51 percent to 49 percent vote.[2]

Many employer plans and other private group plans offer family coverage that cover qualified dependents of the primary member. Some plans have discontinued family coverage.[3] When family coverage is offered, it is usually limited to spouses, minor dependents, dependent students below a specified age and/or disabled dependents.[4] Under single person policies, babies are sometimes not automatically covered.[5] State law often requires automatic coverage of newborns, but such requirements do not apply to ERISA plans due to preemption.

Loss of employment generally results in loss of coverage by the employer's health plan, subject only to the Consolidated Omnibus Budget Reconciliation Right Act (COBRA) continuation rights.[6] Similarly, covered dependents have COBRA continuation rights. This includes the ex-spouse after a divorce. In 2002, a federal appellate court addressed a case in which the divorce decree required the husband to purchase COBRA coverage for the wife. He failed to do so and instead misrepresented to the plan that she was still his wife. When the plan discovered this, it sued him for common law fraud.

---

1   CAL. LAB. CODE §§ 2120 et seq.; *Calif. employer mandate becomes law,* AM. MED. NEWS, Oct. 20, 2003, 9.

2   V. Colliver, *Proposition 72; Health cost issue won't fade away,* SAN FRANCISCO CHRONICLE, Nov. 4, 2004, C1; *see also* Zaremberg v. Superior Court, 115 Cal. App. 4th 111, 8 Cal. Rptr. 3d 723 (1st Dist. 2004) [unsuccessful attempt to block vote].

3   *See* V. Fuhrmans, *Company health plans try to drop spouses,* WALL ST. J., Sept. 9, 2003, D1; J. Peter, *Budget language appears to eliminate family health coverage for state employees,* AP, Mar. 6, 2003 [MA budget proposal].

4   *E.g.,* Ramsey v. Colonial Life Ins. Co., 12 F.3d 472 (5th Cir. 1994).

5   *E.g.,* Gilley v. Protective Life Ins. Co., 17 F.3d 775 (5th Cir. 1994) [insured under single person policy sought coverage of baby, but under policy no coverage until day baby released from hospital].

6   29 U.S.C. §§ 1161-1168; Branch v. G. Bernd Co., 955 F.2d 1574 (11th Cir. 1992) [election of COBRA coverage retroactively covers intervening care].

The court affirmed a judgment against the ex-husband for over $100,000 for the amount that had been paid for the wife's treatment.[7]

Some employer plans are also open to retired persons. Some plans have reduced coverage for retirees.[8] In 2004, the Equal Employment Opportunity Commission (EEOC) issued a preliminary ruling that employers were permitted to cut benefits when retirees qualified for Medicare, and this did not constitute age discrimination. In 2005, a federal court struck down the rule as a violation of the Age Discrimination in Employment Act.[9]

There are some public and private plans that are open to a broader range of individuals.[10] These policies must be structured or priced to deal with the risk of having a disproportionate enrollment of persons with higher costs.[11] To avoid higher prices, these policies generally exclude coverage for illnesses that exist at the time of enrollment. Some states have legislated open enrollment periods, during which time Managed Care Organizations (MCOs) must accept individual applicants for coverage regardless of their health status.[12]

Some states have programs that offer insurance to high risk persons who cannot be covered by the private insurance market. However, unless the programs are subsidized, the cost to enrollees can be prohibitive.[13]

Any sponsor or individual seeking coverage needs to assess the plan to determine whether it can deliver what it states. There are many fraudulent health plans that fail to provide coverage.[14]

---

[7] Trustees of Aftra Health Fund v. Biondi, 303 F.3d 765 (7th Cir. 2002).

[8] M. Freudenheim, *Companies limit health coverage of many retirees*, N.Y. TIMES, Feb. 3, 2004, A1.

[9] AARP v. EEOC, 2005 U.S. Dist. LEXIS 5078 (E.D. Pa.); R. Pear, *Agency to allow insurance cuts for the retired*, N.Y. TIMES, Apr. 23, 2004, A1.

[10] *E.g.*, R. Imrie, *Doyle signs bill to help farmers, others buy health insurance*, AP, Dec. 12, 2003 [Wis. law creates five regional health insurance purchasing cooperatives for farmers, small businesses, and self-employed workers]; *Humana introduces health coverage for individuals*, PR NEWSWIRE, June 11, 2002; S. Jordan, *Mutual ending its individual health policies: Citing rising costs and more rules, the Omaha-based insurer will drop coverage for 50,000 people this year*, OMAHA WORLD-HERALD, Feb. 13, 2002, 1d.

[11] *See* T. Lieberman, *Individual insurance: a game of risk*, L.A. Times, Sept. 15, 2003, pt. 6, 3.

[12] *E.g.*, ARK. STAT. ANN. § 23-76-115; COLO. REV. STAT. § 10-16-408; IDAHO CODE § 41-3919; MINN. STAT. § 62D.10 (1996); OHIO REV. CODE ANN. § 1742.12.

[13] *See Insurance program for high-risk patients facing money woes*, AP, Feb. 22, 2002 [IND.]; *State's high risk health insurance sees premium increase*, AP, Sept. 29, 2003 [29 percent in Neb.]; J.B. Finkelstein, *State high-risk pools fail to deliver affordable premiums*, AM. MED. NEWS, Sept. 15, 2003, 7.

[14] *See* R. Pear, *Inquiry finds sharp increase in health insurance schemes*, N.Y. TIMES, Mar. 3, 2004, A12 [GAO report]; *Report finds increase in illegal health insurance plans alarming*, BEST WIRE, Aug. 28, 2003 [Commonwealth Fund report — four plans left nearly 100,000 people with $85 million in unpaid bills]; C. Windham, *Bogus health insurance is growing*, WALL ST. J., Aug. 28, 2003, D15.

ENROLLMENT. In most plans, qualified persons are not automatically covered. They generally must enroll in the plan to be covered.

DISENROLLMENT. Some payment denials are based on a determination that the individual is not covered by the plan, without ever reaching the issue of whether the individual's condition or the proposed services are covered. Some misrepresentations by the insured on the application form can void all coverage.[15] Loss of employment or dependency status generally results in loss of coverage by the employer's health plan, subject only to COBRA continuation rights discussed previously. When the employer changes insurance carriers, the old plan no longer covers the employees.[16]

10-2 How Is Utilization Managed?

All managed care organizations and many other third-party payers use techniques to manage utilization and discourage the provision of medical care deemed to be "unnecessary" or "inappropriate."

Until the late 1990s, the primary focus of utilization management was on influencing physician behavior through techniques such as capitation, gatekeepers, selective contracting, and utilization review. There was an intense public and resulting political backlash against the impact of many of these techniques. The primary focus shifted to techniques aimed at influencing patient behavior, such as benefit design, variable copayments and coinsurance, and incentives to manage their own care with the support of medical and disease management programs.[17] However, when expenditures began to rise again, some of the older physician-focused efforts began to be selectively reestablished in some markets.[18]

It is expected that there will continue to be efforts to control utilization in an effort to keep the costs of health plans within the reach

---

[15] *E.g.*, Time Ins. Co. v. Bishop, 245 Va. 48, 425 S.E.2d 489 (1993).

[16] *E.g.*, Decatur Mem. Hosp. v. Connecticut Gen. Life Ins. Co., 990 F.2d 925 (7th Cir. 1993).

[17] *See* J.C. Robinson, *Reinvention of health insurance in the consumer era*, J.A.M.A., Apr. 21, 2004, 1880.

[18] *See* G. Mays, G. Claxton & J. White, *MarketWatch: Managed care rebound? Recent changes in health plans' cost containment strategies*, HEALTH AFFAIRS, Aug. 11, 2004 [http://content.healthaffairs.org/cgi/content/full/hlthaff.w4.427/DC1;accessed Sept. 1, 2004; reintroduced prior authorization for selected services and although seldom denied, discourages requests; concurrent review of hospital stays; retrospective review of practice patterns with profiling; no gatekeepers; disease and case management; tiered provider networks; incentive-based provider payments based on measures of quality and efficiency; no return of capitation; increasing consumer cost-sharing requirements].

of the employers and individuals. Accounting rule changes in mid-2004 require businesses to more precisely account for the future costs of health care commitments.[19] This will put more pressure on businesses to find ways creditably to contain their future commitments.

This section examines some of the older and newer techniques and some related issues, including copayments, coinsurance, and/or deductibles (10-2.1); permitted providers (10-2.2); access to permitted providers, including preauthorization requirements (10-2.3); provider incentives (10-2.4); coverage exclusions and mandates (10-2.5); and case or disease management (10-2.6). Perceived abuses in the area of utilization control have resulted in legislation in many states that increase access to providers (10-2.2 and 10-2.3) and mandate some coverage (10-2.5). Care must be taken in communicating denials of coverage to individuals (10-2.7). Some managed care organizations attempt to reduce utilization by promoting healthy behaviors (10-2.8).

10-2.1 Copayments, Coinsurance, and Deductibles

Most non-HMO health plans involve copayments, coinsurance, or deductibles, which providers almost always have the responsibility to collect. Many HMO plans now require copayments. A *copayment* is a fixed portion of each bill that the patient must pay. For example, the patient might have to pay $10 for each office visit to a doctor or the first $10 of every prescription. *Coinsurance* is the payment of a percentage of each bill. For example, the patient would have to pay 20 percent of every hospital bill, with the plan paying the balance. A *deductible* is the amount that the patient must pay before the plan pays anything. For example, the patient might have to pay $200 in covered medical bills before the plan starts paying any of the bills. Sometimes the deductible does not have to be met before the plan starts paying for some services, typically doctor's visits. Usually, the copayments and coinsurance do not count toward the deductible.

Copayments, coinsurance, and deductibles accomplish at least two purposes. First, these payments reduce the cost of insurance or at least the growth in the cost of the insurance so that in theory more employers and individuals can afford to have insurance.[20] Second,

---

[19] R. Pear, *Rules to expose long-term cost of health plans*, N.Y. TIMES, June 21, 2004, A1.

[20] *See* S. Greenhouse, *Deal saves city $100 million a year in health costs*, N.Y. TIMES, Dec. 19, 2003, B1 [New York City labor deal involving higher copayments].

these payments make users more cost conscious so that they control their own utilization.[21] There is a concern that the payments may deter some persons from seeking some needed services. There has been some employee resistance to introducing or increasing copayments, coinsurance, deductibles, or the employee portion of the health insurance premium.[22]

The biggest legal problem with coinsurance has been that some payers have said that the coinsurance was a certain percentage and then have calculated the amount based on full charges of the provider, not based on the discounted payments the provider contracted with the payer to accept. Thus, the payer pays a smaller percent of the total actual payment. These practices have been challenged as overcharges by the payers. After focusing on the plan documents in each case, courts have found the practice permitted by some plan documents and not permitted by others.[23] Plans have settled some of the cases.[24] In 1999, the United States Supreme Court ruled that beneficiaries in Nevada could go forward with a suit against an insurance company that allegedly misrepresented to its insured its methods of applying discounts received from a hospital.[25] The beneficiaries alleged that the insurance company had violated the Racketeer Influenced and Corrupt Organizations (RICO) Act through a pattern of illegal activities that included mail, wire, radio, and television fraud.

Many insurers have returned to basing coinsurance on a usual and customary schedule of charges rather than the contracted rate. As long as this is properly disclosed to the insured persons, the lia-

---

[21] *See* D.E. Rosenbaum, *Do some pay too little for health care?* N.Y. Times, Oct. 26, 2003, 3WK [impact of insurance on utilization, making workers more cost conscious]; L. Landro, *Consumer responsibility rises with costs*, Wall St. J., May 8, 2003, D3 [pressure on consumers to curb heath spending].

[22] *See* R. Kaiser & D. Alexander, *Health care No. 1 cause of labor strife*, Chicago Trib., Oct. 12, 2003, § 1, 14.

[23] *E.g.*, Hoover v. Blue Cross & Blue Shield of Alabama, 855 F.2d 1538 (11th Cir. 1988) [practice permitted]; McConocha v. Blue Cross & Blue Shield of Ohio, 898 F. Supp. 545, 551 (N.D. Ohio 1995) [breach of fiduciary duty not to disclose practice]; *see also* Alves v. Harvard Pilgrim Health Care, Inc., 204 F. Supp. 2d 198 (D. Mass. 2002) [permissible for copayment to exceed actual cost to plan].

[24] *E.g.*, Rosen v. Blue Cross, No. C93-843 Z (W.D. Wash. Apr. 28, 1994), *as discussed in* 3 H.L.R. 601 (1994) [settlement of suit alleging insurer did not pass on savings from rates negotiated with providers in calculating copayments]; *In re* Humana Health Ins. Co. of Florida (D.O.I Case No. 92-L-013JEH, order to show cause filed 1/10/92; Dept. of Legal Affairs Investigative Case No. 92-H-14-91), *as discussed in* 3 H.L.R. 764 (1994) [$6.25 million settlement of overcharges to patients treated at Humana hospitals due to copayments being calculated based on gross, not net, hospital bill].

[25] Humana Inc. v. Forsyth, 525 U.S. 299 (1999).

bility described can be avoided. It is prudent for hospitals to avoid agreeing to collect coinsurance based on full charges unless the plan has disclosed this arrangement clearly to the insured.

Some providers waive some copayments, coinsurance, and deductibles. This is appropriate in some cases, especially when based on financial need. It is especially problematic for elective services because it defeats the goal of promoting cost consciousness in seeking health care services. Some states prohibit providers from waiving copayments, coinsurance, and deductibles.[26] Medicare policy is discussed in Chapter 9.

10-2.2 Permitted Providers

One approach to managing care has been to control access to providers by limiting which providers can be used. Many managed care organizations use a closed panel of providers and authorize going outside the panel only when covered services are needed that cannot be provided by the panel. In a 1997 case, a federal appeals court held that insured persons have no right under ERISA to services of a specific physician.[27] Thus, the insured must look to state law for any rights to gain access to specific providers.

Plans give several reasons for limiting care to a panel. For example, a panel is more efficient to administer; it easier to track a smaller number of providers to assure that plan standards are being met. There is a wide range of practice styles among physicians;[28] a plan that uses more efficient providers can be more cost competitive. As plans are being held liable for the actions of providers, they need to be more selective in which providers they use to minimize their liability exposure. Plans are often able to negotiate better prices due to the number of their patients who will be using the provider or who will not be using the provider if the contract is awarded to another provider.[29]

---

[26] *E.g.*, Parrish v. Lamm, 758 P.2d 1356 (Colo. 1988) [upholding law]; Annotation, *Validity of state statute prohibiting health providers from the practice of waiving patient's obligation to pay health insurance deductibles or copayments, or advertising such practice*, 8 A.L.R. 5th 855.

[27] Maltz v. Aetna Health Plans of N.Y., 114 F.3d 9 (2nd Cir. 1997).

[28] *See* Editorial, *Health care's weird geography*, N.Y. Times, Oct. 25, 1997, A18 [Wennberg's Dartmouth studies of regional variations]; S. Gilbert, *Discrepancy in cataract surgery*, N.Y. Times, June 11, 1997, B10 [different rates of use].

[29] *See Pension fund drops hospitals from plan*, N.Y. Times, May 20, 2004, C5 [California public employee program (CalPERS) dropped 38 hospitals].

TIERED NETWORKS. Some plans classify participating providers into tiers by their performance on various cost and quality measures. When patients select providers who are designated as better performers by the plan, the patient is charged a smaller copayment or is given other financial incentives. The specific cost and quality measures remain controversial.[30]

ANY WILLING PROVIDER LAWS. Some states have responded to the concerns about provider access to patients and patient access to providers by passing "any willing provider" laws. These laws require MCOs to offer contracts to any provider willing to meet their criteria.[31] MCOs and purchasers of their services have expressed concern that this destroys the ability to offer less expensive coverage by selecting a small panel of efficient providers that can be efficiently monitored. Providers excluded from the panels and some consumer groups have expressed concern about the loss of continuity of care when patient-provider relationships are disrupted when patients are limited to a small panel.

In 2003, the United States Supreme Court ruled that ERISA does not preempt state any willing provider laws because the laws regulate insurance.[32] Even when any willing provider laws apply, providers who refuse to accept the economic terms offered by the plan are not "willing" and have no right to demand participation on their own terms.[33] Some courts strictly construe state any willing provider laws to apply only to the types of providers expressly listed in the law. In 2000, a Tennessee appellate court ruled that a provider of human infusion therapy was not included.[34] Any willing provider laws can still be challenged on other grounds.[35]

---

[30] *See* J. Freed, *Insurers try a new way to steer patients toward favored docs*, AP. May 20, 2005; R. Kazel, *Tiered physician networks pit organized medicine vs. United*, AM. MED. NEWS, Mar. 7, 2005, 1.

[31] *See* A.L. Jiranek & S.D. Baker, *Any willing provider laws: Regulating the health care provider's contractual relationship with the insurance company*, 7 THE HEALTH LAWYER (Wint. 1994-95), at 1.

[32] Kentucky Ass'n of Health Plans, Inc. v. Miller, 538 U.S. 329 (2003).

[33] *E.g.*, Blue Cross & Blue Shield v. St. Mary's Hosp., 245 Va. 24, 426 S.E.2d 117 (1993); HCA Health Servs. of Va., Inc. v. Aetna Life Ins. Co., No. 92-574-A (E.D. Va. June 16, 1994), *as discussed in* 3 H.L.R. 143 (1994) [hospital exclusion from PPO resulted from unsuccessful good faith negotiations, did not violate any willing provider law].

[34] Reeves-Sain Med., Inc. v. Blue Cross Blue Shield of Tenn., 40 S.W.3d 503 (Tenn. App. 2000).

[35] *E.g.*, Prudential Ins. Co. v. National Park Med. Ctrs., 2004 U.S. Dist. LEXIS 2906 (E.D. Ark.); *State's 'any willing provider' law on hold again by federal district court*, H.L.R., Mar. 18, 2004, 392 [stay pending appeal issued Mar. 10, 2004)]; J. Jefferson, *Arkansas Senate passes new version of any-willing-provider law*, AP, Feb. 8, 2005 [injunction still in effect].

In 2005, an HMO's agreement with a pharmacy benefit manager (PBM) was challenged by a community pharmacy. A federal district court held that the agreement overcompensated the PBM to the detriment of other pharmacies participating in the network and that this violated the any willing provider law since they were not offered the same arrangement.[36]

POINT-OF-SERVICE OPTION. Some states have mandated that a *point-of-service* (POS) option be available to enrollees in MCOs.[37] Under a POS option, the covered person may elect to receive services from a nonparticipating provider, usually at a higher cost to the covered. POS plans are becoming more popular, especially with employers who have employees residing outside the service area of the provider networks available in traditional HMO plans.

DESELECTED PROVIDERS. When a provider ceases to be included in a MCO (sometimes called *deselection*), the continuing care of his or her patients may become an issue. This concern was first raised with regard to pregnant patients. It has been recognized to include many other types of patients, including those with life-threatening conditions. In response, a number of states have enacted laws mandating coverage of continuing care for a specified period of time (generally 60 to 120 days) for certain types of patients when a provider leaves a health plan.[38] In general, the patients covered under these statutes are those who are pregnant, have a life-threatening condition, or are under active treatment for a particular illness or injury. Some states also require coverage of continued access to primary physicians for the duration of the plan year.

Another avenue of attack on the deselection of provider has been challenges by the deselected providers. California and New Jersey, which tend to give physicians more procedural protections in other contexts than most states, have found a right to a fair hearing before a physician can be dropped from a MCO. In 2000, the California Supreme Court ruled that a MCOs could not enforce its contractual provision for termination without cause; physicians were entitled to common law fair procedure that could not be

---

[36] J.E. Pierce Apothecary, Inc. v. Harvard Pilgrim Health Care, Inc., 365 F. Supp. 2d 119 (D. Mass. 2005).

[37] *E.g.*, GA. CODE § 33-21-29; IDAHO CODE title 41, ch. 39; MD. CODE ANN. § 19-710.2; MONT. CODE ANN. § 33-31-102; 1997 N.J. LAWS ch. 192; 1995 N.Y. ALS § 504.

[38] *E.g.*, 1997 ARK. ACTS 1196; 1997 COLO. SESS. LAWS ch. 238; 1997 MINN. LAWS 237; N.J. ADMIN. CODE § 8:38; 1994 VA. ACTS ch. 851.

waived.[39] In 1997, a federal court found that New Jersey would grant seven psychologists who had been dropped from a network without cause the right to pursue their claims that the termination violated state public policy and fundamental fairness.[40] Some other courts have found that providers with no-cause termination contracts may still have rights. In 1996, the New Hampshire Supreme Court ruled the common law implied a covenant of good faith and fair dealing that applied to deselection, so that the MCO could not terminate without cause, entitling the provider to review of the termination decision.[41] In addition, in some cases deselected physicians have obtained reinstatement in settlement of their claims.[42]

Other courts have refused to override contracts permitting termination without cause. In 1994, a federal court dismissed a suit by five deselected physicians against a MCO. In 1996, a federal appellate court upheld the decision.[43]

Some states have enacted legislation requiring written notification when a provider is terminated or not renewed.[44] Some states have statutes requiring a hearing in some circumstances.[45]

The tendency toward restricting the ability of plans to control who is providing services appears to be in conflict with the expanding liability being imposed on plans for the actions of providers discussed later in this chapter.

---

[39] Potvin v. Metropolitan Life Ins. Co., 22 Cal. 4th 1060, 997 P.2d 1153, 95 Cal. Rptr. 2d 496 (2000).

[40] New Jersey Psychological Ass'n v. MCC Behavioral Care Inc., 1997 U.S. Dist. LEXIS 16338 (D. N.J.).

[41] Harper v. Healthsource New Hampshire, Inc., 674 A.2d 962 (N.H. 1996).

[42] *E.g.*, Napoletano v. CIGNA Healthcare, No. 94-0705-357 (Conn. Super. Ct. 1998), *as discussed in* 7 H.L.R. 1365 (1998) [agreement to reinstate nine deselected physicians in settlement of lawsuit]; Napoletano v. Cigna Healthcare, 238 Conn. 216, 680 A.2d 127 (1996), *cert. denied*, 520 U.S. 1103 (1997) [beneficiary-plaintiffs had reasonable expectation that, as long as their physicians continued to meet credentialing criteria and did not meet other reasons for discharge, they would continue to be providers at least for remainder of one-year provider contracts; no preemption].

[43] Texas Med. Ass'n v. Aetna Life Ins. Co., No. 94-0288 (S.D. Tex. Aug. 24. 1994), *aff'd*, 80 F.3d 153 (5th Cir. 1996); *see also* Grossman v. Columbine Med. Group, 12 P.3d 269 (Colo. App. 1999) [rejecting claims that a doctor's termination without cause from an independent practice association is against public policy].

[44] *E.g.*, Cal. Health & Safety Code § 1373.65; Conn. Gen. Stat. § 38a-478(h); Mo. Rev. Stat. § 354.609(2); Tex. Ins. Code art. 3.70-3C; *see* Lewis v. Individual Practice Ass'n of Western N.Y., Inc., 187 Misc. 2d 812, 723 N.Y.S.2d 845 (Sup. Ct. 2001) [applying N.Y. statute]; L.C. Fentiman, *Patient advocacy and termination from managed care organizations. Do state laws protecting health care professional advocacy make any difference?* 82 Neb. L. Rev. 508 (2003).

[45] *E.g.*, N.Y. Pub. Health Law § 4406-d(2).

10-2.3 Access to Permitted Providers

In the past, many MCOs required prior approval before patients could access some permitted providers. This approval had to be obtained from an assigned primary care provider (often called a gatekeeper) or from a central approval authority, depending on the nature of the service being authorized. This technique has become less common, although it is being reintroduced on a more focused basis for selected services.

GATEKEEPER. Some MCOs require that patients be assigned to a primary care physician (PCP) and allow access to medical specialists only with approval and referral by the PCP. Critics of such requirements claim that the PCP system raises unreasonable obstacles to obtaining specialty care. A few states have responded by passing statutes requiring direct access to specialists or allowing specialists to be designated a PCP.[46] In particular, direct access to obstetricians/gynecologists has been the subject of considerable state legislative activity.[47]

Many MCOs have abandoned or relaxed these gatekeeper requirements to make their products more attractive in competitive markets.[48]

PRIOR APPROVAL. Some MCOs pay for hospitalization and certain procedures only if prior approval is obtained from the plan. These prior approval requirements have generally been upheld.[49] Many plans have reduced the scope of services that require prior approval, but there is some indication that the requirement may be returning for some high cost services. In 2004, one plan announced that it was going to require justification for nonemergency advanced imaging tests.[50]

CONFIRMATION OF COVERAGE. It is prudent to obtain confirmation of coverage and necessary approvals before nonemergency care is provided. In emergencies, federal law forbids providers from delaying medical screening or emergency treatment to make inquiries concerning insurance coverage.[51] However, these restrictions do not

---

[46] *E.g.*, ARK. CODE ANN. § 23-99-301-305; KY. REV. STAT. § 304.17A; MONT. CODE ANN. § 39-71-116; N.J. ADMIN. CODE § 8:38-6.2.

[47] *E.g.*, ALA. ACT § 671; 1997 ARK. ACTS § 1196; CAL. HEALTH & SAFETY CODE §§ 1367.69, 1367.695; CONN. ACTS § 95-199; FLA. STAT. §§ 409.9122, 641.19, 408.701; GA. CODE ANN. § 33-24-58; IDAHO CODE title 41, § 3915; 215 ILL. COMP. STAT. § 5/356r; IND. CODE § 27-8-24.7; MINN. STAT. ch. 62Q.52; UTAH CODE ANN. § 31A-22-623.

[48] *See* R. Kazel, *Managed care easing gatekeeper hassles*, AM. MED. NEWS, Jan. 20, 2003; R. Winslow, *Oxford to give more control to specialists*, WALL ST. J., Mar. 25, 1997, B1.

[49] *E.g.*, City of Hope Nat'l Med. Ctr. v. HealthPlus, Inc., 156 F.3d 223 (1st Cir. 1998).

[50] *Insurer will require doctors to justify imaging tests*, AP, Feb. 27, 2004.

[51] 42 U.S.C. § 1395dd(h).

apply to plans. Several states have adopted laws to make it more difficult for MCOs to avoid paying for emergency care.[52] Plans may be
liable for refusing to provide confirmation of coverage.[53]

EFFECT OF CONFIRMATION OF COVERAGE. Courts have disagreed on whether a MCO or other third-party payer is bound by a
confirmation of coverage. Some courts hold that oral representations
cannot vary the terms of the plan.[54] One federal appellate court
upheld a HMO's denial of heart transplant coverage even though (1)
the patient had joined the HMO only after obtaining oral confirmation of coverage and (2) the denial was not made until after the procedure had been performed.[55] Other courts hold that insurers
cannot refuse to pay for services after verifying coverage.[56] The
Florida Supreme Court ruled that an insurer can be stopped from
denying coverage after confirming coverage if (1) there is detrimental reliance on the confirmation and (2) refusal to enforce coverage
would sanction fraud or other injustice.[57] The detrimental reliance
requirement can mean that the hospital would have to show it would
not have admitted the patient or given the service if there had been
no confirmation. In states that enforce coverage confirmations, careful documentation of what was confirmed is necessary.[58] If the
insurer merely confirmed that the group existed or that the patient
was a member of the group, the insurer may not necessarily have
confirmed that a particular procedure was covered.

One federal court went a step further. The plan gave preadmission certification subject to review for preexisting conditions. The

---

[52] *See* L. Page, *Emergency physicians protest HMO denials of payment*, AM. MED. NEWS,
June 15/22, 1998, 16 [Md. had first prudent lay person law in 1993, complaint with insurance
department of continued noncompliance].

[53] *E.g.*, Mimbs v. Commercial Life Ins. Co., 832 F. Supp. 354 (S.D. Ga. 1993) [deny dismissal of
claim that insurer breached its duty by refusing to confirm coverage, so patient delayed
opportunity for cardiac bypass surgery].

[54] *E.g.*, Healthsouth Rehab. Hosp. v. American Nat'l Red Cross, 101 F.3d 1005 (4th Cir. 1996); *see
also* Charter Canyon Treatment Ctr. v. Pool Co., 153 F.3d 1132 (10th Cir. 1998) [employer may
retrospectively review precertified hospitalization, decline payment when plan so provides].

[55] Inman v. HMO Colo., Inc., No. 88-1625 (10th Cir. Jan. 3, 1989), *as discussed in* 17 HEALTH L.
DIG. (Mar. 1989), at 13.

[56] *E.g.*, St. Joseph's Hosp. v. Reserve Life Ins. Co., 154 Ariz. 307, 742 P.2d 808 (1987); *accord*
Hermann Hosp. v. National Standard Ins. Co., 776 S.W.2d 249 (Tex. Ct. App. 1989); Cypress
Fairbanks Med. Ctr. v. Pan American Life Ins. Co., 110 F.3d 280 (5th Cir. 1997), *cert. denied*,
522 U.S. 862 (1997) [hospital provided services based on insurer confirmation of plan coverage; may sue insurer for negligent misrepresentation of coverage, deceptive and unfair trade
practices].

[57] Crown Life Ins. Co. v. McBride, 517 So. 2d 660 (Fla. 1987).

[58] *E.g.*, Thomas v. Gulf Health Plan, Inc., 688 F. Supp. 590 (S.D. Ala. 1988) [precertification of
bone marrow harvesting did not stop denial of coverage for high dose chemotherapy with
bone marrow transplantation].

court ruled that the plan could not later deny coverage on the basis of a preexisting condition that it could have determined from medical records available when the initial certification was given.[59]

State law requirements that plans abide by coverage confirmations are generally preempted by ERISA. In the past, some federal courts found exceptions,[60] but most recent cases have confirmed preemption.[61]

EFFECT OF PROVIDER ASSURANCES TO PATIENTS. Providers should avoid assuring patients that procedures are covered by insurance unless they are willing to forgo payment if the insurer does not pay. A Georgia appellate court case arose when a physician tried to collect a bill after an insurer refused to pay.[62] The patient claimed the physician had stated the procedure would be covered by insurance and refused to pay. The patient had signed a document promising to pay if the insurer did not. The court decided that the patient had to pay, not because of the document, but because the patient had conducted an investigation of the insurance coverage so there was no reliance on the physician's statements.

10-2.4 Provider Incentives

Some MCOs include provisions in their contracts with health care providers that, directly or indirectly, reward a provider for controlling utilization through, for example, bonuses or increased net revenues shared by the provider. Capitated payments inherently contain an incentive for decreasing utilization because provider reimbursement is based on the number of enrollees, rather than the volume or type of services provided. Concern that such incentives might influence providers to limit necessary services has led a number of states to enact legislation regulating such financial incentives.[63]

Most federal appellate courts that have addressed the issue have concluded that MCOs do not have a duty to disclose these incentives

---

[59] McDaniel v. Blue Cross & Blue Shield, 780 F. Supp. 1363 (S.D. Ala. 1991), *aff'd*, 977 F.2d 599 (11th Cir. 1992).

[60] *E.g*, Lordmann Enters., Inc. v. Equicor, Inc., 32 F.3d 1529 (11th Cir. 1994); The Meadows v. Employers Health Ins. Co., 47 F.3d 1006 (9th Cir. 1995); Cypress Fairbanks Med. Ctr. Inc. v. Pan-American Life Ins. Co., 110 F.3d 280 (5th Cir.1997), *cert. denied*, 522 U.S. 862 (1997).

[61] *E.g.*, Cicio v. Doe, 321 F.3d 83 (2d Cir. 2003); Griggs v. E.I. DuPont de Nemours & Co., 237 F.3d 371, 378 (4th Cir. 2001); Carlo v. Reed Rolled Thread Die Co., 49 F.3d 790 (1st Cir. 1995).

[62] Lozier v. Leonard, 173 Ga. App. 697, 327 S.E.2d 815 (1985).

[63] CAL. HEALTH & SAFETY CODE § 1348.6; ME. REV. STAT. ANN. title 24-A, 4303 (3-B); N.H. REV. STAT. ANN. § 420-J: 8; *State laws banning physician financial incentives*, 7 H.L.R. 1625 (1998).

to patients.[64] However, in 1997, one federal appellate court did a find a duty to disclose in the circumstances of the case.[65]

In 1997, a federal court in Virginia ruled that ERISA preempts state law challenges to HMO financial incentives for physicians to limit care.[66] However, in a Texas case, the state and individual physicians attacked the incentive features of a plan. In a series of settlements during 1997 and 1998, the plan first agreed to disclose its incentives, then removed the disputed incentive features, and made payments to the physicians for the income lost while the incentives were in place.[67]

In 1996, the Health Care Financing Administration issued final regulations concerning physician financial incentives, including requirements that MCOs must disclose in general incentives used by the MCO itself and its subcontractors to any Medicare beneficiary or Medicaid recipient upon request.[68]

10-2.5 Coverage Exclusions and Mandates

Insurance coverage for individual services is denied on a wide variety of grounds. After reviewing possible Americans with Disabilities Act (ADA) constraints on variations in coverage, this section surveys some of those grounds and related issues.

AMERICANS WITH DISABILITIES ACT (ADA). In structuring or changing the structure of plans, nondiscrimination laws need to be considered. Several plans tried to limit their coverage of care for HIV-positive patients by capping benefits. It was first determined that this did not violate ERISA, which gives employers great latitude in changing benefit plans.[69] However, it was then found to vio-

---

[64] *E.g.,* Horvath v. Keystone Health East, Inc., 333 F.3d 450 (3d Cir. 2003); Ehlmann v. Kaiser Found. Health Plan, 198 F.3d 552 (5th Cir. 2000).

[65] Shea v. Esensten, 107 F.3d 625 (8th Cir. 1997), *cert. denied,* 522 U.S. 914 (1997); *see also* Drolet v. Healthsource, Inc., 968 F. Supp. 757 (D. N.H. 1997) [misrepresentation in subscriber agreement breeched duty].

[66] Lancaster v. Kaiser Found. Health Plan, 958 F. Supp. 1137 (E.D. Va. 1997).

[67] *E.g., In re* Harris Methodist Tex. Health Plan, Inc., No. 9702104 (Tex. Dist. Ct. 124th Jud. Dist. settlement Feb. 21, 1997), *as discussed in* 6 H.L.R. 332 (1997) [settlement with state attorney general requires HMO to disclose physician income reduced if they make too many referrals to specialists]; Hubner v. Harris Health Plan, No. 236-169856-97 (Tex. Dist. Ct. 236th Dist. settlement Sept. 26, 1997), *as discussed in* 6 H.L.R. 1533 (1997) [plan agreed to pay physician straight monthly capitation without bonuses or withholds]; (settlement Dec. 12, 1997), *as discussed in* 7 H.L.R. 30 (1998) [HMO to pay doctors despite pharmacy overrun]; (settlement Feb. 9, 1998), *as discussed in* 7 H.L.R. 290 (1998) [confidential settlement concerning incentives].

[68] 61 FED. REG. 69,034 (Dec. 31, 1996).

[69] McGann v. H. & H. Music Co., 946 F.2d 401 (5th Cir. 1991), *cert. denied,* 506 U.S. 981 (1992) [ERISA does not bar employer from reducing AIDS benefits from $1,000,000 to $5,000 where plan allowed changes].

late the federal Americans with Disabilities Act.[70] In 1998, another federal appellate court disagreed and found that the Americans with Disabilities Act did not apply to benefit plans.[71] In that case, an enrollee in an insurance company sued the company over denial of coverage for a heart transplant.

There are two fundamental legal disagreements between the appellate courts that lead to this disagreement. The first disagreement concerns what is a public accommodation. The courts agree that if there is a requirement of no disability discrimination in health plans it must flow from Title III of the ADA that prohibits discrimination in public accommodations. The courts that find that benefit plans are not covered say that a public accommodation must be a physical place,[72] while those that say benefit plans are covered say that a service can be a public accommodation.[73] The second disagreement concerns whether the ADA mandates equality of treatment between persons with different disabilities. Courts that find no such mandate have ruled that it is not a violation of the ADA to provide different coverage for different disabilities.[74]

To the extent not preempted by ERISA, state nondiscrimination laws also need to be observed in structuring plans.[75]

PREEXISTING CONDITION. In some health plans, payment is not made for treatment of conditions that exist at the time the person begins coverage.[76] These exclusions are less common in employer plans in an effort to preserve portability when employers

---

[70] Carparts Distribution Ctr., Inc. v. Automotive Wholesaler's Ass'n, 37 F.3d 12 (1st Cir. 1994).

[71] Lenox v. Healthwise of Ky., 149 F.3d 453 (6th Cir. 1998).

[72] *E.g.*, Parker v. Metropolitan Life Inc., 121 F.3d 1006 (6th Cir. 1997) (en banc), *cert. denied*, 522 U.S. 1084 (1998) [disability plan differences permitted]; Doe v. Mut. of Omaha Ins. Co., 179 F.3d 557 (7th Cir. 1999) (ADA does not regulate content of products or services sold in places of public accommodation); McNeil v. Time Ins. Co., 205 F.3d 179 (5th Cir. 2000) (Title III of ADA prohibits denying disabled the full and equal enjoyment of business's goods and services, not content and type of goods or services), *cert. denied*, 531 U.S. 1191 (2001); Chabner v. United of Omaha Life Ins. Co., 225 F.3d 1042 (9th Cir. 2000) (Title III of ADA does not address terms of policies insurance companies sell).

[73] *E.g.*, Carparts Distribution Ctr., Inc. v. Automotive Wholesalers Ass'n, 37 F.3d 12 (1st Cir. 1994).

[74] *E.g.*, Lenox v. Healthwise of Ky., 149 F.3d 453 (6th Cir. 1998); Krauel v. Iowa Methodist Med. Ctr., 95 F.3d 674 (8th Cir. 1996); McNeil v. Time Ins. Co., 205 F.3d 179 (5th Cir. 2000) (plan that caps benefits for AIDS does not violate Title III of ADA); Doe v. Mutual of Omaha Ins. Co., 179 F.3d 557 (7th Cir. 1999) (same), *cert. denied*, 528 U.S. 1106 (2000); *see also* Modderno v. King, 317 U.S. App. D.C. 255, 82 F.3d 1059 (D.C. Cir. 1996) (plan that caps mental disability benefits does not violate Section 504 of Rehabilitation Act), *cert. denied*, 519 U.S. 1094 (1997).

[75] *E.g.*, Bankers Life & Casualty Co. v. Peterson, 263 Mont. 156, 866 P.2d 241 (1993) [exclusion of normal pregnancy from individual major medical insurance policy violates state sex discrimination law].

[76] *E.g.*, Bullwinkel v. New England Mut. Life Ins. Co., 18 F.3d 429 (7th Cir. 1994); Drury v. Blue Cross/Blue Shield of Missouri, 943 S.W.2d 834 (Mo. Ct. App. 1997).

change plans and employees change jobs. They are more common in individual policies. In some plans, the preexisting condition exclusion ceases to apply if no treatment is required for the preexisting condition during the first year under the plan. State law can forbid preexisting condition exclusions in plans,[77] but such laws generally do not apply to ERISA plans.

HIPAA, which is not preempted by ERISA, limits the period during which a group health plan can deny coverage for a preexisting condition to twelve months (eighteen months for "late enrollees") and further reduces that period by any "creditable coverage" under a previous health plan. HIPAA also defines preexisting condition to include only those conditions treated or diagnosed within six months of enrollment and to exclude pregnancy.

CRIMINAL ACTIVITIES. Some policies exclude coverage for injuries that occur during criminal activities. One federal court ruled that this could be applied to deny coverage for injuries that occurred while driving under the influence of alcohol.[78] Some policies expressly exclude coverage for alcohol-related injuries.[79] This has had the unfortunate effect of causing some providers to hesitate to test for alcohol.[80] In 2005, a New Jersey appellate court ruled that a plan could not deny coverage for drunk drivers.[81]

EXCLUSION OF SPECIFIED PROCEDURES. Plans generally exclude coverage for most cosmetic procedures.[82] Some plans also exclude complications arising from cosmetic surgery.[83] Surgical treatments for weight loss are widely excluded.[84]

Medical plans generally exclude coverage for most dental procedures. There are disputes over the scope of the exclusion.[85] There

---

[77] *E.g.*, American Republic Ins. Co. v. Superintendent of Ins., 647 A.2d 1195 (Me. 1994), *cert. denied*, 514 U.S. 1035 (1995).

[78] Chapter v. Monfort of Colo., Inc., 20 F.3d 286 (7th Cir. 1994); *Drunken drivers may find insurance won't pay the bills for their injuries*, WALL ST. J., July 6, 1995, B1.

[79] *E.g.*, Bishop v. National Health Ins. Co., 344 F.3d 305 (2d Cir. 2003) [intoxication clause enforced].

[80] *See* R. Zimmerman, *Why trauma units seldom test patients for alcohol, drugs,* WALL ST. J., Feb. 26, 2003, B1; T. Albert, *AHA hits laws impeding screening of drunk patients,* AM. MED. NEWS, Jan. 5, 2004, 8.

[81] Walcott v. Allstate New Jersey Ins. Co., 376 N.J. Super. 384, 870 A.2d 691 (App. Div. 2005).

[82] S. Gilbert, *More insurers balk on breast reconstruction*, N.Y. TIMES, Oct. 16, 1996, B6; *but see* N. Jeffrey, *Corrective or cosmetic? Plastic surgery stirs a debate,* WALL ST. J., June 25, 1998, B1.

[83] *E.g.*, Century Med. Health Plan, Inc. v. North Shore Med. Ctr., Inc., 688 So. 2d 97 (Fla. 3d DCA 1997) [HMO did not cover emergency care for complications from noncovered cosmetic surgery].

[84] *See* R. Kazel, *Insurers trim bariatric surgery coverage*, AM. MED. NEWS, Apr. 5, 2004, 1.

[85] *E.g.*, Blair v. Metropolitan Life Ins. Co., 974 F.2d 1219 (10th Cir. 1992) [treatment of traumatic temporal mandibular joint injury by dentist not excluded].

are dental plans that are offered either with medical plans or as a freestanding option.

There has been extensive litigation concerning exclusion of coverage of transplant procedures, usually the issue is either medical necessity or the experimental exclusion that has already been discussed. Some plans expressly exclude or restrict transplant procedure coverage.[86] However, in 2000, one court ruled that terms of a plan should be interpreted from the perspective of the average person; an exclusion for tissue transplant did not exclude peripheral stem cell rescue.[87]

Some patients have challenged the exclusion of alternative treatments. In 2003, a HMO settled a class action suit by agreeing to make refunds for alternative treatments.[88]

LIMITATION OR EXCLUSION OF MENTAL HEALTH COVERAGE. In the past, many health plans provided different coverage for mental health services than for other medical and surgical services. The Mental Health Parity Act restricts some of these differences, but the law sunsets, so that it does not apply to services furnished on or after December 31, 2004.[89] Questions have been raised about whether it has been effective.[90]

OUT-OF-PANEL NONEMERGENCY CARE. Plans that have closed panels generally pay for emergency services by providers outside the panel. There are frequently disputes over what constitutes an emergency.[91] There is occasional adverse publicity when specialized nonemergency out-of-area care is not approved.[92] Point-of-service plans were developed in part to provide an answer to this

---

[86] *E.g.*, Mire v. Blue Cross & Blue Shield, 43 F.3d 567 (11th Cir. 1994) [policy covered procedure for specific diseases not including this disease].

[87] Simkins v. Nevadacare, Inc., 229 F.3d 729 (9th Cir. 2000); *see also* Lubeznik v. HealthChicago, Inc., 268 Ill. App. 3d 953, 644 N.E.2d 777 (1st Dist. 1994) [exclusion of organ transplants did not exclude bone marrow transplants].

[88] *HMO agrees to make refunds to thousands of its members for alternative treatments*, AP, Feb. 12, 2003.

[89] 42 U.S.C. § 300gg-5; 62 FED. REG. 66,932 (Dec. 12, 1997) [interim final rules on parity of coverage for mental health].

[90] R. Pear, *Insurance plans skirt requirement on mental health*, N.Y. TIMES, Dec. 26, 1998, A1 [replacing dollar limits with numerical limits on visits, days, etc.].

[91] *E.g.*, Tabor v. Prudential Ins. Co., 830 F. Supp. 510 (E.D. Mo. 1993) [coverage for out-of-network cancer surgery performed where dependent student was in college properly denied because not emergency]; *see also BCBS to pay state agency $1.8 million in emergency room claims payment case*, H.L.R., Jan. 1, 2004, 22 [admitted violating state laws on payments for emergency room charges due to failure to update claims processing system; 146,000 claims involving $17 million mishandled; all mishandled claims were repaid].

[92] *E.g.*, *Parents fight to have child's brain surgery in Texas*, AP, Mar. 27, 2003.

problem; under such plans patients are free to seek nonemergency care out-of-panel, but must bear more of the cost.

MEDICAL NECESSITY. Medicare, Medicaid, and most private plans cover only medically necessary care. A frequent basis for denial of coverage is that the care lacks medical necessity.[93] There is judgment involved in these determinations, and in most plans the administrator is given discretion to make the determinations.[94] Courts will usually overturn such decisions only if they are arbitrary and capricious. When the administrator is also the insurer who is at risk for the cost, some courts find that there is a conflict of interest, so that a less deferential standard is used to review the medical necessity decisions.[95]

Those involved in making medical necessity determinations have been sued for malpractice and on other grounds with mixed results. This is discussed later in this chapter. In an effort to avoid being sued for judgment calls, some plans adopt rules expressly excluding specific treatments.

In 1998, the Pennsylvania Supreme Court held that physicians can challenge denials based on review by an insurer that found a lack of medical necessity.[96]

There are substantial variations in medical necessity determinations for Medicare. Regional carriers do not agree, which is one of the ways that Medicare fails to be nationally uniform.[97]

MEDICAL APPROPRIATENESS. Sometimes care that is otherwise medically necessary is denied on the grounds that it is not medically appropriate. For example, a federal appellate court upheld the denial of liver transplant on the grounds that it was not medically appropriate in light of the patient's history, including hepatitis B.[98]

LIKELIHOOD OF SUCCESSFUL CLINICAL OUTCOME. The Health Care Financing Administration (HCFA) limited lung transplant coverage to approved programs that have patient selection cri-

---

[93] *E.g.*, Farley v. Benefit Trust Life Ins. Co., 979 F.2d 653 (8th Cir. 1992) [denial affirmed, not medically necessary]; Annotation, *What services, equipment, or supplies are "medically necessary" for purposes of coverage under medical insurance*, 75 A.L.R. 4TH 763.

[94] *E.g.*, Blue Cross & Blue Shield of Va. v. Keller, 450 S.E.2d 136 (Va. 1994) [proper exercise of administrative discretion in medical necessity review of psychiatric hospitalization].

[95] *E.g.*, Florence Nightingale Nursing Serv., Inc. v. Blue Cross & Blue Shield, 41 F.3d 1476 (11th Cir.), *cert. denied*, 514 U.S. 1128 (1995).

[96] Rudolph v. Pennsylvania Blue Shield, 553 Pa. 9, 717 A.2d 508 (1998).

[97] C. Culhane, *Medicare denial rates vary widely: Carriers inconsistent in judging medical necessity*, AM. MED. NEWS, Apr. 18, 1994, 3.

[98] Barnett v. Kaiser Found. Health Plan, Inc., 32 F.3d 413 (9th Cir. 1994).

teria for determining suitable candidates based on critical medical need and a "strong likelihood of a successful clinical outcome."[99]

In 1998, a federal appellate court found that a private plan was arbitrary and capricious when it denied physical therapy to a multiple sclerosis patient based on its position that such patients could not be helped by such therapy. The court required a case-by-case determination by the plan.[100]

EXPERIMENTAL EXCLUSION. Most plans have some exclusion for research or experimental procedures.[101] These exclusions have frequently been used to deny payment for new expensive procedures. Experimental exclusions have also been used to deny coverage for cancer clinical trials even when they offer the most effective or only promising treatment option for patients. Sometimes all associated care is also denied coverage.[102] This has especially been a problem with the use of new drugs and devices and with the new uses of old drugs and devices, as discussed in Chapter 3.

There appears to be an inconsistency between the strict standard of scientific, controlled, statistical proof of safety and efficacy applied to drugs and devices and the absence of any apparent such standard applied to the broad range of alternative treatments that some plans are beginning to cover.[103]

Denials of coverage have led to malpractice suits.[104] In addition, in 1993, the Texas Attorney General sued a plan after it denied coverage for certain cancer coverage on the grounds it was research.

---

[99] 60 FED. REG. 6,537 (Feb. 2, 1995); *HCFA announces new lung transplant payment policy*, AM. MED. NEWS, Mar. 20, 1995, 5.

[100] McGraw v. Prudential Ins. Co., 137 F.3d 1253 (10th Cir. 1998).

[101] *E.g.*, Martin v. Blue Cross & Blue Shield, 115 F.3d 1201 (4th Cir. 1997), *cert. denied*, 522 U.S. 1029 (1997) [not abuse of discretion to deny coverage for experimental cancer therapy]; Graham v. Medical Mut. of Ohio, 130 F.3d 293 (7th Cir. 1997) [plan can deny coverage of experimental chemotherapy]; Turner v. Fallon Community Health Plan, Inc., 127 F.3d 196 (1st Cir. 1997), *cert. denied*, 523 U.S. 1072 (1998) [no ERISA damage claim for denied coverage of bone marrow transplant for cancer]; Healthcare America Plans Inc. v. Bossemeyer, 166 F.3d 347 (10th Cir. 1998) [denial of coverage for high-dose chemotherapy breast cancer treatment as experimental not ERISA violation]; Annotation, *Propriety of denial of medical or hospital benefits for investigative, educational, or experimental medical procedures pursuant to exclusion contained in ERISA-covered health plan*, 122 A.L.R. FED. 1.

[102] *E.g.*, Loyola Univ. of Chicago v. Humana Ins. Co., 996 F.2d 895 (7th Cir. 1993) [upholding denial of insurance coverage for all treatment associated with artificial heart implant, Jarvik-7]; *contra* Doe v. Group Hospitalization & Med. Servs., 3 F.3d 80 (4th Cir. 1993) [proper to exclude coverage of transplant, but not related chemotherapy].

[103] *E.g.*, *Health insurers embrace eye-of-newt therapy*, WALL ST. J., Jan. 30, 1995, B1.

[104] *See* Cicio v. Doe, 321 F.3d 83 (2d Cir. 2003) [ERISA preempts misrepresentation and delay claims, but not claims of malpractice by medical director who allegedly denied coverage of requested treatment under experimental exclusion and approved coverage of treatment not requested].

The suit claimed that the plan had violated state law by misrepresenting its policies. The suit was settled with the plan agreeing to pay for such treatment.[105]

In response to what has been perceived as denials of coverage for care that represents the only chance for recovery for patients with life-threatening illnesses, some states have attempted to increase the availability of experimental treatment through legislation. These statutes have mandated coverage of certain treatments,[106] required external review of experimental treatment denials,[107] or provided guidelines for coverage that otherwise might be excluded.[108]

DRUG FORMULARIES AND OFF-LABEL USE. The use of drug formularies — lists of covered drugs — is widespread among MCOs and other health care providers, as a means to control drug utilization and make sure that patients receive effective drug therapies.

Off-label use of a drug (the use of a drug approved by the FDA for indications other than those approved by the FDA) is an accepted practice in the nonmanaged care setting. Some MCOs have tried to exclude coverage for off-label uses.[109] Other MCOs require prior authorization for some drugs in a effort to curtail off-label use. To ensure that MCOs allow appropriate off-label use and do not employ unnecessarily restrictive formularies, many states have enacted laws requiring MCOs to disclose the use of formularies and/or to have procedures available to enrollees to apply to have a nonformulary drug covered.[110] Off-label use is discussed further in Chapter 3.

ELIGIBILITY REQUIREMENTS. Some plans deny coverage for certain services when specified eligibility requirements are not met. For example, when a state plan provided attendant care only to persons who were mentally alert, a federal appellate court upheld denying such care to a person who was not mentally alert.[111]

---

105 *Texas v. Prudential Ins. Co.*, No. CA A-93-CV-658-SS (W.D. Tex. settlement Mar. 21, 1994), *as discussed in* 3 H.L.R. 384 (1994); *see also Disability law used to order treatment*, WALL ST. J., July 28, 1995, B3 [federal appellate court found employer in violation of ADA for adopting health plan that excluded experimental breast cancer treatment; company, not insurer, ordered to pay for treatment].

106 *E.g.*, MINN. STAT. § 62A.309, subdiv. 2.

107 *E.g.*, CAL. HEALTH & SAFETY CODE § 1370.4; CAL. INS. CODE § 10145.3.

108 *E.g.*, R.I. GEN. LAWS §§ 27-18-36.2, 27-19-32.2, 27-20-27.2, 27-41-41.2.

109 *E.g.*, I.V. Services of Am., Inc. v. Trustees of Am. Consulting Engineers Council of Ins. Trust Fund, 136 F.3d 114 (2d Cir.1998) [health plan provision limiting drug coverage to FDA approved use of drugs did not unambiguously preclude prescribed off-label drug uses].

110 *E.g.*, ARIZ. REV. STAT. § 20-1076; 1997 CONN. ACT 99; IDAHO CODE title 41, ch.39; 1997 LA. ACTS 238.

111 Easley by Easley v. Snider, 36 F.3d 297 (3d Cir. 1994) [requirement complies with ADA because allowing surrogates would not be a reasonable accommodation].

CAP ON BENEFITS. Some plans place a lifetime limit on the dollar amount of coverage.[112] When that maximum is exceeded, no services are covered.

FEDERALLY MANDATED BENEFITS. Several federal laws mandate uniform coverage nationwide for some services.

Mastectomy Provisions. A provision of the federal Omnibus Consolidated and Emergency Supplemental Appropriations Act of 1998[113] requires health plans and insurers that cover mastectomies to cover reconstructive breast surgery as well. However, only the federal government can enforce the law; private individuals cannot use it as a basis for suit.[114]

A number of states have also enacted legislation requiring health plans to cover inpatient hospitals stays of specified lengths following a mastectomy. Generally, these laws require coverage of a stay no less than forty-eight hours following surgery, with possible coverage of a longer stay as recommended by the attending physician.

Inpatient Care after Childbirth. A federal law, the Newborns and Mothers Health Protection Act of 1996[115] mandates that group health plans (including plans regulated under ERISA) must pay for inpatient hospital coverage for mothers and newborns for a minimum of forty-eight hours following normal vaginal deliveries and ninety-six hours following caesarean sections. If the attending physician and mother agree, an earlier discharge is permitted. A majority of the states have similar laws.[116]

The impact of these laws has been questioned. Studies indicate that shorter stays can be safe and that these laws are making insurance more costly.[117]

In 2001, a New York appellate court ruled that a HMO fulfilled its responsibility by making coverage available and was not responsible

---

[112] *See* In Home Health, Inc. v. Prudential Ins. Co., 101 F.3d 600 (8th Cir. 1996) [no ERISA preemption of state action against insurer for negligently failing to inform provider that insured had passed lifetime benefits maximum]; J. Havemann, *Reeve's new role: health care activist*, MIAMI HERALD [FLA.], Feb. 2, 1996, 1A [seeking removal of lifetime cap on catastrophic coverage].

[113] 29 U.S.C. § 1185b, 42 U.S.C. §§ 300gg-6, 300gg-52.

[114] Howard v. Coventry Health Care of Iowa, Inc., 293 F.3d 442 (8th Cir. 2002).

[115] 29 U.S.C. § 1185; 42 U.S.C. §§ 300gg-4, 300gg-51.

[116] Z. Liu, W.H. Dow & E.C. Norton, *Effect of drive-through delivery laws on postpartum length of stay and hospital charges*, 23 J. HEALTH ECON., Jan., 2004, 129.

[117] *See* J.M. Madden et al., *Effects of a law against early postpartum discharge on newborn follow-up, adverse events, and HMO expenditures*, 347 NEW ENG. J. MED. 2031 (2002); *but see* E. Meara et al., *Impact of early newborn discharge legislation and early follow-up visits on infant outcomes in a state Medicaid population*, 113 PEDIATRICS 1619 (2004).

for assuring the mother and baby stayed for the entire period; it was not responsible for the providers' alleged malpractice in premature discharge.[118]

Mental Health Benefit Parity Act of 1996. The Mental Health Benefit Parity Act of 1996[119] requires group health plans (including plans regulated under ERISA) to offer mental health coverage with annual and lifetime monetary limits equal to those applied to medical and surgical service coverage. Mental health benefits cannot be capped if medical benefits are not capped, with certain exemptions. The law sunsets and does not apply to services provided on or after December 31, 2004.

STATE-MANDATED BENEFITS. There are many state-mandated benefits. One study in 2004 found 1,823 state insurance mandates.[120] Some of these mandates are the result of complaints of small numbers of constituents.[121] Some states have recognized that mandated benefits make it impossible to offer inexpensive alternative benefit plans.[122] In 2003, one state enacted a four-year moratorium on adding new mandates.[123] Efforts to exempt alternative benefit plans from mandates often encounter intense lobbying campaigns by the providers of the mandated benefits.[124]

Some religious plans have challenged the applicability of mandates for services that are contrary to their religious beliefs. These efforts have been unsuccessful. In 2004, the California Supreme Court ruled that religious organizations must comply with the state law requiring inclusion of prescription contraceptives in their employee health insurance coverage.[125]

---

[118] Jones v. U.S. Healthcare, 282 A.D.2d 347, 723 N.Y.S.2d 478 (1st Dept. 2001).

[119] 29 U.S.C. § 1185a; 42 U.S.C. § 300gg-5.

[120] *Study finds 1,823 insurance mandates for state-regulated health insurers*, H.L.R., Aug. 12, 2004, 1195.

[121] *See* J.B. Finkelstein, *States steer away from broad health benefit mandates*, AM. MED. NEWS, Sept. 1, 2003, 11 [description of process by which laws get passed].

[122] M. Andrews, *Paying a price for pared-down health plans*, N.Y. TIMES, June 15, 2003, 9BU [state mandated insurance benefits v. laws permitting bare bones policies]; J. Hancock, *Legislated health benefits cause loss of essential care*, BALTIMORE SUN, Mar. 20, 2002, 1C.

[123] *Moratorium on insurance mandates receives final approval*, AP, June 22, 2003 [LA].

[124] *E.g.*, P. Brinkman, *800 chiropractors at Capitol protest an insurance bill*, WIS. ST. J., Feb. 19, 2004, B1 [Wis. legislature considering bill to permit chambers of commerce to offer insurance program that does not include benefits mandated for other plans, including chiropractic services]; M. Pommer, *Health plan bill appears to be dead*, CAPITOL TIMES (Madison WI), Feb. 19, 2004, 3A.

[125] Catholic Charities of Sacramento, Inc. v. Superior Court, 32 Cal. 4th 527, 85 P.3d 67, 10 Cal. Rptr. 3d 283 (2004).

When state administrative agencies exceed their authority in adding mandated benefits, challenges can succeed. In 2002, a California appellate court ruled that a state agency did not have authority to mandate that plans cover an erectile dysfunction drug.[126]

PROVIDERS HAVE NO DUTY TO ADVOCATE FOR BENEFITS. It is the responsibility of the patient to understand and deal with the limitations on and qualifications for benefits. Many providers voluntarily assist their patients and advocate for them, but providers do not have a duty to do so. In 2001, a federal appellate court rejected an attempt to add this to the providers' duties.[127]

10-2.6 Case or Disease Management

Many MCOs are using case or disease management in an effort to assure appropriate utilization and follow-up.[128] This technique usually involves close following of individual cases to promote coordination among primary care and specialty care, the following of proper steps in a timely fashion to optimize outcome and reduce delays, and consideration of alternatives, so that they can be pursued where appropriate. This can involve close contact with patients as well as providers.[129] An important aspect often is to assure that patients obtain appropriate follow-up care and use their medications as prescribed. Sometimes this can involve adjusting aspects of the coverage for specific chronic diseases to promote current utilization that will reduce future more expensive utilization.[130]

10-2.7 Communicating Denials to Individuals

Care must be taken in communicating denials of coverage to individuals. One provider sued a plan administrator for defamation for

---

[126] Kaiser Found. Health Plan, Inc. v. Zingale, 99 Cal. App. 4th 1018, 121 Cal. Rptr. 2d 741 (3d Dist. 2002).

[127] Pryzbowski v. U.S. Healthcare, Inc., 245 F.3d 266 (3d Cir. 2001).

[128] *See* L. Landro, *Disease management: Pro and con*, WALL ST. J, Oct. 20, 2004, D4; G. Ruffenach, *Miracle cure?* WALL ST. J., Aug. 9, 2004, R5 [Medicare disease management]; J.M. Jacobson, *A sheep in wolf's clothing? The legal confusion between care management and managed care*, HEALTH L. DIG., July 2001; *See also* R. Kazel, *Evidence still out on disease management as cost saver*, AM. MED. NEWS, Oct. 27, 2003, 11 [early studies indicated value, but evidence still limited].

[129] *See* A.D. Marcus, *Careful, your HMO is watching*, WALL ST. J., June 17, 2003, D1 [monitoring patients, contacting them to get more tests or see specialists].

[130] *E.g.,* V. Fuhrmans, *A radical prescription*, WALL ST. J., May 10, 2004, R3 [company slashed amount employees pay for diabetes and asthma drugs causing dramatic reduction in health costs].

the wording of the notice to the patient of denial. The suit was unsuccessful because the provider did not overcome the qualified privilege for such communications.[131] However, care should be taken in such communications to avoid acting outside the privilege.

In 1997, a federal appeals court held that a health plan subject to ERISA must provide in writing reasons for denying benefits to an insured and must ask for any necessary information before making its decision.[132] In 2003, the same court ruled that it would show judicial deference to discretionary decisions of plan administrators only when they make a stated decision; there would be no deference to denials that occurred merely by the passage of the review time period.[133]

10-2.8 Promoting Healthy Behavior

Some employers and plans try to promote healthier behavior in an effort to reduce illness and the related health care and other business costs of illness.[134] In some cases, employees have recognized that the bad habits of their coworkers are contributing to the increase in their own out-of-pocket health care costs.[135] These programs have received mixed receptions depending on their focus.[136]

10-3   What Are the Appeal Rights from Adverse Utilization Determinations?

Some states have enacted laws that give patients the right to an external independent review of coverage denial decisions.[137] In 2002, the United States Supreme Court ruled that state laws requir-

---

131 Gulf South Med. & Surgical Inst. v. Aetna Life Ins. Co., 39 F.3d 520 (5th Cir. 1994).

132 Booton v. Lockheed Med. Benefit Plan, 110 F.3d 1461 (9th Cir. 1997).

133 Jebian v. Hewlett-Packard Co., 349 F.3d 1098 (9th Cir. 2003), *accord* Gilbertson v. Allied Signal, Inc., 328 F.3d 625 (10th Cir. 2003).

134 *See* J. Bennett, *HMOs try 'frequent jogger points,'* WALL ST. J., Sept. 25, 2003, D4.

135 *See* T. Aeppel, *Ill will: Skyrocketing health costs start to pit worker vs. worker,* WALL ST. J., June 17, 2003, A1.

136 *See* D. Costello, *Bosses assign a new task: Stay well; In an effort to lower costs, more employers are taking a hands-on approach to workers' health. Such efforts aren't always welcome,* L.A. TIMES, Nov. 17, 2003, pt. 6, 1.

137 *E.g.*, 1998 MD. LAWS chs. 111, 112; MICH. STAT. ANN. § 14.5(21088); MINN. STAT. ch. 62Q.105 (1996); N.M. ADMIN. CODE title 13, § 10.13 (1997); 1998 TENN. PUB. ACTS ch. 952; *see also* L. Berman-Sandler, *Independent medical review: expanding legal remedies to achieve managed care accountability,* 13 ANN. HEALTH L. 233 (Wint. 2004); T. Richmond, *Review panels reverse 42 percent of health insurance decisions,* AP, June 11, 2003 [WI, 2002 data].

ing access to independent review are not preempted by ERISA.[138] However, in 2004, the Hawaii Supreme Court ruled that its state external review law was preempted by ERISA.[139]

However, external reviewers cannot rewrite the insurance contract. In 2002, a California trial judge ruled that a state reviewer cannot require a plan to cover a medically necessary drug that is excluded for the contract.[140]

The National Commission on Quality Assurance, an accreditation body for HMOs, requires HMOs seeking its accreditation to provide an appeal to an independent third party for final resolution of disputes, after a patient has exhausted the HMO's internal appeals process.

10-4 When Can Third-party Payers Be Liable for the Consequences of Their Decisions?

MCO actions have been attacked through malpractice suits, state administrative procedures,[141] racketeering suits,[142] and other ways.

Staff model HMOs, in which the individual practitioners providing patient care are employees of the HMO, may be held liable for the negligent acts of their employees under *respondeat superior*. (This and other theories of tort liability are discussed in more detail in Chapter 11.) Courts are still struggling, however, with the extent to which MCOs should be liable for the consequences of errors of providers who participate through a contractual relationships with the MCO, for MCO selection of such participating providers and for MCO decisions not to authorize hospitalization or other treatment.

In 2004, the United States Supreme Court ruled that ERISA preempts malpractice and most other state law claims concerning

---

[138] Rush Prudential HMO, Inc. v. Moran, 536 U.S. 355 (2002).

[139] Hawaii Management Alliance Ass'n v. Insurance Comm'r, 106 Haw. 21, 100 P.3d 952 (2004); HAW. REV. STAT. § 432E-6.

[140] L. Rapaport, *California judge rules against state regulators in health insurance case*, SACRAMENTO BEE, Jan. 16, 2002.

[141] *E.g.*, B. McCormick, *When coverage decisions threaten care*, AM. MED. NEWS, Feb. 20, 1995, 1 [disciplinary case against Ariz. HMO medical director stopped by lawsuit filed by HMO against licensing board; first attempt to sanction doctor who denied coverage for a service in a managed care setting]; J. Johnsson, *Dad's protests lead to record fine against California HMO*, AM. MED. NEWS, Dec. 12, 1994, 1 [$500,000 state fine for quality violations, endangering life of patient by denying specialty referral].

[142] *E.g.*, Taylor v. Hender, 116 Or. App. 142, 840 P.2d 1331 (1992) [insurers retained experts to evaluate chiropractors to assist in controlling costs; no state RICO claim stated against experts, no inference of fraudulent scheme or artifice].

coverage and treatment-related decisions against MCOs.[143] Thus, MCOS regulated by ERISA generally cannot be sued under state law for its coverage and treatment-related decisions. The only exception is that a MCO can be sued for the malpractice of treating health care providers who are employees of the MCO.

When ERISA does not bar such claims, plaintiffs still must bring their claims under an acceptable theory of liability in order to recover damages from a MCO. If the alleged act of negligence is committed by an employee of the MCO, the MCO can be held liable under the theory of *respondeat superior*. In addition, a Pennsylvania appeals court, in a 1998 decision, held that HMOs can be subject to corporate liability; the patient alleged negligence by a HMO's telephone triage center.[144]

However, most claims against MCOs involve practitioners who are not employed by the MCO but rather contract with the MCO to provide health care to enrollees. Many theories of vicarious liability or agency used against hospitals (see Chapter 11) have been used against such MCOs. Sometimes participating physicians have been found to be apparent agents.[145] At least one court has found that participating physicians who are paid on a capitation basis are actual agents.[146] Other courts have required more than a participating provider agreement to establish apparent agency.[147]

Similar to the evolution of the law concerning hospitals, there has been an effort to impose liability on MCOs for providers who are neither employees nor apparent agents based on negligent selection or failure to deselect a provider when problems become known or should have been discovered. MCOs have sought to avoid all

---

143 Aetna Health, Inc. v Davila, 542 U.S. 200 (2004); Land v. Cigna Healthcare, 381 F.3d 1274 (11th Cir. 2004); L. Greenhouse, *Justices limit ability to sue health plans*, N.Y. TIMES, June 22, 2004, A1.

144 Shannon v. McNulty, 718 A.2d 82 (Pa. Super. Ct. 1998).

145 *E.g.*, Schleier v. Kaiser Found. Health Plan, 277 U.S. App. D.C. 415, 876 F.2d 174 (1989) [HMO liable for negligence of independent contractor, consulting physician]; Boyd v. Albert Einstein Med. Ctr., 377 Pa. Super. 609, 547 A.2d 1229 (1988) [participating physicians may be ostensible agents of HMO]; Jones v. Chicago HMO Ltd. of Ill., 301 Ill. App. 3d 103, 703 N.E.2d 502 (1st Dist. 1998) [aggressive marketing campaign, lack of choice of providers created question concerning physicians' apparent authority to act for HMO]; Petrovich v. Share Health Plan, 188 Ill. 2d 17, 719 N.E.2d 756 (1999) [sufficient evidence for trial on whether HMO liable for treating physicians under apparent, implied authority].

146 Dunn v. Praiss, 256 N.J. Super. 180, 606 A.2d 862 (App. Div. 1992); Physician settled and HMO avoided contribution, 139 N.J. 564, 656 A.2d 413 (1995).

147 *E.g.*, Raglin v. HMO Ill., Inc., 230 Ill. App. 3d 642, 595 N.E.2d 153 (1st Dist. 1992) [physician in IPA model HMO not employee or apparent agent so HMO not liable for alleged malpractice]; Chase v. Independent Practice Ass'n, 31 Mass. Ct. App. 661, 583 N.E.2d 251 (1991) [HMO not liable for negligence of contract physician].

responsibility for selection and retention of providers. In 1989, the Missouri Supreme Court ruled that a HMO had a duty to conduct a reasonable investigation of the credentials and reputation of participating physicians.[148]

MCOs have sought to avoid all responsibility for their coverage decisions based on versions of the theory that patients and providers are still free to seek and provide care at their own expense; the MCO's denial did not cause the failure to obtain timely treatment. In 1986, a California court ruled that a state reviewer could not be liable for the complications a patient suffered when the reviewer authorized only half of the additional hospital days requested by the treating physician because the treating physician had the responsibility to make the discharge decision.[149] The efforts to avoid liability have not been entirely successful. A California jury awarded an $89 million verdict against a HMO for denial of coverage for bone marrow transplantation for a breast cancer patient. The case was later settled for $5 million.[150]

Texas enacted a law that allows an individual to sue a MCO for damages caused by the MCO's failure to exercise ordinary care when making treatment decisions. However, in 2004, the United States Supreme Court ruled that the Texas law was preempted by ERISA, and it cannot be applied to plans regulated by ERISA.[151]

In 1997, the Wisconsin Supreme Court held that the tort of bad faith applies to all HMOs making out-of-network benefit decisions.[152] The tort of bad faith has traditionally been applied to insurance companies in making coverage decisions. The court held that when HMOs are making out-of-network decisions, the HMOs are acting as insurers and are subject to the tort of bad faith, distinct from a claim of medical malpractice.

The area of MCO liability will likely continue to be unsettled, as patients and their attorneys seek to find ways of recovering damages from MCOs that they perceive are making unreasonable or unfair treatment decisions. There is some evidence that in many states patients may find courts sympathetic to their claims.

---

[148] Harrell v. Total Health Care, 781 S.W.2d 58 (Mo. 1989).

[149] Wickline v. State, 183 Cal. App. 3d 1175, 228 Cal. Rptr. 661 (2d Dist. 1986).

[150] B. McCormick, *Managed care posing new liability risks, insurers warn*, AM. MED. NEWS, June 13, 1994, 3.

[151] Aetna Health Inc. v Davila, 542 U.S. 200 (2004).

[152] McEvoy v. Group Health Coop. of Eau Claire, 213 Wis. 2d 507, 570 N.W.2d 397 (1997).

Discussion Points

1. How do persons qualify for coverage?
2. How are out-of-pocket expenses (copayments, coinsurance, and deductibles) used to manage utilization?
3. How do plans manage utilization by controlling permitted providers?
4. How do plans control access to permitted providers?
5. How do plans use provider incentives to manage utilization?
6. What are some coverage exclusions used by plans? What are the legal restrictions of such exclusions?
7. How do plans use case and disease management to manage utilization?
8. Discuss the scope of rights to appeal adverse plan coverage decisions.
9. When can plans be liable for coverage decisions?

CHAPTER ELEVEN

Civil Liability

Objectives

The objective of this chapter is to provide an overview of when health care providers may be subject to civil liability. The reader will learn about liability for negligent torts, liability for intentional torts, major defenses to such suits, strict liability for products, responsibility for payment for liability, types of insurance, tort reform proposals, and examples of tort liability for health care professionals.

Everyone involved in health care delivery is acutely aware of the potential for patients or their families to make legal claims for money because of injuries they believe were caused by malpractice or other wrongful conduct. A basic understanding of liability principles can help minimize claims and facilitate proper handling of claims.

Civil liability is the liability imposed other than through criminal law. Civil liability can be divided into liability that is based on contract, liability based on torts, and other forms of liability that are based on government statutes and regulations. *Tort liability* is the liability that is imposed by the common law and some statutes for injuries caused by breaches of duties not based on contractual agreement. Liability based on contract is discussed in Section 1-5.

Tort liability is almost always based on fault; that is, something was done incorrectly or something that should have been done was omitted. This act or omission can be intentional or can result from negligence. In some exceptional circumstances, there is strict liability for all consequences of certain activities regardless of fault.

This chapter addresses the following questions:

11-1. What must be proved to establish liability for negligence torts?

11-2. What are intentional torts, and how do they differ from negligent torts?

11-3. What are the major defenses to liability suits for torts?

11-4. What are the special strict liability rules for products liability?

11-5. Who is responsible for paying for liability?

11-6. What types of insurance are available?

11-7. What are some of the ways that have been proposed and/or implemented to deal with the periodic malpractice crisis?

11-8. What are some examples of the tort liability of health care providers?

11-1 What Must Be Proved to Establish Liability for Negligence Torts?

The most frequent basis for liability of health care professionals and institutions is the negligent tort. Fortunately, negligence by itself is not enough to establish liability. The negligence must cause an injury. Four elements must be proved to establish liability for negligent torts: (1) duty, that is, what should have been done; (2) breach of duty, as in deviation from what should have been done; (3) injury; and (4) causation — injury directly and legally caused by the deviation from what should have been done.

There is a "fifth element" that the courts do not discuss, but that health care providers should remember: Someone must be willing to make a claim. Health care providers who maintain good relationships with their patients before and after incidents are less likely to be sued. If a staff member suspects that an incident has occurred, the persons responsible for institutional risk management should be notified promptly so that steps can be taken to minimize the chance of a claim.

This section discusses the following questions:

11-1.1. When does a health care provider have a duty to an individual?

11-1.2. What is the duty (standard of care), and how is it proved?

11-1.3. What constitutes a compensable injury?

11-1.4. How is legal causation proved?

11-1.5. When does the *res ipsa loquitur* exception apply?

11-1.1 When Does a Health Care Provider Have a Duty to an Individual?

The first element that must be proved in any negligence suit is the *duty*. Duty has two aspects. First, it must be proved that a duty was owed to the person harmed. Second, the scope of that duty, sometimes called the *standard of care*, must be proved.

In general, the common law does not impose a duty on individuals to come to the rescue of persons for whom they have no other responsibility.[1] Under the common law rule, a person walking down the street has no legal obligation to come to the aid of a heart attack victim unless (1) the victim is the person's dependent; (2) the person contributed to the cause of the heart attack; (3) the person owns or operates the premises where the attack occurred; or (4) the person has a contractual obligation to come to the victim's aid, for example, by being on duty as a member of a public emergency care team.

DUTIES TO PATIENTS. In most health care cases, it is not difficult to establish a duty based on the patient's admission to the institution or professional relationship with the individual practitioner. When a person is denied admission, there can be a question whether a duty was ever created. In addition, complex questions about whether a relationship has been established can arise from consultations, telephone calls, and other interactions. These issues are discussed in Chapter 6.

DUTIES TO NONPATIENTS. Courts disagree on when health care providers have duties to nonpatients. A few courts have prohibited all liability to nonpatients for the effects of the diagnosis and treatment of the patient. For example, the Texas Supreme Court held that a physician owes no duty to third parties outside of the physician-patient relationship for failing to properly diagnose and treat a patient.[2] Other courts have examined specific situations.

Injuries by Patients. Several courts have considered whether health care providers should be liable to nonpatients who are injured by a patient.

Several courts permit suits by persons injured in automobile accidents that are caused by patients who were prescribed or

---

[1] Annotation, *Duty of one other than carrier or employer to render assistance to one for whose initial injury he is not liable*, 33 A.L.R. 3D 301.
[2] Van Horn v. Chambers, Tex., 970 S.W.2d 542 (Tex.1998).

administered drugs. In 2002, the West Virginia Supreme Court permitted a suit when a patient who had negligently been prescribed controlled substances caused an automobile accident.[3] An Oregon appellate court ruled the entity that negligently prescribed the drug Xanax could be liable for the death of two children in an automobile accident with the person under the influence of the drug.[4] In 1997, the Indiana Supreme Court found that a physician who failed to monitor a patient's condition or warn of danger may be liable for the resulting death of a third person.[5] In that case, a patient was involved in a fatal automobile accident after receiving an immunization and experiencing a fainting spell in his physician's office. However, in 1999, the Pennsylvania Supreme Court decided that an ophthalmologist could not be held liable for a death in an automobile accident caused by his patient.[6]

Attempts have been made to hold psychiatrists liable to the estates of persons murdered by their patients. Liability has been imposed for failure to warn when the patient has made a credible threat. See the discussion in Section 8-6.3. Liability has sometimes been imposed for failure to take steps to detain some mental patients. See the discussion in Sections 6-6.2 and 7-7. However, generally liability has not been imposed for alleged malpractice in treatment of the patient.[7]

Injuries to Persons Observing Patient Care. Courts have considered whether health care providers should be liable when family members or others who are observing treatment faint, fall, or are injured in other ways. Courts have uniformly found no duty to observers, realizing that providers should be focusing their attention on the patient and the consequence of imposing liability would be to force providers to exclude observers.[8] For example, the Illinois Supreme Court ruled in 1990 that a hospital had no duty to a nonpatient bystander in the emergency room unless the person had

---

3 Osborne v. U.S., 211 W. Va. 667, 567 S.E.2d 677 (2002).

4 Zavalas v. State, Dep't of Corrections, 861 P.2d 1026 (Ore. Ct. App. 1993), *rev. denied*, 319 Or. 150, 877 P.2d 86 (1994).

5 Cram v. Howell, 680 N.E.2d 1096 (Ind. 1997).

6 Estate of Witthoeft v. Kiskaddon, 557 Pa. 340, 733 A.2d 623 (1999).

7 *Judge drops psychiatrist from lawsuit over 1996 Penn State University killing*, AP, Aug. 9, 2003.

8 *See* Fitzgerald v. Porter Mem. Hosp., 523 F.2d 716 (7th Cir. 1975) [husband may be excluded from delivery room].

been invited to participate in the treatment.[9] In 2003, the Connecticut Supreme Court agreed, finding no duty to prevent an observer from fainting.[10]

Parents Accused of Abuse. Parents accused of abuse have sought to establish liability based on reports by health care providers. In addition to the fact that most such reports are protected by statutory immunity for child abuse reports, most courts have found that the health care providers caring for the children owe no duty to their parents. For example, in 2000, the Pennsylvania Supreme Court adopted this rule.[11] However, some states prioritize prevention of child abuse and parental rights differently. In 2004, a Florida court permitted a psychologist to be sued for negligent interference with parental rights.[12]

Spread of Contagious Disease from Patient. Courts have addressed when providers can be liable to persons who receive contagious diseases from patients. Generally, the only duty to the public at large is to make required reports to public health authorities. Sometimes there is a duty to a nonpatient who has a special relationship to the provider or the patient. Thus, there is generally a duty to advise the immediate caregivers, such as parents of minor patients who live in their home. In some states, this duty is further circumscribed by special confidentiality laws for some diseases, such as HIV/AIDS. In 2003, the highest court of New York applied these principles to conclude that no duty of care was owed to the friend of a patient treated for infectious meningitis; there was no liability when she contracted the disease.[13]

11-1.2 What Is the Duty (Standard of Care), and How Is It Proved?

After existence of a duty is established, the scope of the duty must be established. This aspect is sometimes called the obligation to conform to the *standard of care*. The standard of care for health care institu-

---

[9] O'Hara v. Holy Cross Hosp., 137 Ill. 2d 332, 561 N.E.2d 18 (1990); *see* Annotation, *Liability of hospital for injury to person invited or permitted to accompany patient during emergency room treatment,* 90 A.L.R. 4TH 478.

[10] Murillo v. Seymour Ambulance Assoc., 264 Conn. 474, 823 A.2d 1202 (2003).

[11] Althaus by Althaus v. Cohen, 562 Pa. 547, 756 A.2d 1166 (2000).

[12] Welker v. Southern Baptist Hosp., 864 So. 2d 1178 (Fla. 1st DCA 2004).

[13] McNulty v. City of New York, 100 N.Y.2d 227, 792 N.E.2d 162, 762 N.Y.S.2d 12 (2003).

tions is usually the degree of reasonable care the patient's known or apparent condition requires. Some states extend the standard to include the reasonable care required for conditions the institution should have discovered through exercise of reasonable care. Usually the standard for individual health care professionals is what a reasonably prudent health care professional engaged in a similar practice would have done under similar circumstances. A judge or jury will make the determination based on one or more of the following: (1) expert testimony, (2) common sense, or (3) written standards.

The standard of care is one of the important factors that determine the number of malpractice claims and the cost of defense and liability. Thus, the standard of care is one of the elements that should to be reexamined. This section discusses current law. Reexamination is left for Section 11-7.1.

EXPERT TESTIMONY. The technical aspects of care must be proved through expert testimony, usually by other health professionals. When expert testimony is required and the plaintiff has no expert, the case is dismissed.

Qualifications of Experts. As part of tort reform, some states have limited who may qualify to testify as an expert.[14] These qualifications usually focus on the credentials of the proposed expert but sometimes also look at the person's experience.

Scientific Basis for Testimony. In the 1993 case of *Daubert v. Merrell Dow Pharmaceuticals*, the United States Supreme Court established stricter standards concerning expert testimony in federal courts.[15] The *Daubert* standards focus on the quality of the scientific basis for the expert opinion. The *Daubert* standards apply to expert testimony about standard of care.[16]

Consequences of Testimony. Generally, experts are immune from civil liability for their testimony. However, several courts have ruled that expert witnesses may by sued by the persons who retained them when their performance of litigation services is allegedly deficient. In those states, witness immunity provides protection only from suits by the opposition or third parties.[17]

---

[14] *E.g.*, FLA. STAT. § 766.102(2)(c); Payne v. Caldwell, 796 S.W.2d 142 (Tenn. 1990) [upheld requirement that an expert be licensed in the state or contiguous state for full previous year].

[15] Daubert v. Merrell Dow Pharmaceuticals, Inc., 509 U.S. 579 (1993); Kumho Tire Co. v. Carmichael, 524 U.S. 936 (1999) [*Daubert* also applies to nonscientific experts].

[16] *E.g.*, Schneider v. Fried, 320 F.3d 396 (3d Cir. 2003).

[17] Marrogi v, Howard, 805 So. 2d 1118 (La. 2002); M. Hoenig, *Suing unreliable experts*, N.Y. L. J., Mar. 11, 2002, 3.

In addition to impact on professional reputation, there are other potential consequences for questionable testimony. In some jurisdictions, physicians and other licensed professionals may be disciplined under licensing laws for false or misleading testimony.[18] In 2002, the North Carolina Medical Board revoked a surgeon's license for his expert testimony. A court reinstated the license. On review, the Board suspended the surgeon's license for one year.[19]

Some professional societies also discipline members.[20]

In 2004, a Florida trial judge ordered that a particular physician never appear as an expert in that court again. The physician filed a civil rights action challenging the order. A state appellate court upheld dismissal of the case.[21]

Use of Provider's Own Testimony. Sometimes the health care provider's out-of-court statements can be used against the provider as an admission; care must be taken in what is said or written after an incident.[22] In 2000, the Alaska Supreme Court permitted the defendants interrogatory answers to be used to establish the duty.[23]

This made it difficult for providers to apologize to patients for bad outcomes or to be candid about the cause of the outcome. A few states have passed laws that bar the use of apologies in malpractice cases. At least one state, Colorado, has a law that extends this protection so that even an admission of fault cannot be used against the provider in a malpractice suit.[24]

In some circumstances, courts will compel health care providers to act as involuntary expert witnesses, but most courts either preclude this or strictly limit when it may occur.[25]

---

[18] Deatherage v. Washington State Examining Bd. of Psychology, 134 Wash. 2d 131, 948 P.2d 828 (1997) [expert witness does not have absolute immunity from professional discipline]; D. Gianelli, *Nonexpert witnesses raise delegates' ire*, AM. MED. NEWS, Jan. 4, 1999, at 7 [AMA seeking disciplinary actions against doctors who provide fraudulent testimony].

[19] *N.C. board suspends license for neurosurgeon's expert testimony*, AP, Nov. 22, 2003.

[20] *E.g.*, L. Page, *Expert witness watchdog; Amid complaints, AANS defenders say the program is necessary, fair*, MODERN PHYSICIAN, Aug. 1, 2003, 26.

[21] D. Christensen, *Appeals court lets stand judges ban of surgeon as expert witness*, BROWARD DAILY BUSINESS REV., June 15, 2000, A1; Gervin v. Andrews, 826 So. 2d 504 (Fla. 4th DCA 2002) [affirming dismissal of 1983 action challenging exclusion].

[22] *E.g.*, Brookover v. Mary Hitchcock Mem. Hosp., 893 F.2d 411 (1st Cir. 1990) [father could testify that nurse said after fall of son that son should have been restrained; admissible as a vicarious admission].

[23] D.P. v. Wrangell Gen. Hosp., 5 P.3d 225 (Alaska 2000).

[24] COLO. REV. STAT. § 13-25-135 (2004); *Hospitals with unexpected outcomes explore alternatives to 'deny and defend,'* H.L.R., Feb. 3, 2005, 143.

[25] *E.g.*, Glenn v. Plante, 2004 WI 24, 676 N.W.2d 413; *contra*, Giventer by Giventer v. Rementeria, 181 Misc. 2d 582, 693 N.Y.S.2d 878 (Sup. Ct. 1999) [defendant can be compelled to give expert testimony].

COMMON SENSE. Nontechnical aspects of care can be proved by nonexperts. Some courts will permit juries to use their own knowledge and common sense when the duty is considered common knowledge. For example, in 1992, an Iowa court decided that protecting a disoriented patient from falling was a nontechnical aspect.[26] It is questionable whether this is still supportable in light of legal restrictions on use of restraints and the professional judgment that must be used in choosing between restraints and alternative fall prevention techniques. In 1992, a Texas court ruled that expert testimony was not required to establish negligence in assigning a nurse to duty where evaluation forms disclosed unsatisfactory performance including sleeping on the job.[27] In 2001, a Minnesota court decided that it was common knowledge how a paramedic would locate a home to respond to an emergency call.[28]

Courts frequently reject attempts to apply this exception to avoid the need for an expert. In 2001, a New Jersey court decided that reading patient slides was not a matter of common knowledge.[29]

WRITTEN STANDARDS. Some courts will look to written standards, such as licensure regulations, institutional rules, and accreditation standards, to determine the standard of care. When these written standards are permitted as proof, they are used in one of three ways: (1) as evidence the jury can consider in determining the standard of care without any supporting expert testimony;[30] (2) as evidence the jury can consider in determining the standard of care, but only if there is also expert testimony confirming that the published standard states the actual standard of care;[31] and (3) as presumptively the standard of care that the jury must accept unless the defendant can prove otherwise.[32]

---

[26] *E.g.*, Cockerton v. Mercy Hosp. Med. Ctr., 490 N.W.2d 856 (Iowa Ct. App. 1992) [fall during x-ray exam; failure to use restraint straps is routine nonmedical care]; *see also* Dimora v. Cleveland Clinic Found., 683 N.E.2d 1175 (Ohio Ct. App. 1996).

[27] St. Paul Med. Ctr. v. Cecil, 842 S.W.2d 808 (Tex. Ct. App. 1992).

[28] Blatz v. Allina Health Sys., 622 N.W.2d 376 (Minn. App. 2001).

[29] Lucia v. Monmouth Med. Ctr., 341 N.J. Super. 95, 775 A.2d 97 (App. Div. 2001).

[30] *E.g.*, Peacock v. Samaritan Health Servs., 159 Ariz. 123, 765 P.2d 525 (Ct. App. 1988) [internal hospital protocol for safeguarding psychiatric patients].

[31] *E.g.*, Van Iperen v. Van Bramer, 392 N.W.2d 480 (Iowa 1986) [JCAHO drug monitoring standard]; Gallagher v. Detroit McComb Hosp. Ass'n, 171 Mich. App. 761, 431 N.W.2d 90 (1988) [internal hospital rules].

[32] *E.g.*, Hastings v. Baton Rouge Gen. Hosp., 498 So. 2d 713 (La. 1986).

Statutes and Regulations. Statutes or governmental regulations can be used to establish the standard of care.

When a law requires an action in order to benefit other individuals or forbids an action in order to protect other individuals, a violation is generally considered *negligence per se*. An individual who is harmed by a violation need only prove (1) the law is intended to benefit the class of persons of which the individual is a member, (2) the law was violated, (3) the injury is of the type the law was intended to prevent, and (4) the injury was caused by the violation. Some states limit the defenses that can be used.[33] Some states limit the applicability of negligence per se further. For example, Wisconsin additionally requires that the legislature demonstrate a clear and unambiguous intent that the statute be a basis for the imposition of civil liability.[34]

A Maryland court found a hospital liable for injuries that resulted from failure to comply with a hospital licensing regulation requiring segregation of sterile and nonsterile needles.[35] The patient had a liver biopsy with a needle that was suspected to be nonsterile and required postponement of other therapy and immediate treatment to prevent infection from the needle. This was the type of patient and harm the regulation was designed to address. In 2001, a California court ruled that it was negligence per se to violate a state regulation requiring reasonable efforts to assure that infants are given a blood test to detect the presence of neural tube defects.[36]

When the statute or regulation is intended to benefit the general public, a violation is generally not considered negligence per se; the jury may consider the regulation in determining the standard of care. In 2001, a Florida court decided that violation of a statute requiring physicians to have clinical privileges in order to practice in a hospital was not negligence per se because it was for the protection of the general public.[37]

Institutional Rules. Some courts allow institutional rules to be used to establish the standard of care. For example, in 1975, the highest court of New York ruled that the hospital could be liable for injuries due to failure to raise the patient's bed rails when the hospital

---

[33] 57A AM. JUR.2D *Negligence* §§ 716-803.
[34] Leahy v. Kenosha Mem. Hosp., 118 Wis. 2d 441, 348 N.W.2d 607 (App. 1984); Cooper v. Eagle River Mem. Hosp., 270 F.3d 456 (7th Cir. 2001).
[35] Suburban Hosp. Ass'n v. Hadary, 22 Md. App. 186, 322 A.2d 258 (1974).
[36] Galvez v. Frields, 88 Cal. App. 4th 1410, 107 Cal. Rptr. 2d 50 (2d Dist. 2001).
[37] Lingle v. Dion, 776 So. 2d 1073 (Fla. 4th DCA 2001).

had a rule requiring bed rails to be raised for all patients over the age of fifty.[38] In 2001, a Florida court ruled that internal polices could be introduced into evidence but that they were not conclusive on the standard of care.[39] Some courts that allow policies to be used in this way permit the defendant to prove unwritten exceptions. In 1994, the New Jersey Supreme Court ruled that the standard of care was established by a hospital policy providing that no patient should be left unattended on an emergency room stretcher with the side rails down but allowed defense experts to explain that the policy would not be violated if the physician was satisfied the patient was competent and capable of self-care.[40] Other courts do not permit institutional rules to be used for this purpose. For example, in Wisconsin, the internal procedures of private organizations do not set the standard of care for negligence cases. They are relevant only when it is otherwise shown that substantially all of the industry has essentially the same safety regulation.[41] Similarly, in Virginia, a person cannot fix the standard of the duty owed to others by adopting private rules; evidence of internal policies is inadmissible in evidence either for or against a litigant who is not a party to the rules.[42]

Especially in states that allow institutional rules to establish the standard of care, it is important for staff members to be familiar with and act in compliance with the institutional rules and policies applicable to their areas of practice. If the rules are impossible to follow, steps should be taken to modify them instead of ignoring them.

Eliminating all rules is not a solution because failure to adopt necessary rules can be a violation of the standard of care. In Michigan, a hospital was found liable for an infection transmitted by a transplanted cornea because the hospital did not have a procedure to assure that the relevant medical records of the proposed donor were reviewed prior to the transplant.[43] In 1990, a federal court found that failure to have procedures for determining if products had been recalled was an administrative issue that did not require expert testimony.[44]

---

[38] Haber v. Cross County Hosp., 37 N.Y.2d 888, 378 N.Y.S.2d 369, 340 N.E.2d 734 (1975).

[39] Moyer v. Reynolds, 780 So. 2d 205 (Fla. 5th DCA 2001).

[40] Tobia v. Cooper Hosp. Univ. Med. Ctr., 136 N.J. 335, 643 A.2d 1 (1994).

[41] Johnson v. Misercordia Community Hosp., 97 Wis. 2d 521, 294 N.W.2d 501 (Ct. App. 1980); Cooper v. Eagle River Mem. Hosp., 270 F.3d 456 (7th Cir. 2001).

[42] Pullen v. Nickens, 310 S.E.2d 452, 456 (Va. 1983); Klein v. Boyle, 1993 U.S. App. LEXIS 27628 (4th Cir. 1993).

[43] Ravenis v. Detroit Gen. Hosp., 63 Mich. App. 79, 234 N.W.2d 411 (1975).

[44] Pearce v. Feinstein, 754 F. Supp. 308 (W.D. N.Y. 1990).

Accreditation Standards. Some states permit accreditation standards to be used to establish the standard of care for accredited hospitals. For example, in 1997, a Texas court decided that standards of the Joint Commission on the Accreditation of Healthcare Organizations (JCAHO) concerning anesthesia practice could be considered but were not determinative.[45] As pointed out in the discussion on institutional rules, some states do not permit privately developed standards to be used to establish the standard of care.

Reference Books. Most courts permit some reference books to be used to establish the standard of care, but only when there is expert testimony that the material in the book is the standard of care. For example, in 2000, the highest court of New York applied this rule to the *Physician's Desk Reference* (PDR), which describes uses of drugs.[46] However, one state uses the PDR as an independent standard of care and permits courts to disregard expert evidence of actual practice.

In 2000, the Pennsylvania Supreme Court decided that treatises could be used only to help explain an expert's opinion. They are not an independent source of standards.[47]

Clinical Guidelines. The development of medical practice guidelines, practice parameters, clinical protocols, and other guidelines for clinical decision-making may introduce a new dimension to the role of written standards.[48] The goal is for compliance with the guidelines to preclude suits or assure their successful defense. At least one medical society sponsored insurer required compliance with guidelines by its insured physicians.[49] Others have developed

---

[45] Denton Reg. Med. Ctr. v. LaCroix, 947 S.W.2d 941 (Tex. Ct. App. 1997).

[46] Spensieri v. Lasky, 94 N.Y.2d 231, 723 N.E.2d 544, 701 N.Y.S.2d 689 (1999); *accord,* Bissett v. Renna, 142 N.H. 788, 710 A.2d 404 (1998); Morlino v. Medical Ctr. of Ocean Cty., 152 N.J. 563, 706 A.2d 721 (1998); *contra,* Fournet v. Roule-Graham, 783 So. 2d 439 (La. App. 2001) [liability can be based on PDR even when only expert testimony is that PDR does not reflect practice].

[47] Aldridge v. Edmunds, 561 Pa. 323, 750 A.2d 292 (2000).

[48] M. W. Salganik, *Medical mistakes: Finding the cure,* BALTIMORE SUN, May 1, 2005, 1D [care guidelines reduce obstetrics suits]; National Health Lawyers Ass'n, COLLOQUIUM REPORT ON LEGAL ISSUES RELATED TO CLINICAL PRACTICE GUIDELINES (1995); J.C. West, *The legal implications of medical practice guidelines,* 27 J.HEALTH & HOSP.L. 97 (1994); E.B. Hirshfield, *Practice parameters and the malpractice liability of physicians,* 263 J.A.M.A. 1556 (1990); FDA, *Guidance on the recognition and use of consensus standards,* 7 HEALTH L. RPTR. [BNA] 353 (1998) [http://www.fda.gov/cdrh] [hereinafter HEALTH L. RPTR. is cited as H.L.R]; *see also* S.B. Ransom et al., *Reduced medicolegal risk by compliance with obstetrical pathways: A case-control study,* 101 OBSTETRICS & GYNECOLOGY 751 (2003).

[49] L. Oberman, *Risk management strategy: Liability insurers stress practice guidelines,* AM. MED. NEWS, Sept. 5, 1994, 1 [Colorado].

guidelines for a variety of purposes,[50] including the promotion of more efficient practice.[51]

In the 1990s, Maine conducted an experiment with these guidelines as a way to reduce medical malpractice claims. However, by the end of the experiment in 1999, there were no reports of the guidelines being used in any malpractice case or having had any impact on liability costs.[52]

Physicians have expressed concerns that guidelines are of varying quality, are sometimes contradictory, and may not be sufficiently sophisticated to deal with complex situations. Some studies indicate that guidelines can help physicians avoid selecting traditional tests or treatments that are ineffective.[53] Efforts to stop the release of guidelines have generally been unsuccessful.[54] In 1994, one state medical society challenged the process that a managed care entity was using for development of guidelines and was able to reach an agreement for more medical society input.[55]

TWO SCHOOLS OF THOUGHT. The proof of what should have been done can become confused when there are two or more professionally accepted approaches. The *respected minority* or *two schools of thought* rule addresses this situation. If a health care professional follows the approach used by a respected minority of the profession, then the duty is to follow that approach properly. Liability cannot be based on the decision not to follow the majority approach.[56] In 1992, the Pennsylvania Supreme Court limited the use of the doctrine to situations where the alternative has been adopted by a considerable number of respected physicians.[57]

---

[50] *E.g.*, *Internists call clinical practice guidelines effective*, 3 H.L.R. 781 (1994).
[51] *E.g.*, *Half of unstable angina cases could be treated outside hospital, AHCPR says*, 3 H.L.R. 339 (1994) [practice guidelines released Mar. 15, 1994].
[52] ME. REV. STAT. ANN. title 24, § 2971-79, repealed Laws 1999, c. 668; General Accounting Office, MEDICAL MALPRACTICE, MAINE'S USE OF PRACTICE GUIDELINES TO REDUCE COSTS (Oct. 1993), GAO/HRD-94-8; J.M. Finder, *The future of practice guidelines: should they constitute conclusive evidence of the standard of care?* 10 HEALTH MATRIX 67 (Wint. 2000)
[53] *E.g.*, I.G. Steill et al., *Implementation of the Ottawa ankle rules*, 271 J.A.M.A. 827 (1994) [reduced use of ankle radiography].
[54] *E.g.*, Sofamor Danek Group, Inc. v. Clinton, 870 F. Supp. 379 (D. D.C. 1994) [deny injunction of AHCPR release of clinical practice guidelines for lower back pain].
[55] *Illinois Blues, medical society strike agreement over guidelines*, 3 H.L.R. 310 (1994); *see also* L. Oberman, *AMA panel on guidelines sorts good from misguided*, AM. MED. NEWS, Jan. 10, 1994, at 1.
[56] Furey v. Thomas Jefferson Univ. Hosp., 325 Pa. Super. 212, 472 A.2d 1083 (1984); Fraijo v. Hartland Hosp., 99 Cal. App. 3d 331, 160 Cal. Rptr. 246 (2d Dist. 1979) [applied to nursing decision].
[57] Jones v. Chidester, 531 Pa. 31, 610 A.2d 964 (1992); *accord*, Yates v. University of West Virginia Bd. of Trustees, 209 W. Va. 487; 549 S.E.2d 681 (2001).

Because part of the informed consent process is the disclosure of alternative treatments, the physician generally should disclose the alternative treatment to the patient before pursuing a minority approach. Failure to disclose the alternative majority approach could result in liability under the informed consent doctrine discussed in Chapter 7.

LOCALITY RULE. In the past, some courts limited the standard of care of health care institutions and professionals to the practice in the same or similar communities. Under this locality rule, experts testifying on the standard of care had to be from the same or similar communities. The rule was designed to avoid finding rural providers liable for not following the practices of urban medical centers. The rule sometimes made it difficult to obtain expert testimony. Many courts abandoned the rule, permitting any expert to testify when familiar with the relevant standard of care. The jury usually may consider the expert's degree of familiarity with the community in deciding what weight to give the testimony.

Several states as part of their tort reform efforts have enacted statutes that have reinstated some aspects of the locality rule, restricting which physicians can testify as experts.[58]

LEGALLY IMPOSED STANDARDS. Courts sometimes impose a more stringent legal standard not previously recognized by the profession when they find the professional standards to be deficient. For example, in 1974, the Washington Supreme Court established a legal standard that glaucoma tests must be given to all ophthalmology patients, although the universal practice of ophthalmologists was to administer such tests only to patients over age forty and to patients with possible symptoms of glaucoma.[59] The court disregarded the evidence that so few cases would be discovered that expanded testing would not be cost-effective. The court found the ophthalmologist liable for failing to administer the test to a patient under age forty with no symptoms of glaucoma. In another case, in which a woman was killed by a psychiatric patient, the California Supreme Court found liability for the psychiatrist's failure to warn the woman that his patient had threatened to kill her, even though other psychiatrists would have acted in the same manner.[60]

---

[58] *E.g.,* FLA. STAT. §766.102(2)(c).

[59] Helling v. Carey, 83 Wash. 2d 514, 519 P.2d 981 (1974).

[60] Tarasoff v. Regents of Univ. of Cal., 17 Cal. 3d 425, 131 Cal. Rptr. 14, 551 P.2d 334 (1976).

The national standard of peer review of physicians in hospitals was changed by a 1973 California trial court decision.[61] A hospital was found liable for injuries resulting from treatment provided by an independent staff physician because the hospital had not made use of available information that would have alerted it to the surgeon's propensity to commit malpractice. The hospital met all of JCAH's standards in effect at the time the patient was injured, but the court ruled that the hospital should have had a better system of becoming aware of available information and acting on it.

BREACH OF DUTY. After the duty is proved, the second element that must be proved is the breach of this duty — that is, a deviation in some manner from the standard of care. Something was done that should not have been done, or something was not done that should have been done. There is little law related to this element; it is a matter of proving what happened within the rules of evidence. The legal issues relate to the duty against which the proven behavior is measured.

11-1.3 What Constitutes a Compensable Injury?

The third element of the proof of negligence is injury. The person making the claim must demonstrate physical, financial, or emotional injury. In many malpractice cases, the existence of the injury is very clear by the time of the suit, although there still may be disagreement concerning the dollar value of the injury.

One issue that remains controversial is when to allow claims that result only in negligently inflicted emotional injury.

NEGLIGENTLY INFLICTED EMOTIONAL INJURY. Most courts allow suits based solely on negligently inflicted emotional injuries only in limited situations. These injuries usually are compensated only when they accompany physical injuries. Intentional infliction of emotional injury is generally compensated without proof of physical injury. Negligently inflicted emotional injuries are sometimes compensable without accompanying physical injuries. For example, compensation is available in some states when the plaintiff was in the "zone of danger" created by the defendant's negligence — that is, when the plaintiff was actually exposed to risk of injury. A few states also compensate plaintiffs who witness injury to close relatives. A California court permitted a father to sue for his emotional injuries from being

---

[61] Gonzales v. Nork, No. 228566 (Cal. Super. Ct. Nov. 19, 1973), *rev'd on other grounds*, 20 Cal. 3d 500, 573 P.2d 458 (1978).

present in the delivery room when his wife died and from placing his hands on her body after her death and feeling the unborn child die.[62]

This issue has been presented in several cases where persons have had possible exposure to HIV infection or have been erroneously told that they have HIV infection. They claim emotional injury without evidence of actual infection. Courts have reached different conclusions on whether they have a compensable injury.[63]

11-1.4 How Is Legal Causation Proven?

The fourth element is causation. The breach of duty must be proved to have legally caused the injury. For example, when a treatment is negligently administered (which is a breach of duty), a patient may subsequently die (which is an injury), but the person suing must still prove a substantial likelihood that the patient would have lived if the treatment had been administered properly. Causation is often the most difficult element to prove.[64]

Another example is a Texas case concerning a nurse who gave a patient solid food immediately after colon surgery (which is a breach of duty), and eight days later the ends of the sutured colon came apart (which is an injury).[65] Because of the time lag, the patient was not able to prove causation.

In 2001, an Illinois court addressed a case where nurses had not notified the surgeon of the patient's symptoms, which breached their duty. However, the surgeon testified that he was aware of the

---

[62] Austin v. Regents of Univ. of Cal., 89 Cal. App. 3d 354, 152 Cal. Rptr. 420 (4th Dist.1979).

[63] *E.g.*, Majca v. Beekil, 183 Ill. 2d 407, 701 N.E.2d 1084 (1998) [proof of actual exposure to HIV required to claim fear of contracting AIDS]; Natale v. Gottlieb Mem. Hosp., 314 Ill. App. 3d 885, 733 N.E.2d 380 (1st Dist. 2000) [failure to prove actual exposure from use of nonsterile endoscope]; R.J. v. Humana of Fla., Inc., 652 So. 2d 360 (Fla. 1995) [impact rule applies to damages claim for negligent HIV diagnosis claim, so must show emotional distress flows from physical injury of impact; when misdiagnosis results in harmful treatment, treatment may provide impact]; Lubowitz v. Albert Einstein Med. Ctr., 424 Pa. Super. 468, 623 A.2d 3 (1993) [no claim for fear of AIDS due to mistakenly being told exposed to HIV]; Carroll v. Sisters of St. Francis Health Servs., 868 S.W.2d 585 (Tenn. 1993) [no recovery for negligent infliction of emotional distress based on fear of AIDS without showing exposure to HIV virus]; Herbert v. Regents of Univ. of Cal., 26 Cal. App. 4th 782, 31 Cal. Rptr. 2d 709 (2d Dist. 1994) [no claim for emotional distress for HIV fear from needle scratch where HIV chance minimal]; Marchica v. Long Island R. Co., 31 F.3d 1197 (2d Cir. 1994), *aff'g*, 810 F. Supp. 445 (E.D. N.Y.), *cert. denied*, 513 U.S. 1079 (1995) [affirming jury verdict for employee for fear of AIDS after puncture wound].

[64] *E.g.*, Smith v. Sofamor, S.N.C., 21 F. Supp. 2d 918 (W.D. Wis. 1998) [insufficient testimony surgical device caused injury]; Hodges v. Secretary of DHHS, 9 F.3d 958 (Fed. Cir. 1993) [failure to prove causation of death of infant after DPT vaccination]; Campos v. Ysleta Gen. Hosp., Inc., 836 S.W.2d 791 (Tex. Ct. App. 1992) [failure to prove causation of child's death].

[65] Lenger v. Physician's Gen. Hosp., 455 S.W.2d 703 (Tex. 1970).

patient's condition and would not have changed his diagnosis or treatment if contacted with the nurse's information. Thus, the nurse's breach of duty did not cause the patient's injuries.[66]

Causation can be proved in many cases, as illustrated by an Iowa case involving a baby born with Rh blood incompatibility.[67] An outdated reagent was used for blood tests for bilirubin, and the tests erroneously indicated a safe level. When the error was discovered, the high bilirubin level had caused severe permanent brain damage. The hospital and pathologists were liable because accurate tests would have led to timely therapy that probably would have prevented brain damage.

LOSS OF CHANCE. Some courts have adopted a new standard of causation, the *loss of chance* of recovery, making it easier for plaintiffs to win suits.[68] Under this standard, the plaintiff need only show that the breach of the standard led to a loss of chance of recovery or survival, rather than that the breach caused the injury. Initially, this standard of causation required a showing of a loss of chance of recovery/survival of greater than 50 percent.[69] However, in recent years, some courts have allowed claims to proceed in cases where the loss of chance of recovery was less than 50 percent. For example, in 1998, the Iowa Supreme Court allowed a claim for lost chance of survival based on the failure to resuscitate, even when the survival possibility with resuscitation was only 10 percent.[70] Other courts have rejected this change, retaining the traditional proximate cause standard.[71] Virginia adopted a hybrid approach under which a showing of loss of a substantial possibility of survival is sufficient to create a jury question, but the jury must be instructed using the traditional proximate cause instruction.[72]

BREAKING THE CHAIN OF CAUSATION. Sometimes subsequent providers' errors can break the chain of causation.[73] A New

---

[66] Snelson v. Kamm, 319 Ill. App. 3d 116, 745 N.E.2d 128 (4th Dist. 2001), *aff'd in relevant part*, 204 Ill. 2d 1, 787 N.E.2d 796 (2003).

[67] Schnebly v. Baker, 217 N.W.2d 708 (Iowa 1974).

[68] *E.g.*, Lord v. Lovett, 770 A.2d 1103 (N.H. 2001); Delany v. Cade, 255 Kan. 199, 873 P.2d 175 (1994) [may make claim for loss of chance of better recovery, not just loss of chance of survival]; Annotation, *Medical malpractice: "loss of chance" causality*, 54 A.L.R. 4TH 10.

[69] *E.g.*, Wallace v. St. Francis Hosp. & Med. Ctr., 44 Conn. App. 257, 688 A.2d 352 (1997).

[70] Wendland v. Sparks, 574 N.W.2d 327 (Iowa 1998).

[71] *E.g.*, McKain v. Bisson, 12 F.3d 692 (7th Cir. 1993) [applying Indiana law]; Kilpatrick v. Bryant, 868 S.W.2d 594 (Tenn. 1993).

[72] Blondel v. Hays, 241 Va. 467, 403 S.E.2d 340 (1991).

[73] *E.g.*, Dillon v. Medical Ctr. Hosp., 98 Ohio App. 3d 510, 648 N.E.2d 1375 (1993), *appeal dismissed*, 72 Ohio St. 3d 1201, 647 N.E.2d 166 (1995) [hospital not liable, despite negligence of nurses, because causation broken by acts of independent physicians].

York case arose from the suicide of a patient after a transfer.[74] The referring hospital breached its duty by failing to note the patient's suicidal tendencies in the transfer documents sent with the patient. The referring hospital avoided liability because the receiving hospital did not look at the transfer documents until after the patient was discharged. Thus, the transferring hospital's breach had no impact on the outcome.

STANDARDS FOR SCIENTIFIC TESTIMONY ON CAUSATION. As mentioned in Expert Testimony in Section 11-1.2, in 1993, the United States Supreme Court established a stricter standard for the admissibility of scientific testimony in federal courts.[75] The *Daubert* standards focus on the quality of the scientific basis for the expert opinion. This has had a major impact on expert testimony concerning causation. This has made it more difficult to pursue products liability suits claiming that products caused adverse conditions.[76]

Generally, the expert must point to reliable scientific evidence to support an opinion of causation. The observation that one event typically follows another is insufficient.[77] However, in malpractice cases, while recognizing that *Daubert* standards of reliability apply, federal courts are generally somewhat more flexible concerning medical testimony on causation.[78]

11-1.5 When Does the Res Ipsa Loquitur Exception Apply?

One exception to the requirement that the four elements be proved is the doctrine of *res ipsa loquitur*, "the thing speaks for itself." The doctrine was created in an 1863 English case that arose from a barrel flying out of an upper story window and smashing a pedestrian.[79]

---

[74] Rivera v. New York City Health & Hosps. Corp., 72 N.Y.2d 1021, 531 N.E.2d 644, 534 N.Y.S.2d 923 (1988).

[75] Daubert v. Merrell Dow Pharmaceuticals, Inc., 509 U.S. 579 (1993); Kumho Tire Co. v. Carmichael, 524 U.S. 936 (1999 [*Daubert* applies to nonscientific experts].

[76] *E.g.*, Daubert v. Merrell Dow Pharmaceuticals, Inc., 43 F.3d 1311 (9th Cir. 1995), *upon remand from*, 509 U.S. 579 (1993) [expert scientific testimony not admissible to prove Bendectin caused plaintiff's birth defects]; Sorensen v. Shaklee Corp., 31 F.3d 638 (8th Cir. 1994) [affirming summary judgment for manufacturer in suit claiming mental retardation due to alfalfa tablets; proposed expert testimony did not have sufficient scientific validity in light of *Daubert*].

[77] *E.g.*, Washburn v. Merck & Co., 2000 U.S. App. LEXIS 8601 (2d Cir. 2000).

[78] *E.g.*, Sullivan v. U.S. Dept. of Navy, 365 F.3d 827 (9th Cir. 2004) [in medical malpractice, physician causation testimony could meet *Daubert* reliability requirements when backed by textbooks]; *but see* Tanner v. Westbrook, 174 F.3d 542 (5th Cir. 1999) [insufficient evidence of specialized knowledge on causation].

[79] Byrne v. Boadle, 2 H.& C. 722 (Exch. 1863).

When the pedestrian tried to sue the building owner, the owner claimed that the four elements had to be proved. The pedestrian could not find out what went wrong in the building, and the case would have been lost. The court ruled that there should be liability when someone has clearly done something wrong, and the court developed the *res ipsa loquitur* doctrine.

The doctrine applies when the following elements can be proved:

1. The accident is of a kind that does not happen without negligence,[80]
2. The apparent cause is in the exclusive control of the defendants,
3. The person suing could not have contributed to the difficulties,[81]
4. Evidence of the true cause is inaccessible to the person suing, and
5. The fact of injury is evident.

Courts have frequently applied this rule to two types of malpractice cases: (1) sponges and other foreign objects unintentionally left in the body[82] and (2) injuries to parts of the body distant from the site of treatment, such as nerve damage to a hand during a hysterectomy.[83] Some courts have extended the applicability of the rule to some other types of malpractice cases.[84]

Liability is not automatic in these cases. The defendants are permitted to explain why the injury was not the result of negligence.[85] For example, a physician could establish the absence of negligence by proving the sponge was left in the body because the patient had to be closed quickly on an emergency basis to save the patient's life

---

[80] *E.g.*, Robb *ex rel.* Robb v. Anderton, 864 P.2d 1322 (Utah Ct. App. 1993) [not *res ipsa loquitur*, no showing cardiac arrest during surgery would not occur without negligence]; Chism v. Campbell, 553 N.W.2d 741 (Neb. 1996) [not *res ipsa loquitur*, tooth damage during surgery was known inherent risk of general anesthesia]; Leone v. United Health Servs., 282 A.D.2d 860, 723 N.Y.S.2d 260 (3d Dept. 2001). [not *res ipsa loquitur*, only expert could say whether nerve injury during vasectomy could only occur with negligence]; *see also* States v. Lourdes Hosp., 100 N.Y.2d 208, 792 N.E.2d 151 (2003) [expert testimony can be used to establish that damage would not occur without negligence].

[81] *E.g.* Posta v. Chung-Loy, 306 N.J. Super. 182, 703 A.2d 368 (App. Div. 1997) [*res ipsa loquitur* not applicable to hernia one year after surgery, no evidence showing patient's own actions did not cause or contribute].

[82] *E.g.*, Leonard v. Watsonville Commun. Hosp., 47 Cal. 2d 509, 305 P.2d 36 (1956).

[83] *E.g.*, Parks v. Perry, 68 N.C. App. 202, 314 S.E.2d 287 (1984); Wick v. Henderson, 485 N.W.2d 645 (Iowa 1992) [damage to ulnar nerve during gallbladder surgery]; Baczuk v. Salt Lake Reg. Med. Ctr., 8 P.3d 1037 (Utah App. 2000) [pressure injury to site distant from surgery].

[84] *E.g.*, Sanchez v. Bay Gen. Hosp., 116 Cal. App. 3d 678, 172 Cal. Rptr. 342 (4th Dist. 1981); Reilly v. Straub, 282 N.W.2d 688 (Iowa 1979).

[85] *E.g.*, Mulkey v. Tubb, 535 So. 2d 1294 (La. Ct. App. 1988) [adequate explanation of damage to site distant from surgery].

and there was no time for a sponge count. The evidence necessary to avoid liability varies among states because of variation in the degree to which the burden of proof shifts to the defendant in *res ipsa loquitur* cases.

11-2 What Are Intentional Torts, and How Do They Differ from Negligent Torts?

Some actions are considered to be intentional torts. For intentional torts, all that needs to be proven is that the wrongful contact occurred and that it caused injury. For some intentional torts, at least nominal damages are assumed from the occurrence of the action. There is no requirement that a standard of care be proven. There are privileges and other defenses to some intentional torts, but the burden of proving the applicability of these defenses usually belongs to the defendant. In some states, procedural requirements for malpractice cases do not apply to intentional tort cases.[86]

Intentional torts include assault and battery (11-2.1), defamation (11-2.2), false imprisonment (11-2.3), invasion of privacy (11-2.4), intentional infliction of emotional distress (11-2.5), malicious prosecution (11-2.6), and abuse of process (11-2.7).

11-2.1 Assault and Battery

An *assault* is an action that puts another person in apprehension of being touched in a manner that is offensive, insulting, provoking, or physically injurious without lawful authority or consent. No actual touching is required; the assault is the credible threat of being touched in this manner.

If actual touching occurs, then the action is called *battery*. Liability for assault and battery compensates persons for violations of their right to be free from nonconsensual invasions of their person. Assault or battery can occur when medical treatment is attempted or performed without consent or lawful authority.[87] Assault or battery

---

[86] *E.g.,* Darwin v. Gooberman, 339 N.J. Super. 467, 772 A.2d 399 (App. Div. 2001) [affidavit of merit not required for battery claim]; *but see* Williams v. Boyle, 72 P.3d 392 (Colo. App. 2003) [certificate of review required for defamation claim for medical record entry where privilege may apply].

[87] *E.g.,* Bommareddy v. Superior Court, 222 Cal. App. 3d 1017, 272 Cal. Rptr. 246 (5th Dist. 1990), *rev. denied,* 1990 Cal. LEXIS 4989 (Oct. 30, 1990), *disapproved on other grounds,* Central Pathology Serv. Med. Clinic v. Superior Court, 3 Cal. 4th 181, 10 Cal. Rptr. 2d 208, 832 P.2d 924 (1992).

can occur in other circumstances, such as during attempts to restrain patients without lawful authority.

11-2.2 Defamation

Defamation is wrongful injury to a person's reputation. *Libel* is written defamation, and *slander* is spoken defamation. The defamatory statement must be communicated to a third person; a statement is not defamatory if made only to the person impugned. A defamation claim can arise from inappropriate release of inaccurate medical information or from untruthful statements about other staff members.

The defenses to a defamation claim include truth and privilege. A true statement is not defamatory even if it injures another's reputation. Some communications, although otherwise defamatory, are privileged because the law recognizes a higher duty to disclose the particular information to certain persons.

Courts have recognized the importance of communicating information concerning a staff member's performance to appropriate supervisors and officials. Such communications are protected by a "qualified privilege" when they are made in good faith to persons who need to know. This protection means that liability will not be imposed for communications later proved to be false if they were made without malice. Malice is usually found when the communication was made with knowledge of its falsity or with reckless disregard of whether it was false. An example of the qualified privilege is a 1988 New York appellate court decision in which a hospital official's statements to other officials concerning a physician were found to be privileged.[88] Another example is a 1991 Ohio case resulting from a nurse's statements at a nursing technician's predisciplinary hearing.[89] The communication must be made within appropriate channels because discussions with others will not be protected by the qualified privilege. As discussed in Chapter 8, many states have enacted broader statutory privileges or immuni-

---

[88] Murphy v. Herfort, 140 A.D.2d 415, 528 N.Y.S.2d 117 (2d Dept. 1988); *see also, e.g.*, Malone v. Longo, 463 F. Supp. 139 (E.D. N.Y. 1979) [nurse report to supervisor about physician order protected]; Kletschka v. Abbott-Northwestern Hosp., Inc., 417 N.W.2d 752 (Minn. Ct. App. 1988) [performance evaluation protected].

[89] Bartlett v. Daniel Drake Mem. Hosp., 75 Ohio App. 3d 334, 599 N.E.2d 403 (1991).

ties for participants in some peer review activities. These statutes can provide protection from some defamation claims. As discussed in Chapter 8, many states prohibit use of some peer review committee proceedings and reports in any civil suit, which in effect may make it impossible to pursue most defamation cases for statements within the peer review process.[90]

In 2003, a Colorado court addressed a case in which a patient challenged a medical record entry that said that she was experiencing a mental health disorder. The court decided that entries in the medical record could be defamatory, but that there was a qualified privilege for medical record entries.[91]

11-2.3 False Imprisonment

False imprisonment is the unlawful restriction of a person's freedom. Holding persons against their will by physical restraint, barriers, or even threats of harm can constitute false imprisonment if not legally justified. Claims of false imprisonment can arise from patients who are being detained inappropriately or from patients who are challenging their commitment for being mentally ill.[92] Health care institutions generally have common law authority to detain patients who are disoriented.[93] All states have a legal procedure to obtain authorization to detain some categories of persons who are mentally ill, engage in substance abuse, or are infected with contagious diseases. When relying on these state statutes, care should be taken to follow the specified procedures. In 1998, an Illinois appeals court ruled that a person could sue for false imprisonment when committed in violation of a time limit in state law.[94] When patients are oriented, competent, and not legally committed, staff should avoid detaining them unless authorized by institutional policy or by an institutional administrator. There are few situations in which institutions are justified in authorizing detention of such patients.

---

[90] *E.g.*, Feldman v. Glucoft, 522 So. 2d 798 (Fla. 1988), *appeal after remand*, 580 So. 2d 866 (Fla. 3d DCA) [no evidence extrinsic to proceedings alleged, judgment for defendants affirmed), *rev. denied*, 591 So. 2d 181 (Fla. 1991), *cert. denied*, 503 U.S. 960 (1992).

[91] Williams v. Boyle, 72 P.3d 392 (Colo. App. 2003).

[92] *E.g,* Skobin v. County of Los Angeles, 2004 Cal. App. Unpub. LEXIS 7617 (2d Dist.).

[93] *E.g.*, Boles v. Milwaukee County, 150 Wis. 2d 801, 443 N.W.2d 679 (App. 1989).

[94] Arthur v. Lutheran Gen. Hosp., Inc., 295 Ill. App. 3d 818, 692 N.E.2d 1238 (1st Dist. 1998).

11-2.4 Invasion of Privacy

Claims for *invasion of privacy* can arise from unauthorized release of information concerning patients. Not all releases of information are intentional torts that violate the right of privacy. For example, in 1982, the Minnesota Supreme Court found that even though the patient had requested that information not be released, it was not an invasion of privacy to disclose orally that the patient had been discharged from the hospital and that she had given birth when the information was disclosed in response to a direct inquiry concerning that patient at a time near her stay in the hospital.[95] Even when a disclosure is not an intentional tort, the disclosure can violate state or federal laws and regulations; generally providers should attempt to avoid release of discharge and birth information when the patient requests nondisclosure.

Sometimes information such as a child abuse or contagious disease report is required to be disclosed by law. These disclosures (discussed in Chapter 8) are not an invasion of privacy because they are legally authorized.

11-2.5 Intentional Infliction of Emotional Distress

Intentional infliction of emotional distress is another intentional tort that includes outrageous conduct causing emotional trauma. This tort is easy to avoid by remembering to treat patients and their families in a civilized fashion, but such treatment was apparently forgotten in the following examples of this tort.

In a 2001 North Carolina case, the court decided that a physician could be sued for distributing to other local doctors a list of names and addresses of the jurors, witnesses, and plaintiffs who had found a codefendant physician liable in a malpractice case.[96] In a Tennessee case, a hospital staff member gave a woman the body of her newborn baby preserved in a jar of formaldehyde.[97] In an Ohio case, a physician sent repeated checkup reminders to a deceased patient's family who had sued him for malpractice in her death.[98]

---

[95] Koudski v. Hennepin County Med. Ctr., 317 N.W.2d 705 (Minn. 1982).

[96] Burgess v. Busby, 544 S.E.2d 4 (N.C. Ct. App. 2001).

[97] Johnson v. Woman's Hosp., 527 S.W.2d 133 (Tenn. Ct. App. 1975).

[98] McCormick v. Haley, 37 Ohio App. 2d 73, 307 N.E.2d 34 (1973).

In an Illinois case, statements had allegedly been made in a public area of a hospital accusing family members of trying to kill a patient when they were seeking to discontinue life support. The court concluded that this provided a basis for a jury to impose liability for intentional infliction of emotional distress.[99]

However, in 2003, a Georgia court affirmed dismissal of a case when a woman who had miscarried discovered the fetus in her bloody clothes that a nurse had returned to her on discharge. The Court found that there was emotional distress caused by finding the fetus but that there was no evidence that the nurse's conduct had been intentional or reckless. At worst they had been negligent, and there was no intentional tort.[100]

11-2.6 Malicious Prosecution

Some unjustifiable or harassing litigation constitutes an intentional tort called *malicious prosecution.*

A plaintiff alleging malicious prosecution must prove that (1) the other person filed a suit against the plaintiff, (2) the suit ended in favor of the plaintiff, (3) there was no probable cause for filing the suit, and (4) the other person filed the suit because of malice. It is rare for health care entities to be sued for malicious prosecution. It is unusual for malicious prosecution suits to be successful.[101] A Michigan trial court permitted a jury to find Blue Cross liable for malicious prosecution of a provider. Blue Cross had reported to law enforcement officials that a dentist had filed claims for which he was not entitled to reimbursement. The dentist was acquitted when prosecuted, and he sued for malicious prosecution, claiming that Blue Cross knew that his billing was permitted. In 1995, an appellate court upheld the liability of Blue Cross, but in 1998, the Michigan Supreme Court reversed, finding that Blue Cross could not be liable.[102] The court found that private entities that had reported possible crimes to law enforcement could not be liable because the prosecution was initiated in the sole discretion of the prosecutor and

---

[99] Gragg v. Calandra, 297 Ill. App. 3d 639, 696 N.E.2d 1282 (2d Dist. 1998).

[100] Roddy v. Tanner Med. Ctr., 262 Ga. App. 202, 585 S.E.2d 175 (2003).

[101] *E.g.*, Nicholson v. Lucas, 26 Cal. Rptr. 4th 778, 26 Cal. Rptr. 2d 778 (5th Dist. 1994) [dismissal of dentist's claim that initiation of medical staff proceedings was malicious prosecution].

[102] Matthews v. Blue Cross & Blue Shield, 456 Mich. 365, 572 N.W.2d 603 (1998).

state police had conducted an independent investigation supporting probable cause to believe a crime had been committed. In 1990, a New York court found that a hospital had not committed malicious prosecution by having a patient's son arrested for criminal trespass after he became disruptive. Dismissal of the prosecution by the prosecutor in the interest of justice did not constitute the suit ending in favor of the son, and the second requirement for a malicious prosecution suit was not met.[103] In 1999, a federal appellate court ruled that a physician could not bring a malicious prosecution claim against a management company that had unsuccessfully sued him for defamation for writing a critical article.[104]

After winning malpractice suits, some physicians have sued the patient and/or the patient's attorney for malicious prosecution. Generally, public policy favors giving people an opportunity to present their case to the courts for redress of wrongs; the law protects them when they act in good faith upon reasonable grounds in commencing either a civil or a criminal suit. Few countersuits have been successful.[105]

11-2.7 Abuse of Process

Some other misuses of the legal system constitute intentional torts called *abuse of process*. A plaintiff alleging abuse of process must prove that (1) a legal process, for example, a notice of suit, subpoena, notice of deposition, or garnishment, was used against the plaintiff; (2) the use was primarily to accomplish a purpose for which it was not designed; and (3) the plaintiff was harmed by this misuse. Suits asserting abuse of process are rarely successful.[106]

---

[103] Macleay v. Arden Hill Hosp., 164 A.D.2d 228, 563 N.Y.S.2d 333 (3d Dept. 1990); *but see,* Steele v. Breinholt, 747 P.2d 433 (Utah Ct. App. 1987) [nursing home visitor arrested for criminal trespass charges presented jury question on malicious prosecution].

[104] Schwartz v. Coastal Physician Group, Inc., 172 F.3d 63 (without op.), 1999 U.S. App. LEXIS 2844 (10th Cir.).

[105] Dutt v. Kremp, 894 P.2d 354 (Nev. 1995); Spencer v. Burglass, 288 So. 2d 68 (La. Ct. App. 1974); *but see* Bull v. McCluskey, 96 Nev. 706, 615 P.2d 957 (1980); Miller v. Rosenberg, 196 Ill. 2d 50, 749 N.E.2d 946 [law making malicious prosecution suits easier is constitutional]; *Doctor sued for malpractice fights back with suit of his own,* AP, June 7, 2000 [Ky. jury award doctor $72,000].

[106] *E.g.,* Garrett v. Fisher Titus Hosp., 318 F. Supp. 2d 562 (N.D. Ohio 2004); Hanson v. Hancock County Mem. Hosp., 938 F. Supp. 1419 (N.D. Iowa 1996).

11-3 What Are the Major Defenses to Liability Suits for Torts?

There are several possible defenses to liability suits for torts.

1. When a claim has been litigated, a second suit is usually barred by *res judicata* or *collateral estoppel*.
2. When a claim has been settled, usually a suit is barred by the *release* obtained in the settlement.
3. There are time limits within which most suits must be brought, and a suit that is too late is barred by the *statute of limitations*.
4. Some persons are granted *immunity* from some suits.
5. Persons can sign *exculpatory contracts* that grant contractual immunity, but usually these are not permitted in health care settings.
6. Persons can sign *arbitration agreements*, so that they cannot sue but use the arbitration process.
7. The claimants own conduct can sometimes bar liability or reduce the amount of liability due to *contributory negligence* or *comparative negligence*.
8. In some states, there are *damage caps* that limit the amount of liability.

RES JUDICATA AND COLLATERAL ESTOPPEL. As discussed in Chapter 1, sometimes lawsuits are barred by the fact that they deal with matters that have been litigated before. For example, a Maryland court ruled that a physician's unsuccessful defamation suit against a hospital barred a new suit against nurses for the same conduct.[107] However, the Ohio Supreme Court ruled that a successful malpractice claim during life does not bar a wrongful death claim after death.[108]

RELEASE. Another defense is release. When a claim is settled, the claimant usually signs a release. When a release has been signed, it will generally bar a future suit based on the same incident. Sometimes release of one defendant will release other defendants. A Maryland court ruled that releasing a pathologist released the hospital.[109] However, the North Dakota Supreme Court held that

---

[107] Deleon v. Slear, 328 Md. 569, 616 A.2d 380 (1992).
[108] Thompson v. Wing, 70 Ohio St. 3d 176, 637 N.E.2d 917 (1994); *accord*, Schwarder v. United States, 974 F.2d 1118 (9th Cir. 1992).
[109] Anne Arundel Med. Ctr., Inc. v. Condon, 102 Md. App. 408, 649 A.2d 1189 (1994); *contra*, JFK Med. Ctr., Inc. v. Price, 647 So. 2d 833 (Fla. 1994) [continuation of wrongful death malpractice suit against passive tortfeasor after settlement with active tortfeasor not barred].

releasing a physician's employer from liability in a medical malpractice action did not also release the physician.[110]

In the past, some courts permitted agreements where a settling defendant retained a financial interest in the plaintiff's recovery and remained a party in the trial. The Texas and Florida Supreme Courts declared such agreements to be void as violations of public policy.[111]

Releases on behalf of minors are often later attacked by the minors,[112] and special attention needs to be focused on complying with state requirements to make such releases binding. In some states, it may be necessary to obtain court approval of a settlement on behalf of a minor.[113]

STATUTE OF LIMITATIONS. All states have laws, generally called *statutes of limitations,* which limit the time in which suits may be filed. Suits are barred after the time has expired. The time limit varies depending on the nature of the suit and the applicable state law. States have adopted different definitions of when the time starts, including (1) the time the incident occurs,[114] (2) the time the injury is discovered,[115] (3) the time the cause of the injury is or should have been discovered, and (4) the time the patient ceases receiving care from the negligent provider.[116] Some courts have had trouble accepting formulas that can result in the claim being cut off

---

[110] Keator v. Gale, 1997 N.D. 46, 561 N.W.2d 286 (1997).

[111] Elbaor v. Smith, 845 S.W.2d 240 (Tex. 1992); Dosdourian v. Carsten, 624 So. 2d 241 (Fla. 1993); Annotation, *Validity and effect of "Mary Carter" or similar agreement setting maximum liability of cotortfeaser and providing for reduction or extinguishment thereof relative to recovery against nonagreeing cotortfeaser,* 22 A.L.R. 5TH 483.

[112] *E.g.*, Mitchell v. Mitchell, 963 S.W.2d 222 (Ky. Ct. App. 1998) [release to settle personal injury claim of emancipated and married 17-year-old was void due to incapacity]; *but see* Zivich v. Mentor Soccer Club, Inc., 82 Ohio St. 3d 367, 696 N.E.2d 201 (1998) [exculpatory agreement in favor of volunteers and sponsors of nonprofit sports activity signed by mother of 7-year-old was enforceable against both parents and child].

[113] *E.g.*, Bowden v. Hutzel Hosp, 252 Mich. App. 566, 652 N.W.2d 529 (2002) [settlement remanded to trial court to hold hearing on the minor's best interests before approval]; Ott v. Little Co. of Mary Hosp., 273 Ill. App. 3d 563, 652 N.E.2d 1051 (1st Dist. 1995) [trial judge did not abuse discretion in approving $2 million settlement for minor over objections of parents].

[114] *E.g.*, Nelson v. American Red Cross, 307 U.S. App. D.C. 52, 26 F.3d 193 (1994) [suit for death from HIV barred by statute of limitations, which started when blood given not when AIDS appeared]; Weiss v. Rojanasathit, 975 S.W.2d 113 (Mo. 1998) [rejecting theory of continuing tort; holding statute of limitations period begins to run from date of occurrence of alleged negligent act]; Charter Peachford Behavioral Health Sys., Inc. v. Kohout, 233 Ga. App. 452, 504 S.E.2d 514 (1998) [statute of limitations in claim of misdiagnosis of mental illness began to run when misdiagnosis occurred, not when misdiagnosis recognized].

[115] *E.g.*, Katz v. Children's Hosp., 28 F.3d 1520 (9th Cir. 1994) [under California law, time period started when harm experienced].

[116] *See* Tullock v. Eck, 311 Ark. 564, 845 S.W.2d 517 (1993) [limiting continuous treatment doctrine]; Anderson v. George, 717 A.2d 876 (D.C. App. 1998) [continuous treatment doctrine applies to medical malpractice cases in District of Columbia].

before the potential plaintiff is aware of the injury,[117] but other courts have accepted this result.[118]

The rules are complicated in many states. For example, in Florida, medical malpractice cases must be filed within two years from when the incident should have been discovered, but no more than four years after the incident unless fraudulent concealment or intentional misrepresentation by the provider prevents discovery within the four years, which extends the time to within two years from when the incident should have been discovered, but no more than seven years after the incident.[119] Other states extend the time when there is fraudulent concealment or intentional misrepresentation.[120] Which time limit applies can itself be the subject of litigation. For example, in 1997, the South Dakota Supreme Court ruled that the two-year malpractice statute of limitations applied to a claim for failure to notify of problems associated with a jaw implant, rather than the longer statute of limitations for fraud, as asserted by the plaintiff.[121]

The time limit can be quite long, especially for injuries to children. In many states, the time period for suits by minors does not start until they become adults.[122] This means that suits arising out of care of newborns may be filed eighteen or more years later. Some states have special rules for minors that do not extend the period to adulthood but give minors more time than adults.[123]

---

[117] *E.g.*, McCollum v. Sisters of Charity, 799 S.W.2d 15 (Ky. 1990) [violates state constitution to cut off claim before it could be discovered]; Marin v. Richey, 674 N.E.2d 1015 (Ind. Ct. App. 1997) [finding unconstitutional a two-year statute of limitations requiring injured plaintiff to sue before she reasonably could have learned of injury].

[118] *E.g.*, Doe v. Shands Teaching Hosp. & Clinics, Inc., 614 So. 2d 1170 (Fla. 1st DCA 1993) [statute of limitations for medical malpractice constitutional even for those who could not have known of injury before time limit].

[119] FLA. STAT. § 95.11(4)(b).

[120] *E.g.*, Roberts v. Francis, 128 F.3d 647 (8th Cir. 1997) [physician's nondisclosure of removal of ovary was fraudulent concealment extending time]; McDonald v. United States, 843 F.2d 247 (6th Cir. 1988) [reassurances of complete recovery can extend time]; Muller v. Thaut, 230 Neb. 244, 430 N.W.2d 884 (1988) [fraudulent concealment].

[121] Bruske v. Hille, 1997 S.D. 108, 567 N.W.2d 872.

[122] *E.g.*, IOWA CODE § 614.8; Annotation, *Medical malpractice statutes of limitation minority provisions*, 62 A.L.R. 4TH 758; *see also* Barnes v. Sabatino, 205 Ga. App. 773, 423 S.E.2d 686 (1992) [17-year-old not covered by special rule for minors which applied only to persons under age 5]; *contra*, FLA. STAT. § 95.11(4)(b) [minors subject to same time limit as adults]; Plummer v. Gillieson, 44 Mass. App. Ct. 578, 692 N.E.2d 528 (1998) [minors subject to same time limit as adults].

[123] *E.g.*, WIS. STAT. § 893.56; Partin v. St. Francis Hosp., 296 Ill. App. 3d 220, 694 N.E.2d 574 (1st Dist. 1998) [statute of limitations baring claims of minors after eight years constitutional].

IMMUNITY. Sovereign immunity, charitable immunity, and various statutory immunities may be available in some situations.

Governmental hospitals are generally protected by *sovereign immunity* and cannot be sued unless the immunity has been waived. Some state courts have ruled that only governmental functions, not proprietary functions, are protected by sovereign immunity. Most courts have ruled that governmental hospitals are governmental functions.[124]

The federal government and many states have enacted laws, usually called *tort claims acts*, that partially waive sovereign immunity and permit claims against governmental entities, but only if certain procedures are followed. These laws often also place limits on the liability.[125] If a governmental hospital purchases liability insurance or establishes a liability trust fund, some courts find that sovereign immunity is waived to the extent of the insurance or trust fund.[126] A Minnesota court decided that the waiver applied even when the insurer was insolvent and unable to pay, but the Minnesota Supreme Court reversed the decision, limiting the waiver to collectible insurance.[127] In some states, sovereign immunity also protects employees.[128]

---

[124] *E.g.*, Hyde v. University of Mich. Bd. of Regents, 426 Mich. 223, 393 N.W.2d 847 (1986) [public general hospital is governmental function]. Public hospitals were later removed by statute in Michigan. McCummings v. Hurley Med. Ctr., 433 Mich. 404, 446 N.W.2d 114, 117 n. 3 (1989).

[125] *E.g.*, Allen v. State, 535 So. 2d 903 (La. Ct. App. 1988) [$500,000 cap on damages applied]; Eldred v. North Broward Hosp. Dist., 498 So. 2d 911 (Fla. 1986) [$50,000 cap on damages applied]; *but see* Condemarin v. University Hosp., 775 P.2d 348 (Utah 1989) [$100,000 cap on governmental hospital liability unconstitutional].

[126] *E.g.*, Fields v. Curator of Univ. of Mo., 848 S.W.2d 589 (Mo. Ct. App. 1993) [sovereign immunity waived by purchase of liability insurance]; Green River Dist. Health Dep't v. Wigginton, 764 S.W.2d 475 (Ky. 1989) [sovereign immunity waived to extent of liability insurance]; *but see* Hillsborough County Hosp. v. Taylor, 546 So. 2d 1055 (Fla. 1989) [malpractice trust fund does not waive sovereign immunity]; *contra*, Lawrence v. Virginia Ins. Reciprocal, 979 F.2d 1053 (5th Cir. 1992) [community hospital sovereign immunity protected from punitive damages even when insurance covered such damages]; Sambs v. City of Brookfield, 66 Wis. 2d 296, 224 N.W.2d 582 (1975) [insurance waives caps only when insurance policy precludes the insurer from asserting the cap].

[127] Pirkov-Middaugh v. Gillette Children's Hosp., 479 N.W.2d 63 (Minn. Ct. App. 1991), *rev'd*, 495 N.W.2d 608 (Minn. 1993).

[128] *E.g*, Higgins v. Medical Univ. of S.C., 486 S.E.2d 269 (S.C. Ct. App. 1997) [physicians protected by sovereign immunity]; Joplin v. University of Mich. Bd. of Regents, 173 Mich. App. 149, 433 N.W.2d 830 (1988), *aff'd on remand*, 184 Mich. App. 497, 459 N.W.2d 70 (1990) [physicians protected by sovereign immunity]; Jaar v. University of Miami, 474 So. 2d 239 (Fla. 3d DCA 1985) [physicians protected]; DeRosa v. Shands Teaching Hosp., 504 So. 2d 1313 (Fla. 1st DCA 1987) [resident physicians protected]; Canon v. Thumudo, 430 Mich. 326, 422 N.W.2d 688(1988) [nurses protected]; *see also* D. Holthaus, *County agrees to shield ob/gyns from liability*, 62 Hosps. (July 20, 1988), at 42 [physicians made county agents so protected by $500,000 liability limitation]; *but see* Cooper v. Bowers, 706 S.W.2d 542 (Mo. Ct. App. 1986) [physician not protected]; Keenan v. Plouffe, 482 S.E.2d 253 (Ga. 1997).

As discussed in Chapter 1, the common law doctrine of *chari-table immunity* has been overruled by nearly all courts. However, a few states have reestablished some charitable immunity by statute.[129] This charitable immunity is generally waived to the extent of any liability insurance purchased by the hospital.[130]

Some states have extended statutory immunity to other activities. Good Samaritan laws that protect some emergency services are an example. In a few states, these laws also protect physicians who provide some emergency care in hospitals.[131] Some courts are hostile to these immunities and interpret them very narrowly even when applied to emergency medical service personnel.[132]

EXCULPATORY CONTRACT. An exculpatory contract is an agreement not to sue or an agreement to limit the amount of the suit. This is different from a release because it is signed before the care is provided. While some courts will enforce these agreements in other contexts,[133] they have consistently refused to enforce these contracts concerning health care services on the grounds that they

---

[129] *E.g.*, Lazerson v. Hilton Head Hosp., 312 S.C. 211, 439 S.E.2d 836 (1994) [statutory $200,000 limit on liability of charitable organizations is constitutional]; Endres v. Greenville Hosp. System, 312 S.C. 64, 439 S.E.2d 261 (1993) [after settlement with child at maximum under charitable immunity law, affirmed summary judgment barring parent from collecting derivative maximum again]; Marsella v. Monmouth Med. Center, 224 N.J. Super. 336, 540 A.2d 865 (App. Div. 1988) [$10,000 cap on damages against nonprofit hospitals]; English v. New England Med. Ctr., 405 Mass. 423, 541 N.E.2d 329 (1989), *cert. denied*, 493 U.S. 1056 (1990) [statutory $20,000 cap on liability of nonprofit institutions upheld]; *but see* Chandler v. Hospital Auth., 500 So. 2d 1012 (Ala. 1986) [charitable immunity statute violated state constitution because it applied to too few hospitals].

[130] *E.g.*, Johnese v. Jefferson Davis Mem. Hosp., 637 F. Supp. 1198 (S.D. Miss. 1986) [charitable immunity waived by insurance]; *but see* Ponder v. Fulton-DeKalb Hosp. Auth., 256 Ga. 833, 353 S.E.2d 515, *cert. denied*, 484 U.S. 863 (1987) [self-insurance plan did not waive charitable immunity].

[131] *E.g.*, McIntyre v. Ramirez, 109 S.W.3d 741 (Tex. 2003) [physicians can be protected in hospital in some circumstances]; Hirpa v. IHC Hosps., Inc., 948 P.2d 785 (Utah 1997) [Good Samaritan law applies to hospital-employed physicians who respond to in-hospital immunity without pre-existing duty]; Johnson v. Matviuw, 176 Ill. App. 3d 907, 531 N.E.2d 970 (1st Dist. 1988) [applied to gratuitous hospital emergency care with no preexisting duty]; Kearns v. Superior Ct., 204 Cal. App. 3d 1325, 252 Cal. Rptr. 4 (2d Dist.1988) [applied to emergency assistance in surgery]; Annotation, *Construction and application of "Good Samaritan" statute*, 68 A.L.R. 4TH 294; *but see* Velazquez v. Jiminez, 172 N.J. 240, 798 A.2d 51 (2002) [hospital emergency department physicians not protected]; Deal v. Kearney, 851 P.2d 1353 (Alaska 1993) [Good Samaritan immunity does not apply when there is preexisting duty to provide aid].

[132] *E.g.*, De Tarquino v. Jersey City, 352 N.J. Super. 450, 800 A.2d 255 (App. Div. 2002) [EMT has no immunity for failure to document vomiting since documentation is not part of treatment in N.J.]; Morrell v. Aetna Ambulance Service, Inc., 2002 Conn. Super. LEXIS 3252 (unreported) [EMT has no immunity for feeding turkey sandwich to patient because feeding is not part of emergency services in Connecticut].

[133] *E.g.*, Deboer v. Florida Offroaders Driver's Ass'n, 622 So. 2d 1134 (Fla. 5th DCA 1993) [exculpatory contract protected sponsor of racing event from liability to spectator hit by car while crossing track].

are against public policy.[134] In 2000, the Wyoming Supreme Court enforced an exculpatory agreement concerning a sports medicine clinic. Recreational sports activities have been the area where most courts have enforced such agreements. Even though the man had joined the clinic on doctor's orders, the court saw it more as a recreational activity than as a health care service.[135]

ARBITRATION AGREEMENT. When there is a binding agreement to arbitrate a claim, the claim cannot be taken to court unless the right to arbitration is waived. The arbitration process specified in the agreement must be followed. Usually the dispute is submitted to one or more arbitrators who decide whether any payment should be made and, if so, how much. A valid arbitration decision has the same effect as a court judgment and can be enforced using the same procedures. Courts will generally refuse to accept the case except for limited review of the completed arbitration process. Generally, courts can set aside arbitration decisions only for limited reasons, such as failure to follow proper procedures or bias of the arbitrator.[136]

However, in 1995, the United States Supreme Court ruled that, unless the parties clearly agree to arbitrate the scope of the arbitration, courts should resolve disagreements over whether a particular issue is within the scope of the agreed arbitration.[137]

Under the common law, agreements to arbitrate are not valid unless signed after the dispute arises; statutes were necessary to validate agreements to arbitrate future disputes. Several states enacted statutes authorizing binding agreements to arbitrate future malpractice disputes.[138] Some states specify that certain elements

---

134 *E.g.*, Cudnik v. William Beaumont Hosp., 207 Mich. App. 378, 525 N.W.2d 891 (1994) [exculpatory contract unenforceable]; Tatham v. Hoke, 469 F. Supp. 914 (W.D. N.C. 1979), *aff'd without op.*, 622 F.2d 584, 587 (4th Cir. 1980) [agreement to limit all claims to $15,000 unenforceable]; Annotation, *Validity and construction of contract exempting hospital or doctor from liability for negligence to patient*, 6 A.L.R. 3D 704. For a discussion of the difference between exculpatory, indemnity, hold harmless, and related clauses under Pennsylvania law, *see* Vahal Corp. v. Sullivan Assocs., Inc., 44 F.3d 195 (3d Cir. 1995), *reh'g denied* (en banc), 48 F.3d 760 (3d Cir. 1995).

135 Massengill v. S.M.A.R.T. Sports Med. Clinic, P.C., 996 P.2d 1132 (Wyo. 2000).

136 *E.g.*, Neaman v. Kaiser Found. Hospital, 9 Cal. App. 4th 1170, 11 Cal. Rptr. 2d 879 (2d Dist. 1992), *modified*, 10 Cal. App. 4th 293 (1992) [award in favor of hospital vacated and remanded for new panel of arbitrators because "neutral" third arbitrator failed to disclose prior substantial business relationship with hospital].

137 First Options of Chicago, Inc. v. Kaplan, 514 U.S. 938 (1995).

138 Annotation, *Arbitration of medical malpractice claims*, 24 A.L.R. 5TH 1; Morris v. Metriyakool, 418 Mich. 423, 344 N.W.2d 736 (1984) [state arbitration act constitutional].

must be included in the agreement, such as the right to withdraw for a specified time. The laws differ on which health care providers are eligible to enter arbitration agreements. When the agreement does not satisfy the statutory requirements, it is not enforceable.[139]

There is a Federal Arbitration Act (FAA) that authorizes agreements to arbitrate future disputes concerning transactions that affect interstate commerce.[140] When the FAA applies, it preempts state law so that arbitration agreements can be enforced notwithstanding state common law or statutory restrictions. Courts have found exceptions to FAA preemption for some claims and some remedies.[141]

Some courts have found health care arbitration agreements to be enforceable under the FAA. For example, in 2003, the Alabama Supreme Court found that receipt of Medicare funds was interstate commerce so that an arbitration agreement in a nursing home admission agreement could be enforced.[142]

Some cases have addressed who must sign the arbitration agreement. In 1976, the California Supreme Court upheld the application to an individual employee of an arbitration agreement in a group medical contract negotiated between an employer and a health maintenance organization.[143] In 1985, a California appellate court ruled that an arbitration agreement in a group medical contract also applied to the spouse, children, and heirs of the employee.[144] In 2002, a California appellate court ruled that the next of kin's authority to make medical decisions did not include the authority to sign a binding arbitration agreement unless it was pursuant to a

---

[139] *E.g.*, Colorado Permanente Med. Group v. Evans, 926 P.2d 1218 (Colo. 1996).

[140] 9 U.S.C. §§ 1 – 16.

[141] *E.g.*, Cruz v. Pacificare Health Syss., 30 Cal. 4th 303, 66 P.3d 1157, 133 Cal. Rptr. 2d 58 (2003) [some public injunctions not subject to arbitration, exception to FAA preemption]; Broughton v CIGNA Healthplans, 21 Cal. 4th 1066, 988 P.2d 67, 90 Cal. Rptr. 2d 334 (1999) [injunctive relief portion of a deceptive advertising claim under state Consumers Legal Remedies Act (CLRA) is inarbitrable, but action for damages under CLRA is fully arbitrable; exception to FAA preemption]; Zolezzi v. Pacificare, 105 Cal. App. 4th 573, 129 Cal. Rptr. 2d 526 (4th Dist. 2003) [McCarran-Ferguson Act blocks FAA preemption of state law health plan arbitration requirements, Medicare law does not preempt for Medicare+Choice plans]; Allen v. Pacheco, 71 P.3d 375 (Colo. 2003) [McCarren Ferguson blocks FAA preemption of state law on arbitration of health plan claims].

[142] McGuffey Health & Rehab. Ctr. v. Gibson, 864 So. 2d 1061 (Ala. 2003); *but see* St. Jude Hosp. v. Associated Claims Management, 2002 Cal. App. Unpub. LEXIS 11201 (4th Dist.) [failure to prove interstate commerce affect].

[143] Madden v. Kaiser Found. Hosp., 17 Cal. 3d 699, 131 Cal. Rptr. 882, 552 P.2d 1178 (1976).

[144] Herbert v. Superior Court, 169 Cal. App. 3d 718, 215 Cal. Rptr. 477 (2d Dist. 1985); *accord,* Ling Wo. Leong v. Kaiser Found. Hosp., 71 Haw. 240, 788 P.2d 164 (1990) [newborn covered by arbitration agreement in father's health plan].

power of attorney.[145] In 2003, a Florida court enforced a nursing home arbitration agreement signed by a person with a power of attorney.[146] However, in 2003, Alabama enforced an arbitration agreement signed by the patient's friend.[147]

In 1997, the California Supreme Court ruled that the party seeking arbitration in a medical malpractice case can waive the right to arbitration by undue delay in selection of arbitrators or by fraudulent conduct.[148]

Generally, arbitration only binds the parties to the arbitration and those making claims though the parties. For example, in 1998, a California appellate court ruled that after a hospital successfully opposed being included in arbitration that the resolution of the arbitration involving the physician did not bar a separate suit against the hospital.[149]

Arbitration is favored by some health care providers and patients because it is faster and less costly than litigation. It is a less formal process than litigation, avoiding adverse publicity and the complex rules of litigation that can promote adversarial positions. Others are opposed to arbitration because they prefer having their disputes decided by a jury using procedures with which attorneys are more familiar. Some providers believe they have a better chance of avoiding any payment, while some patients believe that if they win that they will be awarded a larger payment by a jury. However, arbitration can result in substantial payments by providers.[150]

Efforts to make arbitration mandatory can be controversial. In 2003, Utah passed a law permitting providers to require patients to sign arbitration agreements or select other providers. When a large provider implemented the requirement, there were protests on the

---

145 Pagarigan v. Libby Care Ctr., Inc., 99 Cal. App. 4th 298, 120 Cal. Rptr. 2d 892 (2d Dist. 2002).

146 Gainesville Health Care Ctr., Inc. v. Weston, 857 So. 2d 278 (Fla. 1st DCA 2003).

147 McGuffey Health & Rehab. Ctr. v. Gibson, 864 So. 2d 1061 (Ala. 2003).

148 Engalla v. Permanente Medical Group, 15 Cal. 4th 951, 938 P.2d 903, 64 Cal. Rptr. 2d 843 (1997); L. Prager, *Kaiser will turn over arbitration to neutral party*, AM. MED. NEWS, Feb. 2, 1998, 3; J. Appleby, *Los Angeles law firm to oversee arbitration for Kaiser Permanente*, CONTRA COSTA TIMES [CA], Nov. 11, 1998; Saint Agnes Med. Ctr. v Pacificare, 31 Cal. 4th 1187, 82 P.3d 727, 8 Cal. Rptr. 3d 517 (2003) [discussion of what constitutes waiver of arbitration, no waiver found].

149 Orrick v. San Joaquin Community Hosp., 62 Cal. App. 4th 1466, 73 Cal. Rptr. 2d 757 (5th Dist. 1998).

150 D.E. Beeman, *Kaiser loses ruling in newborn's death*, PRESS ENTERPRISE (Riverside CA), Dec. 28, 2002, B1 [arbitrator awards $1 million, reduced to $250,000 under MICRA; Kaiser lost 84 of 228 arbitration cases from 1999 through 2001, with awards ranging from $2,500 to $5.6 million and averaging $207,571].

steps of the state capitol building. In 2004, the law was amended so that arbitration could not be required.[151]

CONTRIBUTORY NEGLIGENCE. One difficult problem of health care law is the extent to which patients are to be held accountable for their own conduct. Persons express a desire to exercise autonomy, claiming the right to decide what risks they will take. When those risks materialize, they frequently seek to escape the consequences and find someone else to pay the resulting costs. In the past, courts tended to hold patients more accountable for their conduct. Courts have weakened this accountability without giving providers power to control patient behavior. To the contrary, increasingly patient autonomy is being respected, and restrictions are placed on provider ability to control patient behavior. The right balance between provider accountability and patient accountability has not yet been found.

In the past, in most states, when the patient did something wrong that contributed to the injury to such a degree that the health care provider was not responsible for the damage, the patient was said to be contributorily negligent. This was a complete defense to a claim of a negligent tort. Examples of contributory negligence included the following:

1. The patient fails to follow clear orders and does not return for follow-up care,[152]
2. The patient fails to seek follow-up care when the patient knows of or suspects a problem,[153]
3. The patient walks on a broken leg,[154]
4. The patient gets out of bed and falls,[155]

---

[151] *Utah's largest health network won't see patients who don't sign arbitration agreement,* AP, Nov. 27, 2003 [notices sent to patients requiring arbitration agreements]; *Demonstrators protest mandatory arbitration,* AP, Jan. 20, 2004 [protests on Utah state capitol steps]; M. Thiessen, *Groups launch education effort in light of new medical arbitration law,* AP, May 3, 2004 [health care providers can no longer refuse service to patients who do not choose to sign a binding arbitration agreement].

[152] *E.g.,* McGill v. French, 333 N.C. 209, 424 S.E.2d 108 (1993); Gruidl v. Schell, 166 Ill. App. 3d 276, 519 N.E.2d 963 (1st Dist. 1988); Roberts v. Wood, 206 F. Supp. 579 (S.D. Ala. 1962); Annotation, *Medical malpractice: patient's failure to return, as directed, for examination or treatment as contributory negligence,* 100 A.L.R. 3d 723; Wilmot v. Howard, 39 Vt. 447 (1867) [neglect, refusal to obey instructions, follow the treatment prescribed].

[153] E.g., Chudson v. Ratra, 76 Md. App. 753, 548 A.2d 172 (1988).

[154] *E.g.,* Shurey v. Schlemmer, 140 Ind. App. 606, 223 N.E.2d 759, *rev'd,* 249 Ind. 1, 230 N.E.2d 534 (1967) [jury must determine whether contributory negligence].

[155] *E.g.,* Jenkins v. Bogalusa Commun. Med. Ctr., 340 So. 2d 1065 (La. Ct. App. 1976).

5. The patient lights a cigarette in bed when unattended,[156]
6. The patient deliberately gives false information that leads to the wrong antidote being given for a drug overdose,[157] and
7. The patient refuses to take antibiotics during the hospital admission.[158]

The success of this defense depended on the intelligence and degree of orientation of the patient. A patient who did not appear able to follow orders could not be relied on to follow orders; contributory negligence was not a successful defense against a claim by such a patient.[159]

Contributory negligence is still a complete defense in a few states. However, in most states, it has been replaced with comparative negligence (discussed in the next section) or is no longer a complete defense to a malpractice case so that it only reduces the damages that can be awarded. The defendant is not responsible for the portion of the damages that result from the contributory negligence.[160]

COMPARATIVE NEGLIGENCE. A majority of the states have abandoned the all-or-nothing contributory negligence rule. Instead, they apply comparative negligence, which means that the percentage of the cause due to the patient is determined and the patient does not collect that percentage of the total amount of the injury.[161] Some states that have adopted the comparative negligence rule have retained one feature of the contributory negligence rule so that the patient cannot collect anything if the patient is determined to be responsible for 50 percent or more of the cause.[162] While the majority rule is that negligent actions cannot be used to reduce liability for intentional torts,[163] there are few cases where such a comparison has been permitted.[164]

---

[156] *E.g.*, Seymour v. Victory Mem. Hosp., 60 Ill. App. 3d 366, 376 N.E.2d 754 (2d Dist. 1978).

[157] *E.g.*, Rochester v. Katalan, 320 A.2d 704 (Del. 1974).

[158] Elbaor v. Smith, 845 S.W.2d 240 (Tex. 1992).

[159] *E.g.*, Cowan v. Doering, 111 N.J. 451, 545 A.2d 159 (1988).

[160] *E.g.*, McDonnell v. McPartlin, 92 Ill. 2d 505, 736 N.E.2d 1074 (2000); Love v. Park Lane Med. Ctr., 737 S.W.2d 720 (Mo. 1987).

[161] *E.g.*, Isern v. Watson, 942 S.W.2d 186 (Tex. Civ. App. 1997) [jury found patient 35 percent responsible for leg amputation, did not return to emergency room or seek medical care for two days].

[162] *E.g.*, Jensen v. Intermountain Health Care, Inc., 679 P.2d 903 (Utah 1984); *contra*, Hoffman v. Jones, 280 So. 2d 431 (Fla. 1973).

[163] 57A Am. Jur. 2d *Negligence* § 1165.

[164] *E.g.*, Veazey v. Elmwood Plantation Assocs., Ltd., 625 So. 2d 675 (La. Ct. App. 1993), *aff'd*, 646 So. 2d 866 (La. 1994), *withdrawn by publisher & reported at* 1994 La. LEXIS 2889 (La. Nov. 30, 1994), *concurring op.*, 650 So. 2d 712 (La. 1995); Comer v. Gregory, 365 So. 2d 1212 (Miss. 1978).

Patients with mental illnesses have sought to be absolved from accountability. However, courts have generally looked at the nature of the mental illness and held individuals accountable to the extent of their capacity.[165]

Other categories of patients have also sought to avoid accountability. Most courts examine the extent of their capacity. However, a few courts have absolved some categories of patients from all responsibility regardless of actual capacity. In 1994, the New Jersey Supreme Court ruled that aged and infirm patients cannot be allocated any responsibility for injuries that result from self-damaging conduct in health care institutions.[166]

Failure to follow instructions and failure to return for follow-up examinations is still frequently a basis for assigning some of the fault to the patient.[167]

Most courts have ruled that actions of the patient prior to the provider's malpractice are not to be considered in apportioning responsibility.[168]

DAMAGE CAPS. Some states have placed statutory limits on the amount that can be awarded in all malpractice suits. Courts have disagreed on the constitutionality of such limits. In 1976, the Illinois Supreme Court declared damage caps to be a violation of the constitutional requirement of equal protection because it could find no rational justification for treating those injured by medical malpractice differently from those injured by other means.[169] In 1980, the Indiana Supreme Court declared damage caps to be constitutional because the need for a risk-spreading mechanism to assure the continued availability of health services provided a rational justification.[170] Generally, when there is a valid state cap on damages, it

---

[165] *E.g.*, Jankee v. Clark County, 2000 WI 64, 235 Wis. 2d 700, 612 N.W.2d 297 [mental hospital patient held to standard of sane person when he could control his conduct through medication]; Sheron v. Lutheran Med. Ctr., 18 P.3d 796 (Colo. App. 2000) [suicidal person can be negligent].

[166] Tobia v. Cooper Hosp. Univ. Med. Ctr., 136 N.J. 335, 643 A.2d 1 (1994).

[167] *E.g.*, Faulk v. Northwest Radiologists, P.C., 751 N.E.2d 233 (Ind. App. 2001).

[168] *E.g.*, Mercer v. Vanderbilt Univ., 134 S.W.3d 121 (Tenn. 2004); Estate of Shinholster v. Annapolis Hosp., 255 Mich. App. 339, 660 N.W.2d 361 (2003).

[169] Wright v. Central DuPage Hosp. Assn., 63 Ill. 2d 313, 347 N.E.2d 736 (1976). The Illinois Supreme Court again struck down damage caps in 1997. Best v. Taylor Machine Works Co., 179 Ill. 2d 367, 689 N.E.2d 1057 (Ill. 1997); *accord*, Morris v. Savoy, 61 Ohio St. 3d 684, 576 N.E.2d 765 (1991).

[170] Johnson v. St. Vincent Hosp., 273 Ind. 374, 404 N.E.2d 585 (1980); *accord*, Duke Power Co. v. Carolina Environmental Study Group, Inc., 438 U.S. 59 (1978) [Congress may cap damages for nuclear reactor incidents]; Pulliam v. Coastal Emergency Servs., 257 Va. 1, 509 S.E.2d 307 (1999) [cap on malpractice awards constitutional]; Scholtz v. Metropolitan Pathologists, P.C., 851 P.2d 901 (Colo. 1993).

applies to most federal suits, including EMTALA suits[171] and federal Tort Claims Act suits.[172]

Many states have damage caps that apply only to governmental providers. These caps are based in sovereign immunity or public policy concerning preservation of public funds. These caps are generally found to be constitutional.[173]

11-4 What Are the Special Strict Liability Rules for Products Liability?

The major exception to the requirement that liability be based on fault occurs when liability is based on breach of implied warranties or on strict liability in tort. In this area of the law, liability based on contract and liability based on tort overlap. The implied warranties of merchantability and fitness for a particular use are based on contract. These warranties form the basis for finding liability without fault for many of the injuries caused by the use of goods and products. Normally the seller is liable for the breach of the warranties, but in some situations persons who lease products to others have also been found liable.

Strict liability applies to injuries caused by the use of a product that is unreasonably dangerous to a consumer or user and that reaches the user without substantial change from the condition in which it was sold. Usually the manufacturer or seller of the product is liable. Strict liability in tort does not require a contractual relationship between the seller and the person injured to establish the liability of the seller. Some courts have extended strict liability to persons who furnish goods or products without a sale. Health care providers are generally considered to be providing services, not selling or furnishing products; health care providers have seldom been found liable for breach of warranties or strict liability. However, plaintiffs have made numerous efforts to convince courts to apply these principles to make it easier to establish liability. These efforts have arisen out of services involving blood transfusions (11-4.1), drugs (11-4.2), radiation (11-4.3), and medical devices (11-4.4).

---

[171] *E.g.*, Power v. Arlington Hosp. Ass'n, 42 F.3d 851 (4th Cir. 1994).

[172] *E.g.*, Lozada v. United States, 974 F.2d 986 (8th Cir. 1992).

[173] *E.g.*, Wis. Stat. §§ 893.80 & 893.82; Anderson v. City of Milwaukee, 208 Wis. 2d 18, 559 N.W.2d 563 (1997).

11-4.1 Blood Transfusions

One known risk of a blood transfusion is the transmission of diseases such as serum hepatitis. In 1954, a New York court ruled that blood transfusions were a service, not a sale, so that hospital liability for diseases conveyed by the blood could not be based on breach of warranties or strict liability.[174] However, courts in several other states began applying these product liability principles to blood transfusions.[175] Legislatures in many states enacted statutes intended to reverse these court decisions.[176] Some of the statutes state that providing blood is a service, not a sale. Other statutes expressly forbid liability based on implied warranty or strict liability. The second type of statute provides somewhat more protection because a court that chooses to ignore the public policy decisions of the legislature embodied in the first type of statute could still impose liability on the hospital by extending the applicability of strict liability to services.[177] These immunity statutes have been found constitutional.[178] Health care providers can still be liable for negligence in administering blood transfusions. Immunity statutes in some states also apply to some other services, such as tissue transplantation.

11-4.2 Drugs

Efforts to use implied warranties or strict liability to impose liability on hospitals for the administration of drugs have generally been unsuccessful. For example, a Texas appellate court refused to apply these product liability principles to the administration of a contaminated drug.[179] In 1992, a Pennsylvania court ruled that a hospital was not a merchant when it dispensed a drug incidental to the service of healing, and it was not liable under implied warranties for an allergic reaction.[180]

---

[174] Perlmutter v. Beth David Hosp., 308 N.Y. 100, 123 N.E.2d 792 (1954).

[175] *E.g.*, Shortess v. Touro Infirmary, 508 So. 2d 938 (La. 1988) [hospital strictly liable for blood with undetectable form of hepatitis]; Cunningham v. MacNeal Mem. Hosp., 47 Ill. 2d 443, 266 N.E.2d 897 (1970).

[176] *E.g.*, Weishorn v. Miles-Cutter, 721 A.2d 811 (Pa. Super. Ct. 1998), *aff'd*, 560 Pa. 557, 746 A.2d 1117 (2000) [state blood shield law also protects commercial suppliers from strict liability, breach of warranty].

[177] *See* Hoven v. Kelbe, 79 Wis. 2d 444, 256 N.W.2d 379 (1977) [rejecting extension of strict liability to medical services].

[178] *E.g.*, Samson v. Greenville Hosp. Sys., 295 S.C. 359, 368 S.E.2d 665 (1988); McDaniel v. Baptist Mem. Hosp., 469 F.2d 230 (6th Cir. 1972).

[179] Shivers v. Good Shepard Hosp., 427 S.W.2d 104 (Tex. Civ. App. 1968).

[180] Stephenson v. Greenberg, 421 Pa. Super. 1, 617 A.2d 364 (1992).

11-4.3 Radiation

In 1980, the Illinois Supreme Court reversed a lower court's application of strict liability principles to X-ray treatment.[181] The court ruled that the issue in the case was the decision to use a certain dosage. The X-rays themselves were not a defective product; so strict liability in tort was not applicable.

11-4.4 Medical Devices

Most courts have not applied implied warranties or strict liability in tort to hospitals for injuries due to medical devices.[182] For example, a California court ruled that the hospital was the user, not the supplier, of a surgical needle that broke during an operation.[183] Similarly, in 1994, an Indiana court ruled that products liability law does not apply to a hospital where a pacemaker is implanted.[184] In 1998, a Washington court held that a hospital that furnished a spinal implant cannot be held liable for selling a defective product, concluding that the transaction was a provision of services, not a sale of goods.[185] However, this position is not unanimous. In 1984, the Alabama Supreme Court ruled that a hospital was liable based on the implied warranty of fitness for intended use when a suturing needle broke and remained in a patient's body.[186] The court viewed the hospital as a merchant, not a user. Even when the health care provider is viewed as only a user, the provider may still be liable

---

[181] Dubin v. Michael Reese Hosp., 83 Ill. 2d 277, 415 N.E.2d 350 (1980), *rev'g*, 74 Ill. App. 3d 932, 393 N.E.2d 588 (1st Dist. 1979); *see also* Nevauex v. Park Place Hosp., 656 S.W.2d 923 (Tex. Ct. App. 1983) [no strict liability for burns from cobalt radiation therapy].

[182] *E.g.*, Brandt v. Boston Scientific Corp, 204 Ill. 2d 640, 792 N.E.2d 296 (2003) [implantation of device is service, not sale]; Royer v. Catholic Med. Ctr., 144 N.H. 330, 741 A.2d 74 (1999) [implantation of prosthetic knee is service, not sale]; *In re* Breast Implant Product Liability Litigation, 331 S.C. 540, 503 S.E.2d 445 (1998); Rolon-Alvarado v. San Juan, 1 F.3d 74 (1st Cir. 1993) [provider not strictly liable for latent defect in endotracheal tube manufactured by third party]; Hoff v. Zimmer, Inc., 746 F. Supp. 872 (W.D. Wis. 1990); North Miami Gen. Hosp. v. Goldberg, 520 So. 2d 650 (Fla. 3d DCA 1988) [hospital not strictly liable for burn from grounding pad]; Hector v. Cedars-Sinai Med. Ctr., 180 Cal. App. 3d 493, 225 Cal. Rptr. 595 (2d Dist. 1986) [hospital not strictly liable for pacemaker]; Annotation, *Liability of hospital or medical practitioner under doctrine of strict liability in tort, or breach of warranty, for harm caused by drug, medical instrument, or similar device used in treating patient*, 65 A.L.R. 5TH 357; *see also* Parker v. St. Vincent Hosp., 1996 NMCA 70, 919 P.2d 1104, 1107, 122 N.M. 39 [rejecting products/services distinction, but declining to extend strict liability on policy grounds].

[183] Silverhart v. Mount Zion Hosp., 20 Cal. App. 3d 1022, 98 Cal. Rptr. 187 (1st Dist. 1971).

[184] St. Mary's Med. Ctr., Inc. v. Casko, 639 N.E.2d 312 (Ind. Ct. App. 1994).

[185] McKenna v. Harrison Mem. Hosp., 92 Wash. App. 119, 960 P.2d 486 (1998).

[186] Skelton v. Druid City Hosp. Bd., 459 So. 2d 818 (Ala. 1984).

based on negligence, and the manufacturer of the equipment may be liable based on implied warranties or strict liability in tort.

The one major exception was Missouri. Missouri permitted strict liability cases against providers[187] until 2000, when the Missouri Supreme Court ruled that they were not permitted.[188]

Some courts may not view certain items supplied by health care providers as integral to the provider's service. In 1981, a Texas court found that a hospital could be strictly liable for supplying a hospital gown that was not flame-retardant because it was not integrally related to supplying services.[189]

Some implied warranty and strict liability claims concerning medical devices are preempted by the federal medical device laws.[190] In 1996, the United States Supreme Court ruled that some claims were not preempted.[191] The exact contours of which claims are preempted are not entirely resolved.[192]

11-5 Who Is Responsible for Paying for Liability?

Liability can be divided into personal liability, liability for employees and agents, and institutional liability. Individual staff members are personally liable for consequences of their own acts. Employers can be liable for the consequences of the job-related acts of their employees or agents even when the employer is not at fault personally. Institutions can also be liable for the consequences of breaches

---

[187] Bell v. Poplar Bluff Physicians Group, 879 S.W.2d 618 (Mo. Ct. App. 1994).

[188] Budding v. SSM Healthcare Sys., 19 S.W.3d 678 (Mo. 2000).

[189] Thomas v. St. Joseph Hosp., 618 S.W.2d 791 (Tex. Civ. App. 1981).

[190] 21 U.S.C. § 360c.

[191] Medtronic, Inc. v. Lohr, 518 U.S. 470 (1996) [for device "substantially equivalent" to devices that preexisted MDA and exempt from the rigorous premarketing approval review, MDA does not preempt the plaintiff's state common law claims for defective design, defective manufacture, failure-to-warn, and failure to comply with FDA standards; MDA may preempt state law tort claim, claim based on state statute, regulation, but federal, state requirements must specifically apply to particular medical device, state requirement must add to or be different from federal requirement]; Buckman Co. v. Plaintiffs' Legal Comm., 531 U.S. 341 (2001) [common law claims of fraud on FDA preempted by MDA, tort claims alleging violations of FDCA preempted].

[192] *E.g.*, Horn v. Thoratec Corp., 376 F.3d 163 (3d Cir. 2004) [state defective design claims preempted]; Brooks v. Howmedica, Inc., 273 F.3d 785 (8th Cir. 2001) (en banc) [failure to warn claim preempted]; Martin v Medtronic, Inc., 254 F.3d 573 (5th Cir. 2001), *cert. denied*, 534 U.S. 1078 (2002) [state product liability claims are preempted by MDA]; Whitson v. Safeskin Corp., Inc., 313 F. Supp. 2d 473 (M.D. Pa. 2004) [implied warranty claims related to latex gloves preempted]; *In re* St. Jude Medical, Inc. Silzone Heart Valves Products Liability Litigation. 2004 U.S. Dist. LEXIS 148 (D. Minn.) [failure to warn claims not preempted].

of duties owed directly to patients and others, such as the duties to maintain buildings and grounds, maintain equipment, and select and supervise employees and medical staff.

The section addresses the following questions:

11-5.1. When is an employer liable for the acts of an employee?
11-5.2. When are individuals liable for their own acts?
11-5.3. When is there liability for the acts of an agent?
11-5.4. When is their institutional liability independent of the acts of individuals?
11-5.5. When is a managed care organization liable for the acts of providers?

When a judgment is entered, whoever is responsible for payment should either arrangement to pay the award or take steps to prohibit collection of the award during appeals. Otherwise, traditional means of collecting debts may be used. In 1989, an attorney who had won a $1.7 million malpractice award against a hospital which had not been paid arranged for police to seize computers, desks, and other hospital property not involved in direct patient care. After the property was loaded on trucks, the hospital promptly paid.[193]

11-5.1 When Is an Employer Liable for the Acts of an Employee?

RESPONDEAT SUPERIOR. Employers are liable for the consequences of their employees' activities within the course of employment for which the employee is liable. This legal doctrine is called *respondeat superior*, which means "let the master answer." The employer need not have done anything wrong. For example, if a nurse employed by a hospital injures a patient by giving the wrong medication, the hospital can be liable even if the nurse was properly selected, properly trained, and properly assigned the responsibility.

SCOPE OF EMPLOYMENT. Employers are liable under *respondeat superior* only for actions of employees within the scope of their employment. Courts differ on what acts are within the scope of employment. Many courts follow the rule that intentional torts are not within *respondeat superior* unless the employee is acting in the furtherance, no matter how misguided, of the employer's busi-

---

[193] *Lawyer hauls off hospital assets in dispute over malpractice award*, MOD.HEALTHCARE, July 28, 1989, 69.

ness.[194] In 1993, a Georgia court ruled that a hospital was not liable for the lethal injection of five patients by a nurse employee because the nurse was pursuing her own interests.[195] In 1994, a federal court ruled that an employing physician was not liable for the disclosure of confidential medical information by a nurse and her daughter nurse assistant where they were not authorized to make the disclosure and did not make it in work time or space.[196] Courts disagree on when an employer is liable for sexual misconduct by employees.[197]

BORROWED SERVANT AND DUAL SERVANT. In some situations, health care providers may not be liable for the consequences of the negligent acts of nurses and other employees because of the *borrowed servant doctrine*. In some states, when an employer delegates its right to direct and control the activities of an employee to an independent staff physician who assumes responsibility, the employee becomes a borrowed servant. The physician, rather than the employer, is then liable under *respondeat superior* for the acts of the employee.[198] Courts in many states do not apply the doctrine when an employee continues to receive substantial direction from the hospital through its policies and rules. Thus, the trend appears to be toward abandoning the borrowed servant doctrine[199] or replacing it with a *dual servant doctrine* under which both the physician and the hospital are liable under *respondeat superior* for the acts of the employee.[200]

PHYSICIAN EMPLOYEES. Usually hospitals and other health care institutions are not liable for the negligent acts of independent staff physicians.[201] When the physician is an employee of the hospital, the

---

[194] *E.g.*, Rice v. Nova Biomedical Corp., 38 F.3d 909 (7th Cir. 1994), *cert. denied*, 514 U.S. 1111 (1995).

[195] Lucas v. Hospital Auth. of Dougherty County, 193 Ga. App. 595, 388 S.E.2d 871 (1989).

[196] Jones v. Baisch, 40 F.3d 252 (8th Cir. 1994).

[197] Thompson v. Everett Clinic, 71 Wash. App. 548, 860 P.2d 1054 (1993) [clinic not liable for sexual misconduct by employee physician with male patient during examination]; P.S. v. Psychiatric Coverage, Ltd., 887 S.W.2d 622 (Mo. Ct. App. 1994) [sexual relations with patient not within scope of employment, clinic not liable]; *contra*, Morin v. Henry Mayo Newhall Mem. Hosp., 29 Cal. App. 4th 473, 34 Cal. Rptr. 2d 535 (2d Dist. 1994) [hospital liable under *respondeat superior* for sexual misconduct of ultrasound technician]; Samuels v. Southern Baptist Hosp., 594 So. 2d 571 (La. Ct. App. 1992), *cert. denied*, 599 So. 2d 316 (La. 1992) [hospital liable for sexual assault by employee nursing assistant during working hours on premises because reasonably incidental to employee's performance of his duty]; Annotation, *Liability of hospital or clinic for sexual relationships with patients by staff physicians, psychologists, and other healers*, 45 A.L.R. 4TH 289.

[198] *E.g.*, Krane v. St. Anthony Hosp. Sys., 738 P.2d 75 (Colo. Ct. App. 1987).

[199] *E.g.*, Lewis v Physicians Ins. Co., 2001 WI 60, 243 Wis. 2d 648, 627 N.W.2d 484; Holger v. Irish, 316 Or. 402, 851 P.2d 1122 (1993).

[200] *E.g.*, Somerset v. Hart, 549 S.W.2d 814 (Ky. 1977) [surgeon, hospital both liable for nurse's instrument count].

[201] *E.g.*, Menzie v. Windham Commun. Mem. Hosp., 774 F. Supp. 91 (D. Conn. 1991); Reed v. Good Samaritan Hosp. Ass'n, 453 So. 2d 229 (Fla. 4th DCA 1984).

hospital can be liable under *respondeat superior* for the physician's acts.

Some courts consider some independent physicians to be employees. The criteria for finding an employment relationship focus on whether the hospital has a right to control the time, manner, and method of the physician's work.[202] Some courts require significant control to find an employment relationship. For example, a Georgia appellate court declined to find an emergency room physician to be an employee despite scheduling, billing, and other control features of the agreement between the physician and the hospital.[203] The court focused on the contract provision that the hospital would exercise no control over the physician's methods of running the emergency room. However, other courts are more liberal in applying the criteria. For example, an Arizona court found a hospital to be the employer of a nonsalaried radiologist based on the hospital's legal right to control the professional performance of medical staff members, exclusiveness of the contract, hospital's role as billing agent, and patient's lack of choice in selecting a radiologist.[204] The court declined to be bound by a statement in the hospital admission form, signed by the patient, acknowledging that the radiologist was an independent contractor and not a hospital employee.

11-5.2 When Are Individuals Liable for Their Own Acts?

Individual staff members are personally liable for consequences of their own acts. Individual liability is nearly always based on the principle of fault. To be liable, the person must have done something wrong or must have failed to do something he or she should have done.

The supervisor is not the employer. *Respondeat superior* does not impose liability on managers and supervisors.[205] Supervisors are liable only for the consequences of their own acts or omissions. The employer can also be liable for those acts or omissions under *respondeat superior*.

---

[202] *E.g.*, Linkous v. United States, 142 F.3d 271 (5th Cir. 1998) [dismissal of claim against U.S. because physician in Army hospital was independent contractor, not government employee, insufficient control].

[203] Overstreet v. Doctor's Hosp., 142 Ga. App. 895, 227 S.E.2d 213 (1977).

[204] Beeck v. Tucson Gen. Hosp., 18 Ariz. App. 165, 500 P.2d 1153 (1972).

[205] Maldonado v. Frio Hosp. Ass'n, 25 S.W.2d 274 (Tex. App. 2000) [management company is not employer of hospital employees].

Employer liability is for the benefit of the injured person, not for the benefit of the employee. The employer does not have to provide the employee with liability protection. *Respondeat superior* permits the plaintiff to sue the employer, the employee, or both. If the employee is individually sued and found liable, the employee must pay. If, as often occurs, the employee is not individually sued, then the employer must pay. The employer may sue the employee to get the money back.[206] The repayment is called *indemnification*. As part of settlements, hospitals sometimes assign their right of indemnity against physicians or others to the plaintiff.[207] However, indemnification is seldom sought except from employees with substantial insurance.

11-5.3 When Is There Liability for the Acts of an Agent?

AGENCY. Hospitals and other health care institutions can be held liable for the consequences of their agents' acts in a fashion similar to their being held liable for their employees' acts. For example, a federal district court found a hospital liable for a radiologist's negligence in not promptly relaying to the treating physician the results of a X-ray examination.[208] The court ruled that prompt reporting was an administrative responsibility and that the physician was functioning as an agent of the hospital when relaying the report.

PARTNERSHIP/JOINT VENTURE. Partners are considered agents of each other, and partners are liable for the torts committed by other partners in carrying out partnership activities. A *joint venture* is a kind of partnership. Health care institutions are liable for actions of physicians within the scope of partnerships or joint ventures with those physicians. In 1987, a Florida appellate court expanded the definition of joint venture to include a hospital contract with an anesthesiologist, imposing liability on the hospital for the anesthesiologist's malpractice.[209] In 1998, the Georgia Supreme

---

[206] *E.g.*, St. John's Reg. Health Ctr. v. American Cas. Co., 980 F.2d 1222 (8th Cir. 1992) [indemnity from nurse's liability insurer].

[207] *E.g.*, Deal v. Kearney, 851 P.2d 1353 (Alaska 1993).

[208] Keene v. Methodist Hosp., 324 F. Supp. 233 (N.D. Ind. 1971).

[209] Arango v. Reykal, 507 So. 2d 1211 (Fla. 4th DCA 1987); *contra,* Underwood v. Holy Name of Jesus Hosp., 289 Ala. 216, 266 So. 2d 773 (1972); *see* R. Miller, *Joint venture: another theory of hospital liability for physicians,* 5 Hosp. L. Newsletter (Sept. 1988), at 5; *see also,* Suarez Matos v. Ashford Presbyterian Comm. Hosp., 4 F.3d 47 (1st Cir. 1993) [granting staff privileges along with sharing profits was joint enterprise under Puerto Rican law which could make hospital liable for pathologist's reporting of tumor as benign although he knew it was not].

Court ruled that on-call arrangements do not make physicians joint venturers for imputation of liability purposes.[210]

Some health care providers refer to themselves as partners in advertising when they are not really partners. Some lawyers advise against this terminology to remove this as a basis for courts to misinterpret the relationship. Fortunately, in 2001, when this was litigated in Connecticut, an appellate court ruled that use of the term *partner* in advertising did not create a partnership.[211]

APPARENT OR OSTENSIBLE AGENCY. Some courts refuse to examine the details of the hospital-physician relationship. Instead they consider how the relationship appears to patients. If the hospital appears to be offering physician services, the physician is considered a hospital agent under the doctrine of *apparent* or *ostensible agency*. For example, the Michigan Supreme Court found a physician to be the hospital's ostensible agent because the patient did not have a patient-physician relationship with the physician independent of the hospital setting.[212] The physician, who was a member of the medical staff, had assisted in the patient's treatment. The court ruled that there was sufficient evidence that the hospital had appeared to provide the physician for the patient. The court noted that there was no evidence that the patient had been given any notice that the physician was an independent contractor. Thus, hospitals may find it helpful to give patients notice.[213] However, even signed acknowledgments may not be sufficient in some states.[214]

---

[210] Rossi v. Oxley, 269 Ga. 82, 495 S.E.2d 39 (1998); *accord,* Freyer v. Albin, 5 P.3d 329 (Colo. App. 1999) [surgeons not in joint venture for operation]; Blackburn v. Columbia Med. Ctr., 58 S.W.2d 263 (Tex. App. 2001) [joint venture not shown].

[211] Davies v. General Tours, Inc., 63 Conn. App. 17, 774 A.2d 1063 (2001).

[212] Greve v. Mt. Clemens Gen. Hosp., 404 Mich. 240, 273 N.W.2d 429 (1978); *accord,* Creech v. Roberts, 908 F.2d 75 (6th Cir. 1990), *cert. denied,* 499 U.S. 975 (1991); Gilbert v. Sycamore Mun. Hosp., 156 Ill. 2d 511, 622 N.E.2d 788 (1993) [hospital liable for acts of physician at hospital regardless of status as independent contractor unless patient knew or should have known he was independent contractor]; Clark v. Southview Hosp. & Family Health Ctr., 68 Ohio St. 3d 435, 628 N.E.2d 46 (1994) [same]; *see also,* Pamperin v. Trinity Mem. Hosp., 144 Wis. 2d 188, 423 N.W.2d 848 (1988); Boyd v. Albert Einstein Med. Ctr., 377 Pa. Super. 609, 547 A.2d 1229 (1988) [HMO may be liable for ostensible agent].

[213] *E.g.*, Baptist Mem. Hosp. Sys. v. Sampson, 969 S.W.2d 945 (Tex. 1998) [hospital not liable for emergency room physician's negligence, no affirmative act to create appearance of agency, reasonable efforts to inform patients by posting signs, patients signed consent form disclosing status]; James v. Ingalls Mem. Hosp., 299 Ill. App. 3d 627, 701 N.E.2d 207 (1st Dist. 1998) [disclaimer in treatment form signed by patient disclosing independent contractor status precludes hospital liability for doctor]; Holmes v. University Health Serv., Inc., 205 Ga. App. 602, 423 S.E.2d 281 (1992) [residents provided by medical college not apparent agents of hospital, especially where decedent had signed document acknowledging that physician was not employee or agent of hospital].

[214] *E.g.*, Beeck v. Tucson Gen. Hosp., 18 Ariz. App. 165, 500 P.2d 1153 (1972).

Some states limit the scope of the doctrine by requiring that the plaintiff prove actual reliance on the apparent agency before imposing liability on the institution. In 2000, an Illinois court ruled that there was no reliance when the patient went to the hospital on his private physician's orders.[215]

Some hospitals address their liability exposure for physicians' actions by including in physician contracts indemnity or "hold harmless" clauses in which the physician agrees to indemnify the hospital for such losses. These clauses do not bar patients from collecting from the hospital, but they provide a basis for seeking reimbursement from physicians and their insurers.

A few hospitals have statutory immunity from liability for the acts of physicians, and liability based on apparent agency cannot be imposed.[216]

11-5.4 When Is There Institutional Liability Independent of the Acts of Individuals?

Institutions can be liable for the consequences of breaches of duties owed directly to the patient.[217] Two examples of these duties — the maintenance of buildings and grounds and the selection and maintenance of equipment — are discussed following in this chapter. Proper selection and supervision of employees is a third duty, discussed in Chapter 4. Proper selecting and monitoring of medical staff are increasingly being recognized as institutional duties. They are discussed in Chapter 5.

In 1978, a Washington appellate court imposed another form of institutional liability. A hospital was found liable for the treatment provided in an emergency room by an independent professional corporation because the emergency services were an *inherent function* of the hospital's overall enterprise for which the hospital bears some responsibility.[218] Liability was not based on *respondeat superior*, ostensible agency, negligent selection, or negligent monitoring of the medical staff. Similarly, in 2000, the South Carolina Supreme Court held that a hospital has a *nondelegable duty* to

---

[215] Butkiewicz v. Loyola Univ. Med. Ctr., 311 Ill. App. 3d 508, 724 N.E.2d 1037 (1st Dist. 2000).

[216] *E.g.*, Wis. Stat. § 233.17.

[217] *E.g.*, Thompson v. Nason Hosp., 527 Pa. 330, 591 A.2d 703 (1991).

[218] Adamski v. Tacoma Gen. Hosp., 20 Wash. App. 98, 579 P.2d 970 (1978); *accord* Griffin v. Matthews, 36 Ohio App. 3d 228, 522 N.E.2d 110 (1987).

render competent emergency room services and may be liable for the negligent actions of emergency room physicians, even though the admissions form stated that emergency room physicians were independent contractors, not employees.[219] In 2003, Alaska refused to extend the scope of nondelegable duties to the operating room.[220] In 2003, an Ohio appellate court refused to apply corporate liability for having a medical residency training program.[221]

Kansas abolished such liability by a statute that bars all liability for licensed medical facilities for professional services of professionals who are not employees or agents.[222]

OFF-PREMISES LIABILITY. Some patients have sought to hold hospitals liable for the actions of medical staff members in their private practice off hospital premises. Nearly all courts have rejected these attempts.[223] One exception is a 1988 Massachusetts decision that a hospital employee could sue the hospital for a rape by a medical staff member during a house call in his private practice.[224] The hospital was aware of prior complaints about the physician's sexual conduct, had given him a verbal warning, and had required a chaperon to be present when he visited female patients in the hospital. Apparently the hospital's liability was based on the court's belief that it should have terminated the physician's privileges or taken other disciplinary measures that would have come to the employee's attention.

11-5.5 When Is a Managed Care Organization Liable for the Acts of Providers?

Courts are still struggling with the extent to which managed care entities should be liable for the consequences of errors of participating providers, for their selection of participating providers, and for their decisions not to authorize hospitalization or other treatment. Some employer-sponsored plans have sought to avoid all such liability

---

219 Simmons v. Tuomey Reg. Med. Ctr., 341 S.C. 32, 533 S.E.2d 312 (2000); *contra*, Baptist Mem. Hosp. Sys. v. Sampson, 969 S.W.2d 945 (Tex. 1998) [no nondelegable duty for emergency room].
220 Fletcher v. South Peninsula Hosp., 71 P.3d 833 (Alaska 2003).
221 Sullins v. University Hosps., 2003 Ohio 398 (App Ct.)
222 KAN. STAT. ANN. § 65-442(b); McVay v. Rich, 255 Kan. 371, 874 P.2d 641 (1994) [statute bars patient claim against hospital for negligently extending clinical privileges to nonemployee physician].
223 *E.g.*, Pedroza v. Bryant, 101 Wash. 2d 226, 677 P.2d 166 (1984).
224 Copithorne v. Framingham Union Hosp., 401 Mass. 860, 520 N.E.2d 139 (1988).

by asserting ERISA preemption. Managed care entities have sought to avoid all responsibility for errors by participating providers who are not employees or apparent agents of the managed care entity. Liability of managed care entities is also reviewed in Chapter 10.

11-6 What Types of Insurance Are Available?

OCCURRENCE/CLAIMS-MADE. In the past, most professional liability insurance was on an occurrence basis, which means that a policy purchased for a specific year covered all future claims arising out of incidents during the policy period. Since the 1970s, many professional liability insurance policies have been written on a claims-made basis, which means that a policy purchased for a specific year covers only the claims that are made during that year that arise from incidents after a retroactive date specified in the policy. Thus, to have coverage for future claims, an additional policy needs to be purchased. This can be a renewal policy with a retroactive date covering incidents in the prior period, or it can be a reporting endorsement, often called a "tail" policy, which covers future claims arising from incidents during the period covered by the prior policy without covering any new incidents.

Sometimes when providers elect not to buy tail coverage, before expiration of the old policy, they send the insurer a list of all the potential claims of which they are aware so that a "claim" will be made during the policy period. In 1992, the New Hampshire Supreme Court ruled that these were valid claims triggering coverage.[225] It was not necessary for the claims to come from the patient.

INSTITUTIONAL COVERAGE. Hospitals and other employers frequently provide insurance coverage for their employees. Usually this coverage does not apply to activities outside the scope of employment. Sometimes this coverage is required by statute. Sometimes it is the result of collective bargaining or individual contracts with employees. Sometimes it is a voluntary benefit provided by the employer.

Hospitals sometimes offer malpractice coverage for non-employee physicians. There have been questions whether this is permitted by federal law. In some contexts, it is possible that providing

---

[225] Concord Hosp. v. New Hampshire Med. Malpractice J. U. A., 63 A.2d 1384 (N.H. 1993).

free coverage would violate either the Stark law or the Medicare antikickback law. An Advisory Opinion issued by the HHS Inspector General in 2004 approved a proposal to subsidize the malpractice insurance for four community obstetricians.[226] The analysis concluded that the arrangement would potentially violate the antikickback law if there were the requisite intent, but the OIG elected not to enforce the law in the case. The analysis depended in large part on the fact that the proposal almost fit into the safe harbor for subsidies of obstetrical malpractice coverage for those providing primary care in health professional shortage areas.[227] Thus, it does not appear to signal receptivity to malpractice premium subsidies.

JOINT UNDERWRITING ASSOCIATIONS. Some states have created agencies sometimes called *joint underwriting associations* that will sell insurance coverage to providers when the commercial market does not offer coverage.

PUNITIVE DAMAGES. States disagree on whether punitive damages may be covered by insurance. Some states permit coverage, while others forbid coverage.[228] Some states permit coverage for some types of punitive damages, but not others. For example, in 2001, an Ohio appellate court ruled that insurance could not cover punitive damages that were awarded upon a finding of malicious, willful, or intentional conduct but that the insurance company had to pay statutory punitive damages that was not based on proof of this type of conduct.[229]

MANUFACTURER PROGRAMS. Faced with the reluctance of physicians to prescribe drugs that frequently lead to litigation, manufacturers have occasionally adopted special programs where they agreed to pay the legal costs and settlements or verdicts against physicians sued for prescribing the drugs.[230] However, these programs predated the HHS OIG focus on malpractice subsidies as kickbacks. It is not clear that these programs would be permitted today.

---

[226] HHS OIG, Advisory Opinion 04-11 (Sept. 9, 2004) [http://oig.hhs.gov/fraud/docs/advisory opinions/ 2004/ao0411.pdf [accessed Sept. 18, 2004].

[227] 42 C.F.R. § 1001.952(o).

[228] *E.g.*, Johnson & Johnson v. Aetna Cas. & Sur. Co., 285 N.J. Super. 575, 667 A.2d 1087 (App. Div. 1995).

[229] *E.g.*, The Corinthian v. Hartford Fire Ins. Co., 143 Ohio App. 3d 392, 758 N.E.2d 218 (2001).

[230] *E.g.*, *Upjohn, in move to back halcion drug, will pay physicians' legal costs in suits*, WALL ST. J., Nov. 27, 1991, at B2 [promise to pay legal costs and settlements or verdicts of physicians sued for prescribing halcion, similar to Eli Lilly program for prozac in summer of 1991]; *Beware of offers of indemnity*, 327 NEW ENG. J. MED. 819 (1992).

11-7 What Are Some of the Ways That Have Been Proposed and/or Implemented to Deal with the Periodic Malpractice Crisis?

The cumulative effect of the number of malpractice cases and the cost of individual cases has resulted in a substantial increase in the cost of malpractice insurance and, in some areas of the country, has occasionally reduced availability of malpractice insurance at any price. When malpractice protection has been unavailable or the cost has been too high, access to services can be adversely impacted when services become unavailable in some areas.[231] This is illustrated by the closure of a trauma center in Las Vegas, Nevada, in the beginning of July 2002, until insurance coverage could be arranged for the physicians.[232] When health care continues to be available, the cost to patients and third-party payers increases in some cases to cover the liability costs. This is illustrated by the threat in 2004 by some Connecticut obstetricians to impose a $500 surcharge on all obstetrical cases. They did not implement the surcharge when payers increased their reimbursement rates.[233]

This periodic malpractice insurance crisis has led nearly every state to review and revise its laws concerning tort suits and/or malpractice coverage. States are confronted with the difficult questions of what standard can realistically be expected and afforded, what events should be compensated and how they should be determined, and what compensation can reasonably be afforded and how shall it be determined. Underlying these issues are many questions, including how to deal with the anger of patients and families at bad outcomes regardless of their cause, how to deal with the ongoing medical costs of persons who are not restored to access to the employment-based health care insurance system, how to maintain access to health care services for all, how to make health care professions attractive career options, and how to promote improvement in health care outcomes. Thus, the issues go beyond the direct insurance and cost issues.

---

[231] *See* D.P. Kessler, W.M. Sage & D.J. Becker, *Impact of malpractice reforms on the supply of physician services*, J.A.M.A., June 1, 2005, 2618.

[232] *See* W. Booth, *Las Vegas trauma center closes as doctors quit; surgeons cite rising costs of malpractice insurance, lawsuits — a growing national problem*, WASH. POST, July 4, 2002, A2; A. Wagner, *UMC trauma center in Las Vegas to reopen Saturday*, AP, July 12, 2002.

[233] *Ob/Gyns say they'll surcharge deliveries to make up insurance costs*, AP, May, 18, 2004; *Doctors opt out of surcharge plan*, AP, Sept. 14, 2004.

Although some changes have had an effect on the availability of insurance and its cost, in many states it is not clear whether they have provided a solution. Periodically there are times when aggregate payments have dropped, but the payments remain substantial. The cause of the drops is difficult to assess. There is still substantial dispute concerning the indirect effect of tort liability on the cost of health care through defensive medicine and other practices.[234]

These tort reforms can be grouped into (1) changes in the standard of care (11-7.1); (2) changes in dispute resolution mechanisms (11-7.2); (3) changes in the amount of the award and how it is paid (11-7.3); (4) changes in the statute of limitations that sets the time in which the suit must be brought (11-7.4); and (5) other tort reform changes (11-7.5). These reforms have received a mixed reception in the courts. Courts have disagreed on whether these reforms violate various state and federal constitutional provisions. When reforms are enacted to apply only to health care providers, there is often litigation over whether a particular type of provider is protected by the law.[235]

Some states have attempted to address the issue through malpractice coverage reform (11-7.6). This has included state-sponsored coverage, facilitation of development of new private coverage, and mandated coverage as a condition of licensure.

Another fundamental problem of health care law is the degree to which the malpractice system disrupts the provision of health care and traumatizes health care providers. The discovery process in litigation can be extremely burdensome as attorneys search for every detail concerning the patient's treatment and any basis to attempt to hold the provider to a higher standard. It consumes a great deal of provider time in preparation and participation in depositions and other discovery, reducing time available to care for other patients and administer the institution. Courts seldom exercise any effective control over this process; court intervention is available to stop only

---

[234] *See* D.M. Studdert et al., *Defensive medicine among high-risk specialist physicians in a volatile malpractice environment*, J.A.M.A., June 1, 2006, 2609.

[235] *See* Annotation, *Medical malpractice: who are 'health providers,' or the like, whose actions fall within statutes specifically governing actions and damages for medical malpractice*, 12 A.L.R. 5TH 1 (1993); Weinstock v. Groth, 629 So. 2d 835 (Fla. 1993) [psychologist not health care provider under Florida tort reform law]; Perez v. Bay State Ambulance & Hosp. Rental Service, Inc., 413 Mass. 670, 602 N.E.2d 570 (1992) [ambulance company not health care provider so not subject to panel review].

the most abusive misuse. Some plaintiffs' attorneys expressly threaten burdensome discovery in an effort to induce settlement.

The traumatizing of health care providers is another significant result. While some plaintiffs' attorneys are very professional in their approach, others seek to demonize defendants. In some cases, this may in part be a response to demands of angry clients, but it also appears to be rewarded by the litigation system when judges and juries award large amounts. This is one of the reasons that some providers have been interested in exploring alternate systems that do not reward the traumatizing of providers.[236] Some argue that providers should be subjected to trauma in retaliation for the trauma that the patient experienced. Even in cases where this impetus may need to be accommodated, it is not clear why this retaliation should be tied into the compensation system.

11-7.1 Standard of Care

As discussed in Section 11-1.2, the standard of care for health care institutions is usually the degree of reasonable care the patient's known or apparent condition requires. Some states extend the standard to include the reasonable care required for conditions the institution should have discovered through exercise of reasonable care. Usually the standard for individual health care professionals is what a reasonably prudent health care professional engaged in a similar practice would have done under similar circumstances.

Most tort reform that has actually been adopted has focused on elements of the malpractice process other than the standard of care. This is understandable because of the difficulty in articulating a different workable standard. However, part of the underlying problem with the tort system is the use of a standard of care that is ultimately unachievable.

The ultimate risk of adopting an unachievable standard for purposes of tort law is that no one will be able to afford to provide the service, except for those who have immunity from liability. This is a still theoretical risk for most areas of health care but is already a reality for obstetrical care in some regions.

There is a potential for improving the quality and outcomes of health care services, but the malpractice system does not appear to

---

[236] D. Shapiro, *Beyond the blame: A no-fault approach to malpractice*, N.Y. TIMES, Sept. 23, 2003, D6 [the trauma of malpractice suits].

be the best way to pursue it. Most providers are committed to processes for reducing errors and improving processes. A tremendous amount has been learned and implemented. Unfortunately, the tort system usually impedes this process, rather than supporting it. It diverts time, resources, and attention from process improvement. It discourages the open information flow that can identify and resolve issues because that information flow is used as a basis for imposing liability.[237]

Likewise, society needs to find a better way to provide a safety net for those with substantial needs so that their major recourse is not the malpractice system. It is understand why the standard of care evolves to impose liability in more situations when the alternative is persons without a means to address their needs.

How does the existing system work? In most cases, there are competing expert opinions concerning the standard, and the jury or judge attempts within their capability to evaluate the opinions and select among them. This process perforce is colored by the drama of the rest of the case.

However, the process does allow a judge or jury to impose as the standard what any one qualified expert is willing to testify is the standard. If there is such testimony on the record, there is often little that appellate courts can do about aberrant findings, except to find a basis to disqualify the expert or find a procedural error that permits the ordering of a new trial. Legislatures and courts have tried to contain the misuse of the process by controlling who can testify and permitting professional licensing boards to discipline professionals whose testimony is aberrant.

The process by which the standard is determined continues to have a bigger impact on the standard in each case than the words that are used to articulate the standard.

Litigation focuses almost solely on the outcome for the individuals who are parties to the litigation. Until the appellate level, the process seldom takes into account the impact on others. This makes it very difficult to establish standards that appropriately balance the competing societal interests in cost of health care, access to health care, and quality of health care.

In order to balance cost, access, and quality, society — through government, institutions, and professional groups — will need to

---

[237] *See also* A. Robeznieks, *JCAHO: liability crisis is a barrier to patient safety,* Am. Med. News, Feb. 28, 2005, 13.

find ways to establish achievable standards that the average professional and institution can achieve on a daily basis. The standards need to permit striving for higher levels of achievement without having liability imposed for the effort.

The standards need to take into account the limitations of the humans who are involved in the process. Standards need to take into account the short time frames within which many medical decisions must be made and the fact that they must be made when there is still uncertainty about the patient's condition. Standards need to take into account the uncertainty regarding medical practice. Notwithstanding the efforts to promote evidence-based medicine, the evidence does not exist for a large part of medical practice. Much of medicine is still based on experience and professional judgment. Where there is evidence, it is often overwhelming in volume. There is no way for an individual to keep track of all of it, even in one specialty. The complex literature review that is sometimes done to establish the standard of care for a malpractice case draws upon a scope of information that no individual can realistically be expected to have mastered.

There are several ways that the changes in the effective standard of care have been addressed directly or indirectly by courts or legislators.

DESCRIPTION OF STANDARD. At least one court has expressly stated that an error of judgment can be within the standard of practice and does not automatically constitute negligence.[238]

The two schools of thought doctrine discussed in Section 11-1.2 can limit the jury's ability to select a standard articulated by one expert when another expert says that what was done was within the standard.

It is possible to convince courts to change the articulated standard of care without legislation. For example, in 1998, the highest court of New York overruled the special high standard of care imposed on common carriers. For over one hundred years, common carriers had been held to the duty of the highest care. The court ruled that they would be held to same general negligence standard of reasonable care under all the circumstances as other businesses.[239]

---

[238] Ezell v. Hutson, 105 Wash. App. 485, 20 P.3d 975 (2001); *contra,* Shumaker v. Johnson, 571 So. 2d 991 (Ala. 1990) [rejecting good faith error of judgment defense].

[239] Bethel v. New York City Transit Auth., 92 N.Y.2d 348, 703 N.E.2d 1214, 681 N.Y.S.2d 201 (1998).

LEVEL OF PROOF. One state requires the standard of care to be proven by clear and convincing evidence in some cases rather than the preponderance of the evidence standard usually used in civil cases.[240] The difference is discussed in Section 7-1.2. The practical effect of this difference is that it permits the trial judge or the appellate court more latitude to find that there was not sufficient evidence to support the jury's decision.

SCRUTINY OF SUPPORT FOR THE EXPERT'S OPINION. As discussed in Section 11-1.2, there is increasing judicial scrutiny of the scientific basis for an expert's opinion, applying the *Daubert* standard. Although the *Daubert* standard has been applied to standard of care testimony, it is difficult to apply the standard, and it is not clear what impact it will have on malpractice cases.

EXPERTS. States have specified the qualifications of experts using such factors as specialty, geographic location, and limits on the time spent serving as an expert.[241] This is discussed in Section 11-1.2.

CONSENSUS PROCESSES. Texas has a governmental process to review and approve consent forms. Maine experimented with using clinical guidelines. This is discussed in Section 11-1.2. There have been proposals to use surveys of providers to establish the standard of care.[242]

This section is an invitation to consider how an appropriate standard could be articulated and applied.

11-7.2 Dispute Resolution Mechanisms

Most malpractice claims are either settled or dropped. Litigation is very expensive, disruptive, and uncertain. However, even when cases are settled or dropped, the cost of the litigation to get the case to that point can be burdensome and traumatic.

In an effort to reduce the burden of litigation, alternate dispute resolution mechanisms have been adopted in some states. Screening

---

[240] Harvest v. Craig, 202 Ariz. 529, 48 P.3d 479 (App. Ct. 2002) [upholding statute that requires clear and convincing evidence in some malpractice cases arising out of births - ARIZ. REV. STAT. § 32-1473].

[241] *E.g.*, FLA. STAT. § 766.102(2)(c); Payne v. Caldwell, 796 S.W.2d 142 (Tenn. 1990) [upheld requirement that expert has been licensed in state or contiguous state for previous year]; Butphin v. Platt, 720 S.W.2d 455 (Tenn. 1986) [medical experts must be from Tennessee or contiguous states]; Dekker v. Magic Valley Medical Center, 115 Idaho 322, 766 P.2d 1213 (1988) [expert barred from testifying because statutory standard not met].

[242] *E.g.*, A. Hartz et al., *Physician surveys to assess customary care in medical malpractice cases*, 17 J. GEN. INT. MED. 546 (2002).

panels have been adopted with limited success. Arbitration has been pursued. Administrative systems have been proposed but have not been adopted.

SCREENING PANELS. Some states enacted laws that require all malpractice claims to be screened by a panel before a suit can be filed.[243] These screening panels were designed to promote settlement of meritorious claims and abandonment of frivolous claims. Some states have abandoned the use of screening panels.[244]

A few courts have held the panels unconstitutional as an infringement of state constitutional rights to access to the courts.[245] The Florida Supreme Court declared the state's medical mediation requirement unconstitutional on the ground that it violated due process by being arbitrary and capricious in operation because of its ten-month limitation on the mediation process with no procedure to extend the limit.[246]

Most courts have upheld the required use of screening panels since plaintiffs still have the right to sue after the screening process is completed.[247] However, state courts vary in how broadly they interpret the scope of cases subject to screening.[248]

Federal courts require plaintiffs to complete any state-required screening process before pursuing a state malpractice claim in federal court.[249]

State law varies on the ways the results of such screening panels can be used in a subsequent suit.[250]

---

[243] *See* Annotation, *Validity and construction of state statutory provisions relating to limitations on amount of recovery in medical malpractice claim and submission of such claims to pretrial panel*, 80 A.L.R. 3D 583.

[244] *See* Eby v. Kozarek, 153 Wis. 2d 75, 450 N.W.2d 249 (1990).

[245] *E.g.*, Hoehm v. State, 756 P.2d 780 (Wyo. 1988); Bernier v. Burris, 113 Ill. 2d 219, 497 N.E.2d 763 (1986); State *ex rel.* Cardinal Glennon Mem. Hosp. v. Gaertner, 583 S.W.2d 107 (Mo. 1979).

[246] Aldana v. Holub, 381 So. 2d 231 (Fla. 1980).

[247] *E.g.*, Keyes v. Humana Hosp. Alaska, Inc., 750 P.2d 343 (Alaska 1988); Paro v. Longwood Hosp., 373 Mass. 645, 369 N.E.2d 985 (1977); Johnson v. St. Vincent Hosp., Inc., 273 Ind. 374, 404 N.E.2d 585 (1980); Cha v. Warnick, 476 N.E.2d 109 (Ind. 1985), *cert. denied*, 474 U.S. 920 (1985).

[248] *E.g.*, Winoma Mem. Found. v. Lomax, 465 N.E.2d 731 (Ind. Ct. App. 1984) [screening not required for slip and fall case]; Brown v. Rabbitt, 300 Md. 171, 476 A.2d 1167 (1984) [screening required for express contract to cure].

[249] *E.g.*, Daigle v. Maine Med. Ctr., Inc., 14 F.3d 684 (1st Cir. 1994) [affirming judgment for hospital after findings of prelitigation hearing panel used in accordance with Maine law].

[250] *See* McGee v. Bonaventura, 605 N.E.2d 792 (Ind. Ct. App 1993) [unanimous opinion of malpractice panel in favor of surgeon coupled with plaintiff's failure to provide rebutting expert testimony entitled surgeon to judgment as a matter of law]; Wright v. Carter, 604 N.E.2d 1236 (Ind. Ct. App. 1992) [expert evidence not necessary to defeat summary judgment motion by radiologist sued for portion of needle left in body in biopsy despite unanimous medical review panel opinion of no violation of standard of care].

ARBITRATION. Some states passed laws to facilitate arbitration as an alternative to litigation. Arbitration is used extensively in some areas. Arbitration is discussed in Section 11-3.

ADMINISTRATIVE SYSTEMS. There have been proposals to create an administrative system to determine whether there should be payment and, if so, the amount in all malpractice cases.[251] This would replace the courts and arbitration. Appeals to the courts would be allowed only in limited circumstances. No state has enacted such a system. Courts in many states would probably view such a system as a violation of the right under the state constitution to access to the courts. In those states, an amendment to the state constitution may be necessary before such a law would be possible.

The definition of the grounds for entitlement to payment under any administrative system would need to be carefully written. Under the law applicable to Veterans Affairs (VA) hospitals, veterans can claim disability through an administrative process. In 1994, the United States Supreme Court ruled that a claim for disability benefits from the VA does not require any fault of the VA hospital.[252]

New Zealand has an administrative system for health care compensation. Numerous studies and articles have described the effects of that system.[253]

In 2003, the governor of Massachusetts and the Harvard School of Public Health began developing a plan for a pilot project to use tribunals of administrative law judges to determine whether compensation should be awarded and to set the amount in accordance with a schedule.[254]

A few states have offered administrative systems for some types of claims but generally have not made them binding on the claimant. For example, the Florida Birth-Related Neurological Injury Compensation Act provides for an administrative law judge to determine whether the claim is compensable and the amount of the compensation. In order to obtain payment from the fund, the award must be accepted. However, the claimant is free to litigate if

---

[251] *E.g.*, P.R. McGinn, *Vermont MDs push tort system revamp: medical negligence bill calls for administrative system*, AM.MED.NEWS, Apr. 28, 1989, 3.

[252] Brown v. Gardner, 513 U.S. 115 (1994).

[253] *E.g.*, E.K. Solender, *New Zealand's no-fault accident compensation scheme has some unintended consequences: a caution to U.S. reformers*, 27 INT'L LAW. 91 (1993).

[254] R. Ranalli, *Malpractice plan would limit trials*, BOSTON GLOBE, Nov. 13, 2003, A1.

dissatisfied with the outcome.[255] This system has been criticized by providers.[256]

11-7.3 Amount and Payment of Award

The amount and payment of the award have been modified by (1) imposing ceilings on the award, (2) abolishing the collateral source rule, (3) authorizing periodic payments, and (4) modifying joint and several liability.

There is another development in tax law that may put upward pressure on the amount of awards. In 2005, the United States Supreme Court ruled that the plaintiff must pay income taxes on the entire amount of any award, including the portion paid to the attorney. The payment to the attorney is not deductible, except when a special law applies that permits deduction of lawyers fees in some employment discrimination cases. This will mean that plaintiffs will be able to keep a smaller portion of the amount awarded.[257]

CEILINGS ON AWARDS. Limitations on the amount that can be awarded in a malpractice suit have been one of the most controversial approaches to tort reform. Several states have enacted limits.[258]

A 1993 study by the Congressional Office of Technology Assessment reported that damage caps were one of the most effective means of reducing malpractice costs.[259] A 2004 study by the Rand Corporation concluded that the California damage cap had cut payouts by 30 percent and that this comprised a 15 percent reduction in payments to patients and a 60 percent reduction in payments to the patients' attorneys.[260]

In 1978, the United States Supreme Court ruled that Congress could place caps on damages.[261] The case involved liability for nuclear reactors. Although Congress has considered proposals to

---

[255] FLA. STAT. § 766.304.

[256] *E.g.*, S. Martin, *NICA - Florida Birth-Related Neurological Injury Compensation Act: four reasons why this malpractice reform must be eliminated,* 26 NOVA L. REV. 609 (2002).

[257] C.I.R. v. Banks, 125 S. Ct. 826 (U.S. 2005).

[258] *See* Annotation, *Validity and construction of state statutory provisions relating to limitations on amount of recovery in medical malpractice claim and submission of such claims to pretrial panel,* 80 A.L.R.3D 583; R. Zimmerman & J.T. Hallinan, *As malpractice caps spread, lawyers turn away some cases,* WALL ST. J., Oct. 8, 2004, A1.

[259] OTA, IMPACT OF LEGAL REFORMS ON MEDICAL MALPRACTICE COSTS (Oct. 27, 1993).

[260] R.L. Rundle, *Malpractice cap helps out doctors,* WALL ST. J., July 13, 2004, D4; *see also Study says caps lower premiums,* AM. MED. NEWS, Feb. 9, 2004, 16 [Health Affairs].

[261] Duke Power Co. v. Carolina Environmental Study Group, Inc., 438 U.S. 59 (1978).

cap liability in malpractice cases, it has not enacted such a cap, leaving the matter to the states.

State courts have disagreed on the constitutionality of such limits under state constitutions.[262] For example, in 1976, the Illinois Supreme Court declared ceilings to be an unconstitutional violation of equal protection because it could find no rational justification for treating those injured by medical malpractice differently from those injured by other means.[263] An example of a state that upheld caps is Indiana. In 1980, the Indiana Supreme Court declared ceilings to be constitutional because it found a rational justification in the need for a risk-spreading mechanism for malpractice liability at a reasonable cost to assure the continued availability of health services.[264] In 2003, the highest court of Massachusetts upheld applying the state's cap on liability of charitable corporations to a charitable hospital.[265] Also in 2003, the Nebraska Supreme Court upheld a malpractice damage cap.[266]

In at least one state, the constitutional objection was addressed by an amendment to the constitution. In 2003, Texas voters approved a constitutional amendment permitting caps in suits against health care providers.[267]

Generally, where there is a valid state cap on damages, it applies to most federal suits, including EMTALA suits and Federal Tort

---

262 See K.A. Olson, *Survey of constitutional arguments in medical malpractice award limit cases*, 23 J. HEALTH & HOSP. L. 328 (1990).

263 Wright v. Central DuPage Hosp. Ass'n, 63 Ill. 2d 313, 347 N.E.2d 736 (1976); *accord*, Morris v. Savoy, 61 Ohio St. 3d 684, 576 N.E.2d 765 (1991) [statutory damage cap unconstitutional]; Sofie v. Fibreboard Corp., 112 Wn. 2d 636, 771 P.2d 711 (1989); Reynolds v. Porter, 760 P.2d 816 (Okla. 1988); Smith v. Department of Ins., 507 So. 2d 1080 (Fla. 1987) [unconstitutional].

264 Johnson v. St. Vincent Hosp., Inc., 273 Ind. 374, 404 N.E.2d 585 (1980); *accord*, Scholtz v. Metropolitan Pathologists, 851 P.2d 901 (Colo. 1993) [cap on noneconomic damages constitutional]; Adams v. Children's Mercy Hosps., 832 S.W.2d 898 (Mo. 1992) [cap on damages constitutional]; Butler v. Flint Goodrich Hosp., 607 So. 2d 517 (La. 1992) [cap on medical malpractice judgments not violation of equal protection]; Samsel v. Wheeler Transp. Servs., Inc., 244 Kan. 726, 771 P.2d 71 (1989); Boyd v. Bulala, 877 F.2d 1191 (4th Cir. 1989) [Virginia cap on damages upheld]; Etheridge v. Medical Center Hosps., Inc., 237 Va. 626, 376 S.E.2d 525 (1989) [cap on total damages upheld]; Franklin v. Mazda Motor Corp., 704 F. Supp. 1325 (D. Md. 1989) [cap on noneconomic damages upheld]; Williams v. Kushner, 524 So. 2d 191 (La. Ct. App. 4th Cir. 1988) [cap upheld]; Fein v. Permanente Medical Group, 38 Cal. 3d 137, 695 P.2d 665, 211 Cal. Rptr. 368 (1985), *appeal dismissed*, 474 U.S. 892 (1985) [cap on noneconomic damages upheld].

265 Conners v. Northeast Hosp. Corp., 439 Mass. 469, 789 N.E.2d 129 (2003).

266 Gourley v. Nebraska Methodist Health Sys., Inc., 265 Neb. 918, 663 N.W.2d 43 (2003).

267 R. Blumentahl, *Cap on suits vs. doctors is approved in Texas vote*, N.Y. TIMES, Sept. 15, 2003, A12.

Claims Act suits.[268] The state caps apply when federal courts try malpractice cases under state law. The state caps also apply to suits against the United States when federal law specifies that state law should be followed.[269]

One difficulty with state caps is that they sometimes can be bypassed by bringing suit in another state. When a provider does business in another state and the malpractice claims arises out of that business, it is subject to the law of the state where the malpractice occurred. In 1979, the United States Supreme Court ruled that even a state cap on liability of the state did not have to be recognized by other states in which the state engaged in business.[270] A Nevada governmental entity was sued in California for actions in California, and the Nevada damages cap did not apply to a suit in California. A few states recognize some caps of other states. In 1989, the Illinois Supreme Court ruled that Illinois courts should recognize other states' limits on the liability of state agencies.[271] However, this has not been extended to other caps on damages.

Sometimes patients from other states try to bring suit in their home state against out-of-state providers for services provided in the other state. It is usually difficult to obtain jurisdiction over the out-of-state provider, and the suit gets dismissed.[272] However, occasionally the provider has engaged in enough business in the state where the suit is brought to permit obtaining jurisdiction. Then the court must decide which state's law will govern. In most cases, the law of the state where the services were provided is applied.[273] However, in some cases, the law of the state where the suit is brought is applied so that the provider loses the benefit of its state cap.

---

[268] *E.g.*, Power v. Arlington Hosp. Ass'n, 42 F.3d 851 (4th Cir. 1994) [EMTALA claim subject to state damages cap]; *but see* Root v. New Liberty Hosp. Dist., 209 F.3d 1068 (8th Cir. 2000) [while acknowledging applicability of damage caps to EMTALA, rejects that complete sovereign immunity applies].

[269] *E.g.*, Lozada v. U.S., 974 F.2d 986 (8th Cir. 1992) [state cap applicable to Federal Tort Claims Act (FTCA) suit despite contention hospital did not meet requirements as qualified health care provider]; Carter v. U.S., 982 F.2d 1141 (7th Cir. 1992) [U.S. protected in FTCA suit by Indiana malpractice damage cap].

[270] Nevada v. Hall, 440 U.S. 410 (1979).

[271] Schoeberlein v. Purdue Univ., 129 Ill. 2d 372, 544 N.E.2d 283 (1989).

[272] *E.g.*, O'Brien v. Hackensack Univ. Med. Ctr., 305 A.D.2d 199, 760 N.Y.S.2d 425 (1st Dept. 2003) [no NY jurisdiction over NJ hospital]; Townsend v. University Hospital - University of Colorado, 83 S.W.3d 913 (Tex. App. 2002) [Internet communications, acceptance of referrals not sufficient business for jurisdiction]; Smith v. Gottlieb, 2002 U.S. Dist. LEXIS 15343 (N.D. Ill) [no jurisdiction over University of Wisconsin Hospitals and Clinics Authority].

[273] *E.g.*, Bledsoe v. Friedman, 270 U.S. App. D.C. 308, 849 F.2d 639 (1988) [requiring D.C. resident suing Md. provider for care in Md. to follow Md. law].

There have been repercussions for some courts that have invalidated limits. In May 1988, the Texas Supreme Court struck down the state cap on noneconomic damages.[274] Texas judges must be periodically approved by the voters. In the November 1988 election, the justices that had dismantled the tort reform law were removed.[275] In 1990, the court upheld a cap on damages.[276]

In June 1988, the Kansas Supreme Court struck down the state cap on malpractice damages.[277] The legislature scheduled hearings on a state constitutional amendment. In March 1989, the court ruled that it would uphold a cap on noneconomic damages in nonmedical cases, and the constitutional amendment effort was dropped.[278]

COLLATERAL SOURCE RULE. Under the common law the defendant must pay for the entire cost of the plaintiff's injuries even if the plaintiff has already received some compensation from other sources, such as insurance. This is called the *collateral source* rule. Several states abolished the collateral source rule, and the amount of compensation the plaintiff receives from other sources is deducted from the amount the defendant owes. This process has been declared constitutional by several courts,[279] but a few courts have disagreed.[280]

When the collateral source rule applies, it often inflates the amount awarded in unexpected ways. For example, in 2001, the Wisconsin Supreme Court ruled that an injured person could recover the full charges for the medical services received even though his health care insurer had actually paid much less for the services.[281] The court viewed the medical expenses as a measure of damages rather than as an expense to be reimbursed through the tort system. In 2003, a Florida appellate court ruled that a medical expense award was properly reduced to the amount actually paid for the services.[282]

---

[274] Lucas v. U.S., 757 S.W.2d 687 (Tex. 1988).

[275] L. Page, *TMA-backed coalition ousts court majority*, Am. Med. News, Nov. 18, 1988, 7.

[276] Rose v. Doctors Hosp., 801 S.W.2d 841 (Tex. 1990).

[277] Kansas Malpractice Victims Coalition v. Bell, 243 Kan. 333, 757 P.2d 251(1988).

[278] S. Hillen, *Kansas backs limits for pain, suffering*, Am. Med. News, Apr. 21, 1989, 22; Samsel v. Wheeler Transp. Servs., Inc., 244 Kan. 726, 771 P.2d 71 (1989); P.R. McGinn, *Kansas MDs await ruling on award cap*, Am. Med. News, Oct. 13, 1989, 1.

[279] *E.g.*, Bernier v. Burris, 113 Ill. 2d 219, 497 N.E.2d 763 (1986); Rudolph v. Iowa Methodist Medical Center, 293 N.W.2d 550 (Iowa 1980).

[280] *E.g.*, Coburn v. Augustin, 627 F. Supp. 983 (D. Kan. 1985).

[281] Koffman v. Leichtfuss, 2001 WI 111, 246 Wis. 2d 31, 630 N.W.2d 201; *accord,* Rose v. Via Christi Health Sys., Inc., 276 Kan. 539, 78 P.3d 798 (2003) [recovery of full charges even where Medicare paid lower rate].

[282] Goble v. Frohman, 848 So. 2d 406 (Fla.2d DCA 2003).

PERIODIC PAYMENT. Under the common law, the plaintiff is entitled to payment of court judgments in a single lump sum. One advantage of settling cases involving large liabilities is that the parties can agree to periodic payments that are easier for the defendant to pay. Some states have passed laws authorizing courts to direct that large judgments be paid by periodic payments. The courts have not agreed on whether these laws are constitutional.[283]

Some courts may have inherent authority to structure payout of awards to the beneficiary provided the full amount has been paid by the person found liable. Thus, a federal appellate court ruled that there was inherent authority to place an award for a child in a reversionary trust over the objections of the parents who had a conflict of interest.[284]

JOINT AND SEVERAL LIABILITY. Under the common law when several defendants are found liable, each is liable for the entire amount. The plaintiff can select from whom to try to collect. Thus, for example, when a rider was injured on a ride at Walt Disney World and the jury allocated responsibility 14 percent to the rider, 85 percent to his accompanying fiancé, and 1 percent to Walt Disney World, the rider was permitted to collect 86 percent from Walt Disney World.[285] Under contributory negligence principles, he was not permitted to collect the remaining 14 percent due to his personal fault.

Moreover, under the common law the defendant who pays is not permitted in most cases to recover reimbursement from the other defendants even if they have greater responsibility.[286]

Some states have modified these harsh rules by statute.[287]

---

[283] *E.g.*, Desiderio v. Ochs, 100 N.Y.2d 159, 791 N.E.2d 941, 761 N.Y.S.2d 576 (2003) [uphold applying structured settlement law even when it might exceed jury award]; Bernier v. Burris, 113 Ill. 2d 219, 497 N.E.2d 763 (1986) [constitutional]; American Bank & Trust Co. v. Community Hosp., 36 Cal. 3d 359, 683 P.2d 670, 204 Cal. Rptr. 671 (1984) [constitutional]; *contra,* Smith v. Myers, 181 Ariz. 11, 887 P.2d 541 (1994) [periodic payment statute unconstitutional limit on remedies]; Kansas Malpractice Victims Coalition v. Bell, 243 Kan. 333, 757 P.2d 251 (1988).

[284] Hull v. U.S., 971 F.2d 1499 (10th Cir. 1992).

[285] Walt Disney World v. Wood, 515 So. 2d 198 (Fla. 1987).

[286] *E.g.*, Florida Patient's Compensation Fund v. St. Paul Fire & Marine Ins. Co., 535 So. 2d 335 (Fla. 4th DCA 1988).

[287] Fla. Stat. §768.81 [joint and several liability modified], §768.31 [contribution permitted]; *see also* Smith v. Dep't of Ins., 507 So. 2d 1080 (Fla. 1987) [§768.81 constitutional]; Fabre v. Marin, 623 So. 2d 1182 (Fla. 1993) [§768.81(3) not ambiguous; entry of judgment on basis of percentage fault means judgment must be based on percentage of total fault regardless of whether others responsible could have been joined as defendants]; Freyer v. Albin, 5 P.3d 329 (Colo. App. 1999) [physician not liable for acts of another physician unless employee, partner, joint venturer, or acting in concert].

11-7.4 Statute of Limitations

The statute of limitations specifies the time in which suits must be filed or forever barred. Some states have shortened this time. Prior to the malpractice crisis amendments of the 1980s, nearly all states permitted minors to wait to file suit until they became adults. Some tort reform acts limit minors to a specific number of years after the right to sue accrues. While some courts have upheld these laws, other courts have found them to violate state constitutions.[288]

Some states have redefined when the time begins as another way to shorten the time. In most states, the time begins when the patient discovers an injury that may be due to someone else's negligence.[289] Courts have disagreed on whether limits that start on the date of the incident are enforceable.[290]

Such limits can bar the suit before the patient knows there is a basis to sue. In some cases, such as unwanted births after negligent sterilizations, the injury may not occur until many years after the incident.

11-7.5 Other Tort Reform

Other tort reform amendments have:

1. Limited the grounds for suits based on lack of informed consent,[291]
2. Restricted contingency fees for lawyers or given courts the authority to modify them,[292]

---

[288] *E.g.*, Baird v. Loeffler, 69 Ohio St. 2d 533, 434 N.E.2d 194 (1982) [one-year limit upheld]; Douglas v. Hugh A. Stallings, M.D., Inc., 870 F.2d 1242 (7th Cir. 1989) [upheld requirement that minors injured when less than six years old sue by age eight]; *contra,* Stahler v. St. Luke's Hosp., 706 S.W.2d 7 (Mo. 1986) (en banc) [minors have right to wait until becoming adults to sue]; Barrio v. San Manuel Div. Hosp., 143 Ariz. 101, 692 P.2d 280 (1984) [unconstitutional to require minors injured when less than seven years old to sue by age ten].

[289] *E.g.*, Hershberger v. Akron City Hosp., 34 Ohio St. 3d 1, 516 N.E.2d 204 (1987).

[290] *E.g.*, Carr v. Broward County, 541 So. 2d 92 (Fla. 1989) [suit can be barred before discovery possible]; McDonald v. Haynes Medical Laboratory, Inc., 192 Conn. 327, 471 A.2d 646 (1984) [suit can be barred before injury occurs]; *contra,* Hardy v. VerMeulen, 32 Ohio St. 3d 45, 512 N.E.2d 626 (1987) [suit cannot be barred before discovery]; Shessel v. Stroup, 253 Ga. 56, 316 S.E.2d 155 (1984) [suit cannot be barred before injury occurs].

[291] *E.g.*, Fla. Stat. § 768.46.

[292] *E.g.*, Iowa Code §147.138; Newton v. Cox, 878 S.W.2d 105 (Tenn. 1994) [upholding cap on contingent fees in medical malpractice cases]; *see also* Walters v. National Ass'n of Radiation Survivors, 473 U.S. 305 (1985); National Ass'n of Radiation Survivors v. Derwinski, 994 F.2d 583 (9th Cir. 1992), *cert. denied,* 510 U.S. 1023 (1993) [upholding $10 limit on fees veteran can pay attorney for assistance in VA claim, but note Congress removed the $10 limit in 1988 in Pub. L. No. 100-687, 102 Stat. 4105, for later claims]; Beck v. Secretary of HHS, 924 F.2d 1029 (D.C. Cir. 1991) [attorney in successful Vaccine Act claim limited to fees provided in Act].

3. Prohibited asking for a specific amount of money in the suit,[293]
4. Prohibited punitive damages[294] or required part of punitive damage awards to be paid to the state,[295]
5. Required notices of intent to sue,[296] and
6. Required an affidavit of merit from a expert to be attached to the suit.[297]

11-7.6 Malpractice Coverage Reform

Some states have tried to address the cost or unavailability of malpractice insurance coverage by facilitating the development of new insurers, developing state-run systems, and subsidizing the cost of insurance directly or indirectly.

NEW INSURERS. In some states, state Joint Underwriting Authorities provide insurance to some providers who cannot obtain insurance in the private market.

Some states established other malpractice insurance plans.[298]

In Nevada, some physicians were made part-time faculty members so that they could be covered by the state university self-insurance fund and be protected by its cap on damages.[299]

GOVERNMENTAL PAYMENT SYSTEMS. Some states have insurance systems that pay part of any malpractice award. These laws have generally been upheld, including the requirement that all health

---

[293] *E.g.*, Iowa Code § 619.18; *contra,* White v. Fisher, 689 P.2d 102 (Wyo. 1984) [unconstitutional]; *but see* Boothe v. Lawrence Hosp., 188 A.D.2d 435, 591 N.Y.S.2d 412 (1st Dept. 1992) [only sanction for violation was striking offensive reference].

[294] *E.g.*, Williams v. Chicago Osteopathic Med. Ctr., 173 Ill. App. 3d 125, 527 N.E.2d 409 (1st Dist. 1988); Shackleford v. State, 534 So. 2d 38 (La. Ct. App. 1988).

[295] *E.g.*, Fla. Stat. § 768.73; *Punitive damages tax falls short as New York state revenue source,* Wall St. J., Nov. 13, 1992, B10.

[296] *E.g.*, Hardy v. New York City Health & Hosps. Corp, 164 F.3d 789 (2d Cir. 1999) [EMTALA suit must comply with state notice of claim requirement]; Patry v. Capps, 633 So. 2d 9 (Fla. 1994) [acknowledged receipt of hand-delivered notice is sufficient despite statutory requirement of certified mail]; Boyd v. Becker, 627 So. 2d 481 (Fla. 1993) [90-day presuit period began on mailing not receipt, so suit untimely].

[297] *E.g.*, Horizons/CMS Healthcare Corp., Inc. v. Fischer, 111 S.W. 3d 67 (Tex. 2003) [nurse's expert report did not satisfy requirement, so case properly dismissed]; Mosberg v. Elahi, 80 N.Y.2d 941, 605 N.E.2d 353, 590 N.Y.S.2d 866 (1992) [dismissal mandated where affidavit of merit not filed]; Williams v. Boyle, 72 P.3d 392 (Colo. App. 2003) [dismissal for failure to attach certificate of review]; Estate of Cassara by Cassara v. State, 853 F. Supp. 273 (N.D. Ill. 1994) [dismissal for failure to comply with state law requirement of attached affidavit of professional attesting to reasonable and meritorious case]; *see also* Witte v. Azarian, 369 Md. 518, 801 A.2d 160 (2000) [interpreting statute that bars professional witnesses who spend more than 20 percent of their time directly involved in testimony in personal injury claims].

[298] *E.g.*, *Insurers see Nevada malpractice agency as temporary fix,* AP, Mar. 15, 2002 [state run malpractice insurance agency].

[299] *See* J. Babula, *Trauma center faces new threat,* Las Vegas Rev.-J., Mar. 21, 2002, 1A.

care providers contribute to the fund[300] and the requirement that the administrative procedure associated with the system be followed.[301]

The federal government established the National Childhood Vaccine Injury Act to pay for injuries caused by certain vaccination programs.[302]

SUBSIDIES. Some states have provided subsidies directly. For example, Nevada used state funds to start a malpractice plan.[303] Other subsidies were provided through changing the timing of physician assessments.[304]

11-8 What Are Some Examples of the Tort Liability of Health Care Providers?

This section reviews the application of those principles to specific situations that have resulted in suits against hospitals and health care professionals, illustrating the scope of the duty of hospitals and their staff members to patients and others.

HOSPITALS. Hospital liability can be based on (1) a violation by an employee of employee's duties or (2) a violation of the hospital's duties. Hospital liability for injuries caused by an employee's violation of the employee's duties is based on the doctrine of *respondeat superior* discussed previously in this chapter.

Whenever individual health care professionals function as hospital employees or agents, their liability exposure also constitutes

---

[300] *E.g.*, King v. Virginia Birth-Related Neurological Injury Compensation Program, 410 S.E.2d 656 (Va. 1991) [constitutional to require physicians to contribute to fund]; McGibony v. Florida Birth-Related Neurological Injury Comp. Plan, 564 So. 2d 177 (Fla. 1st DCA 1990) [no fault compensation plan not violation of due process or equal protection rights of physicians who were required to contribute; lawful to delegate to Department of Insurance power to increase assessments on actuarial sound standard]; Johnson v. St. Vincent Hosp., Inc., 273 Ind. 374, 404 N.E.2d 585 (1980); Meier v. Anderson, 692 F. Supp. 546 (E.D. Pa. 1988).

[301] *E.g.*, Turner v. Hubrich, 656 So. 2d 970 (Fla. 5th DCA 1995) [Birth-Related Neurological Injury Compensation Act, Fla. Stat. §§ 766.301–766.316, provides exclusive administrative remedy against participating providers if they give notice of their participation to patients prior to services; claimant allowed to amend to claim lack of notice].

[302] *See* Schindler v. Secretary of DHHS, 29 F.3d 607 (Fed. Cir. 1994); Patton v. Secretary of DHHS, 25 F.3d 1021 (Fed. Cir. 1994); Weddel v. Secretary of DHHS, 23 F.3d 388 (Fed. Cir. 1994); Whitecotton by Whitecotton v. Secretary of HHS, 17 F.3d 374 (Fed. Cir. 1994).

[303] *See supra*, note 298.

[304] *E.g., Pennsylvania Gov. Schweiker directs immediate steps to provide temporary relief to PA physicians facing costly malpractice insurance; decision removes burden of paying both primary insurance and CAT fund surcharge simultaneously*, PR Newswire, Dec. 28, 2001; *Pennsylvania regulator seeks med-mal surcharge freeze*, Best-Wire, Jan.11, 2002; *Pennsylvania Governor signs med-mal bill into law*, BestWire, Mar. 20, 2002 [discounts on surcharges].

hospital liability exposure. Many hospital duties are not based on *respondeat superior.* To prove liability for injuries caused by breaches of these duties, it is not necessary to show that an individual staff member breached a duty; it is sufficient to show a breach of the hospital's duty. Areas in which hospitals have an independent duty include (1) maintenance of the physical condition of the buildings and grounds, (2) selection and maintenance of equipment, and (3) selection and supervision of staff.

Physical Condition of the Buildings and Grounds. The hospital must exercise reasonable care in maintaining its buildings and grounds in a reasonably safe condition. An accident alone is not enough to establish liability. State or local regulations may establish standards, and injuries resulting from violations of those standards can lead to liability. When regulatory standards have not been violated, hospitals generally are liable only when the plaintiff proves that the hospital's employees or agents created a condition likely to cause injury or that they knew or should have known of a condition likely to cause injury and failed to take action to provide warning or correct the condition. For example, in 2002, a New York court held that a hospital was not liable to a visitor who slipped and fell on a french fry on the floor of the hospital cafeteria. There was no evidence that the french fry had been there long enough for the hospital to have constructive notice of its presence so that it could correct the condition.[305]

The hospital must exercise the same reasonable care as any other business that regularly invites the public onto its grounds and into its buildings. Hospital buildings and grounds should also be designed and maintained to meet the special needs of the infirm and disabled persons using hospital facilities. The hospital is generally not liable for injuries caused by a dangerous condition when the injured person was aware of the condition, was able to avoid the risk of injury, and, nevertheless, chose to ignore the risk. For example, in a Texas case the antenna wire for a television in a patient's room was in a place where it could be tripped over. The patient had been aware of the wire and had walked around the set to avoid the wire several times during her stay. On the day of her discharge, she chose to step over the wire and tripped. The hospital won the suit because the danger was open and obvious and the

---

[305] Mulvihill v. Good Samaritan Hospital (N.Y. Sup. Ct. 2002), N.Y.L.J., April 16, 2002, 20.

patient had the ability to avoid it.[306] However, the North Carolina Supreme Court ruled that a hospital visitor was not responsible for watching for a three-inch rise in the sidewalk when there were diversions such as low-hanging tree branches and uneven illumination.[307] Suits have arisen out of accidents involving, for example, elevators,[308] broken steps,[309] slippery materials on the floors,[310] defective carpet,[311] automobiles in the parking lot,[312] and malfunction of automatic gates and doors.[313]

Courts have disagreed on the extent to which a hospital must protect persons on hospital premises from crimes by persons unassociated with the hospital. The California Supreme Court ruled that a hospital had a duty to protect persons in its parking lot in a high crime area, and it could be liable to a physician shot by a robber.[314] A Georgia court ruled that injuries to a hospital employee who was attacked in the hospital parking lot arose out of her employment so she could only pursue a claim under the workers' compensation law.[315] The Louisiana Supreme Court ruled that a nurse's employer

---

[306] Charrin v. Methodist Hosp., 432 S.W.2d 572 (Tex. Civ. App. 1968); *accord*, Collum v. Jackson Hosp. & Clinic, Inc., 374 So. 2d 314 (Ala. 1979); Spann v. Hosp. Auth. of Calhoun County, 208 Ga. App. 494, 430 S.E.2d 828 (1993) [nurse's aid].

[307] Pulley v. Rex Hosp., 326 N.C. 701, 392 S.E.2d 380 (1990).

[308] *E.g.*, Shoemaker v. Rush-Presbyterian-St. Luke's Med. Ctr., 187 Ill. App. 3d 1040, 543 N.E.2d 1014 (1st Dist. 1989); J.A. Lozano, *Family of doctor killed in elevator accident at Houston hospital files wrongful death lawsuit*, AP, Aug. 29, 2003 [portion of head of resident physician cut off when elevator doors closed].

[309] *E.g.*, DeKalb County Hosp. Auth. v. Theofanidis, 157 Ga. App. 811, 278 S.E.2d 712 (1981); *see* Annotation, *Hospital's liability to visitor injured as result of condition of exterior walks, steps, or grounds*, 71 A.L.R. 2D 427.

[310] *E.g.*, Calvache v. Jackson Mem. Hosp., 588 So. 2d 28 (Fla. 3d DCA 1991); Burwell v. Easton Mem. Hosp., 83 Md. App. 684, 577 A.2d 394 (1990); Gales v. United States, 617 F. Supp. 42 (W.D. Pa. 1985); *see* Annotation, *Hospital's liability to visitor injured by slippery, obstructed, or defective interior floors or steps*, 71 A.L.R. 2D 436.

[311] Pierson v. Sharp Mem. Hosp., Inc., 216 Cal. App. 3d 340, 264 Cal. Rptr. 673 (4th Dist. 1989).

[312] *E.g.*, Lovell v. St. Paul Fire & Marine Ins. Co., 310 Ark. 791, 839 S.W.2d 222 (1992); Chernov v. St. Luke's Hosp. Med. Ctr., 123 Ariz. 521, 601 P.2d 284 (1979); *see* Annotation, *Liability of owner or operator of parking lot for personal injuries caused by movement of vehicles*, 38 A.L.R. 3D 138.

[313] *E.g.*, McHenry v. Utah Valley Hosp., 724 F. Supp. 835 (D. Utah 1989), *aff'd*, 927 F.2d 1125 (10th Cir.), *cert. denied*, 502 U.S. 894 (1991) [gate]; McDonald v. Aliquippa Hosp., 414 Pa. Super. 317, 606 A.2d 1218 (1992) [doors]; *see* Annotation, *Liability of owner or operator of business premises for injuries from electronically operated door*, 99 A.L.R. 2D 725.

[314] Isaacs v. Huntington Mem. Hosp., 38 Cal. 3d 112, 211 Cal. Rptr. 356, 695 P.2d 653 (1985); *see* Annotation, *Parking facility proprietor's liability for criminal attack on patron*, 49 A.L.R. 4TH 1257.

[315] Maxwell v. Hospital Auth., 202 Ga. App. 92, 413 S.E.2d 205 (1991); *see* Annotation, *Workers' compensation law as precluding employee's suit against employer for third person's criminal attack*, 49 A.L.R. 4TH 926.

was not liable for her injuries from being stabbed by an unknown person as she exited a hospital elevator where there had been no prior similar accidents and nothing could have prevented assault.[316]

Numerous cases have arisen out of sexual assaults on patients and others. Courts have disagreed on the standard for determining when the hospital should be liable. The Alabama Supreme Court ruled that hospitals were responsible for protecting anesthetized patients from sexual assault even by trespassers.[317] A California court ruled that a hospital could be liable for the sexual assault of a disabled patient if it was shown to have provided inadequate supervision and security.[318] The Oregon Supreme Court ruled that a hospital could be liable for the sexual assault of a patient by an employee only if negligent retention or supervision of the employee was shown. The hospital did not have an independent direct duty to the patient in Oregon, and the act was outside the scope of employment under state law.[319]

Selection and Maintenance of Equipment. Hospitals have an obligation to furnish reasonably adequate equipment for use in the diagnosis and treatment of patients. Problems can arise when hospitals do not have needed equipment, when needed equipment is not available, or when equipment has not been properly inspected and maintained.

When a hospital does not have the equipment reasonably necessary for the treatment of certain conditions, patients with these conditions should be advised of the hospital's limitations, and arrangements should be made for transfer to another hospital with the necessary equipment unless the patient or the patient's representative makes an informed decision to decline the transfer. In a 1977 case, a woman had delivered a stillborn baby because the fourteen-bed obstetrical clinic she entered for delivery did not have the facilities for a Caesarean delivery.[320] The court found the clinic

---

[316] Mundy v. Dep't of Health & Human Resources, 620 So. 2d 811 (La. 1993).

[317] Young v. Huntsville Hosp., 595 So. 2d 1386 (Ala. 1992); *accord*, K.M.H. v. Lutheran Gen. Hosp., 230 Neb. 269, 431 N.W.2d 606 (1988) [direct hospital duty independent of *respondeat superior*].

[318] Andrea N. v. Laurelwood Convalescent Hosp., 13 Cal. App. 4th 1992, 16 Cal. Rptr. 2d 894 (2d Dist. 1993) [not citable in Cal.]; *accord*, Gregory by Gregory v. State, 195 A.D.2d 1030, 601 N.Y.S.2d 720 (4th Dept. 1993) [supervision adequate].

[319] G.L. v. Kaiser Found. Hosps., Inc., 306 Or. 54, 757 P.2d 1347 (1988).

[320] Hernandez v. Smith, 552 F.2d 142 (5th Cir. 1977); *see* Annotation, *Hospital's liability to patient for injury allegedly sustained from absence of particular equipment intended for use in diagnosis or treatment of patient*, 50 A.L.R. 3D 1141.

liable because it admitted the woman without having the necessary facilities or warning her of the limited nature of the facilities. In a California case, a hospital was found liable for injuries to a patient with third-degree burns who was kept for nearly two months in a hospital that did not have the equipment to care for the patient's burns.[321] The court ruled that the hospital had a duty to transfer the patient to another hospital with the necessary equipment. When a patient is reluctant to accept transfer, the most prudent practice is still to encourage transfer, rather than relying on refusal. A federal appellate court ruled that a VA hospital was not negligent for failing to have a lung scan machine and that timely arrangements had been made for transfer to a hospital that had the machine; the United States was not liable for the patient's death.[322]

Hospitals are generally not required to provide the latest equipment. For example, in a Louisiana case, a hospital was found not liable for having older equipment to cut sections of tissue for diagnosis instead of having more modern equipment that could cut thinner sections for a more accurate diagnosis.[323] Several experts testified that the older equipment was widely accepted and produced satisfactory results. A woman whose breast was removed due to misdiagnosis of malignancy was not awarded compensation.

Sometimes equipment might not be available for use due to system design problems or hospital staff failure to plan to have the proper equipment in the area. For example, in a North Carolina case, a hospital was found liable for the death of a patient due to delay in reintubation because the emergency cart was not stocked with the needed laryngoscope blade.[324] The Georgia Supreme Court decided that a hospital could be liable when its employees supplied incorrect parts for cataract equipment which caused a malfunction that injured the eye.[325] In a Texas case, the hospital was found liable for a patient's death because oxygen was unavailable after she was transferred to a private room.[326] A wall plug in the room supplied oxygen, but the equipment accompanying the patient required a wall plug of a different shape. The design problem was the lack of standardization of wall plugs. Portable oxygen equipment could

---

[321] Carrasco v. Bankoff, 220 Cal. App. 2d 230, 33 Cal. Rptr. 673 (2d Dist. 1963).
[322] Ducharme v. United States, 850 F.2d 27 (1st Cir. 1988).
[323] Lauro v. Travelers Ins. Co., 261 So. 2d 261 (La. Ct. App.).
[324] Dixon v. Taylor, 111 N.C. App. 97, 431 S.E.2d 778 (1993).
[325] Lamb v. Chandler Gen. Hosp., Inc., 262 Ga. 70, 413 S.E.2d 720 (1992).
[326] Bellaire Gen. Hosp. v. Campbell, 510 S.W.2d 94 (Tex. Civ. App. 1974).

have supplied the necessary oxygen, but none had accompanied the patient. In 2000, an Illinois court found a hospital liable for not having infant blood pressure equipment available.[327]

A hospital must also exercise reasonable care in inspecting and maintaining equipment. Equipment should be periodically inspected, and discovered defects should be remedied. However, the hospital does not guarantee that the equipment will function properly during customary use. Liability for injuries due to defects in equipment generally depends on whether the defect is latent (hidden) or patent (visible). The user of equipment is generally liable for injuries due to use of equipment with patent defects. The owner of the equipment is generally liable for injuries due to use of equipment with latent defects detectable through reasonable inspections that were not performed. The manufacturer or seller of the equipment is generally liable when the equipment has a latent defect, such as a flaw in the metal, the owner could not detect through reasonable inspections.

For example, an Alabama case addressed a patient who was injured because of a defect in an electrical-surgical instrument used in the removal of skin for grafting.[328] A bent spring caused the removal of too thick a patch of skin. The bent spring could have been detected only by the instrument for inspection. The court found the hospital, but not the surgeon who had used the instrument, liable for the injuries. If the bent spring had been visible to the surgeon without dismantling, the surgeon would have been liable. When equipment users are hospital employees, the hospital can be liable under the doctrine of *respondeat superior* for their failure to detect patent defects. If hospital employees switch equipment that the physician has already inspected, the hospital can also be liable for resultant injuries. An Ohio case concerned a surgeon who examined a cauterizing machine and then left the operating room.[329] While he was gone, a hospital employee substituted another machine that appeared so similar that the surgeon did not

---

[327] Suttle v. Lake Forest Hosp., 315 Ill. App. 3d 96, 733 N.E.2d 726 (1st Dist. 2000).

[328] South Highlands Infirmary v. Camp, 279 Ala. 1, 180 So. 2d 904 (1965); *see* Annotation, *Hospital's liability to patient for injury sustained from defective equipment furnished by hospital for use in diagnosis or treatment*, 14 A.L.R. 3D 1254.

[329] Clary v. Christiansen, 54 Ohio Abs. 254, 83 N.E.2d 644 (Ct. App. 1948); *see* Annotation, *Malpractice: attending physician's liability for injury caused by equipment furnished by hospital*, 35 A.L.R. 3D 1068.

notice the switch. The patient was burned during the surgery due to a defect in the machine. The surgeon was found not to be liable.

When the hospital or physician knows that the equipment is defective, it is easier to establish liability because the defect is clearly patent. In an Oklahoma case, the employer was found liable for an employee's use of equipment that was clearly malfunctioning.[330] The employee knew the electrotherapy machine was malfunctioning, but instead of turning off the machine and seeking assistance, she continued to use the machine until the patient was burned. In an Iowa case, a surgeon was found liable for a patient's infection resulting from contaminated sutures because he knew they were contaminated when he used them.[331] An earlier patient had become infected through use of sutures from the same supply.

At least one state has adopted a minority position that hospitals may be liable for some defects that are not detectable. A 1975 New Jersey case involved a surgical device that broke with a piece lodging in the patient's spine.[332] The break was due either to improper twisting by the surgeon or to a flaw in the metal that could not be detected by the inspections normally conducted by hospitals. The jury found that neither the physician nor the hospital had been negligent. The appellate court ordered a new trial at which either the physician or the hospital had to be found responsible.

Selection and Supervision of Staff. A hospital can be liable for failing to exercise reasonable care in selecting and supervising its staff and in setting staffing levels.[333] This liability applies to both professional and nonprofessional staff. Hospitals have a responsibility to evaluate the credentials of applicants for jobs. When a state license is required, the hospital should determine that the applicant has the license, but checking the license alone is usually not a sufficient check of the applicant's background and qualifications. The hospital should also provide appropriate training, supervision, and evaluation. In 1997, a Texas appeals court found a hospital liable for the negligence of unsupervised certified registered nurse anesthetists.[334] When evaluations indicate problems, appropriate action

---

[330] Orthopedic Clinic v. Hanson, 415 P.2d 991 (Okla. 1966).

[331] Shepard v. McGinnis, 251 Iowa 35, 131 N.W.2d 475 (1964).

[332] Anderson v. Somberg, 67 N.J. 291, 338 A.2d 1, *cert. denied*, 423 U.S. 929 (1975).

[333] *See* Annotation, M*edical malpractice: hospital's liability for injury allegedly caused by failure to have properly qualified staff,* 62 A.L.R. 4TH 692; Annotation, *Hospital's liability for injury resulting from failure to have sufficient number of nurses on duty,* 2 A.L.R. 5TH 286.

[334] Denton Reg. Med. Ctr. v LaCroix, 947 S.W.2d 941 (Tex. Ct. App. 1997).

should be taken. A Texas court ruled that expert testimony was not required to establish negligence in the supervising and assigning of a nurse, where the employee evaluation forms indicated an unsatisfactory rating over three months before the incident.[335] These issues are discussed in more detail in Chapter 4.

The hospital also has a responsibility to exercise reasonable care in credentialing and monitoring members of the medical staff, as discussed in Chapter 5. The potential for hospital liability for acts of physicians is discussed earlier in this chapter.

GOVERNING BODY AND ADMINISTRATOR. Members of the governing body have seldom been found personally liable for the activities of the hospital or for their own activities related to the hospital. Their liability exposure is discussed in Chapter 2. Administrators have been found liable for negligently supervising their subordinates, for entering contracts outside their authority, and for breaching duties imposed by statute. This liability exposure is discussed in the Liability part of Sections 2-3 and 11-5.2.

MANAGERS AND SUPERVISORS. Managers and supervisors are not the employers of staff they supervise. Thus, *respondeat superior* does not impose liability on supervisors for the acts or omissions of staff they supervise. Managers and supervisors are liable only for the consequences of their own acts or omissions. The manager or supervisor is usually a hospital employee, and the hospital can be liable under *respondeat superior* for the acts or omissions of supervisors.

The liability of a supervising nurse for the actions of supervised nurses was discussed in a California case involving a needle left in a patient's abdomen during surgery.[336] The patient sued the physicians, hospital, and supervising nurse. The court dismissed the suit against the supervising nurse because she had done nothing wrong. She had assigned two competent nurses to assist with the surgery, and she had not been present. Therefore, she had no opportunity to intervene. The court ruled that *respondeat superior* did not apply to the nursing supervisor because she was not the employer.

The actions that can lead to liability of supervising health care professionals are discussed in more detail in a New Jersey

---

[335] St. Paul Med. Ctr. v. Cecil, 842 S.W.2d 808 (Tex. Ct. App. 1992).
[336] Bowers v. Olch, 120 Cal. App. 2d 108, 260 P.2d 997 (2d Dist. 1953).

court decision.[337] The case involved a surgeon who had ordered a resident physician to remove a tube being used to extract the patient's gastric contents. The patient's esophagus was perforated during the removal. The court ruled that the supervising surgeon was not liable for the resident's acts. The court said that the supervising surgeon could be liable only if (1) it was not accepted medical or hospital practice to delegate the particular function to someone with the resident's level of training, (2) he knew or should have known the individual resident was not qualified to perform the task with the degree of supervision provided, (3) he had been present and able to avoid the injury, or (4) he had a special contract with the patient that he did not fulfill. Since none of these circumstances was present, the supervising surgeon was not liable. In some states, the courts apply a different legal doctrine to supervising physicians. The borrowed servant and dual servant doctrines are discussed earlier in this chapter.

A Canadian case provides another illustration of the potential liability of supervising nurses.[338] The court found both the supervising nurse and her hospital employer liable for injuries to a woman who was not observed often enough in a postanesthesia recovery room. The patient had surgery without complications and was transferred to the postanesthesia recovery room. The hospital had provided two nurses for the area, which the court accepted as adequate staffing, but the supervising nurse permitted the other nurse to leave the area for a coffee break just before three patients were admitted to the area. One of the patients suffered a respiratory obstruction that was not observed until the lack of oxygen caused permanent brain damage. The court ruled that the supervising nurse was liable for permitting the other nurse to leave the area at a time when she knew that the operating schedule would result in several admissions to the unit. The court stated that even if she had not known the operating schedule, she would still be liable for not knowing the aspects of the schedule that applied to the staffing needs of the area she supervised. Since the supervising nurse also provided direct nursing care to the patients in the area, she was also liable for failing to observe the patient more frequently. The court ruled that the nurse who left the area would also have been liable if she had been included in the

---

[337] Stumper v. Kimel, 108 N.J. Super. 209, 260 A.2d 526 (App. Div. 1970); *see* Annotation, *Liability of one physician or surgeon for malpractice of another*, 85 A.L.R. 2D 889.
[338] Laidlaw v. Lions Gate Hosp., 8 D.L.R. 3d 730 (B.C. Sup. Ct. 1969).

suit because she should have known the aspects of the operating schedule that applied to the staffing needs of the area in which she worked.[339] The hospital was also liable for the acts of both nurses under the doctrine of *respondeat superior.*

In a New York case, a patient who was disoriented had been found on a balcony outside a second-story window.[340] After the patient was returned to the hospital room, the physician told the staff to arrange to have the patient watched. The charge nurse called the patient's family to tell them to arrange to have someone watch the patient. The family said someone would be at the hospital in ten to fifteen minutes. When the family member arrived, the patient had fallen out of the window and was severely injured. The hospital was found liable for failing to move the patient to a secure room, apply additional restraints, or find someone to watch the patient for fifteen minutes. One charge nurse, one new registered nurse in orientation, one practical nurse, and one aide were working in a unit with nineteen patients. The court found that all except the aide had been engaged in routine duties that could have been delayed for fifteen minutes and that the aide had been permitted to leave for supper during the period. The court said that this finding was evidence that staffing was sufficient to provide continuous supervision for a patient in known danger for fifteen minutes. The failure of the supervising nurse to allocate the time of the available staff properly was one of the grounds for hospital liability. The general principles discussed in this section also apply to other supervising health care professionals.

In 1994, a federal court decided that there had been failure to supervise assistants adequately at an air force medical center where the supervision had consisted of a random review of a ten percent sample of the records of their care.[341]

In summary, a supervisor can be liable if:

1. The supervisor assigns a subordinate to do something the supervisor knows or should know the subordinate is unable to do;

---

[339] *See also* Husher v. Commissioner of Ed., 188 A.D.2d 739, 591 N.Y.S.2d 99 (3d Dept. 1992) [nurse guilty of professional misconduct by leaving unit without proper coverage after agreeing to stay, knowing of nursing shortage, and not giving reasonable notice of leaving].

[340] Horton v. Niagara Falls Mem. Med. Ctr., 51 A.D.2d 152, 380 N.Y.S.2d 116 (4th Dept. 1976).

[341] MacDonald v. United States, 853 F. Supp. 1430 (M.D. Ga. 1994).

2. The supervisor does not supervise a subordinate to the degree the supervisor knows or should know the subordinate needs;

3. The supervisor is present and fails to take action when possible to avoid the injury; or

4. The supervisor does not properly allocate the time of available staff.

NURSES. A professional nurse is usually held to the standard of care generally observed by other competent nurses under similar circumstances.[342] The standard of care applicable to nursing students is not different from the standard for professional nurses. States vary on the standard of care expected of nurses in specialties that overlap with the scope of practice of physicians. In some states, such nurses are held to the standard of physicians. For example, a Louisiana decision ruled that when a person assisting a physician performs a task deemed to be medical in nature, such as removal of a cast with a saw, the person is held to the standard of care applicable to a physician.[343] Other states have recognized a distinct standard of care for such nurses. For example, a Texas ruling held nurse specialists to the standard of care observed by those in the same specialty under similar circumstances.[344] In 1985, the California Supreme Court ruled that nurse practitioners should not be held to the standard of care of a physician even when performing functions that overlap with the physician's scope of practice.[345] In 2004, the Illinois Supreme Court ruled that in most cases the standard of care for nurses had to be established by testimony of other nurses; testimony by physicians did not establish the standard of care.[346]

Duty to Interpret and Carry Out Orders. Nurses have a duty to interpret and carry out orders properly. Nurses are expected to know basic information concerning the proper use of drugs and procedures they are likely to be ordered to use. When an order is

---

[342] *E.g.*, Deese v. Carroll City County Hosp., 203 Ga. App. 148, 416 S.E.2d 127 (1992); Cox v. Board of Hosp. Managers, 467 Mich. 1, 651 N.W.2d 356 (2002) ["the skill and care ordinarily possessed and exercised by practitioners of the profession in the same or similar localities"]; *see* Annotation, *Nurse's liability for her own negligence or malpractice*, 51 A.L.R. 2D 970.

[343] Thompson v. Brent, 245 So. 2d 751 (La. Ct. App. 1971).

[344] Webb v. Jorns, 473 S.W.2d 328 (Tex. Civ. App. 1971), *rev'd on other grounds*, 488 S.W.2d 407 (Tex. 1972).

[345] Fein v. Permanente Med. Group, 38 Cal. 3d 137, 211 Cal. Rptr. 368, 695 P.2d 665, *appeal dismissed*, 474 U.S. 842 (1985).

[346] Sullivan v. Edward Hosp., 209 Ill. 2d 100, 806 N.E.2d 645 (2004).

ambiguous or apparently erroneous, the nurse has a responsibility to seek clarification from the ordering physician. This will almost always result in correction or explanation of the order. In the unusual situation in which the explanation does not clarify the appropriateness of the order, the nurse has a responsibility to inform nursing, hospital, or medical staff officials designated by hospital policy who can initiate review of the order and, if necessary, other appropriate action. Pending review, if the drug or procedure appears dangerous to the patient, the nurse should decline to carry out the order, but should immediately notify the ordering physician. Hospitals should have established procedures for nurses to follow when they are not satisfied with the appropriateness of an order. Frequently this procedure will involve notification of a nursing supervisor who will then contact appropriate medical staff officials. Hospital administration may occasionally need to become involved to resolve individual issues.

A North Dakota case arose when a child was born with severe brain damage after a nurse's alleged failure to place the mother on a fetal heart monitor in accordance with her physician's instructions.[347] In a 1973 California case, a hospital was found liable for the death of a patient because a nurse had failed to follow the physician's order to check the patient's vital signs every thirty minutes and had failed to notify the physician when the patient's condition became life threatening.[348] In a New York case, a nurse and a hospital were held liable for the scalding of a young tonsillectomy patient by water that was served as part of his meal by a nurse, contrary to the dietary instructions ordered by the attending physician.[349] A hospital was sued in a New York case for the blindness of an infant caused by too much oxygen when a nurse gave six liters per minute instead of the four liters per minute ordered by the physician.[350] The hospital presented evidence that six liters per minute was within the range of permissible dosages. The court found this evidence irrelevant because the nurse had not been given authority to deviate from the physician's order and, thus, had breached her duty to the patient. The court ordered a lower court

---

[347] Nelson v. Trinity Med. Ctr., 419 N.W.2d 886 (N.D. 1988).
[348] Cline v. Lund, 31 Cal. App. 3d 755, 107 Cal. Rptr. 629 (1st Dist. 1973).
[349] Striano v. Deepdale Gen. Hosp., 54 A.D.2d 730, 387 N.Y.S.2d 678 (2d Dept. 1976).
[350] Toth v. Community Hosp., 22 N.Y.2d 255, 292 N.Y.S.2d 440, 239 N.E.2d 368 (1968).

to reconsider the case to determine whether the blindness had been caused by breach of duty.

A physician must, however, make the order known to the nurse by putting it in the medical records or informing the nurse directly. There can be no liability for not following orders given privately to the patient.[351]

Nurses are sometimes given authority to adjust within guidelines the amounts of some drugs or other substances being given to patients. The nurse then has the added responsibility to exercise appropriate judgment in making those adjustments. In many states, there are legal limits on the discretion that can be delegated concerning some drugs and substances. As with all delegations, the physician should provide appropriate guidance and delegate this responsibility only to nurses who are able to make the required judgments. In 1979, a California court recognized the appropriateness of delegating to a nurse the decision concerning when a prescribed pain medication was needed.[352] The patient suffered cardiopulmonary arrest and died soon after pain medication was given. The court ruled that it was appropriate for the trial court to give the jury two special instructions usually used only for physicians because the case involved a nurse who was exercising delegated independent judgment. One instruction emphasized that perfection was not required; therefore, liability could not be based on a mere error in judgment by a nurse who possessed the necessary learning and skill and who exercised the care ordinarily exercised by reputable nurses under similar circumstances. The standard applied was the conduct of nurses, not physicians. The other instruction emphasized that when there is more than one recognized method of treatment, it is not negligent to select one of the approved methods that later turns out to be wrong or not to be favored by certain other practitioners. The court upheld the jury verdict in favor of the nurse and the hospital.

Nurses cannot assume that orders have remained unchanged from previous shifts. They have a duty to check for changes in orders. A Delaware case addressed a female patient who had been receiving a drug by injection.[353] The physician wrote an order changing the mode of administration from injection to oral. When a

---

[351] *E.g.*, Hering v. McShane, 145 A.D.2d 683, 535 N.Y.S.2d 227 (3d Dept. 1988).

[352] Fraijo v. Hartland Hosp., 99 Cal. App. 3d 331, 160 Cal. Rptr. 246 (2d Dist. 1979).

[353] Larrimore v. Homeopathic Hosp. Ass'n, 54 Del. 449, 181 A.2d 573 (1962).

nurse prepared to give an injection, the patient objected and referred the nurse to the physician's new order. The nurse told the patient that the patient was mistaken and gave the medication by injection. The nurse's conduct was held to be negligent. The court permitted the jury to find the nurse negligent by applying ordinary common sense, and expert testimony was not necessary to prove the standard of care.

A Louisiana case focused on the nurse's responsibility to obtain clarification of an apparently erroneous physician order.[354] The order was incomplete and subject to misinterpretation. Believing the dosage to be incorrect, the nurse asked two other physicians whether the medication should be given as ordered. The physicians did not interpret the order as the nurse did, and they said the order did not appear out of line. The nurse did not contact the attending physician and administered the misinterpreted dosage, resulting in the patient's death. The nurse was found liable for failing to contact the attending physician before giving the medication. The physician who wrote the ambiguous order was also found liable.

Duty to Monitor Patients and Communicate Significant Changes. Nurses have a duty to monitor patients. Nurses are expected to distinguish abnormalities in the patient's condition and determine whether nursing care is a sufficient response or whether a physician or others may be required. The nurse has a responsibility to inform the physician promptly of abnormalities that may require physician attention.[355] In a Kansas case, a nurse and a hospital were sued because a woman was injured during delivery of a baby without physician attendance.[356] The nurse had refused to call the physician despite clear signs of imminent delivery; the nurse and the hospital were found liable. In a West Virginia case, the court ruled that the hospital could be found liable for the death of a patient when the nurse failed to notify the physician of the patient's symptoms of heart failure for six hours.[357] In 1992, a New Mexico court affirmed a jury verdict against a hospital based on a finding

---

[354] Norton v. Argonaut Ins. Co., 144 So. 2d 249 (La. Ct. App. 1962).
[355] *E.g.*, Rampe by Rampe v. Commun. Gen. Hosp., 241 A.D.2d 817, 660 N.Y.S.2d 206 (3d Dept. 1997) [nurse breached duty to notify physician of decelerations in heart rate, but no proof this caused injuries]; Gill v. Foster, 157 Ill. 2d 304, 626 N.E.2d 190 (1993) [nurse breached duty by failing to tell doctor of patient's complaints of pain at discharge, but not cause of injury because doctor already knew of pain]; McMillan v. Durant, 439 S.E.2d 829 (S.C. 1993).
[356] Hiatt v. Groce, 215 Kan. 14, 523 P.2d 320 (1974).
[357] Duling v. Bluefield Sanitarium, Inc., 149 W.Va. 567, 142 S.E.2d 754 (1965).

that the negligence of the nurses in determining whether a woman was in labor influenced the physician's decision to deliver a baby prematurely.[358]

Observations should be properly documented. In an Illinois case, the hospital was sued for the loss of a patient's leg.[359] The patient had been admitted for treatment for a broken leg. The admitting physician wrote an order to "watch condition of toes" and testified at trial that routine nursing care required frequent monitoring of a seriously injured patient's circulation even in the absence of a physician order. The patient developed irreversible ischemia in his leg, requiring its amputation. The nursing notes for the seven-hour period prior to discovery of the irreversibility of the ischemia did not reflect any observations of circulation. The jury was permitted to conclude that absence of entries indicated absence of observations. Thus, the nurse and the hospital could be liable even if the nurse had actually made the observations. It is as important to document no change as it is to document changes. A hospital and a physician were sued in a 1963 California case for damage to a patient's leg from infiltration of intravenous fluid into tissue.[360] The nurse observed increasing swelling and redness around the intravenous tube that indicated infiltration. She notified the physician several times of the swelling, but he ordered continuation of the intravenous infusions. There was conflicting testimony at the trial concerning (1) whether the nurse had communicated the seriousness of the swelling when it became markedly worse and (2) whether the nurse had authority to discontinue an intravenous infusion without a physician order. The court overturned the trial court decision in favor of the hospital and the physician and ordered a new trial so that a jury could determine these issues. This case illustrates the importance of clearly communicating changes in the patient's condition and clearly defining the authority of nurses to discontinue harmful therapy.

If the physician fails to respond appropriately when notified that a patient is in a dangerous situation, then the nurse is confronted with the same situation as when the physician has not adequately explained an apparently erroneous order. The nurse has a responsibility to inform nursing, hospital, or medical staff officials desig-

---

[358] Lopez v. Southwest Comm. Health Servs., 114 N.M. 2, 833 P.2d 1183 (Ct. App. 1992).
[359] Collins v. Westlake Commun. Hosp., 57 Ill. 2d 388, 312 N.E.2d 614 (1974).
[360] Mundt v. Alta Bates Hosp., 223 Cal. App. 2d 413, 35 Cal. Rptr. 848 (1st Dist. 1963).

nated by hospital policy who can initiate review of the situation and, if necessary, take other appropriate action. This is the way a nurse confronted with the situation in the 1963 California case should respond today if the nurse believes the seriousness of the swelling has been communicated, if the physician neither examines the patient nor orders discontinuance of the procedure, and if the nurse does not have clear authority to discontinue the procedure without an order. In *Darling v. Charleston Community Memorial Hospital*, [361] one reason for the hospital's liability for amputation of the patient's leg was the nurses' failure to inform hospital administration of the progressive gangrenous condition of the patient's leg and the inappropriate efforts of the attending physician to address the condition. No effective alternative channel had been established for direct nursing notification of the medical staff and for appropriate medical staff intervention. The court found that hospital administration should have been notified so that it could obtain appropriate medical staff intervention. In most hospitals, direct communication channels have been established between nursing administration and medical staff leadership so that direct hospital administration involvement is less frequent. These channels must be used when necessary. In a 1977 West Virginia case, the hospital was found liable for the failure of nurses to comply with the hospital's nursing manual and report the patient's deteriorating condition to the department chairman when the attending physician failed to respond adequately to the patient's worsening condition.[362]

The fact that the nurse believes the physician will not respond does not justify failure to notify the physician and to take other action if the physician does not respond. A California court ruled that two nurses and a hospital could be sued for the death of a woman from severe bleeding from an incision made to assist her in giving birth.[363] Although the nurses believed the patient was bleeding heavily, the physician was not notified until nearly three hours later when the patient went into shock. One nurse explained that she did not call the physician because she did not believe he would respond. The court concluded that she should have notified

---

[361] Darling v. Charleston Commun. Mem. Hosp., 33 Ill. 2d 326, 211 N.E.2d 253 (1965), *cert. denied*, 383 U.S. 496 (1966).

[362] Utter v. United Hosp. Ctr., Inc., 160 W.Va. 703, 236 S.E.2d 213 (1977).

[363] Goff v. Doctors Gen. Hosp., 166 Cal. App. 2d 314, 333 P.2d 29 (3d Dist. 1958).

the attending physician and then notified her superiors if the attending physician did not respond.

As with other negligent tort cases, in order for there to be liability the deviation from the standard of care must be demonstrated to have caused the injury. In 2001, an Illinois appellate court upheld reversing a jury verdict against the hospital employer of a nurse who had not communicated patient changes to the physician because the physician testified that the information would not have changed the care of the patient; the failure to report did not cause the subsequent injuries.[364]

Duty to Supervise Patients. When nurses determine that a patient requires supervision, they have a duty to exercise appropriate judgment and provide appropriate supervision within the constraints of proper physician orders and available resources. In 1992, an Oklahoma court decided that a nurse and hospital could be liable for a patient's slip and fall in the shower while unsupervised after a nurse administered a drug known to cause drowsiness.[365] An Iowa case illustrates that hospitals may have a direct duty to supervise patients in some situations.[366] A patient with a history of fainting spells had a seizure and fell during a shower, breaking her jaw and losing several teeth. An aide was outside the shower room but allowed the patient to enter the shower alone. The court ruled that decisions concerning supervision of patient showers are a matter of routine care, not professional care, so no expert testimony is necessary to establish the standard of care. The jury can apply common sense to determine the reasonable care the patient's known condition requires. The court noted that absence of physician orders requiring close supervision does not insulate the hospital from liability. If subsequent circumstances show a need for change or action, the hospital should make the changes permitted without a physician order and, if further changes are necessary, seek appropriate orders.

Special Duty Nurses. Special duty nurses are held to the same standard of care as other nurses. Because they are not employees of the hospital, the hospital is usually not liable for their actions.[367]

---

364 Snelson v. Kamm, 319 Ill. App. 3d 116, 745 N.E.2d 128 (4th Dist. 2001), *aff'd in pertinent part by*, 204 Ill. 2d 1, 787 N.E.2d 796 (2003).
365 Pierce v. Mercy Health Ctr., Inc., 847 P.2d 822 (Okla. Ct. App. 1992).
366 Kastler v. Iowa Methodist Hosp., 193 N.W.2d 98 (Iowa 1971).
367 *See also* Robinson by Bugera v. Faine, 525 So. 2d 903 (Fla. 3d DCA 1987) [agency not liable for private duty nurse's negligence where she was independent contractor].

Even when hospital rules require special duty nurses, they do not become hospital employees. In some situations, nurses who are called special duty nurses may be considered agents or employees of the hospital, so that the hospital can be liable under *respondeat superior*.[368] Agency or employment is likely to be found when special duty nurses are selected by the hospital, not by the patient or the patient's representatives. Collection of the nurse's bills by the hospital has also been interpreted by some courts to indicate agency.

PHARMACISTS. Pharmacies are highly regulated, and standards of practice are frequently found in federal or state statutes, agency regulations, and municipal or county ordinances. These generally require pharmaceutical services to be provided by or under the direction of a licensed pharmacist. Some states require hospitals to have at least one pharmacist with a special pharmacist license.[369] The JCAHO and other accreditation standards also establish duties.[370] The hospital may be liable for drug-related injuries if it fails to employ a licensed and competent pharmacist.[371]

Court decisions concerning pharmacists also help to define their standard of care. Dispensing the wrong drug clearly can lead to liability. In a 1971 Michigan case, a tranquilizer was dispensed instead of the prescribed oral contraceptive.[372] The patient became pregnant, delivered a child, and sued the pharmacist for damages. Damages were awarded, including child support until the child reached the age of majority.

A hospital must take reasonable steps to assure that drugs are available when they are needed. In a 1969 New York case, the hospital was found liable for the suicide of a patient who exhausted his supply of an investigational psychotropic drug.[373] The drug was not available during a long holiday weekend because it was stored in the research department, which was closed. The drug should have been

---

[368] Emory Univ. v. Shadburn, 180 Ga. 595, 180 S.E. 137 (1935).

[369] *E.g.*, FLA. STAT. § 465.019(5) [consultant pharmacist license].

[370] Joint Commission on Accreditation of Healthcare Organizations, 2005 COMPREHENSIVE ACCREDITATION MANUAL FOR HOSPITALS, MM.4.10, 4.50 [hereinafter cited as 2005 JCAHO CAMH].

[371] Sullivan v. Sisters of St. Francis, 374 S.W.2d 294 (Tex. Civ. App. 1963).

[372] Troppi v. Scarf, 31 Mich. App. 240, 187 N.W.2d 511 (1971); *see* Annotation, *Druggist's civil liability for injuries sustained as a result of negligence in incorrectly filling drug prescription*, 3 A.L.R. 4TH 270.

[373] McCord v. State, Nos. 43405, 43406, and 43407 (N.Y. Ct. Cl. 1969).

stored in the pharmacy, which was open during the weekend. Some investigational drugs are not available outside of approved research projects, and subjects can no longer receive the drug after they complete their involvement in the study. In 1989, a federal district court applied this principle to dismiss a challenge by an AIDS patient to loss of access to a drug when a study was terminated.[374] Another federal court reached the same conclusion in 2005 concerning access to an investigation drug for Parkinson's disease.[375] This limited availability should be disclosed to the subject before the subject enters the study. In this case, the patient was still in the study. At times, certain noninvestigational drugs are not available because of manufacturing, transport, or stocking problems. The hospital is not an insurer that drugs will continue to be available, but it should take reasonable steps to anticipate needs to minimize nonavailability.

Drugs should be properly stored to avoid deterioration and contamination. The skill with which this is ordinarily done is exemplified by the lack of reported cases arising from breaching this duty.

Pharmacists sometimes assume the responsibility to maintain profiles of the drugs patients are being administered, advise physicians concerning drug selection, and review the appropriateness of drug orders. Until 1995, JCAHO stated that the pharmaceutical department should provide drug monitoring services, which could include a drug profile for each patient and review of each patient's drug regimen for interactions, consonant with available resources.[376] In 1995, JCAHO replaced its pharmacy requirements with medication requirements that do not require pharmacists to perform any functions except reviewing prescriptions and orders and performing other duties required by law.[377] The 2005 standards require that the hospital have a mechanism to capture, use, and communicate important patient medication information, including a medication history, and monitor medication effects, but there is no requirement that this be done by the pharmacy.[378]

---

[374] DeVito v. HEM, Inc., 705 F. Supp. 1076 (M.D. Pa. 1989).
[375] Suthers v. Amgen Inc., 2005 U.S. Dist. LEXIS 11119 (S.D. N.Y.).
[376] Joint Commission on Accreditation of Healthcare Organizations, 1994 ACCREDITATION MANUAL FOR HOSPITALS, 162.
[377] Joint Commission on Accreditation of Healthcare Organizations, 1995 COMPREHENSIVE ACCREDITATION MANUAL FOR HOSPITALS, 139-50.
[378] 2005 JCAHO CAMH, MM.1.10, MM.6.10.

Although pharmacists have avoided liability in some cases arising out of these new responsibilities,[379] pharmacists can be liable for failing to fulfill the professional standard of care associated with the responsibilities assumed.[380] While physicians will remain primarily liable for injuries due to negligent prescriptions, pharmacists can be codefendants when they assume the responsibility of review and carry it out negligently.

PHYSICAL THERAPISTS. Most professional liability cases involving physical therapists have dealt with breaches of the duties (1) to follow the physician's instructions, (2) not to subject the patient to excessive therapy, and (3) to supervise the patient properly.

A physical therapist must follow the prescribing physician's instructions unless they are apparently erroneous and dangerous to the patient. In a Florida case, a hospital was found liable for the injuries to a patient who fell while undergoing physical therapy.[381] The physician had ordered that the patient be attended at all times. The therapist left the patient alone in a standing position while getting her a robe. A fall during that short time resulted in a fractured hip. No expert testimony was required to establish the duty to follow the physician's instructions. In 2001, a Louisiana court upheld finding a physical therapist liabile for providing postoperative exercises beyond the scope of the prescription and other deviations from the standard of care. The patient's suture line separated requiring a second surgery.[382]

Physical therapists are expected to be familiar with the appropriate use of the procedures they use. If a physician's order is apparently erroneous, the therapist has a duty to seek modification or clarification from the prescribing physician. In most states, the therapist should not unilaterally initiate different treatment. If the

---

[379] *E.g.*, Morgan v. Wal-Mart Stores, Inc., 30 S.W.3d 455 (Tex. Ct. App. 2000) [no generalized duty to warn patients of potential adverse reactions to prescription drugs]; Mielke v. Condell Mem. Hosp., 124 Ill. App. 3d 42, 463 N.E.2d 216 (2d Dist. 1984) [no liability for not notifying physician of drug interaction discovered by monitoring systems]; Walker v. Jack Eckerd Corp., 209 Ga. App. 517, 434 S.E.2d 63 (1993) [pharmacist has no duty to warn customer or notify physician that drug is being prescribed in dangerous amounts].

[380] *E.g.*, Happel v. Wal-Mart Stores, Inc., 199 Ill. 2d 179, 766 N.E.2d 1118 (2002) [pharmacist duty to warn in some circumstances]; Cottam v. CVS Pharmacy, 436 Mass. 316, 764 N.E.2d 814 (2002); Hooks SuperX, Inc. v. McLaughlin, 642 N.E.2d 514 (Ind. 1994) [pharmacist has duty to cease filling refills when they are being sought at an unreasonably faster rate than prescribed].

[381] South Miami Hosp. v. Sanchez, 386 So. 2d 39 (Fla. 3d DCA 1980); *see* Annotation, *Liability for injuries or death resulting from physical therapy*, 53 A.L.R. 3d 1250.

[382] Pontiff v. Pecot & Assocs. Rehab & Physical Therapy Servs. Inc, 780 So. 2d 478 (La. Ct. App. 2001).

orders are still apparently erroneous after discussion with the prescribing physician and if the ordered therapy is dangerous to the patient, the therapist should decline to provide the prescribed therapy and notify the prescribing physician and the appropriate supervisors, medical staff, or administrative officials in accord with hospital policy.

The physician's orders often give the physical therapist latitude concerning the therapy to be provided. The physical therapist is then generally held to the duty of acting as other physical therapists in good standing would act under the circumstances. In 1976, a Pennsylvania hospital was sued by a patient who fell in the physical therapy room and fractured her leg and arm.[383] The patient was receiving gait training after multiple hip surgeries and was instructed to walk between parallel bars. The patient fell either while between the parallel bars or while using her cane to take a few steps away from the parallel bars. The court ruled that the duty of the physical therapist must be established by expert testimony and that only ordinary care and skill were required, and the physical therapist was not liable for a mere mistake in judgment. The court affirmed a verdict for the hospital.

Physical therapists have been found liable for subjecting patients to excessive therapy. The Kentucky Supreme Court applied *res ipsa loquitur* when a femur was fractured during therapy to prepare the stump of a leg for an artificial leg.[384] The court did not believe bones would fracture while a leg was being lifted and lowered unless someone was negligent. Thus, it did not require expert testimony. The court ruled that the physician could also be liable for failing to provide an adequate explanation of the procedure to the therapist.

Falls are a frequent cause of injuries involving patients receiving physical therapy. Some courts tend to apply *res ipsa loquitur* to cases involving falls, as illustrated by the Kentucky case, while other courts analyze the appropriateness of the attendance given from a professional perspective, as illustrated by the Pennsylvania case. Another example of a professional standard involved an Oregon patient undergoing therapy after hip surgery who became dizzy and fainted just after returning to a tilt table after walking

---

[383] McAvenue v. Bryn Mawr Hosp., 245 Pa. Super. 507, 369 A.2d 743 (1976).
[384] Meiman v. Rehabilitation Ctr., Inc., 444 S.W.2d 78 (Ky. 1969).

between parallel bars.[385] His total hip replacement became dislocated when he fell. The patient's expert witness testified that he should have been given support, including being strapped to the tilt table, as soon as he became dizzy. The court found the hospital liable for the physical therapist's failure to fulfill this duty.

LABORATORIES AND PATHOLOGY. Liability can arise from injuries due to negligent acts associated with laboratory tests and other pathology services. The error can be committed by a laboratory technician, a pathologist, or other staff members. The hospital can become liable under *respondeat superior* when the person who made the error is the hospital's employee or agent. As discussed in the *Respondeat Superior* (11-5.1) and Agency (11-5.3) sections of this chapter, some courts hold hospitals responsible for the acts of physicians, particularly radiologists, pathologists, and emergency room physicians, by considering the physician to be the agent or apparent agent for the hospital.

Liability has arisen from mishandling specimens.[386] In a Texas case, the hospital was found liable for a patient's mental anguish when an eyeball that had been removed because of a tumor was lost by a technician.[387] The technician was washing the eyeball and dropped it into the sink. The eyeball went down the drain and could not be removed; the pathologist could not diagnose whether the tumor was malignant. In a Florida case, the patient was awarded $100,000 from the hospital and a surgeon because the identities of two specimens were confused, resulting in the unnecessary removal of one of the patient's breasts.[388] The surgeon had removed a biopsy specimen from each breast, and the two specimens were put in the same container without labels telling which breast each came from. The pathologist did not attempt to distinguish the two specimens. One specimen was malignant, and the other was not. Because it was impossible to determine which breast had the malignancy, both breasts were removed. The surgeon was liable for failing to instruct the nurses to label the specimens. The hospital was liable for the

[385] Forsyth v. Sisters of Charity, 39 Or. App. 851, 593 P.2d 1270 (1979); *accord*, Hodo v. General Hosps., 211 Ga. App. 6, 438 S.E.2d 378 (1993); *but see* Gilles v. Rehabilitation Inst., 262 Or. 472, 498 P.2d 777 (1972) [no liability because of patient's efforts to thwart therapist from preventing fall].
[386] *But see*, Holdren v. Legursky, 16 F.3d 57 (4th Cir.), *cert. denied*, 513 U.S. 831 (1994) [handling of blood sample at hospital that precluded DNA test did not violate due process].
[387] Mokry v. University of Tex. Health Science Ctr., 529 S.W.2d 802 (Tex. Civ. App. 1975).
[388] Variety Children's Hosp. v. Osle, 292 So. 2d 382 (Fla. 3d DCA 1974).

nurses' failure to label the specimens and for the failure of its pathologist employee to segregate the specimens.

Misreading a specimen can lead to liability. An Ohio hospital was found liable because its pathologist-employee misdiagnosed a frozen section as indicating cervical cancer.[389] After a total hysterectomy (removal of the uterus and cervix) was performed, it was discovered that the patient did not have cancer. Misdiagnosis alone is not enough to establish breach of duty. A diagnosing physician is not expected always to be correct. Most diagnoses are professional judgments. Thus, for there to be liability, the misdiagnosis must be one that a physician in good standing in the same specialty would not have made in the same circumstances.

Using improper techniques or reagents to conduct a test can be a breach of duty. A federal appellate court found a hospital liable because a technician used sodium hydroxide instead of sodium chloride to perform a gastric cytology test.[390] In an Iowa case, a hospital was found liable for using a reagent that was too old.[391] The pediatrician ordered appropriate blood tests for a baby with symptoms of Rh incompatibility, but the old reagent caused the test results to indicate normal blood levels of bilirubin rather than the baby's actual high levels. When the high levels were discovered, it was too late to avoid permanent severe brain damage that probably could have been avoided had therapy been initiated after the initial blood tests.

Errors in testing can also result in liability. A 1992 case involved a military member who had been told that he was HIV-positive as a result of a false-positive test. A federal appellate court ruled that the government could be sued for the failure of the military to inform him after discharge of its discovery of the error.[392] Courts disagree on whether there can be liability for a false-positive HIV test in the absence of receiving unnecessary and harmful treatment in the mistaken belief of having the virus.

---

[389] Lundberg v. Bay View Hosp., 175 Ohio St. 133, 191 N.E.2d 821 (1963); *see* Annotation, *Malpractice in connection with diagnosis of cancer*, 79 A.L.R. 3D 915.

[390] Insurance Co. of N. Am. v. Prieto, 442 F.2d 1033 (6th Cir. 1971), *cert. denied*, 404 U.S. 856 (1971).

[391] Schnebly v. Baker, 217 N.W.2d 708 (Iowa 1974), *overruled in part on other grounds*, Franke v. Junko, 366 N.W.2d 536 (Iowa 1985).

[392] M.M.H. v. United States, 966 F.2d 285 (7th Cir. 1992).

Autopsies and other aspects of handling dead bodies are another area of potential liability arising from pathology services. Dead bodies are discussed in Chapter 15.

In a 1998 case, a New York appeals court held that pathologists owned no duty of care to a surgeon who, based on an initial pathology report that indicated cancerous tissue, performed a mastectomy.[393] When additional pathology reports indicated no malignancy, the surgeon sued the pathologists, alleging that he relied on their misdiagnoses.

RADIOLOGY. Three common problem areas of radiology include radiation injuries, falls and other problems with patient positioning, and errors or delays in diagnosis. There can also be liability for performing radiologic procedures of no beneficial value.[394]

Radiation injuries from excessive radiation or radiation to the wrong body part have resulted in several suits. The application and effect of radiation are not within the knowledge of lay persons, and courts generally require expert proof of how the radiation should have been administered. If the injury is to a body part that was not intended to receive radiation, most courts will apply *res ipsa loquitur*. However, some courts apply *res ipsa loquitur* in all cases involving severe radiation injuries. These courts require the defendant to show the patient was hypersensitive or otherwise explain injuries to avoid liability.

Several cases have addressed the duty to disclose the risk of radiation injuries from therapeutic radiologic procedures. One of the earliest court decisions to apply the requirement of informed consent ruled that a Kansas physician had a duty to inform the patient of the probable consequences of the radioactive cobalt he administered for breast cancer.[395] A federal appellate court ruled that the physician had to disclose the probable consequences and the experimental nature of the therapy he proposed when he planned to give extremely large doses that exceeded the accepted range and were justified only by research papers read at conferences.[396] The responsibility to obtain informed consent is discussed in Chapter 12.

---

[393] Megally v. LaPorta, 253 A.D.2d 35, 679 N.Y.S.2d 649 (2d Dept. 1998).

[394] *E.g.*, Riser v. American Med. Int'l, 620 So. 2d 372 (La. Ct. App. 1993).

[395] Natanson v. Kline, 187 Kan. 186, 354 P.2d 670 (1960).

[396] Ahern v. Veterans Admin., 537 F.2d 1098 (10th Cir. 1976).

When radiologic technologists fail to check patient status adequately, sometimes necessary precautions are not taken for patient protection. When injuries result, liability is likely. In a Louisiana case, the court ruled the hospital could be liable for a patient's broken ankle that was discovered after the patient slumped on an X-ray table.[397] The radiologic technologist had not noticed that the patient was sedated, and the X-ray requisition had not included the brief history required by hospital policy. The technologist had not strapped the patient to the table before raising it. The technologist had a duty to strap the sedated patient. A federal appellate court ruled that the hospital could be sued for the way a radiologic technologist handled a patient.[398] Although the patient was to be x-rayed for suspected neck and spinal injuries from an automobile accident, the radiologic technologist told the patient to scoot onto the table and then twisted the patient's neck to position her, resulting in permanent spinal cord damage. Experts testified the neck should have been immobilized before the patient was moved to the table, and after she was on the table, the machine, not the patient's head, should have been moved to achieve the desired angles.

Misdiagnosis by the physician reading X-ray film or another radiologic test has also led to suits. The radiologist is held to the standard of other physicians. Thus, the misdiagnosis must be more than a mere judgmental error to establish breach of duty. The misdiagnosis must be outside the accepted range of determinations by qualified radiologists under similar circumstances. Even when there is misdiagnosis, liability may be avoided if the misdiagnosis did not cause the injury. In an Iowa case, the court ruled in favor of the radiologists in a suit arising from the loss of a patient's eyesight.[399] The radiologist had not detected a piece of steel in the patient's eye. A second set of X-rays led to the discovery of the piece. The patient was unable to prove that delay in diagnosis had caused the eyesight loss.

Delay in reporting a proper diagnosis can also result in liability. A federal district court decided that an Indiana hospital was liable for the death of a patient due to delay in forwarding a radiologist's report.[400] The patient who had head injuries from a fight was exam-

---

[397] Albritton v. Bossier City Hosp. Comm'n, 271 So. 2d 353 (La. Ct. App. 1972).

[398] Modave v. Long Island Jewish Med. Ctr., 501 F.2d 1065 (2d Cir. 1974).

[399] Barnes v. Bovenmeyer, 255 Iowa 220, 122 N.W.2d 312 (1963).

[400] Keene v. Methodist Hosp., 324 F. Supp. 233 (N.D. Ind. 1971); *see also* Davidson v. Mobile Infirmary, 456 So. 2d 14 (Ala. 1984) [failure to inform treating physician of X-rays showing large number of pills in stomach].

ined by a physician in a hospital emergency room and released. Four skull X-rays were taken. After the release, a radiologist read the X-rays and found a skull fracture. He did not call the physician who had ordered the X-rays. He dictated his report, which was transcribed two days later. The patient was found unconscious after the X-rays had been read. The patient was taken to a hospital where emergency surgery was performed, but he died. The court ruled that the forwarding of reports was the hospital's administrative responsibility and that the physician was a hospital agent when performing that function. Hospitals need a system for promptly reading emergency X-rays and reporting critical X-ray findings.

Radiologists may also be liable for not informing the treating physician that the X-rays ordered are too limited in scope, so that the diagnosis cannot be relied on.[401]

INFECTION CONTROL. Hospitals can be liable for some infections acquired in the hospital.[402] This liability has been based on the hospital's independent duty concerning the physical condition of buildings and grounds and the selection and maintenance of equipment, the hospital's liability under *respondeat superior* for acts of its employees and agents.

In the past, courts found liability for infections when the patient proved the existence of unsanitary conditions in the hospital. Even with improvements in infection control and in determination of infection sources, courts recognize that hospitals cannot guarantee absence of infection and that infections do occur in hospitals for many reasons other than negligence. Thus, most courts require proof of a causal relationship between the alleged injury and a deviation from proper practices.[403] An Ohio court ruled that *res ipsa loquitur* did not apply to a staph infection after a surgical procedure and no break in sterile technique had been identified, and there could be no liability for the infection.[404]

---

[401] *E.g.*, Shuffler v. Blue Ridge Radiology Assocs., 73 N.C .App. 232, 326 S.E.2d 96 (1985).

[402] Annotation, *Hospital's liability for exposing patient to extraneous infection or contagion*, 96 A.L.R. 2D 1205.

[403] Helman v. Sacred Heart Hosp., 62 Wash. 2d 136, 381 P.2d 605 (1963) [hospital liable for staphylococcus infection where nurses failed to take necessary precautions, such as handwashing, to avoid cross-infection from other patient in room who was infected with the same staphylococcus organism]; Wilson v. Stilwill, 411 Mich. 587, 309 N.W.2d 898 (1981) [*res ipsa loquitur* not applicable to hospital infection]; Vogt v. Katz, 745 S.W.2d 221 (Mo. Ct. App. 1987) [failure to clean injection site established claim for infection].

[404] Mahan v. Bethesda Hosp., Inc., 84 Ohio App. 3d 520, 617 N.E.2d 774 (1992).

Some hospital licensing rules specify infection control steps that must be taken, particularly isolation and sterilization procedures. These rules can be used to prove the standard of care. In a Maryland case, a hospital was found liable when it failed to comply with a regulation requiring segregation of sterile and nonsterile needles.[405] A hospital may be held to a higher standard of care than is specified in regulations if other hospitals follow a higher standard.

When hospital employees fail to sterilize equipment properly, the hospital can be liable. In a California case, a hospital was found liable for a nurse 's failure to sterilize a needle before using it to give a patient an injection.[406] The use of presterilized supplies has reduced both the risk to the patient and the hospital's liability exposure in these situations. If a patient is infected by a presterilized item, the manufacturer will usually be liable unless the item was contaminated by negligent conduct of hospital staff or there was a pattern of infection that should have led the hospital to discontinue the supplies. The Iowa case discussed in the Selection and Maintenance of Equipment section (11-8) of this chapter is an example of a pattern of infection from presterilized supplies.

Another aspect of infection control is preemployment and periodic screening of hospital personnel. The Americans with Disabilities Act (ADA), discussed in Chapter 4, limits when preemployment examinations may be given, but examinations are permitted. The ADA does not provide an excuse for not performing necessary examinations. A federal district court found liability for failing to give an employee a preemployment examination before she was assigned to a newborn nursery.[407] The employee had a staphylococcus infection of the same type that was transmitted to a baby. If the hospital becomes aware that a staff member may be infected, it must remove the person from direct and indirect patient contact until the condition is diagnosed and, if the condition is infectious, until the condition is no longer infectious or until appropriate procedures are implemented to preclude infecting others. Other aspects of health screening are discussed in Chapter 4.

Some states require special training for hospital employees concerning HIV and other transmissible diseases.[408] The Occupational

---

[405] Suburban Hosp. Ass'n v. Hadary, 22 Md. App. 186, 322 A.2d 258 (1974).

[406] Kalmus v. Cedars of Lebanon Hosp., 132 Cal. App. 2d 243, 281 P.2d 872 (2d Dist. 1955).

[407] Kapuschinsky v. United States, 248 F. Supp. 732 (D. S.C. 1966).

[408] *E.g.*, FLA. STAT. § 381.0035.

Safety and Health Administration (OSHA) requires employers to follow certain precautions concerning blood borne pathogens, and the Centers for Disease Control (CDC) have provided considerable guidance for handling various diseases.

Hospitals are expected to have a system to monitor their facilities, discover infections, and take appropriate remedial action. The JCAHO standards require such a system.[409] Failure to have an appropriate system could result in liability if a patient's infection could have been prevented by the type of system other hospitals have.

EMERGENCY SERVICES. Emergency services are a source of substantial liability exposure for hospitals and their staff members. The possible bases of liability of the hospital for acts of a physician in the emergency room are discussed earlier in this chapter. The hospital's duty to provide assistance to patients who come to the emergency room and the proper handling of transfers are discussed in Chapter 6. Consent issues are discussed in Chapter 7. This section focuses on issues concerning the examination of the patient.

The responsibility for diagnosis rests with the physician or other independent practitioner. Severely injured patients should generally not be diagnosed over the telephone because of the risk of communication errors. It is best for patients with severe injuries to come to the emergency room. They then need to be given an appropriate medical screening that satisfies the EMTALA requirements, unless they refuse the screening.

A Maryland case illustrates the problem.[410] A person who had been drinking was hit by a car and was thrown through the air. He was brought to an emergency room, and the on-call surgeon was telephoned. The surgeon told the nurse to admit the patient and x-ray him in the morning. Since the hospital was full, the patient was placed in the hall outside the nursing station. His condition deteriorated, and he died within three hours of entering the hospital. The autopsy found a lacerated liver and a badly fractured leg and pelvic area, with bone fragments penetrating the peritoneal cavity. The physician and nurses contradicted each other concerning the information exchanged over the telephone. The physician was found liable because he failed to examine the patient personally, and the

---

[409] 2005 Joint Commission CAMH, IC.1.10 – IC.6.30.
[410] Thomas v. Corsco, 265 Md. 84, 288 A.2d 379 (1972).

hospital was found liable because the nurses failed to notify the physician of the deterioration of the patient's condition.

Emergencies are not always apparent. All patients should be treated as having emergencies until they are determined not to have emergency problems. The most obvious aspect of the patient's condition frequently is not the most critical. Several cases have arisen from emergency personnel assuming that drunkenness is the only problem and overlooking more serious problems. In a Florida case, a young man was brought unconscious to an emergency room.[411] A superficial examination indicated he was drunk, and he was turned over to police. He was later found dead in his cell with broken ribs piercing his thoracic cavity. The court ruled that a jury could find responsibility to make a thorough examination of an unconscious patient and to take a history from those accompanying the patient. A history would have uncovered the fact that the patient was found lying on a lawn after a suspected fall from twenty-three feet.

Existing records should be examined when time permits. In a 1974 Louisiana case, a man had chest pains and called his physician, who advised him to go to the emergency room.[412] The physician alerted the emergency room, ordered an electrocardiogram (EKG), and told the emergency room staff to advise him of the outcome. The emergency room physician was not notified of the call; he ordered an EKG and, without comparing it to prior EKGs, decided there was no heart attack. He sent the patient home with medication and instructions to call if he got worse. The personal physician was not called. The patient got worse and was later admitted for cardiac care. The court said the emergency room physician could be sued for his misdiagnosis due to failure to compare the EKG to prior EKGs. This case also illustrates the importance of involving a physician, when available, who knows the patient. Another reason to examine prior records is that distraught patients may forget information, such as allergies. However, reliance can generally be placed on a history from a competent patient. This is illustrated by a Michigan case in which the patient had a fatal allergic reaction to morphine.[413] He had denied allergies to any painkilling drugs. Although records of a prior unrelated stay noted the allergy, the

---

[411] Bourgeois v. Dade County, 99 So. 2d 575 (Fla. 1957).

[412] Fox v. Argonaut Sw. Ins. Co., 288 So. 2d 102 (La. Ct. App. 1974).

[413] Howell v. Outer Drive Hosp., 66 Mich. App. 142, 238 N.W.2d 553 (1975).

court found the hospital not liable. When laboratory and radiologic diagnostic tests are performed on emergency patients, the patients should be advised not to leave until the tests are completed.

GENETIC SCREENING AND TESTING. The increasing ability to identify genes that cause or increase the likelihood of disease has raised many legal issues and created a growing area of potential liability for health care providers.

Both parents and children have sued when negligently conducted tests have led parents to conceive or deliver children with genetic defects. This issue is discussed in Section 14-5.

The duty of a physician to warn relatives of patients found to have genetically transmissible diseases has been the subject of several cases. In a 1995 case, the Florida Supreme Court held that a physician who did not warn a patient that her condition was genetically transferable may be liable to the patient's daughter, who later learned that she had the disease.[414] The court also concluded that the duty to warn of genetically transferable disease may be satisfied by warning the patient. However, in a 1996 case, a New Jersey appeals court held that a physician's duty to warn of genetic disease may extend beyond the patient to immediate family members.[415]

Knowledge of the genetic basis of disease in increasing rapidly, mainly due to the Human Genome project, a government-sponsored program designed to map and sequence the human gene, which completed the first complete sequencing of a human genome in 2003.[416] As more individuals (and their physicians) become aware that they carry genes associated with disease, it is almost certain that litigation related to genetic screening and testing will increase.

Discussion Points

1. What are the four elements of a negligent tort?
2. When does a health care provider have a duty to an individual?
3. How is the scope of the duty proven?
4. How is legal causation proven?
5. What are intentional torts?

---

[414] Pate v. Threlkel, 661 So. 2d 278 (Fla. 1995).

[415] Safer v. Pack, 291 N.J. Super. 619, 677 A.2d 1188 (App. Div. 1996).

[416] *Researchers complete sequencing of human genetic code, opening way for new medicine*, AP, Apr. 14, 2003.

6. What are the major defenses to liability suits?
7. Discuss the use of arbitration as an alternative to litigation.
8. When does strict liability apply in health care settings?
9. When there is liability, who is responsible for making the payment?
10. Discuss respondeat superior.
11. When can an institution be held directly liable?
12. What is the difference between occurrence and claims-made insurance?
13. Discuss the periodic malpractice crisis and attempted solutions — changes in the standard of care, changes in dispute resolution mechanisms, changes in the amount of the award and how it is paid, changes in the time in which suits must be filed, malpractice insurance coverage reform, and other changes.
14. What nursing actions are most likely to lead to liability?

CHAPTER TWELVE

Criminal Law and Civil Penalties

Objectives

The objective of this chapter is to provide an overview of criminal liability and civil penalties. The reader will learn about compliance programs; enforcement agencies; differences between criminal and civil penalties; criminal law; suspension, recoupment, and exclusion from federal programs; civil money penalties; and private lawsuits.

Since the early 1990s, there has been an explosive growth in applying criminal law and civil penalties to health care providers. It is still not clear why there was a fundamental shift in public policy concerning the application of criminal and civil penalty laws to health care professionals and entities. Efforts to reverse the trend have had only limited success. For the foreseeable future, anyone in the health care field needs to recognize that there is a real risk that they and their organizations are being or will be subjected to criminal or civil investigation.

This chapter reviews some of these criminal laws and civil penalties and how they have been applied to health care providers. The sections address compliance programs (12-1); enforcement agencies (12-2); differences between criminal and civil penalties (12-3); criminal law (12-4); suspension, recoupment, and exclusion from federal programs (12-5); civil money penalties (12-6); and private lawsuits (12-7).

12-1 Compliance Programs

The response of most health care entities to this new focus on criminal law has been to develop compliance programs that strive to achieve compliance with the complex governmental requirements.[1] The primary goal is to minimize violations. A secondary goal is to reduce penalties when the government finds violations.[2] The government has provided model compliance programs for hospitals, home health agencies, and other groups.[3]

As part of settlement agreements, some providers have had to agree to establish expensive compliance programs in the form dictated by the government, called Corporate Integrity Agreements.[4]

12-2 Enforcement Agencies

Enforcement efforts have been initiated from at least three sources — federal and state administrative agencies, federal and state prosecutors, and private individuals and organizations. The focus in this section will be on two federal enforcement agencies — the Office of the Inspector General (OIG) of the United States Department of Health and Human Services (HHS) and the United States Department of Justice (DOJ). There is also active state enforcement. Actions by private individuals will be discussed later in the chapter.

OFFICE OF THE INSPECTOR GENERAL. The administrative agency that has been most widely publicized and active in penalizing health care providers has been the Office of the Inspector General of the United States Department of Health Human Services. It has taken a lead in civil enforcement of Medicare, Medicaid, and other civilian health care programs of the federal government. The

---

1   G. Anders, *Hot new job in health care: in-house cop*, WALL ST. J., Sept. 18, 1997, B1.
2   See *Corporate compliance plans may help companies even if problems are found*, 6 HEALTH L. RPTR. [BNA] 746 (1997) [hereinafter HEALTH L. RPTR. cited as H.L.R.]; B. Saunders et al., *Corporate compliance programs; An effective shield against civil penalties*, 1 HEALTH CARE FRAUD RPT. [BNA] 98 (1997) [hereinafter HEALTH CARE FRAUD RPT. cited as H.C.F.R.].
3   OIG documents can be found at http://oig.hhs.gov/fraud/complianceguidance.html; *e.g.*, 63 FED. REG. 8,987 (Feb. 23, 1998) [hospitals]; 70 FED. REG. 4,858 (Jan. 31, 2005) [supplemental guidance for hospitals]; 63 FED. REG. 42,410 (Aug. 7, 1998) [home health agencies]; 65 FED. REG. 14,289 (Mar. 16, 2000) [nursing facilities]; 63 FED. REG. 45,076 (Aug. 24, 1998) [clinical laboratories].
4   For a list of agreements in effect and the text of the agreements, *see* http://oig.hhs.gov/fraud/cias.html.

Department of Defense and Veterans Administration health care systems have separate enforcement agencies.

There have been a series national enforcement plans. For example, Operation Restore Trust started in 1995, and the Comprehensive Plan for Program Integrity started in 1999. In addition, the OIG publishes an annual work plan listing the issues on which it is focusing.[5] This is supplemented by periodic fraud alerts detailing other areas of focus. For example, in 1999, a Special Fraud Alert was issued that detailed the liability of physicians when they falsely certify the need for medical equipment or home health services, and in 2003, another alert was issued concerning contractual joint ventures.[6]

In 1998, the Health Care Financing Administration (HCFA) supplemented the OIG's efforts with two new programs. HCFA began using private subcontractors for enforcement.[7] In addition, as authorized by the Health Insurance Portability and Accountability Act (HIPAA), HCFA began a controversial program of training beneficiaries to act as spies and report suspected violations.[8] Concerns have been expressed about the effects of this program on the relationship of trust necessary for patient care. HCFA has been renamed the Centers for Medicare & Medicaid Services (CMS).

DEPARTMENT OF JUSTICE. The Department of Justice comprises the central office in Washington, D.C., and the United States Attorney's offices in each federal judicial district that function with great autonomy. Federal criminal prosecutions must be brought by DOJ. When the OIG determines that criminal prosecutions should be considered, the case is referred to DOJ. DOJ can also initiate prosecutions on its own.

Most prosecutions are local and focused on individual providers based on a case by case assessment. These prosecutions have in most cases targeted serious violators, for example, those who have been billing for services not provided. This is an essential role in the enforcement of appropriate standards.

However, there have been a few controversial national projects. For example, two of the national programs that were focused on all

---

[5] The work plan can be found at http://oig.hhs.gov/publications/workplan.html.

[6] OIG documents can be found at http://oig.hhs.gov/.

[7] *See* HCFA, *Program Safeguard Contractors (PSC)* [www.hcfa.gov/medicare/mip/pscwebp.2.htm].

[8] 42 U.S.C. § 1395b-5(b); 42 C.F.R. §§ 420.400, 420.405; 63 FED. REG. 31,123 (June 8, 1998); *HCFA to pay seniors for tipping off government to Medicare fraud,* 2 H.C.F.R. 442 (1998); G. Weinreich, *Medicare incentive program: A new fix or another problem?* 2 H.C.F.R. 484 (1998).

hospitals were Operation Bad Bundle and the DRG Three-Day Window Project.

In Operation Bad Bundle, many hospitals in the United States were accused of improperly billing Medicare individually for laboratory tests that should have been grouped together at a lower rate. Despite the conflicting federal instructions and bad data that the prosecutors were using, most hospitals had to settle rather than face financial ruin. An example is given by the congressional testimony of the CEO of an Ohio hospital who described that the hospital was given the choice of either (1) paying $25,000 for overpayments — in 13,496 bills with an average overpayment of $1.85 — plus $25,000 in penalties, plus establishing a corporate compliance program at a cost of $100,000 or (2) trying to prove the billing errors were not fraudulent in court with the risk that, if the hospital were found guilty, it would have to repay three times the overpayment, plus $10,000 per claim, or a total of over $135 million, which was ten times the hospital's annual budget, plus being excluded from Medicare and Medicaid participation. The hospital had to settle regardless of the merits of the case because it could not risk bankruptcy and closure of the hospital. After collecting many such settlements, DOJ recognized that in many cases it was using bad data as the basis for its demands and revised the program.[9]

The DRG Three-Day Window project alleged that hospitals were submitting bills for outpatient services that should be included in the inpatient bill. In 1990, Congress amended the Medicare law to mandate that all outpatient service provided within seventy-two hours before hospital admission could not be billed separately. Interim regulations were issued in 1994, and final regulations were issued in 1998. Notwithstanding the lack of directions, lack of good data, and evidence that hospitals had achieved a high compliance rate, DOJ decided to apply a Zero Tolerance rule retroactively, sending demand letters to hospitals offering the options of settlements based

---

[9] *Close to 5,000 hospitals to be target of IG/DOJ Medicare unbundling project,* 1 H.C.F.R. 83 (1997); *AHA memo to members on Outpatient Lab Unbundling Project* (Feb. 5, 1997), 1 H.C.F.R. 102 (1997); *Tiered settlement agreement model being used in Medicare hospital cases,* 2 H.C.F.R. 238 (1998); *Hospital industry says no legal basis for DOJ's Medicare "unbundling" probe,* 2 H.C.F.R. 337 (1998); *Twenty-five Ohio hospitals to pay $9.4 million in lab unbundling probe,* 2 H.C.F.R. 561 (1998); *Bad data causing prosecutors to retreat from hospital lab billings investigations,* 2 H.C.F.R. 591 (1998); Testimony of James H. Schaum, President and CEO of Allen Memorial Hospital, Oberlin, Ohio, before the House Subcommittee on Commercial and Administrative Law, Committee on the Judiciary (July 23, 1998)[fca.aha.org/testallenmemorial.html].

on the erroneous DOJ information or risking penalties that would bankrupt the hospital. Again, hospitals settled.[10]

These programs lead to a backlash from providers who sought Congressional relief. Legislation was introduced to curtail the use of the threat of fraud penalties for billing errors and disputes. In 1998, the OIG and DOJ issued enforcement guidelines to curtail some of the most abusive approaches. This satisfied some of the Congressional concern, and legislative change was not adopted. After the legislative effort was dropped, questions were raised about the effect of the enforcement guidelines; it is not clear when the extraordinary powers that Congress has granted to these agencies will be used.[11]

Another controversial issue has been whether the practices of federal prosecutors are subject to any external legal ethical standards. In recent years, DOJ has asserted that external legal ethical standards do not apply. Although occasionally a court has disagreed, generally DOJ has not felt bound by external legal ethical standards.[12] In 1998, Congress passed a law mandating that DOJ comply with state legal ethics standards.[13] However, federal courts tend to find that conduct of DOJ does not violate state standards.[14]

In one situation in 2004, DOJ asserted control over an individual United States attorney. It was reported that the attorney had encouraged his staff to find public corruption cases and pursue indictments. He was required to obtain prior approval from his superiors before authorizing any indictments in such cases.[15]

---

[10] 42 U.S.C. § 1395ww(a)(4); 59 Fed. Reg. 1,654 (Jan. 12, 1994) [interim final rule] & 63 Fed. Reg. 6,864 (Feb. 11, 1998) [final rule], codified as 42 C.F.R. § 412.2(c)(5).

[11] *Legislation changing FCA to ease up on hospitals introduced in House*, 2 H.C.F.R. 203 (1998); *DOJ refines enforcement approach in pursuing hospital Medicare fraud*, 2 H.C.F.R. 269 (1998) [use of "contact" letters instead of "demand" letters]; *DOJ refutes charges of prosecuting "honest billing errors"; Industry still cries foul*, 2 H.C.F.R. 403 (1998); *Department of Justice False Claims Guidance* (June 3, 1998), 2 H.C.F.R. 459 (1998); *DOJ offers enforcement guidance; Pressure for FCA legislation deflated*, 7 H.L.R. 975 (1998); *DOJ official addresses confusion surrounding enforcement guidelines*, 2 H.C.F.R. 868 (1998) [backing away from apparent commitments in guidelines]; *see also* Editorial, *About independence*, N.Y. Times, July 4, 2004, 8WK [criticism of unfettered enforcement in pursuit of worthy ends destroying innocent lives through hubris and carelessness].

[12] *E.g.*, United States *ex rel.* O'Keefe v. McDonnell Douglas Corp., 961 F. Supp. 1288 (E.D. Mo. 1997) [DOJ attorneys not exempt from professional responsibility rules concerning ex parte contacts].

[13] Citizens Protection Act of 1998, Pub. L. No. 105-277, § 801 (1998) [codified as 28 U.S.C. § 530B]; United States v. Colorado Supreme Court, 189 F.3d 1281 (10th Cir. 1999) [state rule restricting prosecutorial practice of subpoenaing attorneys to compel evidence about past or present client in criminal proceedings applies to federal attorneys].

[14] *E.g.*, United States v. Whittaker, 268 F.3d 185 (3rd Cir. 2003).

[15] *U.S. attorney questioned*, N.Y. Times, July 17, 2004, A26.

CONFLICTS CREATED BY MULTIPLE ENFORCERS. The existence of multiple independent enforcers makes enforcement more complex for the enforcers and makes dealing or settlement with any one enforcement agency more complex for providers. Consideration must be given to the potential actions by other agencies. Each enforcer can make a commitment concerning only its own enforcement activities. However, anything disclosed to one agency can be shared with others; a deal struck with one agency generally creates the possibility of prosecution or penalties by other agencies. This has also complicated the responses to efforts by many enforcement agencies to encourage self-reporting of detected violations.[16]

Some enforcement agencies have developed cooperative agreements concerning some aspects of their operations.[17] In some cases, it has been possible to achieve resolution of cases with multiple agencies at the same time.

12-3 Differences Between Criminal and Civil Penalties

There is a fundamental difference between criminal penalties and civil penalties. Criminal penalties can only be imposed by courts. Civil penalties can be imposed directly by administrative agencies or by courts, but generally they must follow specified administrative procedures. The government does not have to follow criminal law procedures before it can impose civil penalties.

There is also a fundamental difference in the *burden of proof* the government must meet before imposing penalties. For a criminal conviction, the government must prove its case *beyond a reasonable doubt*. Certainty is not required, but any reasonable doubt must be resolved against the government. For crimes where the maximum prison term is in excess of six months, there is a right to have a jury make the determination of guilt or inno-

---

[16] 63 FED. REG. 58,399 (Oct. 30, 1998); J. Meyer, *The self-disclosure protocol: treading warily under the HHS IG's eye*, 3 H.C.F.R. 304 (1999); for an OIG assessment of self-disclosure, see http://oig.hhs.gov/fraud/cia/docs/assessment.htm (accessed Sept. 4, 2004); for an example of self-disclosure, *see Community Health Systems, Inc. agreement with OIG finalized; Voluntary disclosure and self-audit yields release of liability and $31 million repayment to government*, PR Newswire, Mar. 3, 2000.

[17] *E.g.*, DHHS & DOJ, Fraud and Abuse Control Program as Mandated by the Health Insurance Portability and Accountability Act of 1996 (Jan. 24, 1997).

cence.[18] To impose a civil penalty, the government need only prove its case by a *preponderance of the evidence*, that is, the government need only show that it is more likely than not that the violation occurred. In civil penalty cases, there is no right to a jury trial. However, there is generally a right to judicial review after the administrative process is completed. Civil penalties cannot include imprisonment, but they can include large civil money penalties and exclusion from participation in government programs, such as Medicare and Medicaid.

There is one aspect of proof that surprisingly may be easier in criminal cases than in some civil cases. Most states require expert medical testimony to establish proper medical practice before the imposition of civil tort liability. In criminal cases that depend on whether proper medical practice was followed, some courts have not required expert medical testimony.[19]

The Double Jeopardy Clause of the United States Constitution bars a second criminal prosecution for the same offense. Although "same offense" has a technical definition that leaves open the possibility of a second prosecution in some circumstances,[20] the Double Jeopardy Clause does provide substantial protection. However, in 1997, the United States Supreme Court ruled that a prior civil administrative proceeding that imposed severe monetary penalties and occupational disbarment did not bar a subsequent criminal prosecution.[21]

---

[18] Duncan v. Louisiana, 391 U. S. 145 (1968) [right to jury trial for serious offenses, not petty offenses]; Blanton v. North Las Vegas, 489 U. S. 538 (1989) [offense with maximum sentence of up to six months presumed petty, unless severe additional statutory penalties indicating legislature considered offense serious]; Lewis v. United States, 518 U.S. 322 (1996) [no right to trial by jury when prosecuted for multiple petty offenses even when maximum aggregate sentence exceeds six months].

[19] *E.g.*, Einaugler v. Supreme Court, 109 F.3d 836 (2d Cir. 1997), *application for stay of mandate denied*, 520 U.S. 1238 (1997) [denial of habeas corpus for absence of expert testimony where physician convicted of reckless endangerment for not transferring nursing home patient to hospital more quickly after treatment error]; *but see* United States v. Wood, 207 F.3d 1222 (10th Cir. 2000) [reversing conviction of physician for death of patient, ordering new trial, degree of deviation from standard of care a central issue].

[20] Blockburger v. United States, 284 U.S. 299 (1932); United States v. Dixon, 509 U.S. 688 (1993) [two criminal laws provisions not "same offense" if each contains element not included in other].

[21] Hudson v. United States, 522 U.S. 93 (1997) [disavowing United States v. Halper, 490 U.S. 435 (1989)]; United States v. Lippert, 148 F.3d 974 (8th Cir. 1998) [double jeopardy does not bar fine after conviction, applying *Hudson*]; *see also* Smith v. Doe, 538 U.S. 84 (2003) [retroactive application of sex offender registration law not violation of *ex post facto* prohibition since not punitive].

12-4 Criminal Law

This section is divided into five subsections. Some aspects of criminal investigations are discussed (12-4.1). In this section, criminal penalties for three areas are discussed — health care decisions (12-4.2); failing to meet billing requirements (12-4.3); and business arrangements Medicare and Medicaid fraud and abuse (12-4.4). The final subsection reviews some other criminal laws used against health care providers (12-4.5), but many other actions such as theft, trespass, sexual contact, or disorderly conduct that are not unique to health care settings are not discussed.

12-4.1 Criminal Investigations

In most circumstances, individuals have a right not to answer questions from criminal investigators. This is part of the right against self-incrimination guaranteed by the Fifth Amendment to the United States Constitution. Thus, in most circumstances, there is an opportunity to seek legal counsel before answering questions. Fifth Amendment protections do not apply to corporations, and disclosure of corporate records can be compelled.

When individuals elect to answer questions from criminal investigators, they must answer truthfully. False responses are a separate crime.[22] In 1998, the United States Supreme Court ruled that even a false denial of guilt was a crime.[23] One federal court has interpreted medical records to be statements to federal officials whenever those records are required by federal law.[24] Thus, some false statements in medical records can also be federal crimes.

Health care organizations may advise staff of the criminal risks of responding and of their right to seek counsel before responding, ask staff to advise them when contacted by investigators, and offer

---

[22] 18 U.S.C. § 1001; United States v. Brown, 151 F.3d 476 (6th Cir. 1998) [affirming conviction for false statements to federal agency as to one defendant, reversing as to other]; M. Morris, *Pharmacist's wife gets one day of probation for making false statement to FBI*, KANSAS CITY STAR, Feb. 8, 2003; *see also* Editorial, *Martha Stewart misgivings*, WALL ST. J., Mar. 8, 2004, A16 [this discourages persons from talking to governmental agents].

[23] Brogan v. United States, 522 U.S. 398 (1998) [no exception to 18 U.S.C. § 1001 for exculpatory "no"]; L. Greenhouse, *Court backs prosecution for false denial of guilt*, N.Y. TIMES, Jan. 27, 1998, A12.

[24] United States v. Rutgard, 116 F.3d 1270 (9th Cir. 1997) [false statements in physician's files can be statements to federal agency in violation of § 1001 when required by Medicare as documentation of medical necessity].

to provide counsel, but they cannot tell their staff not to respond or threaten adverse employment consequences for responding or not reporting contacts.

Investigators have broad powers to use undercover means, including wiretapping and recording of meetings and conversations.[25]

Prosecutors have broad powers to seize or freeze assets prior to conviction.[26] This is permitted even when the seizure does not leave assets for a legal defense.[27] Violating freezes is a separate criminal offense. In 1997, a Florida attorney was indicted for transferring funds that had been frozen.[28]

12-4.2 Criminal Penalties for Health Care Decisions

Criminal law addresses health care decisions in at least three ways. Some cases focus on all health care decisions regardless of outcome. Other cases focus on deaths or significant injuries that result from health care decisions. The third type of case is the rare challenge to intentional end-of-life decisions that is discussed in Chapter 7.

PROSECUTIONS WITHOUT REGARD TO HEALTH CARE OUTCOME. One example of the use of criminal penalties to punish health care decisions without regard to health care outcome is the Medicare law. That law requires that services be medically necessary, meet professionally recognized standards of care, and be supported by evidence in the required form and fashion.[29]

The government takes the position that any Medicare bill is a certification of compliance with these and other Medicare requirements. Thus, it asserts that any bill for a service that does not meet the necessity, quality, and documentation requirements is a fraudulent bill. At least one federal appellate court has decided in the civil

---

[25] *E.g.*, P. Callahan & T.M. Burton, *U.S. Abbott probe involves sting, undercover tapes*, WALL ST. J., July 18, 2003, A3.

[26] *HIPAA's emphasis on parallel proceedings prompts increased use of mail fraud statute*, 1 H.C.F.R. 757 (1997) [power of government to seize assets, destroy business before day in court]; United States v. Oncology Associates, 198 F.3d 489 (4th Cir. 1999); United States v. Sriram, 147 F. Supp. 2d 914 (N.D. Ill. 2001); L. Browning, *$500 million frozen in I.R.S. crackdown in doctors' tax case*, N.Y. TIMES, Nov. 5, 2004, A1; T. Zeller, *U.S. seizes assets of operator of online drug business*, N.Y. TIMES, May 23, 2005, C2; *but see* S.E.C. v. Health-South Corp., 261 F. Supp. 2d 1298 (N.D. Ala. 2003) [dissolving freeze].

[27] *See* United States v. Kirschenbaum, 156 F.3d 784, 1998 U.S. App. LEXIS 24431 (7th Cir.).

[28] United States v. Braxton, No. 97-0352 (S.D. Fla. indictment May 7, 1997); *Attorney indicted for transferring frozen funds*, 1 H.C.F.R. 368 (1997).

[29] 42 U.S.C. § 1320c-5(a).

penalties context that even decisions not to provide elements of care can violate the requirement of meeting professionally recognized standards of care.[30] However, in 2001, a federal appellate court ruled that claims submitted for payment of services that did not meet professional standards of care were not false on that basis alone for False Claims Act purposes.[31]

The cases that have been selected for criminal prosecution so far have generally been egregious deviations from acceptable practice. However, in the jurisdictions where the courts do not limit the use of the False Claims Act, prosecutorial discretion is the only limit that keeps this law from creating a federal criminal law of medical malpractice.

The government has also adopted the position that a Medicare bill is an implied certification on compliance with a variety of other regulatory requirements, so that the False Claims Act can be used to punish violations of other requirements. Some courts have permitted this approach.[32] However, this remains an open issue in other jurisdictions; some courts have expressly declined to decide whether they will permit this approach.[33]

PROSECUTIONS FOR BAD HEALTH CARE OUTCOMES. The law of medical malpractice and professional licensing developed in early America as an alternative to criminal prosecution that had previously been used as the primary means of legal regulation of medical practice. Many prosecutors still exercise their discretion not to apply the criminal law,[34] but this can be difficult especially when elected prosecutors are pressured by families of those injured and by the media. Recently there has been a disturbing return to

---

[30] Corkill v. Shalala, 109 F.3d 1348 (9th Cir. 1996).

[31] United States *ex rel.* Mikes v. Straus, 274 F.3d 687 (2d Cir. 2001).

[32] *E.g.,* United States *ex rel.* Augustine v. Century Health Servs., 289 F.3d 409 (6th Cir. 2002); United States *ex rel.* Barrett v. Columbia/HCA Healthcare Corp., 251 F.3d 28 (D. D.C. 2003) [applying implied certification theory]; *see also* Shaw v. AAA Engineering & Drafting, Inc., 213 F.3d 519 (10th Cir. 2000) [implied certification permitted in non-Medicare case]; Mikes v. Straus, 274 F.3d 687 (2d Cir. 2001) ["implied false certification is appropriately applied only when the underlying statute or regulation... *expressly* states the provider must comply in order to be paid"].

[33] *E.g.,* Harrison v. Westinghouse Savannah River Co., 176 F.3d 776 (4th Cir. 1999); United States *ex rel.* Herarra v. Danka Office Imaging Co., 91 Fed. Appx. 862 (4th Cir. 2004); United States *ex rel.* Willard v. Humana Health Plan, 336 F.3d 375 (5th Cir. 2003).

[34] *E.g., Prosecutor decides against charging doctor,* AP, Nov. 5, 2001 [18-year-old patient died two days after liposuction]; *see also* S.K. Dewan, *When is an accident a crime,* N.Y. Times, Feb. 1, 2003, 12WK [discussion of analogous problem of deciding when to prosecute police for shooting civilian].

the colonial use of criminal law to punish actions within the scope of medical practice.[35]

For example, New York prosecuted and convicted a physician for the death of a nursing home patient. In 1990, the physician had mistakenly ordered administration of feeding solution through the patient's dialysis catheter. When he was notified of the error, he consulted with another physician. There were disputes over what was said in that consultation. The physician eventually transferred the patient to a hospital, where the patient died. The prosecutor took the position that the timing of the transfer constituted criminal reckless endangerment. The jury agreed, and the conviction was upheld on appeal.[36] The federal courts refused to grant relief through habeas corpus.[37] There was considerable controversy in the medical community over the prosecution.[38] In 1997, the state commuted the sentence to community service.[39]

In 1996, a California physician saw an eleven-month-old with diarrhea and vomiting at a small hospital's emergency room. The physician concluded that he could not provide the care the child required; he had the parents drive the child to a tertiary care facility over one hour away because of delays in availability of ambulance service. The baby died. Both a civil liability case and licensing review were initiated. However, in addition, the prosecutor brought criminal charges against the physician, obtaining a grand jury indictment of second-degree murder, involuntary manslaughter,

---

[35] *E.g., Jury convicts anesthesiologist*, N.Y. TIMES, Oct. 24, 1996, C22 [Colorado physician fell asleep during surgery, 8-year-old died, convicted of extreme deviation from standard medical procedures]; United States v. Wood, 207 F.3d 1222 (10th Cir. 2000) [reversing conviction of physician for death of patient, ordering new trial, degree of deviation from standard of care a central issue; discusses cases where physicians have been prosecuted for the outcome of patient care]; J.A. Filkins, *'With no evil intent:' the criminal prosecution of physicians for medical negligence*, 22 J. LEGAL MED. 467 (2001); *see also Nurse pleads guilty to neglect in death of patient*, AP, Jan. 7, 2003 [Fla. nurse anesthetist failed to monitor vital signs during surgery]; *Caregiver sentenced to 90 days in jail for death of patient*, AP, Jan. 23, 2002 [Wis. assisted living facility caregiver left mentally retarded resident in bathtub, drowned].

[36] People v. Einaugler, 208 A.D.2d 946, 618 N.Y.S.2d 414 (2d Dept. 1994) [affirming jury conviction].

[37] Einaugler v. Supreme Court, 918 F. Supp. 619 (E.D. N.Y. 1996), *aff'd*, 109 F.3d 836 (2nd Cir. 1997) [affirming denial of habeas corpus, sufficient evidence to support reckless endangerment, willful patient neglect convictions, expert medical testimony not required; failure to timely hospitalize patient after mistaken order of feeding solution through dialysis catheter; consciously deviated from known standard of care, not punishment for medical judgment], *application for stay of mandate denied*, 520 U.S. 1238 (1997).

[38] *See* E. Fein, *In rare case, a doctor faces time in jail over a medical decision*, N.Y. TIMES, May 17, 1997, 18.

[39] *Doctor in negligence case has his sentence eased*, N.Y. TIMES, June 28, 1997, 20 [sentence commuted to 52 days of community service].

and child endangerment. The trial court permitted the prosecutor to present the case, but at the conclusion of the prosecutor's case, the court dismissed the case and acquitted the physician because there was insufficient evidence.[40]

There has also been a trend toward more prosecutions of physicians for prescribing pain medications.[41] For example, in 1999, a California physician was charged with murder, prescription violations, and fraudulent medical claims after five patients died who he was treating with painkillers. During the trial, the murder charges were withdrawn or dismissed. In 2004, a jury acquitted him of the remaining charges.[42] In some cases, the physicians were clearly outside the scope of accepted practice. In other cases, it was not clearly articulated how those selected for prosecution differed from physicians who regularly deal with patients with severe chronic pain. Thus, in some cases, there has been fear that cautious physicians will reduce their prescription of needed pain medications. Attempts have been made to promulgate guidelines of practices that will not be prosecuted. However, the tension between pain control and drug enforcement practices is likely to continue.

Physicians and nurses have been prosecuted for theft of drugs.[43]

Nursing home officials have been prosecuted for the death of residents. For example, in 2000, a Missouri appellate court upheld the conviction of a nursing home administrator for felony neglect after the death of two residents.[44]

Criminal cases involving deaths of patients are discussed in Section 7-8.5.

---

[40] People v. Schug, No. CR 4514 (Cal. Super. Ct. Lake County Feb. 20, 1998), *as discussed in* 7 H.L.R. 470 (1998); L. Prager, *Keeping clinical errors out of criminal courts*, AM. MED. NEWS, Mar. 16, 1998; *Statement of ACEP President Dr. Nancy Auer re: California criminal trial of Dr. Wolfgang Schug* [Feb. 11, 1998 News Release of Am. College of Emergency Physicians – www.acep.org/press/pi980212.htm — emergency room physicians should not face prison sentences for medical decisions; license discipline, civil malpractice action provide appropriate recourse]; *see also Doctor faces 2nd-degree murder charge in baby's death*, AM. MED. NEWS, Sept. 21, 1998, 9 [Dr. Turner; Washington]; *Murder charge dropped in case against doctor*, N.Y. TIMES, Feb. 2, 1999, A15 [Dr. Turner].

[41] *See DEA v. Doctors*, AM. MED. NEWS, Dec. 1, 2003, 14 [441 actions by DEA in first three quarters of 2003]; A. Barton, *Psychiatrist pleads in drug death*, PALM BEACH POST [Fla.], Dec. 7, 2002, 1C.

[42] R. Vartabedian, *Jury finds doctor not guilty*, L.A. TIMES, May 20, 2004, B6.

[43] *E.g.*, *Nurse accused of drug tampering sentenced to nine years*, AP, Sept. 13, 2003 [Idaho nurse accused of stealing lifesaving medication from hospitalized seizure patient].

[44] State v. Boone Retirement Ctr., Inc., 26 S.W.3d 265 (Mo. App. 2000).

12-4.3 Criminal Penalties for Billing

The aggregate amount of fraud fines has grown dramatically. In the 1990s, there was $3.29 billion in health care fraud fines. From 2000 to 2002, there was $4.2 billion in fines. It is estimated that there was $2 billion in 2003.[45]

MEDICARE FRAUD AND ABUSE. Misrepresentations in Medicare and Medicaid claims and reports are subject to a maximum penalty of $25,000 and/or five years in prison.[46] For example, in 1987, a federal appellate court upheld a Medicaid fraud conviction of a physician for using improper billing codes on claims.[47]

Billing under the provider number of another provider generally constitutes fraud.[48] For some services, a provider must be present when the services are provided in order to bill; billing for services when the provider is not present can constitute fraud.[49]

FALSE CLAIMS ACT. The False Claims Act[50] imposes criminal penalties on anyone who knowingly presents, or causes to be presented, to the United States government a false or fictitious claim for payment. This includes using a false record or statement to get a false or fictitious claim paid. It is not limited to health care; it applies equally to all others who make claims for payment to the government for anything. There does not have to be specific intent to defraud the government; recklessness is enough. If the government suffered damages as a result of the false claim, the defendant can be assessed three times those damages. In addition, a penalty of $5,000 to $10,000 per false claim can be assessed. Providers have been found liable under this Act.[51]

In 1988, a federal appellate court upheld a finding that an ophthalmologist had violated the false claims statute by billing for procedures that were medically unnecessary.[52] One of the grounds for

---

[45] P. Callahan, *Health industry sees a surge in fraud fines,* WALL ST. J., Aug. 18, 2003, B1.

[46] 42 U.S.C. § 1320a-7b.

[47] United States v. Larm, 824 F.2d 780 (9th Cir. 1987), *cert. denied,* 484 U.S. 1078 (1988).

[48] *E.g.,* United States v. Mitrione, 357 F.3d 712 (7th Cir. 2004).

[49] *E.g., Doctor sentenced for health-care billing fraud,* AP, Sept. 26, 2003 [Wash. physician sentenced to five years probation, 1,000 hours community service, $100,000 restitution for noting on chart that he was present during dialysis when he was not].

[50] 31 U.S.C. §§ 3729 – 3731; *see* J.C. West, *The False Claims Act: potential liability for health care providers for fraud and abuse and beyond,* 28 J.H.H.L. 15 (1995).

[51] *E.g.,* United States v. Lorenzo, 768 F. Supp. 1127 (E.D. Pa. 1991).

[52] United States v. Campbell, 845 F.2d 1374 (6th Cir.), *cert. denied,* 488 U.S. 908 (1988) [conviction under 18 U.S.C. §§ 287, 1341].

the lack of medical necessity was the improper way in which the procedures were performed.

In 2001, a federal appellate court ruled that claims submitted for payment of services that did not meet professional standards of care were not false on that basis alone for False Claims Act purposes.[53]

Federal courts generally require that False Claims Act cases identify specific claims. Broad claims of bad practices are generally insufficient.[54]

Improper coding of bills can render them false claims. Enforcement efforts have focused on a few codes where there are significant differences in payment between closely related codes, such as the codes for pneumonia cases. There have been numerous settlements of pneumonia upcoding cases.[55]

12-4.4 Criminal Penalties for Business Arrangements

MEDICARE AND MEDICAID FRAUD AND ABUSE (ANTIKICK-BACK LAW). Providers of services and supplies to Medicare and Medicaid patients are subject to strict antifraud and abuse requirements.[56] Kickbacks, bribes, rebates, and other inducements for referrals of Medicare and Medicaid patients are all felonies. Both paying and receiving inducements are offenses. Payment need not be completed. Solicitations and offers of inducements are also offenses. In addition, the Secretary of Health and Human Services can impose civil penalties, including exclusion from participation in the Medicare and Medicaid programs.

In 1989, a federal appellate court ruled that any payment to induce future referrals can be a violation even if the payment is for actual services.[57] The court decided that a payment for professional services is permitted only if it is wholly and not incidentally attributable to the delivery of goods and services. Also in 1989, another federal appellate court upheld the convictions of an ambulance company and a hospital training director who was paid by the

---

[53] United States *ex rel.* Mikes v. Straus, 274 F.3d 687 (2d Cir. 2001).

[54] *E.g.,* United States *ex rel.* Karvelas v. Melrose-Wakefield Hosp., 360 F.3d 220 (1st Cir. 2004).

[55] *E.g.,* United States v. Shelby Memorial Hosp., No. 02-CV-3094 (C.D. Ill. settlement Jan. 15, 2004), *as discussed in* H.L.R., Jan. 22, 2004, 116 [$1.75 million paid for alleged pneumonia upcoding].

[56] 42 U.S.C. § 1320a-7b.

[57] United States v. Kats, 871 F.2d 105 (9th Cir.1989); *accord,* United States v. Greber, 760 F.2d 68 (2d Cir. 1985), *cert. denied,* 474 U.S. 988 (1985); *see also* United States v. Lipkis, 770 F.2d 1447 (9th Cir. 1985); *but see* United States v. Porter, 591 F.2d 1048 (5th Cir. 1979).

ambulance service for serving as its part-time training consultant.[58] The director served on the hospital committee that wrote specifications, reviewed bids, and recommended contracting with the ambulance company. The court ruled that he did not have to be in a position to make a referral but could violate the statute by being in a position to recommend or arrange a referral.

In 2004, one federal appellate court ruled that payments to a nonmedical company to advertise home health services did not constitute kickbacks even where they were based on the amount of business generated. The business could make not referrals, and no payments were made to those who did make referrals.[59]

In 2001, a drug company paid federal fines of $885 million to settle charges of bribing and paying kickbacks to doctors and hospitals to promote drug sales. Eight drug company employees were criminally charged with similar charges. In 2004, a federal jury acquitted the individuals.[60]

In 2004, a federal court refused to dismiss the indictment of defendants who had offered a federal undercover company free medical supplies to induce the company to buy other enteral products from the defendants.[61]

Willfully and Knowingly. Conviction requires a showing that the violation was willfully and knowingly made. This intent requirement is called a *scienter* requirement. It is often a key element of the defense of these cases,[62] but federal courts have disagreed on what this means.

In 1995, in the first major set back for HHS, the federal Ninth Circuit Court of Appeals ruled that the Hanlester Network had not violated the kickback prohibition through its joint venture laboratory arrangements with physicians.[63] HHS claimed that the payments to the limited partner physicians were to induce referrals. The court interpreted the knowing and willful requirement to mean that it must be proved that the defendants knew the conduct was unlawful and acted with specific intent to disobey the law. Thus, unlike most

---

[58] United States v. Bay State Ambulance & Hosp. Rental Serv., 874 F.2d 20 (1st Cir. 1989).

[59] United States v. Miles, 360 F.3d 472 (5th Cir. 2004).

[60] *Eight acquitted in drug incentives case*, N.Y. Times, July 15, 2004, C2.

[61] United States v. Carroll, 320 F. Supp. 2d 748 (S.D. Ill. 2004).

[62] *Scienter is key in defending accusations of FCA violations*, 1 H.C.F.R. 315 (1997).

[63] Hanlester Network v. Shalala, 51 F.3d 1390 (9th Cir. 1995); *see also* United States *ex rel.* Hochman v. Nackman, 145 F.3d 1069 (9th Cir. 1998) [affirming summary judgment for defendants, failure to show "knowingly" presented false claims].

areas of the law, ignorance of the law was recognized as an excuse. The court relied on a 1994 United States Supreme Court decision that applied this interpretation to the law against structuring currency transactions.[64] Previously this interpretation had been applied by the Court only to federal income tax cases,[65] and other federal courts have been reluctant to expand the scope of those rulings.[66]

Federal courts in other circuits have declined to follow the Hanlester ruling. In 1996, the Eighth Circuit Court of Appeals ruled that the prosecution needed to prove that the defendant knew the conduct was wrongful but did not have to prove that the defendant knew that it violated a legal duty.[67] In 1998, another federal appellate court agreed that it was necessary to prove specific intent to perform an illegal act, but it was not necessary to prove knowledge of which law was being violated.[68]

In 1998, in a nonhealth care case, the United States Supreme Court ruled that a "knowingly and willfully" requirement requires proof that the "defendant acted with an evil-meaning mind, that is to say, that he acted with knowledge that his conduct was unlawful." The Court ruled that knowledge the conduct is unlawful is all that is required; it is not necessary to prove knowledge of which statute is being violated.[69] Later that year a federal appellate court applied the ruling to a Medicare kickback case.[70]

Safe Harbors. The statute expressly states that payments to physicians are not considered kickbacks if the physician is a bona fide employee of the entity making the payment. Regulations have been issued that define other "safe harbors," conduct that will not be considered a violation.[71] There are safe harbors for (1) investment interests,[72]

---

[64] Ratzlaf v. United States, 510 U.S. 135 (1994).

[65] *E.g.*, Cheek v. United States, 498 U.S. 192 (1991).

[66] *E.g.*, United States v. Hilliard, 31 F.3d 1509 (10th Cir. 1994).

[67] United States v. Jain, 93 F.3d 436 (8th Cir. 1996), *cert. denied*, 520 U.S. 1273 (1997) [affirming conviction of psychologist for receiving payment from psychiatric hospital for referral; to show "willful" for Medicare antikickback law, need only prove knew conduct wrongful, not that it violated legal duty; *Hanlester* distinguished as dealing only with administrative debarment proceeding].

[68] United States v. Davis, 132 F.3d 1092 (5th Cir. 1998); *accord*, United States v. Starks, 157 F.3d 833 (11th Cir. 1998).

[69] Bryan v. United States, 524 U.S. 184 (1998).

[70] United States v. Starks, 157 F.3d 833 (11th Cir. 1998) [need not be aware of specific law to knowingly violate law, *Bryan* refutes *Ratzlaf*].

[71] 42 C.F.R. § 1001.952; 56 FED. REG. 35,952 (July 29, 1991); 61 FED. REG. 2,122 (Jan. 25, 1996); 64 FED. REG. 63,504 (Nov. 19, 1999); 64 FED. REG. 63,518 (Nov. 19, 1999); 64 FED. REG. 71,317 (Dec. 21, 1999); 67 FED. REG. 11,928 (Mar. 18, 2002).

[72] 42 C.F.R. § 1001.952(a); OIG Advisory Op. 97-5, 98-19, 03-12, 03-13.

(2) space rental,[73] (3) equipment rental,[74] (4) personal services and management contracts,[75] (5) sale of practice,[76] (6) referral services,[77] (7) warranties,[78] (8) discounts,[79] (9) employees,[80] (10) group purchasing organizations,[81] (11) waiver of beneficiary copayments and deductibles,[82] (12) increased coverage, reduced cost-sharing amounts, or reduced premium amounts offered by health plans,[83] (13) price reductions offered to health plans,[84] (14) practitioner recruitment,[85] (15) obstetrical malpractice insurance subsidies,[86] (16) investments in group practices,[87] (17) cooperative hospital service organizations,[88] (18) ambulatory surgical centers,[89] (19) referral arrangements for specialty services,[90] (20) price reductions offered to eligible managed care organizations,[91] (21) price reductions offered by contractors with substantial financial risk to managed care organizations,[92] (22) ambulance replenishing,[93] and (23) waiver of some

---

[73] 42 C.F.R. § 1001.952(b); United States *ex rel.* Goodstein v. McLaren Reg. Med. Ctr., 202 F. Supp. 2d 671 (E.D. Mich. 2002); OIG Advisory Op. 01-17, 01-21, 03-02, 04-08.

[74] 42 C.F.R. § 1001.952(c); United States v. Carroll, 320 F. Supp. 2d 748 (S.D. Ill. 2004); OIG Advisory Op. 98-18, 04-03.

[75] 42 C.F.R. § 1001.952(d); United States v. Norton, 17 Fed. Appx. 98, 2001 U.S. App. LEXIS 18811 (4th Cir. 2001) (unpub.); Nursing Home Consultants, Inc. v. Lamey, 926 F. Supp. 835 (E.D. Ark. 1996); United States v. Neufield, 908 F. Supp. 491 (S.D. Ohio 1995); OIG Advisory Op. 98-01, 98-04, 98-10, 98-15, 98-16, 98-19, 99-8, 01-01, 01-17, 01-21, 03-02, 03-07, 03-08, 04-08, 04-16, 05-01, 05-02, 05-03, 05-04, 05-05, 05-06.

[76] 42 C.F.R. § 1001.952(e).

[77] 42 C.F.R. § 1001.952(f); OIG Advisory Op. 99-08, 99-11, 00-08.

[78] 42 C.F.R. § 1001.952(g); OIG Advisory Op. 01-08, 02-06.

[79] 42 U.S.C. § 1320a-7b(b)(3)(A); 42 C.F.R. § 1001.952(h); United States *ex rel.* Schmidt v. Zimmer, Inc., 386 F.3d 235 (3d Cir. 2004); United States v. Carroll, 320 F. Supp. 2d 748 (S.D. Ill. 2004); Klaczak v. Consol. Med. Transp., Inc., 2002 U.S. Dist. Lexis 16824 (N.D. Ill.); United States *ex rel.* Bidani v. Lewis, 2001 U.S. Dist. LEXIS 20947 (N.D. Ill.); United States v. Shaw, 106 F. Supp. 2d 103 (D. Mass. 2000); United States *ex rel.* Walsh v. Eastman Kodak Co., 98 F. Supp. 2d 141 (D. Mass. 2000); OIG Advisory Op. 98-02, 98-05, 99-02, 99-03, 99-13, 02-10, 02-13, 04-16.

[80] 42 U.S.C. § 1320a-7b(b)(3)(B); 42 C.F.R. § 1001.952(i); OIG Advisory Op. 98-09, 04-09.

[81] 42 U.S.C. § 1320a-7b(b)(3)(C); 42 C.F.R. § 1001.952(j); OIG Advisory Op. 98-11, 01-06.

[82] 42 U.S.C. § 1320a-7b(b)(3)(D); 42 C.F.R. § 1001.952(k); OIG Advisory Op. 01-07, 03-10.

[83] 42 C.F.R. § 1001.952(l); OIG Advisory Op. 98-05, 99-06, 02-12.

[84] 42 U.S.C. § 1320a-7b(b)(3)(F); 42 C.F.R. § 1001.952(m); OIG Advisory Op. 98-05.

[85] 42 C.F.R. § 1001.952(n); United States *ex rel.* Perales v. St. Margaret's Hosp., 243 F. Supp. 2d 843 (C.D. Ill. 2003); OIG Advisory Op. 01-04.

[86] 42 C.F.R. § 1001.952(o); OIG Advisory Op. 04-11.

[87] 42 C.F.R. § 1001.952(p).

[88] 42 C.F.R. § 1001.952(q).

[89] 42 C.F.R. § 1001.952(r); OIG Advisory Op. 01-21, 02-09, 03-02, 03-05.

[90] 42 C.F.R. § 1001.952(s).

[91] 42 U.S.C. § 1320a-7b(b)(3)(F); 42 C.F.R. § 1001.952(t); 64 FED. REG. 63,504 (Nov. 11, 1999); OIG Advisory Op. 00-04.

[92] 42 U.S.C. § 1320a-7b(b)(3)(F); 42 C.F.R. § 1001.952(u); 64 FED. REG. 63,504 Nov. 11, 1999.

[93] 42 C.F.R. § 1001.952(v); 66 FED. REG. 62979 (Dec. 4, 2001); OIG Advisory Op. 02-02, 02-03.

Part D cost sharing by pharmacies.[94] Each of these safe harbors is subject to detailed requirements. When possible it is safest to stay within them, but many transactions in the actual market place do not fit within the safe harbors. Venturing outside the safe harbors does not mean that the law is necessarily being violated.

Other Administrative Guidance. Several fraud alerts have been issued by the OIG that state that certain conduct is prohibited or suspicious. The fraud alerts address (1) joint venture arrangements, (2) waiver of copayments and deductibles, (3) hospital incentives to physicians, (4) prescription drug marketing, (5) clinical laboratory arrangements, (5) offering of gifts and other inducements to Medicare and Medicaid beneficiaries, and (6) other areas.[95]

Federal courts have been reluctant to provide authoritative guidance as to what conduct is permitted. A federal court refused to decide whether it would be a violation for a physician who admitted patients to a hospital also to own part of the hospital.[96]

Federal administrative agencies also have been reluctant to give authoritative guidance concerning what is permitted under this law. When the federal government approves certain conduct, it is not permitted to prosecute that conduct as fraud and abuse.[97] In 1997, HHS began providing advisory opinions.[98] While relevant opinions should be examined when structuring arrangements because they give some guidance, they are generally worded to minimize the extent to which they provide providers with any legal protection.

STATE LAW. Some states also have laws that forbid kickbacks for referrals[99] or splitting of fees.[100]

STARK LAW (SELF-REFERRAL). Congress has directly prohibited many referrals by a physician to an entity in which the physician or a family member has an ownership interest or other financial rela-

---

[94] 42 U.S.C. § 1320a-7b(b)(3)(G).

[95] 59 FED. REG. 65,372 (Dec. 19, 1994); 67 FED. REG. 55,855 (Aug. 30, 2002).

[96] Bakersfield Commun. Hosp. v. Sullivan, No. 89-1056-TPJ (D. D.C. Aug. 8, 1989), *as discussed in* 17 HEALTH L. DIG. (Sept. 1989), at 15; D. Burda, *Judge refuses to rule on hospital sale*, MOD. HEALTHCARE, Sept. 1, 1989, 7.

[97] *E.g.*, United States v. Levin, 973 F.2d 463 (6th Cir. 1992) [dismissal of fraud, abuse charges against manufacturer for giving gifts to surgeons pursuant to marketing plan approved by HHS, HCFA].

[98] 42 C.F.R. pt. 1008; advisory opinions are available at http://oig.hhs.gov/fraud/advisoryopinions/opinions.html.

[99] *E.g.*, FLA. STAT. §§ 395.0185, 455.237; *see also* Schmidt v. Foundation Health, 35 Cal. App. 4th 1702, 42 Cal. Rptr. 2d 172 (3d Dist. 1995) [illegal kickback for health insurance broker to rebate commission to subscribers].

[100] *E.g.*, FLA. STAT. § 458.331(1)(i).

tionship.[101] This is usually referred to as the Stark law. Initially, these restrictions applied only to referrals for laboratory services,[102] but a 1993 amendment expanded the restrictions effective January 1, 1995, to apply to a wide range of services.[103] This is usually called Stark II. A 1994 technical amendment clarified that not all diagnostic services are covered.[104] There are several safe harbors stated in the statute and the regulations.[105] There are safe harbors for (1) rental of office space,[106] (2) rental of equipment,[107] (3) bona fide employment relationships,[108] (4) personal service arrangements,[109] (5) physician recruitment,[110] (6) isolated transactions,[111] (7) certain arrangements with hospitals,[112] (8) group practice arrangements with hospitals,[113] (9) certain payments by a physician,[114] (10) charitable donations by a physician,[115] (11) nonmonetary compensation up to $300,[116] (12) fair market value compensation,[117] (13) medical staff incidental benefits,[118] (14) risk-sharing arrangements,[119] (15) compliance training,[120] (16) indirect compensation arrangements,[121] (17) referral services,[122] (18) obstetrical malpractice insurance subsidies,[123] (19) professional courtesy,[124] (20) retention payments in underserved areas,[125] (21) communitywide health information

---

[101] 42 U.S.C. § 1395nn; 42 C.F.R. pt. 1003 [civil money penalties].
[102] Pub. L. No. 101-239, § 6204 (1989); Pub. L. No. 101-508, § 4207 (1990).
[103] Pub. L. No. 103-66, § 13562(a) (1993); 66 FED. REG. 856 (Jan. 4, 2001) [Phase I final rule]; 66 FED. REG. 60154 (Dec. 3, 2001) [interim final rule with partial delay]; 69 FED. REG. 16054 (Mar. 26, 2004) [Phase II interim final rule].
[104] Pub. L. No. 103-432, § 152 (1994).
[105] 42 C.F.R. §§ 411.350 - 411.357; United States ex rel. Perales v. St. Margaret's Hosp., 243 F. Supp. 2d 843 (C.D. Ill. 2003).
[106] 42 U.S.C. § 1395nn(e)(1); 42 C.F.R. § 411.357(a).
[107] 42 U.S.C. § 1395nn(e)(1); 42 C.F.R. § 411.357(b).
[108] 42 U.S.C. § 1395nn(e)(2); 42 C.F.R. § 411.357(c).
[109] 42 U.S.C. § 1395nn(e)(3); 42 C.F.R. § 411.357(d).
[110] 42 U.S.C. § 1395nn(e)(5); 42 C.F.R. § 411.357(e).
[111] 42 U.S.C. § 1395nn(e)(6); 42 C.F.R. § 411.357(f).
[112] 42 C.F.R. § 411.357(g).
[113] 42 U.S.C. § 1395nn(e)(7); 42 C.F.R. § 411.357(h).
[114] 42 C.F.R. § 411.357(i).
[115] 42 C.F.R. § 411.357(j).
[116] 42 C.F.R. § 411.357(k).
[117] 42 C.F.R. § 411.357(l).
[118] 42 C.F.R. § 411.357(m).
[119] 42 C.F.R. § 411.357(n).
[120] 42 C.F.R. § 411.357(o).
[121] 42 C.F.R. § 411.357(p).
[122] 42 C.F.R. § 411.357(q).
[123] 42 C.F.R. § 411.357(r).
[124] 42 C.F.R. § 411.357(s).
[125] 42 C.F.R. § 411.357(t).

systems,[126] (22) group practices,[127] (23) some compensation,[128] (24) some ownership or investment interests,[129] (25) some physician services,[130] (26) some in-office ancillary services,[131] (27) services furnished by an organization (or its contractors or subcontractors) to enrollees,[132] (28) academic medical centers,[133] (29) implants furnished by an ASC,[134] (30) EPO and other dialysis-related drugs furnished in or by an ESRD facility,[135] (31) preventive screening tests, immunizations, and vaccines,[136] (32) eyeglasses and contact lenses following cataract surgery,[137] (33) intrafamily rural referrals,[138] (34) investments in publicly-traded securities,[139] (35) investments in mutual funds,[140] (36) investments in some specific providers,[141] and (37) electronic prescribing.[142]

Unlike the Medicare fraud and abuse law, venturing outside those safe harbors violates the law, and there is no requirement to prove the act is knowing or willful.

In 1998, under Congressional mandate HHS began issuing advisory opinions on the applicability of the Stark law to specific arrangements.[143]

A Kansas hospital administrator was sentenced to federal prison for arranging payments to physicians that violated the Stark rules. In 2004, a federal court refused to vacate the conviction.[144]

---

[126] 42 C.F.R. § 411.357(u).
[127] 42 C.F.R. § 411.352; Advisory Opinion No. CMS-AO-98-002.
[128] 42 C.F.R. § 411.354(c).
[129] 42 C.F.R. § 411.354(b).
[130] 42 U.S.C. § 1395nn(b)(1); 42 C.F.R. § 411.355(a).
[131] 42 U.S.C. § 1395nn(b)(2); 42 C.F.R. § 411.355(b); Advisory Op. No. CMS-AO-98-002.
[132] 42 C.F.R. § 411.355(c).
[133] 42 C.F.R. § 411.355(e).
[134] 42 C.F.R. § 411.355(f).
[135] 42 C.F.R. § 411.355(g).
[136] 42 C.F.R. § 411.355(h).
[137] 42 C.F.R. § 411.355(i).
[138] 42 C.F.R. § 411.355(j).
[139] 42 U.S.C. § 1395nn(c); 42 C.F.R. § 411.356(a).
[140] 42 C.F.R. § 411.356(b).
[141] 42 U.S.C. § 1395nn(d); 42 C.F.R. § 411.356(c); Advisory Op. No. CMS-AO-98-001.
[142] 42 U.S.C. § 1395nn(b)(5).
[143] 63 FED. REG. 1,646 (Jan. 9, 1998) [advisory opinion procedures]; No. HCFA-AO-98-001 (Oct. 29, 1998) [ambulatory surgery center can qualify for rural provider exception].
[144] United States v. Anderson, 2004 U.S. Dist. LEXIS 5087 (D. Kans.); *see also* Anderson v. Thompson, 311 F. Supp. 2d 1121 (D. Kan. 2004) [affirming exclusion form Medicare, Medicaid, other federal programs].

12-4.5 Other Criminal Laws

Prosecutors have included claims of bribery, mail or wire fraud, money laundering,[145] filing false tax returns,[146] obstructing justice,[147] witness tampering,[148] embezzlement from an entity providing Medicare/Medicaid services,[149] and other criminal laws in cases against health care providers.[150]

ANTI-BRIBERY ACT. The federal Anti-Bribery Act makes it a federal crime to engage in fraud or bribery involving an organization that receives federal funds.[151] In 2000, the United States Supreme Court decided that receipt of Medicare funds is sufficient to trigger applicability of this law.[152]

MAIL FRAUD/WIRE FRAUD. False claims and other false statements that are sent through the mails can be punished under the mail fraud law.[153] If statements are sent by wire, punishment can be under the wire fraud law.[154] Generally, some tangible harm must be

---

[145] 18 U.S.C. § 1957; United States v. Rutgard, 116 F.3d 1270 (9th Cir. 1997) [proof of violation of § 1957 requires proof of transfer of particular criminal proceeds].

[146] 26 U.S.C. § 7206.

[147] 18 U.S.C. § 1503; United States v. Vaghela, 169 F.3d 729 (11th Cir. 1999) [reversing conviction obstructing justice, affirming other convictions; agreed acts did not meet nexus requirement — the act must have relationship in time, causation, or logic with the judicial proceedings — applying *United States v. Aguilar*, 515 U.S. 593 (1995)].

[148] 18 U.S.C. § 1512; United States v. Mills, 138 F.3d 928 (11th Cir. 1998), *cert. denied*, 525 U.S. 1003 (1998) [affirming conviction of officers of home health company for witness tampering].

[149] 18 U.S.C. § 669, *added by* HIPAA (Pub. L. No. 104-191); United States v. Rector, No. 3:98-CR39WN (S. D. Miss. May 1, 1998) [guilty plea resulted in first conviction under law].

[150] *E.g.*, 18 U.S.C. § 286 [conspiracy to defraud the government with respect to a claim]; 18 U.S.C. § 287 [fictitious or fraudulent claims]; 18 U.S.C. § 371 [conspiracy to commit offense or defraud]; 18 U.S.C. § 494 [contractors, bonds, bids, and public accords]; 18 U.S.C. § 495 [contracts, deeds, and powers of attorney]; 18 U.S.C. § 1001 [statements or entries generally]; 18 U.S.C. § 1002 [possession of false papers to defraud U.S.], *see* United States v. Radetsky, 535 F.2d 556 (10th Cir. 1976), *cert. denied*, 429 U.S. 820 (1976) [conviction for false Medicare billing under 18 U.S.C. §§ 1001, 1002], *overruled in part on other grounds*, United States v. Dailey, 921 F.2d 994 (10th Cir. 1990), *cert. denied*, 502 U.S. 952 (1991); 18 U.S.C. §§ 1961–1963 [racketeer influenced, corrupted organizations (RICO)]; 18 U.S.C.§ 1018 [official certificates, writings]; 18 U.S.C. § 1505 [obstruction of proceedings before departments, agencies, committees]; 31 U.S.C. § 231 [liability of persons making false claims].

[151] 18 U.S.C. § 666.

[152] Fischer v. United States, 529 U.S. 667 (2000).

[153] 18 U.S.C. § 1341; United States v. Woodely, 9 F.3d 74 (9th Cir. 1993) [mail fraud conviction for Medicare claims by nursing home]; United States v. Migliaccio, 34 F.3d 1517 (10th Cir. 1994) [conviction of doctors for mail fraud for sending false CHAMPUS claims reversed and new trial ordered, alleged misrepresentation of surgical procedures performed, inadequate jury instructions]; United States v. Vest, 116 F.3d 1179 (7th Cir. 1997), *cert. denied*, 522 U.S. 1119 (1998) [mail fraud conviction of physician].

[154] 18 U.S.C. § 1343.

demonstrated to convict under these laws.[155] It is not limited to claims to the government. Physicians have been convicted of mail fraud for bills submitted to private insurers.[156]

In 2003, in one of the first criminal prosecutions of a hospital corporation, a Michigan hospital was charged with mail and wire fraud for the submission of bills for medically unnecessary procedures. The case was resolved by the hospital pleading guilty and being placed in federal pretrial diversion with a compliance agreement for three years, the hospital paying a $1 million fine and full restitution to Medicare and private insurers, and some individual defendants pleading guilty to state misdemeanor charges, paying fines and restitution, providing community service, and being placed in federal pretrial diversion.[157]

12-5 Suspension, Recoupment, and Exclusion from Federal Programs

SUSPENSION OR RECOUPMENT OF PAYMENTS. The Centers for Medicare & Medicaid Services has broad powers to suspend payments to providers during investigations of suspected violations. Courts will not review such suspensions.[158]

When CMS chooses not to suspend payments, it generally has broad powers to recoup disputed past payments from current payments.[159] Courts generally will not intervene, even in bankruptcy cases. There is one unusual case in which CMS's predecessor HCFA agreed in a settlement to stop recoupment and to refund recouped funds until the matter could be heard in court.[160]

---

155 *See* United States v. Jain, 93 F.3d 436 (8th Cir. 1996), *cert. denied*, 520 U.S. 1273 (1997) [mail fraud conviction reversed, no evidence any patient experienced tangible harm].

156 *E.g.*, United States v. Hooshmand, 931 F.2d 725 (11th Cir. 1991).

157 *Cases in court*, HEALTH CARE FRAUD & ABUSE, Feb. 13, 2003, 7; G. Martin & B.C. Tanase, *The first criminal prosecution of a hospital: lessons from the United Memorial Hospital case*, presented at the Am. Health Lawyers Ass'n 2003 Annual Meeting in San Antonio, Tex.).

158 *E.g.*, Clarinda Home Health v. Shalala, 100 F.3d 526 (8th Cir. 1996) [no jurisdiction to review suspension of Medicare payments during investigation]; *sees also Feds cite mistakes at State Hospital prior to suicide*, AP, Sept. 27, 2003 [Vt. state hospital participation terminated].

159 See *HCFA changes instructions for suspending payments and recouping overpayments*, 2 H.C.F.R. 407 (1998) [Intermediary Manual Transmittal No. 1745; Carriers Manual Transmittal No. 1604].

160 Fendell v. Shalala, No. 4:97-CV-118-MP (N.D. Fla. settlement agreement June 19, 1997) [HCFA agreed not to recoup from current claims for prior disputed payments]; settlement on Aug. 26, 1998 in which HCFA refunded $2.2 million until hearing, 2 H.C.F.R. 743 (1998).

EXCLUSION. The Department of Health and Human Services has broad powers to exclude any providers who violate false claims, anti-kickback, self-referral, medical necessity, or medical quality requirements from participation in Medicare, Medicaid, and other federal programs. In some cases, exclusion is mandated, and in other cases, it is permissive.[161] When exclusions are permissive, HHS has broad powers to offer corrective action plans in lieu of exclusion and generally does so. Providers who desire to continue in business generally cooperate in developing such plans because failure to do so can result in exclusion.[162] Exclusions generally remain in effect during appeals.[163] Exclusion of most health care organizations is essentially a death penalty. Thus, care must be taken in negotiating settlement of other matters not to inadvertently create a basis for exclusion.

Medicare and Medicaid providers are not permitted to employ or contract with persons or entities that have been excluded. To assist in enforcing this requirement, the OIG maintains a Web site with a list of all who have been excluded.[164] These actions are collected in the Healthcare Integrity and Protection Data Bank.[165]

HHS sometimes reinstates institutional providers after their ownership or management is changed.[166]

12-6 Civil Money Penalties

The Department of Health and Human Services has authority to impose huge civil money penalties for violations of the Medicare and Medicaid fraud and abuse requirements.[167] This includes misrepresentations in claims and reports, kickbacks, and other violations.

---

[161] 42 C.F.R. pts. 1001 (Medicare), 1002 (Medicaid); 62 FED. REG. 67,392 (Dec. 24, 1997) [permissive exclusion guidelines]; 63 FED. REG. 46,676 (Sept. 2, 1998) [IG exclusion rules]; R. Roth & T. Hoffman, *HHS IG makes power play in finding exclusion authority over indirect providers*, 2 H.C.F.R. 797 (1998); 63 FED. REG. 57,918 (Oct. 29, 1998) [modifying IG exclusion rules]; 63 FED. REG. 68,687 (Dec. 14, 1998) [final rule on procedures to impose civil money penalties, assessments, exclusions].

[162] *E.g.*, Corkill v. Shalala, 109 F.3d 1348 (9th Cir. 1996) [affirming three-year exclusion of physician for violating medical necessity, quality requirements; refused to enter corrective action plan].

[163] *E.g.*, Erickson v. United States *ex rel.* D.H.H.S., 67 F.3d 858 (9th Cir. 1995) [reversing injunction of exclusion pending appeal].

[164] *See* http://exclusions.oig.hhs.gov.

[165] 64 FED. REG. 57,740 (Oct. 26, 1999), *codified in* 45 C.F.R. pt. 61.

[166] *E.g.*, *Golden Valley hospital has Medicare reinstated*, AP, May 22, 2002.

[167] 42 U.S.C. § 1320a-7b; 42 C.F.R. pts. 402, 1003 [civil money penalties, assessments]; 42 C.F.R. pts. 400, 1005 [procedures]; 63 FED. REG. 68,687 (Dec. 14, 1998); 65 FED. REG. 24,400 (Apr. 26, 2000); 67 FED. REG. 11,928 (Mar. 18, 2002).

False claims can now result in civil money penalties of up to $10,000 per item or service and, in addition, assessments of up to $25,000 per item or service, plus three times the amount claimed.[168]

Another reason to be careful about fraud and abuse issues is that even when the government chooses not to challenge the arrangement, one of the parties can try to use a violation as a basis for avoiding its responsibilities in the arrangement. Illegality of a contract can be a reason to declare a contract void and unenforceable. One Texas court declared a physician recruitment contract void as an illegal inducement of referrals; when the physician violated the contract by refusing to make required repayments, the hospital could not recover the money it had advanced.[169] A California court ruled that a hospital's free rent office arrangement with a physician was an illegal inducement for referrals, and the hospital could get out of the lease.[170] A federal court in Illinois found that a laboratory management agreement was unenforceable because it was illegal inducement for referrals. Although the court questioned whether there was sufficient proof of willfulness for any crime to have occurred yet, the court ruled that future performance would be willful after the decision in the case was issued.[171] These attacks do not always succeed. A California jury rejected a radiologist's challenge to a marketing agreement with a hospital and required him to pay the fee under the contract.[172]

12-7 Private Lawsuits

QUI TAM SUITS. The False Claims Act permits some individuals to bring suits, called *qui tam* actions, in the name of the United States as "private attorneys general."[173] The individual filing the suit is

---

[168] 42 U.S.C. § 1320a-7a; 42 C.F.R. pts. 402, 1003.

[169] Polk County v. Peters, 800 F. Supp. 1451 (E.D. Tex. 1992).

[170] Vana v. Vista Hosp. Sys., Inc., No. 233623, 1993 WL 597402 (Cal. Super. Ct. Riverside County Oct. 25, 1993). The case settled in 1994, 3 H.L.R. 180 (1994).

[171] Modern Med. Labs., Inc. v. Smith-Kline Beecham Clinical Labs., Inc., No. 92 C 5302 (N.D. Ill. Aug. 16, 1994), *reprinted in* MEDICARE & MEDICAID GUIDE [CCH] ¶42754.

[172] Klaczak v. Consolidated Med. Transport, Inc., 2002 U.S. Dist. LEXIS 16824 (N.D. Ill.) [denying dismissal of qui tam action brought by former employees of transport company alleging ambulance services were provided that were medically unnecessary, kickbacks were paid for referrals]; Anaheim General Hosp. v. Pacific Coast Radiology Med. Group, No. 660926 (Cal. Super. Ct. Oct. 11, 1994); B. McCormick, *Antikickback law no defense for not paying fee*, AM. MED. NEWS, Nov. 14, 1994, at 8.

[173] 31 U.S.C. § 3730(b).

generally called the *relator*. There are specific procedures that must be followed in such cases that give the federal government an opportunity to intervene and take over control of the case. The relator is generally awarded part of any recovery in the suit.[174]

In 2000, the United States Supreme Court decided that the qui tam law is constitutional but also ruled that states and state agencies cannot be sued under the law because they are not included in the definition of "persons" subject to the law.[175] In 2003, the Court ruled that local governments are subject to the law.[176]

WHO MAY FILE SUIT? An individual must be the source of the information that forms the basis of the suit. Generally, a qui tam suit cannot be based on publicly disclosed information, unless the relator was the original source of the information.[177]

Some persons cannot be relators even if they would otherwise be the original source of information. Generally, governmental employees, such as auditors and investigators, under a duty to disclose the information are barred.[178] However, there is no similar barrier to employees of private businesses even when they are employed to achieve compliance; several compliance officers have brought qui tam suits.[179] However, some releases signed by employees or former employers of businesses bar them from bringing qui tam actions against their employers.[180]

---

174 United States *ex rel.* Johnson-Pochardt v. Rapid City Reg. Hosp., 252 F. Supp. 2d 892 (D. S.D. 2003) [relator who had challenged lease arrangement between medical group and hospital awarded 24% of total $6,525,000 settlement].

175 Vermont Agency of Natural Resources v. United States *ex rel.* Stevens, 529 U.S. 765 (2000); *see also* Donald v. University of Ca. Bd. of Regents, 329 F.3d 1040 (9th Cir. 2003) [relators not entitled to part of federal settlement with state agency].

176 Cook County v. United States *ex rel.* Chandler, 538 U.S. 119 (2003).

177 *E.g.*, United States *ex rel.* Paranich v. Sorgnard, 396 F.3d 326 (3d Cir. 2005) [qui tam action precluded, not original source because information released involuntarily pursuant to subpoena]; United States *ex rel.* Reagan v. East Texas Med. Ctr. Reg'l Healthcare Sys., 384 F.3d 168 (5th Cir. 2004) [not original source]; United States *ex rel.* Feingold v. AdminaStar Federal, Inc., 324 F.3d 492 (7th Cir. 2003) [not original source]; United States *ex rel.* Jones v. Horizon Healthcare Corp., 160 F.3d 326 (6th Cir. 1998) [not original source]; United States *ex rel.* Stone v. Am. West Savings Ass'n, No. 3:96-CV-0549-G (N.D. Tex. Oct. 2, 1997) [statements in exchange for immunity not voluntary, so not original source]; Jones v. Horizon Healthcare Corp., No. 94-CV-71573-DT (E.D. Mich. Mar. 11, 1997) [dismissal because plaintiff put information in public domain before informing government].

178 *E.g.*, United States *ex rel.* Biddle v. Board of Trustees, 161 F.3d 533 (9th Cir. 1998) *cert. denied*, 526 U.S. 1066 (1999); United States *ex rel.* Fine v. Chevron, USA, Inc., 72 F.3d 740 (9th Cir. 1995) (en banc); United States *ex rel.* Fine v. MK-Ferguson Co., 99 F.3d 1538 (10th Cir. 1996).

179 For an example, see before 2 H.C.F.R. 888 (1998).

180 *E.g.*, United States *ex rel.* Hall v. Teledyne Wah Chang Albany, 104 F.3d 230 (9th Cir. 1997) [general release by relator to settle employment action with former employer barred qui tam action where government had knowledge of claims]; *but see* United States *ex rel.* Green v. Northup, 59 F.3d 953 (9th Cir. 1995) [some releases will not bar qui tam claims].

GOVERNMENT ROLE. The Department of Justice cannot be compelled to investigate a qui tam case.[181] When the government investigates and chooses to intervene, then the government takes over the control of the case. The government may even dismiss the case despite the objection of the relator.[182] When the government decides not to intervene, it is bound by adverse rulings.[183] There is a disagreement among the courts about the extent to which the government can control settlements by realtors.[184]

RETALIATION. The False Claims Act prohibits retaliation against employees for qui tam claims.[185] The protection can start before the qui tam action is actually filed.[186] The protection does not apply to persons, such as medical staff members, who are not employees.[187]

Discussion Points

1. Discuss compliance programs and Corporate Integrity Agreements.
2. Discuss the agencies that enforce criminal law and civil penalties.
3. What are the differences between criminal penalties and civil money penalties?

---

[181] *See* United States *ex rel.* Baggan v. DME Corp., 1997 WL 305262 (D. D.C. May 27, 1997) [no mandamus to compel DOJ to investigate qui tam case].

[182] *E.g.*, United States *ex rel.* Sequoia Orange Co. v. Baird-Neece Packing Corp., 151 F.3d 1139 (9th Cir. 1998), *cert. denied*, 525 U.S. 1067 (1999) [government may dismiss qui tam suit despite objection from whistleblower].

[183] *E.g.*, *In re* Schimmels, 127 F.3d 875 (9th Cir. 1997) [government bound by adverse ruling against relators in privity].

[184] *See* Searcy v. Philips Electronics N. Am. Corp, 117 F.3d 154 (5th Cir. 1997) [government can veto voluntary settlements of qui tam suits]; *accord,* United States v. Health Possibilities, P.S.C., 207 F.3d 335 (6th Cir. 2000) [realtor may not seek voluntary dismissal without Attorney General's consent]; *contra,* Killingsworth v. Northrup Corp., 25 F.3d 715 (9th Cir. 1994) [government can appeal settlement, but cannot automatically veto after first sixty days].

[185] 31 U.S.C. § 3730(h); *but see* United States *ex rel.* Grandeau v. Cancer Treatment Ctrs., 2004 U.S. Dist. LEXIS 2799 (N.D. Ill.) [retaliation claim dismissed, no evidence termination in any way motivated by defendants' knowledge of protected activity].

[186] *See* United States *ex rel.* Dorsey v. Dr. Warren E. Smith Community Mental Health/Mental Retardation & Substance Abuse Ctrs., 1997 U.S. Dist. LEXIS 9424 (E.D. Pa.) [intracorporate complaint sufficient to trigger protection]; Childree v. UAP/GA AG Chem., Inc., 92 F.3d 1140 (11th Cir. 1996) [protection triggered when FCA action distinct possibility]; United States *ex rel.* Ramseyer v. Century Healthcare Corp., 90 F.3d 1514 (10th Cir. 1996) [to be protected before filing, relator must show discharge results from actions in furtherance of qui tam suit].

[187] *E.g.*, Latham v. Navapache Healthcare Ass'n, No. CIV 96-2547-PHX-EHC (D. Ariz. Sept. 29, 1997) [physician with staff privileges not employee, not protected]; Vessel v. DPS Assocs. of Charleston Inc., 148 F.3d 407 (4th Cir.1998) [independent contractors not protected].

4. What are the consequences of various approaches to respond to criminal investigations?
5. When are the criminal penalties imposed for health care decisions?
6. When are the criminal penalties imposed for billing issues?
7. When are the criminal penalties imposed for provider business arrangements?
8. Discuss the range of safe harbors from the Medicare antikickback law.
9. Discuss the range of safe harbors from the Stark self-referral ban.
10. Discuss the power of the Centers for Medicare & Medicaid Services to suspend or recoup provider payments and to exclude providers from Medicare participation.
11. Discuss the scope of civil money penalties that the Department of Heath and Human Services can impose.
12. Discuss private qui tam suits to enforce the False Claims Act. Who may bring such suits?

CHAPTER THIRTEEN

Antitrust

Objectives

The objective of this chapter is to provide an overview of antitrust laws. The reader will learn about antitrust laws (Sherman Antitrust Act, Clayton Act, and Federal Trade Commission Act); some exemptions from liability; and how the laws are enforced.

Antitrust laws apply to most hospitals and other health care organizations.[1] Federal and state antitrust laws are designed to preserve the private competitive market system by prohibiting various anticompetitive activities. Antitrust suits challenge mergers, exclusive contracts, medical staff privilege denials and terminations, exchanges of price information, and many other actions of health care organizations. These suits are generally very complex and expensive to litigate; courtroom victory can be costly. Organizations need to be aware of potential antitrust problems so that questionable conduct can be either avoided or structured to provide the strongest possible defense.

The primary federal antitrust laws are the Sherman Antitrust Act,[2] the Clayton Act,[3] the Federal Trade Commission Act,[4] and the Robinson-Patman Act.[5]

---

[1] FTC & DOJ, IMPROVING HEALTH CARE: A DOSE OF COMPETITION (July 2004), http://www.usdoj.gov/atr/public/health_care/204694.htm (accessed Sept. 6, 2004).
[2] 15 U.S.C. §§ 1-7.
[3] 15 U.S.C. §§ 12-27, 44.
[4] 15 U.S.C. §§ 41-58.
[5] 15 U.S.C. § 13c.

Federal antitrust laws apply only to actions affecting interstate and foreign commerce, but interstate commerce has been broadly defined by the United States Supreme Court to include intrastate or local activities that have a substantial economic effect on interstate commerce. For example, in 1976, the Supreme Court ruled that Mary Elizabeth Hospital, a forty-nine-bed proprietary hospital operated by Hospital Building Company, was involved in interstate commerce because it purchased $100,000 worth of medicines and supplies from out-of-state vendors and received considerable revenues from out-of-state insurance companies and federal payers.[6] Hospital Building Company had sued a competing hospital, Rex Hospital, which had opposed expansion of Mary Elizabeth Hospital. The Court ruling allowed the trustees of Rex Hospital to be sued under the antitrust laws for an alleged conspiracy to restrain trade by blocking the expansion. However, Rex Hospital ultimately won the suit because a jury found that its actions had been reasonable and good faith participation in the health planning process.[7] In 1991, the Court established a standard for determining affect on interstate commerce that means virtually all health care cases affect interstate commerce.[8] A plaintiff does not have to allege an actual effect on interstate commerce. The court has to look at the impact on other participants and potential participants in the market, not just the impact on the plaintiff. Thus, the revocation of the clinical privileges of an ophthalmologist at one hospital was found to affect interstate commerce.

Some of these laws are aimed at relationships among competitors, called "horizontal" relationships. Other laws are aimed at relationships among different levels of production and distribution, called "vertical" relationships. Most states have parallel antitrust laws that apply to intrastate activities.

One unique aspect of the federal antitrust laws is the existence of two independent federal agencies, the Antitrust Division of the Department of Justice (DOJ) and the Federal Trade Commission (FTC), with overlapping authority to evaluate and attack actions as antitrust violations. As more attention has been focused on this anomaly, these two organizations have developed joint guidelines

---

[6] Hospital Bldg. Co. v. Trustees of Rex Hosp., 425 U.S. 738 (1976).
[7] Hospital Bldg. Co. v. Trustees of Rex Hosp., No. 4048 (E.D. N.C. Dec. 5, 1984), *aff'd*, 791 F.2d 288 (4th Cir. 1986).
[8] Summit Health, Ltd. v. Pinhas, 500 U.S. 322 (1991).

and taken other steps to coordinate their activities,[9] but these competing agencies retain their independent authority.

Both of these agencies give binding advance rulings approving proposed actions.[10] However, a curious anomaly in the antitrust law and weakness of these agencies is that a ruling from them or a settlement with them does not bar a private action by anyone with standing who is dissatisfied with the ruling or settlement.[11]

This chapter discusses the Sherman Antitrust Act (13-1), the Clayton Act (13-2), the Federal Trade Commission Act (13-3), and some of the exemptions from antitrust laws (13-4).

13-1 Sherman Antitrust Act

The Sherman Antitrust Act is aimed at eliminating both restraints of trade and monopolies. Violations of the Act are federal crimes. The federal government and private parties can also obtain injunctive relief from violations. Any person who is injured in business or property by a violation can recover three times his or her actual damages, "treble damages," in a civil suit.[12] The effect of trebling damages is illustrated by an Ohio case in which 1,800 physicians brought a class action against a HMO. In 1988, a jury found the HMO had engaged in price fixing and other violations, causing over $34 million in damages. After trebling, the jury award was over $100

---

9   E.g., Department of Justice & FTC, Statements of antitrust enforcement policy in health care (Aug. 28, 1996), http://www.usdoj.gov/atr/public/guidelines/1791.htm (accessed Sept. 6, 2004) [hereinafter Statements will be cited "as 1996 DOJ/FTC Statements"]; Revised Justice/FTC Enforcement Guidelines for Health Care Industry (Sept. 27, 1994), *reprinted in* 3 HEALTH L. RPTR. [BNA] 1376 (1994) [hereinafter HEALTH L. RPTR will be cited as H.L.R] [hereinafter the Guidelines will be cited as "1994 DOJ/FTC Guidelines"]; *see also* Protocol for coordination in merger investigations between the federal enforcement agencies and state attorneys general (Mar. 11, 1998); *Federal, state antitrust authorities post joint merger investigation protocol*, 7 H.L.R. 445 (1998).

10   http://www.ftc.gov/bc/advisory.htm & http://www.usdoj.gov/atr/public/busreview/letters.htm (accessed Sept. 6, 2004).

11   *E.g., Physicians' group clashes with hospital over standing*, 3 H.L.R. 1646 (1994) [after hospital settled with federal government, physicians sued Santa Cruz, Calif. hospital that had acquired other hospital in town]; Santa Cruz Med. Clinic v. Dominican Santa Cruz Hosp., No. C93 20613 RMW (N.D. Cal. Mar. 28, 1995), *as discussed in* 23 HEALTH L. DIG. (May 1995), at 18 [physicians have antitrust standing to sue over hospital acquisition], 1995 U.S. Dist. LEXIS 21032 (N.D. Cal. Sept. 7, 1995) [partial summary judgment granted for defendants on tying, channeling claims, but denied on exclusive dealing claim].

12   15 U.S.C. §§ 1, 2, 4, 15.

million. The parties settled the suit, with the HMO paying \$37.5 million and agreeing not to appeal.[13]

This section discusses Section 1 (13-1.1) and Section 2 (13-1.2) of the Sherman Antitrust Act.

Physicians bring antitrust suits under Sections 1 and/or 2 of the Sherman Antitrust Act to challenge exclusive hospital contracts with other physicians and other adverse hospital actions concerning their membership on the medical staff or clinical privileges in the hospital. This is discussed in Sections 5-6 and 5-7 in Chapter 5.

13-1.1 Section 1

Section 1 of the Sherman Antitrust Act forbids "every contract, combination . . . or conspiracy, in restraint of trade" in interstate or foreign commerce.[14]

RULE OF REASON. The United States Supreme Court has recognized that a literal reading of this section would forbid virtually all commercial contracts, so the Court has interpreted this section to forbid only unreasonable restraints. This *rule of reason* standard looks at challenged agreements on a case-by-case basis to determine whether they promote or suppress competition.[15] Courts examine the structure of the industry, defendant's operation in that industry, history and duration of the restraint, and reasons for its adoption.

GEOGRAPHIC/PRODUCT MARKET. A plaintiff has the burden of proof to prove what the relevant geographic and product markets are.

The relevant geographic market in hospital cases generally includes the facilities that referring physicians and patients would perceive as attractive alternatives. For many health care services, this usually includes an area of several counties,[16] but can be a smaller or larger area and is generally determined on a case-by-case basis.

---

[13] Thompson v. Midwest Found. Indep. Physician Ass'n, No. C-1-86-744 (S.D. Ohio Mar. 14, 1988) [jury verdict]; 124 F.R.D. 154 (S.D. Ohio Dec. 4, 1988) [settlement approved]; Note that not all IPA HMO arrangements are antitrust violations, *e.g.,* Hassan v. Independent Practice Assocs., P.C., 698 F. Supp. 679 (E.D. Mich. 1988).

[14] 15 U.S.C. § 1.

[15] *E.g.*, Westchester Radiological Assocs., P.C. v. Empire Blue Cross & Blue Shield, 707 F. Supp. 708 (S.D. N.Y.), *aff'd*, 884 F.2d 707 (2d Cir. 1989), *cert. denied*, 493 U.S. 1095 (1990).

[16] *E.g.*, Cogan v. Harford Mem. Hosp., 843 F. Supp. 1013, 1019 (D. Md. 1994); Morgenstern v. Wilson, 29 F.3d 1291 (8th Cir. 1994), *cert. denied*, 513 U.S. 1150 (1995); N. Hershey, *Geographic market definition critical to monopolization claim*, 12 Hosp. L. Newsletter (July 1995), at 5 [discussing *Morgenstern*].

Where a company presently competes does not necessarily determine the relevant market for antitrust purposes.[17] The Department of Justice, Federal Trade Commission, and courts are cognizant that attempts by one company to attempt to engage in anticompetitive behavior, such as raising prices too high, will lead consumers to look more widely for alternatives.[18] Many antitrust cases are dismissed based on the failure to allege a relevant geographic market.[19]

The relevant product market varies depending on the action being challenged.[20] In many hospital merger cases, the relevant product market is acute care hospital services.[21] When individual professionals bring antitrust actions, the services they provide determine the product market. Thus, when an anesthetist challenged an exclusive agreement with an anesthesiology group, the patient market for individual anesthesia services constituted the relevant product market.[22] In some cases, a single brand of a product or service can constitute the relevant product market.[23]

MARKET POWER. In addition to proving the relevant market, a plaintiff must prove the defendant has significant market power, which means the ability to injure customers by curtailing output or raising prices. When this is not proven, Section 1 claims fail.[24]

---

[17] *E.g.*, Morgan, Strand, Wheeler & Biggs v. Radiology, Ltd., 924 F.2d 1484 (9th Cir. 1991).

[18] *E.g.*, DOJ & FTC 1992 Horizontal Merger Guidelines (Apr. 2, 1992), 57 FED. REG. 41,552 (Sept. 10, 1992), *reprinted in* 4 TRADE REG. REP. (CCH) ¶13,103 (1992) [hereinafter "1992 DOJ/FTC Guidelines"]; *In re* Adventist Health System/West, FTC Docket No. 9234 (Apr. 1, 1994) [FTC dismissal of complaint due to failure to address sufficiently where services would be sought in the event of anticompetitive behavior].

[19] *E.g.*, Arani v. TriHealth, Inc., 77 Fed. Appx. 823, 2003 U.S. App. LEXIS 20231 (6th Cir. 2003) [challenge to exclusion from physician panel who interpreted electrocardiograms and Holter Monitor results]; Surgical Ctr. of Hammond, L.C. v. Hospital Serv. Dist No. 1, 309 F.3d 836 (5th Cir. 2002) [exclusion of competing surgical center from managed care contracts].

[20] *E.g.*, Continental Orthopedic Appliances, Inc v. Health Ins. Plan of Greater N.Y., 994 F. Supp. 133 (E.D. N.Y. 1998) [proper product market in antitrust attack on HMO exclusive contract for orthotics not the provision of orthotic services to the HMO's enrollees, orthotics company given opportunity to replead], 40 F. Supp. 2d 109 (E.D. N.Y. 1999) [deny dismissal of claim based on product market of orthotics services to all HMO patients, although reservations about limiting to HMO patients, permitted to proceed with discovery].

[21] *E.g.*, FTC v. University Health, Inc., 938 F.2d 1206 (11th Cir. 1991); *see also* Forsyth v. Humana, Inc., 827 F. Supp. 1498 (D. Nev. 1993) [rejecting attempt to limit market to large for-profit hospitals].

[22] Oltz v. St. Peter's Commun. Hosp., 861 F.2d 1440 (9th Cir. 1988).

[23] E.g., Eastman Kodak Co. v. Image Technical Services, Inc., 504 U.S. 451 (1992).

[24] *E.g.*, Minnesota Association of Nurse Anesthetists v. Unity Hospital, 208 F.3d 655 (8th Cir. 2000) [affirming dismissal of CRNA challenge to exclusive anesthesia contracts with MDs; not boycotts & failure to demonstrate market power]; Ford v. Stroup, 113 F.3d 1234 (*without op.*), 1997 U.S. App. LEXIS 8692 (6th Cir. 1997) [summary judgment for defendants in challenge to exclusive contract for linear accelerator treatment for failure to show market power; market share of 50-55 percent alone not sufficient]; Flegel v. Christian Hosp., Northeast-Northwest, 4 F.3d 682 (8th Cir. 1993); Cogan v. Harford Mem. Hosp., 843 F. Supp. 1013 (D. Md. 1994).

ANTITRUST INJURY. In order to have standing to bring an antitrust suit, the plaintiff must also prove an *antitrust injury*. In 1990, the United States Supreme Court ruled that to be an "antitrust injury" the injury must be attributable to an anticompetitive aspect of the practice under scrutiny and cannot merely be a loss stemming from continued competition.[25] Another way of saying this is that the antitrust law is designed to protect competition in the relevant market, not to protect competitors. Some antitrust cases have been rejected based on the failure of the plaintiff to allege or show more than harm to plaintiff as an individual competitor.

For example, when a radiologist challenged exclusion from an IPA providing services to a HMO and from a hospital staff, the case was dismissed because there was no antitrust injury, since there was no harm to competition. The court found pro-competition reasons for the exclusion and that there was no duty to aid the plaintiff who was a competitor.[26]

In a challenge to the termination of a contract with nurse anesthetists, one federal appellate court ruled that the staffing decisions at a single hospital generally do not constitute an antitrust injury.[27] The court listed many of the cases dealing with staffing decisions at a single hospital. Although the courts used a variety of different reasons, with only a few exceptions the cases found no violation of Section 1. The court could find only one case in which the plaintiff actually prevailed in establishing antitrust liability for the staffing decision at a single hospital and that was due to the finding that the relevant market in a remote area of Montana has only two hospitals.[28]

Similarly, in 2002, a federal district court dismissed a lactation consultant's challenge to exclusion from a hospital; because she actually practiced in other area hospitals, she could not show antitrust injury.[29]

In 1998, a federal court dismissed an antitrust suit by nurse anesthetists claiming that outsourcing constituted monopolization

---

[25] Atlantic Richfield Co. v. USA Petroleum Co., 495 U.S. 328 (1990).

[26] Williamson v. Sacred Heart Hosp., 41 F.3d 667 (*without op.*), 1994 U.S. App. LEXIS 33199 (11th Cir. 1994); *see also* Cogan v. Harford Mem. Hosp., 843 F. Supp. 1013 (D. Md. 1994).

[27] BCB Anesthesia Care v. Passavant Mem. Area Hosp. Ass'n, 36 F.3d 664 (7th Cir. 1994).

[28] Oltz v. Saint Peter's Commun. Hosp., 861 F.2d 1440 (9th Cir. 1988).

[29] Volm v. Legacy Health Sys. Inc., 237 F. Supp. 2d 1166 (D. Or. 2002); Volm v. Legacy Health Sys. Inc., 91 Fed. Appx. 581 (9th Cir. 2004) [upholding jury verdict for Volm on remaining state law claims].

of the anesthesia services market. The court ruled that they had failed to show antitrust injury.[30]

In 2004, a federal district court in New York found sufficient antitrust injury to permit an ambulatory surgery center to pursue a challenge to the exclusive contract of a hospital with a managed care organization.[31]

Challenges to exclusive physician contracts are often barred on the basis of lack of antitrust injury.[32]

EFFICIENT ENFORCER. Courts also ask whether the particular plaintiff is an *efficient enforcer*,[33] which means that the plaintiff has a strong interest in the antitrust goals of promoting competition. Persons who are not efficient enforcers also lack standing to sue.[34]

PER SE VIOLATIONS. When the relevant market, significant market power, and antitrust injury are shown by an efficient enforcer, then the rule of reason is applied, except for the business agreements, which courts have identified as *per se* unreasonable because they are not viewed as having potential redeeming competitive benefits. Courts presume that these agreements are unreasonable, and the plaintiff does not have to prove unreasonableness, which shortens and simplifies some trials. *Per se* violations include price fixing, market division, tie-ins, and boycotts. Losses flowing from *per se* violations are not automatically "antitrust injuries."[35]

Price-fixing. Price-fixing agreements among competitors for the purpose of raising, lowering, or stabilizing prices are *per se* violations. No defense or justification is recognized except for a governmental mandate. The United States Supreme Court ruled that a maximum fee schedule for physicians set by physicians was price-fixing and,

---

[30] Minnesota Ass'n of Nurse Anesthetists v. Unity Hosp., 5 F. Supp. 2d 694 (D. Minn. 1998), *aff'd*, 208 F.3d 655 (8th Cir. 2000).

[31] Rome Ambulatory Surgery Ctr. LLC v. Rome Mem. Hosp., 349 F.2d 389 (N.D. N.Y. 2004).

[32] *E.g.*, Imaging Ctr. v. Western Md. Health Syss., 2004 U.S. Dist. LEXIS 16138 (D. Md.); Kochert v. Greater Lafayette Health Srvs., 2004 U.S. Dist. LEXIS 28059 (N.D. Ind.) [dismissal of antitrust challenge to loss of subcontract to perform anesthesia service in hospital that had exclusive contract with group; no antitrust injury]; Bobcobo v. Radiology Consultants, 305 F. Supp. 2d 422 (D. N.J. 2004) [radiologist failed to show antitrust injury when excluded from exclusive contract].

[33] *E.g.*, Todorov v. DCH Healthcare Auth., 921 F.2d 1438 (11th Cir. 1991); *but see* Ertag v. Naples Commun. Hosp. Inc., 121 F.3d 721 (11th Cir. 1997) [neurology group had standing to challenge hospital decision to permit only radiologists to provide official MRI interpretations].

[34] *E.g.*, Korshin v. Benedictine Hosp., 34 F. Supp. 2d 133 (N.D. N.Y. 1999) [anesthesiologist not efficient enforcer in challenge to exclusive anesthesia contract]; Feldman v. Palmetto Gen. Hosp., Inc., 980 F. Supp. 467 (S.D. Fla. 1997).

[35] Atlantic Richfield Co. v. USA Petroleum Co., 495 U.S. 328 (1990).

thus, a *per se* violation.[36] Most requirements of sellers concerning the price at which their products may be resold are *per se* violations. A seller's nonprice restrictions on resale, such as territorial limits, are generally examined under the rule of reason.[37] One federal court ruled that a discharged anesthesiologist lacked standing to claim that a hospital and an anesthesiology department were engaged in price-fixing because the only injury claimed from the alleged price-fixing was the inability to participate in the scheme.[38] In 1994, the American Medical Association requested approval from the FTC for a proposed program of advisory peer review of physicians' fees. The FTC did not object to some aspects of the proposed program but rejected some aspects as price-fixing.[39]

In 2003, a federal appellate court ruled that in the circumstances of the particular case joint efforts by a consortium of physician and consumer groups to negotiate non-price terms with a health plan did not constitute a conspiracy to fix prices or to boycott.[40]

Attempts by physicians to jointly establish fees to be paid by third-party payers can be price-fixing,[41] unless the group is sufficiently integrated. There has been aggressive enforcement against physician groups that seek to collectively bargain without sufficient integration. This has resulted in numerous consent decrees.[42]

Market Division. Any agreement among competitors to divide up the market is a *per se* violation.[43] For example, if two competing hospitals agree that one will provide obstetrical services, while the other will provide open heart surgery services, this would be a *per se* violation. In 2003, the state of Florida entered a consent judg-

---

[36] Arizona v. Maricopa County Med. Soc'y, 457 U.S. 332 (1982).

[37] Continental T.V. v. GTE Sylvania, Inc., 433 U.S. 36 (1977).

[38] Purgess v. Sharrock, 806 F. Supp. 1102 (S.D. N.Y. 1992).

[39] FTC Advisory Opinion Letter to General Counsel of AMA and the Chicago Medical Society, No. P923506 (Feb. 14, 1994), *as discussed in* 22 HEALTH L. DIG. (Mar. 1994), at 6; B. McCormick, *FTC gives qualified OK to medicine's fee-review plan*, AM. MED. NEWS, Mar. 7, 1994, at 3.

[40] International Healthcare Management v. Hawaii Coalition for Health, 332 F.3d 6000 (9th Cir. 2003).

[41] *See* D. Marx, *Messenger models: what can the agencies do to prevent provider networks from violating the antitrust laws?* HEALTH LAWYERS NEWS, Apr. 2004.

[42] *E.g., In re* SPA Health Org. (FTC consent order June 9, 2003) [network of Texas physicians agreed not to negotiate with payers unless certain qualified arrangements were in place], http://www.ftc.gov/opa/2003/06/southwestphys.htm (accessed Sept. 6, 2004); *In re* Carlsbad Physicians Ass'n, Inc. (FTC consent order May 2, 2003) [agreement to dissolve organization that had been bargaining with health plans on behalf of physicians], http://www.ftc.gov/opa/2003/05/carlsbad.htm (accessed Sept. 6, 2004).

[43] *E.g.*, Palmer v. BRG of Georgia, Inc., 498 U.S. 46 (1990).

ment with two hospitals that had agreed to allocate markets as part of settlement of certificate of need litigation.[44] The judgment barred the hospitals from honoring or entering any allocation agreements.

Tying Arrangements. Under a "tying" arrangement, the seller refuses to sell product A to a customer unless that customer agrees to buy product B from the seller. If three conditions are present, a tying arrangement is generally a *per se* violation: (1) products A and B must be separate, (2) the seller must have sufficient market power to restrain competition in product B, and (3) the arrangement must sufficiently affect commerce.[45] In 1984, the United States Supreme Court found an exclusive hospital contract with an anesthesia group not to be a *per se* violation.[46] Similarly, in 1988, a federal appellate court ruled that an exclusive pathology contract was not an unlawful arrangement because pathology services are not a separate product, but part of hospital services.[47] However, another federal appellate court in the same year found there was a separate demand for anesthesia services, making them a separate product, so that a nurse anesthetist could successfully challenge an exclusive hospital contract with a group of anesthesiologists.[48] The case was viewed as different from the 1984 United States Supreme Court anesthesia case because it involved an alleged conspiracy to eliminate the availability of nurse anesthetist services in the hospital.

Market power in the tying product must be shown to make a claim. In 1998, a federal appellate court ruled that it was not illegal tying for a HMO to require that a pharmacy company use the HMO's subsidiary as third-party administrator in order to obtain approval of more of its pharmacies as providers for the HMO.[49] The court found that the HMO did not exercise sufficient market power in the tying market and that there was no demonstrated harm to competition in the tied market.

There is no illegal tying as long as the buyer is free to choose to buy the two products separately. Discount packages are permitted as long as the products are offered separately.[50] This is especially

---

[44] State v. Hospital Corp. of Am., 2003 Trade Cas. (CCH) ¶ 74,027 (M.D. Fla. Apr. 18, 2003).

[45] *See* Eastman Kodak Co. v. Image Technical Services, Inc., 504 U.S. 451 (1992).

[46] Jefferson Parish Hosp. Dist. v. Hyde, 466 U.S. 2 (1984).

[47] Collins v. Associated Pathologists, Ltd., 844 F.2d 473 (7th Cir.), *cert. denied*, 488 U.S. 852 (1988).

[48] Oltz v. St. Peter's Commun. Hosp., 861 F.2d 1440 (9th Cir. 1988).

[49] Brokerage Concepts, Inc. v. U.S. Healthcare, Inc., 140 F.3d 494 (3d Cir. 1998).

[50] *E.g.*, Northern Pacific Ry. Co. v. United States, 356 U.S. 1 (1958).

true when there is also a market for discount packages in which there is also competition.[51] When dealers of sound systems for cars challenged the inclusion of the sound systems in the price of vehicles, a federal court ruled that there was insufficient market power to trigger the *per se* rule and that the seller could take advantage of market failure due to inadequate consumer information. As long as the seller does nothing to stop comparison shopping, the seller has no duty to promote comparison shopping.[52]

Boycotts. Any agreement among competitors not to deal with anyone outside the group or to deal with them only on certain terms is considered a boycott and a *per se* violation. For example, in a 1942 decision, a federal appellate court found the American Medical Association ethics rules against salaried practice to be a *per se* violation.[53]

Hospitals have been on both sides of boycott claims. Hospitals and others have accused physicians of boycotts of hospitals. An Arizona medical staff settled a claimed boycott of a hospital in 1994 by agreeing not to combine to restrict services to the hospital.[54] In 1994, a federal court ruled that a hospital was not engaged in an illegal boycott by having a policy of sending its patients for radiology services only to another Joint Commission accredited facility, where the former chief of radiology who operated a freestanding radiology clinic failed to show any anticompetitive effects in a relevant market.[55] The chief's contract with the hospital had been terminated when he refused to enter a new agreement limiting his right to compete. In 1993, a federal court ruled that it was not an illegal boycott for a HMO to pay a contracting physician more if he did not do work for competing HMOs, where the exclusivity was not mandatory and could be ended with thirty days notice.[56]

In 1997, a federal appellate court refused to apply the *per se* doctrine in a suit in which a retina specialist claimed a referral agreement between a competitor and an ophthalmologic group was

---

[51] *E.g.*, Nobel Scientific Indust., Inc. v. Beckman Instruments, Inc., 670 F. Supp. 1313 (D. Md. 1986), *aff'd*, 831 F.2d 537 (4th Cir. 1987), *cert. denied*, 487 U.S. 1226 (1988).

[52] Town Sound & Custom Tops, Inc. v. Chrysler Motors Corp., 959 F.2d 468 (3d Cir.), *cert. denied*, 506 U.S. 868 (1992).

[53] American Med. Ass'n v. United States, 76 U.S. App. D.C. 70, 130 F.2d 233 (1942), *aff'd*, 317 U.S. 519 (1943).

[54] *In re* Med. Staff of Good Samaritan Med. Ctr., FTC File No. 901 0032 (settlement Sept. 7, 1994), *as discussed in* 3 H.L.R. 1257 (1994); B. McCormick, *Doctors settle FTC boycott case*, AM. MED. NEWS, Oct. 3, 1994, 10.

[55] Cogan v. Harford Mem. Hosp., 843 F. Supp. 1013 (D. Md. 1994).

[56] U.S. Healthcare, Inc. v. Healthsource, Inc., 986 F.2d 589 (1st Cir. 1993).

a boycott. The court based this on finding that there was historical acceptance of eye care networks that affiliated with only one retina group and the network controlled only fifteen percent of retina referrals, lacking market power to restrain trade. The court then applied a rule of reason analysis to affirm rejection of the claim.[57]

JOINT VENTURES. Usually when two competitors enter a joint venture, the courts will apply a rule of reason analysis because the integration of resources in a joint venture can produce efficiencies and new products. Courts determine whether the restraints on competition resulting from the joint venture are necessary to achieve the permitted purpose. For example, in 1988, a federal district court dismissed a physician's price-fixing antitrust suit against a HMO because (1) the HMO was a legitimate joint venture with a shared risk of loss and a new product and (2) the price agreement was necessary to distribute the revenues and control costs to remain competitive.[58] Attention has been focused on the minimum characteristics necessary to demonstrate sufficient integration.[59] The 1996 joint statements of the DOJ and FTC on antitrust enforcement discuss hospital joint ventures and physician network joint ventures.

INFORMATION EXCHANGE. Exchange of information, especially price information, among competitors can be a violation. Exchange of past price information is less likely to be a violation. In 1993, the DOJ approved a salary survey by an independent contractor that was voluntary and only reported aggregated data at least three months old.[60] Current and prospective salary information generally cannot be directly exchanged. The DOJ successfully challenged exchange of current and prospective nursing salary information among Utah hospitals, resulting in a consent decree in 1994 specifying what conduct would be permitted.[61] Nonprice information has been viewed more leniently except where it appears to be aimed at suppressing competition. The 1996 joint statements of

---

[57] Retina Associates, P.A. v. Southern Baptist Hosp. of Fla., Inc., 105 F.3d 1376 (11th Cir. 1997).

[58] Hassan v. Independent Practice Assocs., P.C., 698 F. Supp. 679 (E.D. Mich. 1988).

[59] *See* 1994 DOJ/FTC Guidelines; *Capitation seen as brightest line in quest for sufficient integration*, 4 H.L.R. 269 (1995).

[60] Business Review Letter from Assistant Attorney General Anne K. Bingaman to Counsel for the New Jersey Hospital Ass'n, DOJ, Antitrust Div. (Feb. 18, 1994), *as discussed in* 22 HEALTH L. DIG. (Mar. 1994), at 9; *New Jersey hospital salary survey satisfies antitrust enforcement guidelines*, 3 H.L.R. 237 (1994).

[61] United States v. Utah Soc'y for Healthcare Human Resources Admin., 1994 U.S. Dist. LEXIS 17531 (D. Utah consent decree Mar. 14, 1994).

the DOJ and FTC on antitrust enforcement discuss exchange of information. FTC and DOJ have issued letters approving additional exchanges of information.[62]

TRADE ASSOCIATIONS. "Self-regulation" by trade associations must be carefully structured. Any suppression or destruction of competition can be a violation. In 1994, an association of Iowa hospitals agreed to a consent decree with the DOJ ending an agreement which limited competitive advertising by the hospital members.[63]

In 1999, the United States Supreme Court vacated and remanded a federal appellate court ruling that a trade association's advertising policy was an unreasonable restraint of trade to the extent that it restricted truthful nondeceptive advertising.[64] The Court ordered the lower court to apply a more extensive examination that gave more consideration to the professional context. On remand, the federal appellate court found the restrictions to be procompetitive and ordered the FTC to dismiss the case.[65]

AGREEMENT. Many violations require the showing of an "agreement" among competitors. An actual agreement need not always be shown. Courts have stated that "interdependent conscious parallelism" among competitors can provide the basis for inferring an agreement.[66] For example, if the dominant health insurer in the area announced that it would not send patients to any hospital unless the hospital stopped accepting patients covered by a competing health insurer and if all the hospitals in the area stopped accepting the competing insurer's patients, an agreement could be inferred from this parallel behavior which cannot be justified by independent business judgment. It would not be necessary to prove any actual communications among the hospitals. However, parallel business behavior is not sufficient when independent business judgment can justify the decisions. For example, if all the hospitals in an area decide independently to stop dealing with a nursing agency that charges more than any other agency or provides unresponsive

---

[62] *E.g.,* Washington State Med. Ass'n. (DOJ letter Sept. 23, 2003), http://www.usdoj.gov/atr/public/busreview/200260.htm (accessed Sept. 6, 2004); PriMed Physicians (FTC letter Feb. 6, 2003), http://www.ftc.gov/bc/adops/030206dayton.htm (accessed Sept. 6, 2004).

[63] United States v. Hospital Ass'n of Greater Des Moines, No. 4-92-70648 (S.D. Iowa settlement Sept. 22, 1992); *Hospitals settle suit alleging anticompetitive ad rules,* AM. MED. NEWS, Oct. 12, 1992, 12.

[64] California Dental Ass'n v. FTC, 526 U.S. 756 (1999), *rev'g,* 128 F.3d 720 (9th Cir. 1997).

[65] California Dental Ass'n v. FTC, 224 F.3d 942 (9th Cir. 2000).

[66] Interstate Circuit, Inc. v. United States, 306 U.S. 208 (1939).

service, the parallel business behavior could be justified by independent business judgment.

CONSPIRACY/ INTRACORPORATE IMMUNITY. Section 1 of the Sherman Antitrust Act requires a conspiracy between separate economic entities. An unincorporated association of otherwise competing physicians can constitute a conspiracy.[67] However, a single integrated entity cannot conspire among itself.[68] Usually a corporation cannot conspire with itself or its employees.[69]

There is disagreement among the federal circuit courts whether the hospital and medical staff are a single entity for antitrust conspiracy purposes or multiple entities that can conspire. At least four circuits have ruled that, when engaged in peer review, the hospital and medical staff are a single entity protected by the intracorporate conspiracy doctrine.[70] One of these circuits has recognized an exception to intracorporate immunity when a physician is acting pursuant to an independent personal stake,[71] while one of the circuits has rejected any such exception.[72] One court indicated that while the hospital could not conspire with its medical staff, the members could conspire among themselves, but since the ultimate decision was by the board of directors, any conspiracy among the

---

[67] Anesthesia Advantage, Inc. v. Metz Group, 708 F. Supp. 1180 (D. Colo. 1989), *rev'd on other grounds*, 912 F.2d 397 (10th Cir. 1990).

[68] Copperweld Corp. v. Independence Tube Corp., 467 U.S. 752 (1984); *e.g.,* HealthAmerica Pa., Inc. v. Sequehanna Health Sys., 278 F. Supp. 2d 423 (M.D. Tenn. 2003) [summary judgment for defendants functioning as a single entity; defendant's alliance had been formed pursuant to a consent decree with the state attorney general in 1994]; *but see* New York *ex rel.* Sptizer v. Saint Francis Hosp., 94 F. Supp. 2d 399 (S.D. N.Y. 2000) [hospitals not sufficiently integrated to be single entity].

[69] *E.g.*, Podiatrist Ass'n, Inc. v. La Cruz Azul De Puerto Rico, Inc., 332 F.3d 6 (1st Cir. 2003) [dismiss challenge to exclusion of podiatrists from standard benefit packages; intracorporate immunity; input by physicians does not show control]; Viazis v. American Ass'n of Orthodontists, 314 F.3d 758 (5th Cir. 2002) [orthodontist suspended from association membership for claims in flyers sent to public promoting his patented orthodontic bracket; dismiss claim of conspiracy to exclude brackets from market; no showing of concerted action].

[70] Oksanen v. Page Mem. Hosp., 945 F.2d 696 (4th Cir. 1991) (en banc), *cert. denied,* 502 U.S. 1074 (1992); Weiss v. York Hosp., 745 F.2d 786 (3d Cir. 1984), *cert. denied,* 470 U.S. 1060 (1985); Nanavati v. Burdette Tomlin Mem. Hosp., 857 F.2d 96 (3d Cir. 1988), *cert. denied,* 489 U.S. 1078 (1989); Potters Med. Ctr. v. City Hosp. Ass'n, 800 F.2d 568 (6th Cir. 1986); Nurse Midwifery Assocs. v. Nibbett, 918 F.2d 605 (6th Cir. 1990), *modified on reh'g,* 927 F.2d 904 (6th Cir.), *cert. denied,* 502 U.S. 952 (1991); Pudlo v. Adamski, 789 F. Supp. 247 (N.D. Ill. 1992), *aff'd without op.*, 2 F.3d 1153, 1993 U.S. App. LEXIS 20,442 (7th Cir. 1993), *cert. denied,* 510 U.S. 1072 (1994).

[71] Oksanen v. Page Mem. Hosp., *supra*, note 70.

[72] Nurse Midwifery Assocs. v. Nibbett, *supra*, note 70; *see also* Chiropractic Ass'n v. Trigon Healthcare, Inc., 367 F.3d 212 (4th Cir. 2004) [in challenge to health plan policies on coverage of chiropractic services, managed care advisory panel and health plan part of single entity, so could not conspire; independent personal stake exception does not apply where no power to bind corporation].

medical staff could not cause antitrust injury.[73] At least two other circuits have ruled that hospitals and their medical staffs are separate entities capable of conspiracy.[74] Other circuits have declined to rule on the issue.[75] To avoid the personal stake exception and to avoid the appearance of a conspiracy, hospitals should limit the involvement of physicians in decisions and recommendations concerning those involved in the same or competing specialties. For example, when a medical staff committee is hearing or considering charges against a cardiac surgeon, other competing cardiac surgeons should not serve on the committee.

13-1.2 Section 2

Section 2 of the Sherman Antitrust Act prohibits monopolizing, attempts to monopolize, and combinations or conspiracies to monopolize any part of interstate or foreign commerce.[76]

Like Section 1, it is necessary to prove a relevant geographic and product market.

MONOPOLY POWER. In addition, to establish a monopolization claim under Section 2, it must be shown that defendants possess monopoly power in the relevant market.[77] However, mere possession of monopoly power is not a violation if it resulted from a superior product, business acumen, or a historical accident. For example, it is not an illegal monopoly to be the sole community hospital when by historical accident only one hospital has been founded or the only competitors have experienced business failure without illegal help from the survivor. Monopoly power is the power to control prices or exclude competition. Courts usually look to market share as a sign of monopoly power.

---

[73] Pudlo v. Adamski, *supra*, note 70.

[74] Bolt v. Halifax Hosp. Med. Ctr., 851 F.2d 1273 (11th Cir.), *vacated*, 861 F.2d 1233 (11th Cir. 1989), *reinstated in part*, 874 F.2d 755 (11th Cir. 1989) (en banc), *after remand*, 891 F.2d 810 (11th Cir.), *cert. denied*, 495 U.S. 924 (1990); Oltz v. St. Peter's Commun. Hosp., 861 F.2d 1440 (9th Cir. 1988).

[75] *E.g.,* Willman v. Heartland Hosp., 34 F.3d 605 (8th Cir. 1994), *cert. denied*, 514 U.S. 1018 (1995); Okusami v. Psychiatric Inst. of Wash., Inc., 959 F.2d 1062 (D.C. Cir. 1992).

[76] 15 U.S.C. § 2.

[77] *E.g.,* United States v. Grinnell Corp., 384 U.S. 563 (1966); *but see* United States v. Dentsply International, Inc., 277 F. Supp. 2d 387 (D. Del. 2003), *appeal docketed*, No. 03-4097 (3d Cir. 2004) [exclusive distributor contracts by manufacturer of over 75 percent of fabricated teeth not a violation because competitors could sell directly to labs, so contracts did not exclude rivals from market].

In 2004, a federal court in Ohio found that an anesthesia group did indeed have monopoly power in the relevant market for anesthesia services. When a hospital declined to enter an exclusive anesthesia agreement with the group, the group entered into agreements with independent physicians in the area that provided for those physicians to use the group's certified registered nurse anesthetists (CRNAs) as their primary source of anesthesia services. The group then refused to provide anesthesia services at the hospital to any physician who had not signed an agreement with the group. The hospital challenged the arrangements.[78]

PURPOSEFUL ACT. Monopolizing requires possession of monopoly power in a relevant market, plus a "purposeful act." A purposeful act is the willful acquisition or maintenance of monopoly power.

ELEMENTS OF A CLAIM. In 1993, the United States Supreme Court ruled that to demonstrate attempted monopolization a plaintiff must prove (1) use of unfair or predatory means, such as boycotts or discriminatory pricing, with (2) specific intent to monopolize, and (3) a dangerous probability of achieving monopoly power. In determining the third element, courts consider (1) the relevant market, both the product and the geographic markets, and (2) market power, that is, the defendant's ability to lessen or destroy competition in that market.[79]

In 2002, a federal appellate court addressed a case in which an ambulatory surgery center challenged several steps that a hospital had taken, including entering an exclusive contract with a managed care organization that precluded use of the surgery center and refusing to enter a transfer agreement. After a trial without a jury, the federal district court had ruled in favor of the hospital. The district court had concluded that attempted monopolization had not been demonstrated because the surgery center had shown neither predatory conduct by the hospital nor a dangerous probability that the hospital would achieve monopoly power in the outpatient surgery market. The district court rejected the conspiracy claim. The parties involved were principal and agent and, thus, were incapable of conspiring with one another. The appellate court affirmed the district court.[80]

---

[78] Defiance Hosp. v. Fauster-Cameron, Inc., 344 F. Supp. 2d 1097 (N.D. Ohio 2004).

[79] Spectrum Sports, Inc. v. McQuillan, 506 U.S. 447 (1993); Copperweld Corp. v. Independence Tube Corp., 467 U.S. 752 (1984).

[80] Surgical Care Ctr. v. Hospital Service Dist. No. 1, 309 F.3d 836 (5th Cir. 2002).

13-2 Clayton Act

Four sections of the Clayton Act are discussed — Section 2 (13-2.1); Section 3 (13-2.2); Section 7 (13-2.3); and Section 4 (13-2.4).

13-2.1 Section 2

Section 2 of the Clayton Act, as amended by the Robinson-Patman Act, forbids certain price discrimination.[81] It is unlawful to discriminate in price between different purchasers when selling commodities of like grade or quality where the effect may be substantially to lessen competition or to injure, destroy, or prevent competition. At least one of the two comparative transactions must cross state lines. The section applies only to commodities, so sales of services and intangibles are not affected, and the section applies only to sales, so leases and consignments are not affected.

Section 2 also prohibits indirect price discrimination through seller-supplied facilities, services, or payments. For example, if the seller provides special promotional advertising for one buyer, this service is indirect price discrimination in favor of that buyer.

The seller is not the only possible violator. A buyer who knowingly induces or receives discriminatory prices also violates Section 2.

EXEMPTIONS. Nonprofit institutions have an exemption for purchases "for their own use."[82] As a result, hospital pharmacies in nonprofit hospitals usually buy drugs from manufacturers at a discount not available to commercial pharmacies. These drugs can be used only "for their own use." In 1976, the United States Supreme Court defined "for their own use" to be limited to the following:

(1)   Treatment of inpatients at the hospital;
(2)   Treatment of admitted emergency patients in the hospital;
(3)   Personal use by outpatients on the hospital premises;
(4)   Personal use away from the premises by inpatients or emergency patients upon their discharge;
(5)   Personal use away from the premises by outpatients;

---

[81] 15 U.S.C. § 13.
[82] 15 U.S.C. § 13c.

(6)   Personal use by hospital employees, students, and their immediate dependents; and

(7)   Personal use by medical staff members and their immediate dependents.[83]

Thus, hospitals must confine their sales of drugs purchased at a discount to these groups to avoid possible civil liability, including treble damages and loss of the valuable discount.

Purchasers who do not qualify include (1) former patients who wish to renew prescriptions given when they were inpatients, emergency facility patients, or outpatients; (2) physicians who are medical staff members and who intend to dispense the drugs in the course of their private practices away from the hospital; and (3) walk-in customers who are not hospital patients. Hospitals should refuse to sell to these groups or set up a separate purchase order system to fill their requests.

FTC staff members have further interpreted the scope of "own use" in staff advisory letters. For example, one letter concluded that contracted workers who were not technically employees could still receive the discounted drugs because they were assigned exclusively to the hospital as their regular place of work.[84]

In 1987, a federal court ruled that drug companies and a hospital could be sued for the hospital's alleged transfer of drugs between its in-house pharmacy and its retail pharmacy.[85]

Governmental entities are also generally exempt from the price discrimination prohibition. However, in 1983, the United States Supreme Court ruled that governmental hospitals must observe the same restrictions on resale of discount drugs that nonprofit hospitals do.[86] In 1984, a federal appellate court ruled that resale of drugs by health maintenance organizations to their own members is "for their own use."[87]

There is no exemption for for-profit hospitals; their purchases must be on the same volume discount basis as generally available to other consumers.

---

[83] Abbott Labs. v. Portland Retail Druggists Ass'n, Inc., 425 U.S. 1 (1976).

[84] Valley Baptist Medical Ctr., http://www.ftc.gov/os/2003/03/030313vbmc.htm (accessed Sept. 6, 2004).

[85] Rudner v. Abbott Labs., 664 F. Supp. 1100 (N.D. Ohio 1987).

[86] Jefferson County Pharmaceutical Ass'n, Inc. v. Abbott Labs., 460 U.S. 150 (1983).

[87] DeModena v. Kaiser Found. Health Plan, Inc., 743 F.2d 1388 (9th Cir. 1984), *cert. denied*, 469 U.S. 1229 (1985).

In 1989, a federal appellate court upheld the fraud conviction of an operator of a shared services organization for obtaining pharmaceuticals at lower prices in excess of the amount needed by qualified member hospitals and selling the surplus to wholesale drug companies.[88]

13-2.2 Section 3

Section 3 of the Clayton Act[89] prohibits sales of commodities that are conditioned on the buyer not dealing with competitors of the seller. Examples include tie-in sales and exclusive dealing arrangements where the effect "may be substantially to lessen competition or tend to create a monopoly" in any line of commerce. Section 1 of the Sherman Antitrust Act prohibits the same conduct not only for commodities, but also for services, intangibles, and real property. Examples of the prohibited conduct are included in the discussion of that section earlier in this chapter.

13-2.3 Section 7

Section 7 of the Clayton Act[90] prohibits acquisitions or mergers where the effect "may be substantially to lessen competition or tend to create a monopoly in any line of commerce in any section of the country." With the rapid growth in some national hospital companies and the consolidation of providers, this section has increasingly been applied to hospitals.

Relevant product and geographic markets must be identified in a manner similar to the analysis under Section 2 of the Sherman Antitrust Act.

Section 7 is preventive, not merely corrective. A reasonable likelihood of substantially lessening competition is sufficient to establish a violation.

MERGER GUIDELINES. The DOJ and FTC issued merger guidelines in 1992 that are not binding on courts but give some direction.[91] In 1994, the DOJ and the FTC issued further guidelines that created a "safety zone" for mergers with older hospitals with fewer than 100

---

[88] United States v. Stewart, 872 F.2d 957 (10th Cir. 1989).
[89] 15 U.S.C. § 14.
[90] 15 U.S.C. § 18.
[91] 1992 DOJ & FTC Guidelines, *supra*, note 18.

beds and an average census of fewer than forty patients.[92] One of the 1996 joint statements of DOJ and FTC addressed hospital mergers.

HERFINDAHL-HIRSCHMAN INDEX. One of the tools that is used is a formula, the Herfindahl-Hirschman Index (HHI), which is a measure of market concentration. The HHI is calculated by adding the squares of the percentage market shares of the entities in the market. For example, if there were twenty competing hospitals and each had 5 percent of the market, the HHI would be 500 [Each of the twenty hospitals contribute 25 (5×5)]. If a merger results in a HHI less than 1,000, the government generally will not challenge the merger, so four of the twenty hospitals in the example could merge into one hospital (HHI = 800) [The merged hospital would have a 20 percent share, contributing 400 (20×20) while the remaining 16 hospitals would each contribute 25 (5×5)]. There are potential significant federal competitive concerns depending on other factors stated in the 1992 guidelines, but there is no presumption of violation if (a) the resulting HHI is from 1,000 to 1,800 and is more than 100 points above the premerger HHI or (b) the resulting HHI is over 1,800 and is 50 to 100 points above the premerger HHI. If the resulting HHI is over 1,800 and is more than 100 points above the premerger HHI, there is a presumption the merger will create or enhance market power.[93] This would occur if the twenty hospitals in the example merged into four hospitals with equal market shares of 25 percent (HHI = 2,500) [Each of the four new hospitals would contribute 625 (25×25)]. This presumption can be overcome by showing efficiencies and other factors.

HOSPITAL MERGERS. Section 7 has been used by both the FTC and the DOJ to attack mergers of hospitals. Section 7 clearly applies to for-profit hospital mergers. For example, in 1986, a federal appellate court upheld a FTC order that a for-profit hospital chain divest itself of two of three hospitals that it owned in the Chattanooga, Tennessee area and notify the FTC in advance of any plan to make a similar acquisition.[94] Generally, when large chains combine, the resulting entity finds itself with too many hospitals in one or more local markets, and the entity has to divest itself of one or more hospitals in those areas.[95] Failure to comply with divestiture orders can

---

[92] 1994 DOJ/FTC Guidelines, Statement 1.

[93] *E.g.,* FTC v. University Health, Inc., 938 F.2d 1206 (11th Cir. 1991) [HHI would increase by over 630 to 3,200].

[94] Hospital Corp. of Am. v. FTC, 807 F.2d 1381 (7th Cir. 1986), *cert. denied*, 481 U.S. 1038 (1987).

[95] *E.g.*, *Columbia, Health Trust will sell 3 Utah sites amid FTC discussions*, WALL ST. J., Feb.17, 1995, B6.

result in substantial civil money penalties.[96] Challenges to mergers can sometimes result in consent decrees that put conditions on the behavior of the resulting organization. For example, in 2000, a court order was obtained to enforce a 1994 Florida consent decree.[97]

There is still a question whether Section 7 applies to nonprofit hospitals. Section 7 applies to (1) persons who acquire shares of stock or capital and (2) persons subject to the jurisdiction of the FTC. Nonprofit companies do not have shares of stock or capital, and Section 7 applies to nonprofit hospitals only if they are subject to the jurisdiction of the FTC. There is a question whether nonprofit hospitals are subject to the jurisdiction of the FTC within the meaning of Section 7; the FTC takes the position that they are. In 1988, the FTC ordered two nonprofit hospitals in Reading, Pennsylvania, to separate.[98] Some courts have agreed. One federal appellate court ruled in 1991 that Section 7 does apply to asset acquisitions by nonprofit hospitals.[99]

The DOJ challenged the proposed merger of two nonprofit hospitals in Rockford, Illinois. In 1989, a federal district court in Illinois enjoined the proposed merger. It found that the merger violated Section 7.[100] The appellate court found Section 7 not applicable to the merger of two nonstock, nonprofit hospitals but upheld barring the merger because it violated Section 1 of the Sherman Antitrust Act.[101] The appellate court indicated that its decision on Section 7 was limited by the way the parties framed the issues. The court indicated its belief that Section 7 would be applicable if the government presented its case correctly.

One other court has found that Section 7 does not apply. The DOJ challenged the proposed merger of two hospitals in Roanoke, Virginia. A federal district court in Virginia ruled in 1988 that Section 7 did not apply to affiliations of nonprofit entities where there

---

[96] *E.g.*, F.T.C. v. Columbia/HCA Healthcare Corp., No. 98 CV 1889 (D. D.C. July 30, 1998), *as discussed in* 7 H.L.R. 1239 (1998) [$2.5 million civil penalty for late divestiture of hospitals]; L. Legnado, *Columbia agrees to pay $2.5 million FTC fine*, WALL ST. J., July 31, 1998, A3.

[97] *Florida, U.S. Department of Justice require hospitals to enter into enforcement order in consent decree case*, NATIONAL ASS'N OF ATTORNEYS GENERAL ANTITRUST REPT., July/Aug. 2000, 5.

[98] McGinn, *A first: FTC tells two nonprofit hospitals to separate*, AM. MED. NEWS, Oct. 7, 1989, 3.

[99] FTC v. University Health, Inc., 938 F.2d 1206 (11th Cir. 1991); *see also* California Dental Ass'n v. FTC, 526 U.S. 756 (1999) [under § 5, FTC has jurisdiction over nonprofit association providing economic benefit to for-profit members].

[100] United States v. Rockford Mem. Corp., 717 F. Supp. 1251 (N.D. Ill. 1989).

[101] United States v. Rockford Mem. Corp., 898 F.2d 1278 (7th Cir. 1990), *cert. denied*, 498 U.S. 920 (1990).

was no exchange of stock or share capital and then in 1989 ruled that the merger did not violate Section 1 of the Sherman Antitrust Act under the rule of reason.[102] In 1989, a federal appellate court affirmed the decision but did not issue an opinion.[103]

In 1989, the FTC began challenging the acquisition of a small hospital in Ukiah, California, by a large hospital chain that owned the other small hospital in the town.[104] The hospitals tried to stop the FTC from proceeding with its complaint on the grounds that the FTC lacked jurisdiction under Section 7, but the federal court refused to rule until after the FTC had made a final ruling on jurisdiction.[105] In 1990, an Administrative Law Judge (ALJ) dismissed the complaint on the grounds of lack of jurisdiction, but the FTC reversed. In 1992, the ALJ again dismissed, but on the basis that the acquisition was not likely to substantially lessen competition when the proper geographic market was considered.[106] In 1994, the FTC affirmed, dismissing the complaint on the basis that there was insufficient evidence to establish the relevant geographic market.[107] Thus, it is unlikely that the jurisdictional issue will protect hospitals from the expense of responding to the FTC.

The FTC continues to challenge acquisitions of nonprofit hospitals.[108] However, it has generally been unsuccessful.[109] In 2002, the FTC Bureau of Competition created a Merger Litigation Task Force to focus on whether consummated mergers had resulted in anti-competitive price increases.[110] In 2004, the FTC launched a challenge to the merger of hospitals in Evanston, Illinois.[111]

---

[102] United States v. Carilion Health Sys., 707 F. Supp. 840 (W.D. Va. 1989).

[103] United States v. Carilion Health Sys., 892 F.2d 1042 (*without op.*), 1989 U.S. App. LEXIS 17,911 (4th Cir.).

[104] Burda, *FTC files complaint against hospital merger*, MOD. HEALTHCARE, Nov. 17, 1989, 4 [challenge to merger in Ukiah, California].

[105] Ukiah Valley Med. Ctr. v. F.T.C., 911 F.2d 261 (9th Cir. 1990).

[106] *In re* Adventist Health Sys./West, FTC Docket No. 9234 (A.L.J. Dec. 9, 1992).

[107] *In re* Adventist Health System/West, FTC Docket No. 9234 (Apr. 1, 1994).

[108] *E.g.*, FTC v. Freeman Hosp., 911 F. Supp. 1213 (W.D. Mo. 1995) [injunction of hospital merger denied].

[109] *See* D. Ho, *Government looks for ways to break losing streak in challenging hospital mergers*, AP, Mar. 28, 2003.

[110] http://www.ftc.gov/opa/2002/08/mergerlitigation.htm (accessed Sept. 6, 2004); R. Abelson, *Merged hospitals gain both power and critics*, N.Y. TIMES, Sept. 26, 2002, C1; R. Abelson, *F.T.C. opens inquiry into hospital merger*, N.Y. TIMES, Nov. 6, 2002, C4 [Poplar Bluff, Mo.].

[111] Evanston Northwest Healthcare Corp, FTC Docket No. 9315 (2004); B. Japsen, *FTC says merger of Chicago hospital operators violated antitrust laws*, CHICAGO TRIB., Feb. 11, 2004; B. Wysocki, *FTC targets hospital merger in antitrust case*, WALL ST. J, Jan. 17, 2005, A1 [seeking to undo acquisition of Highland Park Hospital by Evanston Northwestern Healthcare Corp.].

In April 2005, the hospitals settled a portion of the case dealing with negotiating fees, but the challenge to the merger continued. In October 2005, a FTC administrative law judge ruled that the hospital merger in Evanston violated Section 7 of the Clayton Act and ordered Evanston Northwestern Healthcare Corporation (ENHC) to sell Highland Park Hospital. ENHC appealed, seeking review by the FTC.[112]

13-2.4 Section 4

Section 4 of the Clayton Act[113] gives any person the right to sue for treble damages when injured by violations of the Sherman Antitrust Act or the Clayton Act. There are no criminal sanctions for violations of the Clayton Act, but violations can be enjoined.

13-3 Federal Trade Commission Act

Section 5(a) of the Federal Trade Commission Act[114] prohibits "unfair methods or competition in or affecting commerce and unfair or deceptive acts or practices in or affecting commerce." The FTC has exclusive authority to enforce this section; private individuals cannot use it as a basis for suits. The FTC can also take action to enforce the Sherman Antitrust Act or the Clayton Act, but its authority is not exclusive. Examples of FTC action are included in the discussion of Section 7 of Clayton Act (13-2.3).

The FTC can (1) issue an order to cease and desist from violating antitrust laws, (2) seek a court-imposed fine for a violation of a cease and desist order, (3) seek injunctions of prohibited conduct, and (4) seek court-ordered restitution to consumers and others from violations.

---

[112] *Hospital group settles part of FTC complaint*, AP, Jan. 19, 2005; *Chicago-area doctors settle charges involving collective bargaining of fees*, H.L.R., Apr. 7, 2005, 449 [*In re* Evanston Northwestern Healthcare Corp., FTC Dkt. No. 9315 (Apr. 5, 2005)]; *Judge voids suburban hospital merger*, AP, Oct. 22, 2005) [*In re* Evanston Northwestern Healthcare Corp., FTC Dkt. No. 9315 (Oct. 20, 2005)]; for documents in the Evanston case, *see* http://www.ftc.gov/os/adjpro/d9315/index.htm [accessed Nov. 1, 2005].
[113] 15 U.S.C. § 15.
[114] 15 U.S.C. § 45.

13-4 Exemptions

The United States Supreme Court has made it clear that health care providers are treated in the same way as other industries for antitrust purposes. For example, in 1975, the Court ruled that the learned professions, such as law and medicine, were not exempt from the antitrust laws.[115]

There are several laws and legal principles that do exempt some activities or some actors from antitrust liability. This section discusses six sources of exemptions — the Health Care Quality Improvement Act of 1986 (13-4.1); state action (13-4.2); petitioning government (13-4.3); the business of insurance (13-4.4); the match (13-4.5); and implied exemptions (13-4.6). This section concludes with a warning that exemption from one law may not be exemption from another (13-4.7).

13-4.1 Health Care Quality Improvement Act of 1986

The Health Care Quality Improvement Act of 1986 (HCQIA) extends protection from monetary liability in private suits under the antitrust laws for professional review activities that meet its procedural standards.[116] HCQIA does not protect from suit, governmental actions, or injunctions.[117] HCQIA is discussed in Chapter 5.

13-4.2 State Action

The law has recognized an exemption from antitrust liability for state action. In 1943, the United States Supreme Court ruled that state-compelled activities were immune from antitrust liability to preserve the state's authority to supervise economic activity within the state.[118] The state action doctrine was clarified in 1980 when the Court ruled that state authorization is not enough. The actions must be pursuant to a clearly articulated and affirmatively expressed state policy actively supervised by the state.[119] The doctrine was further

---

[115] Goldfarb v. Virginia State Bar Ass'n, 421 U.S. 773 (1975).
[116] 42 U.S.C. § 11111(a)(1); Annotation, *Construction and application of Health Care Quality Improvement Act of 1986*, 121 A.L.R. FED. 255.
[117] *Id.*
[118] Parker v. Brown, 317 U.S. 341 (1943).
[119] California Retail Liquor Dealers Ass'n v. Midcal Aluminum, Inc., 445 U.S. 97 (1980).

defined in 1985 when the Court ruled that the clearly defined state policy did not have to compel the actions to bring them within the state action immunity.[120] Collective rate-making by motor carriers was found to be protected as state action because the states expressly permitted the rate-making and actively supervised it. On the same day, the Court ruled that active state supervision is not a requirement for exemption when the actor is a municipality, rather than a private individual.[121]

One area of dispute has been whether state medical peer review laws provide the requisite state action to protect hospitals from antitrust liability for their peer review activities. Prior to 1988, several courts found various such laws did provide the requisite state action.[122] In 1988, in a medical peer review case, the United States Supreme Court tightened the active supervision requirement to require that "state officials have and exercise power to review particular anticompetitive acts of private parties and disapprove those that fail to accord with state policy."[123] The case dealt with an Oregon law that did not include any state administrative review of hospital peer review decisions. The defendants argued that the availability of state judicial review was sufficient active supervision. Applying the new standard, the Court decided that the judicial review available in Oregon was not sufficient without ruling that state judicial review could never provide sufficient state supervision. The efforts to obtain state action immunity for these activities have been reduced since it has become clearer that the HCQIA provides significant protection from antitrust liability for medical peer review actions.[124]

Numerous actions by governmental hospitals have been found to be immune under this standard. Statutory authority to acquire other hospitals is sufficient to immunize acquisitions.[125] Statutory authority to own and operate hospitals immunizes acquisitions of other hospi-

---

[120] Southern Motor Carriers Rate Conference, Inc. v. United States, 471 U.S. 48 (1985).
[121] Town of Hallie v. City of Eau Claire, 471 U.S. 34 (1985).
[122] *E.g.*, Marrese v. Interqual, Inc., 748 F.2d 373 (7th Cir. 1984), *cert. denied*, 472 U.S. 1027 (1985).
[123] Patrick v. Burget, 486 U.S. 94 (1988); *see also* Shahawy v. Harrison, 875 F.2d 1529 (11th Cir. 1989) [judicial supervision in Florida insufficient to provide state action immunity for medical staff actions]; FTC v. Ticor Title Ins. Co., 504 U.S. 621 (1992) [state regulatory scheme insufficient to provide immunity for setting prices for title insurance].
[124] *E.g.*, Bryan v. James E. Holmes Reg. Med. Ctr., 33 F.3d 1318 (11th Cir. 1994), *cert. denied*, 514 U.S. 1019 (1995).
[125] FTC v. University Health, Inc., 938 F.2d 1206 (11th Cir. 1991).

tals.[126] In 1994, a federal appellate court found that state action immunity protected the proposed purchase of Cape Coral Hospital by a health care authority created by Florida as a special purpose unit of local government that already owned another hospital in the county and that had authority to acquire other hospitals.[127] However, authority to do business is not sufficient alone to demonstrate a state intent to displace competition.[128] In 1999, a federal appellate court ruled that authority to contract for health services alone was not sufficient to grant a hospital service district immunity when it allegedly entered exclusive contracts with managed care plans that excluded a competing outpatient surgical center.[129]

Governmental hospitals can also have state action immunity from physician challenges to peer review and staffing decisions.[130]

In 1991, the United States Supreme Court ruled that there was no conspiracy exception to the state action immunity.[131]

The Local Government Antitrust Act of 1984[132] extends statutory immunity from antitrust damage claims to local governmental agencies and their employees and agents. This applies to local government hospitals.[133] The law does not provide protection from antitrust suits seeking injunctions, but many of those will be precluded by the state action doctrine.[134]

Several states have passed laws providing a mechanism by which health care providers can apply to obtain state approval and, thus,

---

[126] Askew v. DCH Reg. Health Care Auth., 995 F.2d 1033 (11th Cir. 1993), *cert. denied*, 510 U.S. 1012 (1993).

[127] F.T.C. v. Hospital Bd. of Directors, 38 F.3d 1184 (11th Cir. 1994).

[128] *E.g.*, Lancaster Commun. Hosp. v. Antelope Valley Hosp. Dist., 940 F.2d 397 (9th Cir. 1991), *cert. denied*, 502 U.S. 1094 (1992).

[129] Surgical Care Ctr. of Hammond v. Hospital Serv. Dist No. 1, 171 F.3d 231 (5th Cir. 1999) (en banc); *but see* Jackson v. West Tennessee Healthcare, Inc., 2004 U.S. Dist. LEXIS 4571 (W.D. Tenn.) [state action immunity protected exclusive contract that kept competing hospital out of managed care arrangements].

[130] *E.g.*, Cohn v. Bond, 953 F.2d 154 (4th Cir. 1991), *cert. denied*, 505 U.S. 1230 (1992); Todorov v. DCH Healthcare Auth., 921 F.2d 1438 (11th Cir. 1991); Shaw v. Phelps County Reg. Med. Ctr., 858 F. Supp. 954 (E.D. Mo. 1994); Crosby v. Hospital Auth. of Valdosta, 873 F. Supp. 1568 (M.D. Ga. 1995) [government hospital, its officials protected in medical staff privilege case by state action immunity, Local Government Antitrust Act, and HCQIA].

[131] City of Columbia v. Omni Outdoor Advertising, Inc., 499 U.S. 365 (1991); Bolt v. Halifax Hosp. Med. Ctr., 980 F.2d 1381 (11th Cir. 1993).

[132] 15 U.S.C. §§ 34-36.

[133] *E.g.*, Sandcrest Outpatient Servs., P.A. v. Cumberland County Hosp. Sys., Inc., 853 F.2d 1139 (4th Cir. 1988).

[134] Bloom v. Hennepin County, 783 F. Supp. 418 (D. Minn. 1992) [challenge by physician whose privileges were terminated when he ceased to be employed by group with exclusive contract; Act protected hospital from liability, state action doctrine protected from injunction].

antitrust immunity.[135] Some state approvals have been given under these laws.[136]

13-4.3 Petitioning Government

In two cases, the United States Supreme Court ruled that the antitrust laws do not apply to most activities intended to induce governmental action, such as lobbying.[137] This concept is called the *Noerr-Pennington doctrine* and is based on the right under the First Amendment to petition the government and on a judicial interpretation that lobbying activities are not a restraint of trade. The petitioning must be conducted honestly and for the legitimate purpose of influencing governmental policy. For example, a federal appellate court ruled in 1986 that the Noerr-Pennington doctrine protected a hospital's full use of the administrative process (including delaying tactics and appeals) to challenge a competing hospital's application for a certificate of need for a cardiac surgery program, but the doctrine did not protect misrepresentations to the governmental agency.[138] Efforts that are considered a "mere sham" to suppress competition are not protected. For example, repetitive insubstantial lawsuits might be a mere sham to tie up the competitor so that it cannot make financing or other business arrangements.[139] However, an objectively reasonable effort to litigate is not a sham, regardless of the plaintiff's subjective intent.[140]

---

135 *E.g.*, Antitrust Immunity and Competitive Oversight, Substantive Rules and Procedural Rules (Washington Health Services Comm'n Jan. 26, 1995), *as discussed in* 23 HEALTH L. DIG. (May 1995), at 19; *Little activity seen under state laws granting antitrust immunity*, 4 H.L.R. 303 (1995) [20 states have such laws, but only Minnesota, Maine had approved applications by Dec. 1994; table of laws at 333]; *Health department drafts rules to implement new antitrust immunity*, 4 H.L.R. 434 (1995) [Wyo.]; D. Burda, *Mont. hospitals asking state for immunity*, MOD. HEALTHCARE, Mar. 6, 1995, 36.

136 *E.g., AG approves joint venture between benefits, rival surgical center in Great Falls, Mont.*, 7 H.L.R. 91 (1998); *In re* Inland Northwest Health Servs. (Washington Health Servs. Comm'n Mar. 1995), *In re* Inland Northwest Health Servs. (Wash. Att'y Gen.) (informal op.), *as discussed in* 23 HEALTH L. DIG. (May 1995), at 20.

137 Eastern R.R. President's Conference v. Noerr Motor Freight, Inc., 365 U.S. 127 (1961); United Mine Workers v. Pennington, 381 U.S. 657 (1965); Boulware v. State, 960 F.2d 793 (9th Cir. 1992) [opposition to physician construction of MRI facility].

138 St. Joseph's Hosp. v. Hospital Corp. of Am., 795 F.2d 948 (11th Cir. 1986), *reh'g denied* (en banc), 801 F.2d 404 (11th Cir. 1986); *see also* Kottle v. Northwest Kidney Ctrs., 146 F.2d 1056 (9th Cir. 1998), *cert. denied*, 525 U.S. 1140 (1999) [Noerr-Pennington doctrine protects competitor opposition to issuance of CON].

139 Otter Tail Power Co. v. United States, 410 U.S. 366 (1973).

140 Professional Real Estate Inv., Inc. v. Columbia Pictures Indus., Inc., 508 U.S. 49 (1993).

13-4.4 Business of Insurance

The McCarran-Ferguson Act created a statutory exemption for the "business of insurance" when it is regulated by state law and does not constitute coercion, boycott, or intimidation.[141] The United States Supreme Court has taken a restrictive view of what constitutes the business of insurance entitled to this exemption. For example, in 1979, the Court limited the exemption to the business of insurance, not the business of insurers.[142] It defined the business of insurance as limited to the procedures and activities related to the spreading of risk among policyholders. It held that special reimbursement arrangements between Blue Shield and participating pharmacies were not within the business of insurance, but instead were merely the business of insurers.

13-4.5 The Match

In 2003, some students filed an antitrust challenge to the process by which medical students are matched to first-year residency programs. In early 2004, the federal court dismissed the case as to some defendants but permitted the case to proceed against the remaining defendants. In 2004, Congress passed a law prohibiting antitrust attacks against the graduate medical education matching program through which students completing medical school are matched with first-year house staff positions. After the protective law was passed, the federal court dismissed the suit.[143]

13-4.6 Implied Exemptions

In 1981, the United States Supreme Court ruled that implied exemptions to antitrust laws are not favored and will be applied only to the limited extent necessary to fulfill the purposes of other laws.[144] The Court ruled that the national health planning law which was then in effect did not provide implied protection for an insurer

---

[141] 15 U.S.C. § 1012(b).

[142] Group Life & Health Ins. Co. v. Royal Drug, 440 U.S. 205 (1979).

[143] Jung v. Association of Am. Med. Colleges, 300 F. Supp. 2d 119 (D. D.C. 2004), 339 F. Supp. 2d 26 (D. D.C. 2004) [barred by new law], 226 F.R.D. 7 (D. D.C. 2005) [not permitted to amend complaint]; 15 U.S.C. § 37b.

[144] National Gerimedical Hosp. v. Blue Cross, 452 U.S. 378 (1981).

from antitrust law liability for refusing to deal with a hospital that did not obtain approval from a planning agency for its new building. State law did not require approval. This principle was applied by a federal appellate court in 1984 when it ruled that a certificate of need does not protect a provider from being charged with monopolization.[145] The provider must still comply with all other laws, including antitrust laws.

13-4.7 Scope of Exemptions

When an exemption is found from one antitrust law, other antitrust laws still must be complied with. In 1988, a federal district court ruled that "conduct that is specifically exempted from a particular antitrust law may nonetheless be prohibited by another statute. If that same conduct violates another law, the exemption does not follow."[146]

Discussion Points

1. Discuss liability under the Sherman Antitrust Act.
2. Discuss the rule of reason.
3. Discuss antitrust injury.
4. Discuss per se violations of the Sherman Antitrust Act.
5. Discuss intracorporate immunity.
6. Discuss monopoly power.
7. Discuss liability under the Clayton Act.
8. Discuss the scope of the "own use" exemption from price fixing restrictions for drug purchases by nonprofit institutions.
9. Discuss the federal efforts to challenge hospital mergers.
10. Discuss the Federal Trade Commission Act.
11. Discuss the scope of health care exemptions from antitrust laws.

---

[145] North Carolina *ex rel.* Edmisten v. P.I.A. Asheville, Inc., 740 F.2d 274 (4th Cir. 1984), *cert. denied*, 471 U.S. 1003 (1985).
[146] American Academic Suppliers, Inc. v. Beckley-Cardy, Inc., 699 F. Supp. 152 (N.D. Ill. 1988).

CHAPTER FOURTEEN

Reproductive Issues

Objectives

The objective of this chapter is to provide an overview of some of the legal issues related to reproduction. The reader will learn about contraceptive devices and drugs, sterilization, assisted conception, abortion, and liability for birth of children after negligent sterilizations or failure to inform of genetic risks.

This chapter discusses the reproductive issues of contraception (14-1); sterilization (14-2); assisted conception (14-3); abortion (14-4); and wrongful conception, wrongful birth, and wrongful life suits (14-5).

14-1 Contraception

Numerous contraceptive drugs and devices are available to reduce the probability of pregnancy. The National Center for Health Statistics reported in 2004 that more than 98 percent of women ages fifteen to forty-four who had ever had sex with a male had used at least one contraceptive method. In 2002, 11.6 million women were using an oral contraceptive pill, 10.3 million had been sterilized, and 9 million women and their partners used the condom.[1]

ADULTS. Today few barriers confront an adult who seeks to obtain contraceptives. There are limits on the scope of state regulation of the sale or use of contraceptive drugs and devices.

---

[1] W.D. Moser et al, *Use of contraception and use of family planning services in the United States — 1982–2002*, ADVANCE DATA FROM VITAL AND HEALTH STATISTICS, Dec. 10, 2004, www.cdc.gov/nchs/data/ad/ad350.pdf [accessed June 11, 2005].

States cannot prohibit the use of contraceptives by adults. In 1965, the United States Supreme Court declared a Connecticut law forbidding the use of contraceptives by married persons to be an unconstitutional violation of the right of privacy.[2] In 1972, the Court declared a Massachusetts law forbidding unmarried persons to buy or use contraceptives to be unconstitutional.[3] The Court ruled that married and unmarried adults have the same right to access to contraceptives.

States may regulate sales of contraceptives, but in 1977, the Supreme Court limited the permissible scope of such regulation. The Court invalidated a New York statute prohibiting the distribution of nonprescription contraceptives to persons over the age of sixteen by anyone other than licensed pharmacists, finding it an undue burden on an individual's right to decide whether to bear a child.[4] The Court also invalidated a prohibition on advertising and display of both prescription and nonprescription contraceptives by persons licensed to sell such products.

Prescription contraceptives or those requiring fitted insertion often must be obtained through an authorized individual. Other contraceptives may be purchased without medical involvement. There has been dispute over whether the morning-after pill should be available without physician involvement. In 2003, a FDA expert advisory panel recommended over-the-counter (OTC) status so that a prescription would not be required. In 2004, the FDA rejected the recommendation and continued to require a prescription. In August 2005, in response to a renewed application for OTC status, the FDA again delayed action.[5] An FDA official resigned in protest. In November 2005, the United States Government Accountability Office published a report criticizing the decision making process. In December 2005, Wisconsin announced that it was suing the FDA challenging the approval delay.[6] At least seven states permit pharmacists to dispense the morning-after pill without a physician prescription.[7]

---

[2] Griswold v. Connecticut, 381 U.S. 479 (1965).

[3] Eisenstadt v. Baird, 405 U.S. 438 (1972).

[4] Carey v. Population Servs. Int'l, 431 U.S. 678 (1977).

[5] G. Kolata, *A contraceptive clears a hurdle to wider access,* N.Y. Times, Dec. 17, 2003, A1.

[6] G. Harris, *U.S. rules morning-after pill can't be sold over-the-counter,* N.Y. Times, May 7, 2004, A1.

[7] *New law lets pharmacists dispense morning-after pill without prescription,* Health L. Rptr. [BNA], Mar. 11, 2004, 347 [Maine Ch. 524 signed; five other states have such laws – Alaska, Calif. Hawaii, N.M., Wash.].

Some states mandate that health care providers offer emergency contraception to rape victims.[8] This may be the standard of care in some jurisdictions, even where there is no legislative mandate. In 1989, a California appellate court ruled that a Catholic hospital could be sued for failing to provide a rape victim with access to a "morning after" pill.[9] The hospital took the position that the pill was an abortion so it could refuse to participate. The court ruled that it was birth control, not abortion, so the hospital could be liable if the standard of care in other hospitals was to offer the pill.

MINORS. In some states, minors still face obstacles to obtaining contraceptives. The United States Supreme Court's first comment on a minor's right of access to birth control came in the 1977 case discussed previously.[10] The Court struck down a portion of a New York law that prohibited the sale or distribution of nonprescription contraceptives to minors under sixteen. In 1980, a federal appellate court ruled that minors have a right to obtain contraceptive devices from a county-run family planning center without parental notification or consent.[11] In 1988, a federal district court ruled that a Roman Catholic foster child care agency engaged in unconstitutional state action when it confiscated contraceptive devices and prescriptions of minors placed by the state in its care.[12]

A 1981 federal law required that federally funded family planning projects "encourage family participation" in counseling and decisions about services.[13] The Department of Health and Human Services proposed rules interpreting this to require parental notification after services were initially provided to any minor under age eighteen unless (1) the minor was emancipated under state law or (2) the project director determined that notification would result in physical harm to the minor by a parent or guardian. The proposed rules also required compliance with all state laws concerning notification or consent.[14]

---

[8] D. Crary, *Contraception for rape victims face opposition,* Wis. St. J., Sept. 27, 2003, A3 [three states require hospitals to offer emergency contraception to rape victims (Calif., Wash., and N.M.); New York governor about to sign fourth law].

[9] Brownfield v. Daniel Freeman Marina Hosp., 208 Cal. App. 3d 405, 256 Cal. Rptr. 240 (2d Dist. 1989); *see also* Ark. Att'y Gen. Op. No. 88-380 (Dec. 22, 1988) ["morning-after" pill not an abortion]; *Scant use of morning-after pill is analyzed,* N.Y. TIMES, Mar. 29, 1995, A13.

[10] *Id.*

[11] Doe v. Irving, 615 F.2d 1162 (6th Cir. 1980); *see also* Jane Does v. Utah Dep't of Health, 776 F.2d 253 (10th Cir. 1985).

[12] Arneth v. Gross, 699 F. Supp. 450 (S.D. N.Y. 1988).

[13] 42 U.S.C. § 300(a).

[14] 48 FED. REG. 3,600-36,14 (Jan. 26, 1983).

The rules never took effect because they were blocked by a federal court order.[15] The court ruled that Congress intended to encourage, not require, parental involvement, so the rules exceeded statutory authority. In 1983, a federal district court declared unconstitutional a Utah law requiring parental notification before furnishing contraceptives to minors.[16] However, states may still be able to regulate a minor's access to contraceptives more strictly than would be allowed for adult access to the same materials.

While it is prudent to encourage minors to involve their parents, many minors cannot or will not accept parental involvement. Physicians must then decide whether to prescribe contraceptives in the absence of parental involvement. Physicians who choose to prescribe contraceptives to unemancipated minors face a theoretical possibility of civil liability for battery or malpractice in some states. Several states explicitly authorize minors to consent to these services.[17] Even in states without a minor consent statute, the legal risk is small, especially when the minor is mature.

CONSCIENCE CLAUSES. Some pharmacists have sought to establish the right to refuse to provide prescription contraceptives when they have personal moral objections. In cases of emergency contraception where there is a short time period in which it must be taken, the opportunity to obtain the service can be effectively foreclosed by such refusals. Some states have disciplined pharmacists and pharmacies that have refused to provide such services. A few states have passed legislation permitting pharmacists to refuse this service. Legislation has been proposed in other states to either permit or ban such refusals. The conflict may be eliminated if emergency contraceptives are granted a status that does not require dispensing by a pharmacist.[18]

---

15 Planned Parenthood Fed'n v. Schweiker, 559 F. Supp. 658 (D. D.C. 1983), aff'd, 229 U.S. App. D.C. 336, 712 F.2d 650 (1983); New York v. Heckler, 719 F.2d 1191 (2d Cir. 1983).

16 Planned Parenthood Ass'n v. Matheson, 582 F. Supp. 1001 (D. Utah 1983).

17 E.g., CAL. FAM. CODE § 6925.

18 M. Davey, Illinois pharmacies ordered to provide birth control, N.Y. TIMES, Apr. 2, 2005, A10; G. Ruethling, Illinois pharmacist sues over contraceptive rule, N.Y. TIMES, June 10, 2005, A1; P. Simms, Board: patient need ignored by pharmacist, WIS. ST. J., Apr. 14, 2005, B1 [Wis. pharmacist reprimanded, fined $20,000 costs, ordered to attend classes]; D. Crary, Antiabortion activists broaden efforts, AP, Sept. 15, 2004 [Miss., S.D., Ark. laws]; M. Davey & P. Belluck, Pharmacies balk on after-sex pill and widen fight, N.Y. TIMES, Apr. 19, 2005, A1.

14-2 Sterilization

Sterilization involves the termination of the ability to produce children. Sterilization may be the desired result of a surgical operation or the incidental consequence of an operation to remove a diseased reproductive organ or to cure a malfunction of such an organ. When the reproductive organs are not diseased, most sterilizations are effected by vasectomy for males and tubal ligation for females.

Sterilization can be voluntary (14-2.1) or in some circumstances involuntary (14-2.2).

14-2.1 Voluntary Sterilization

ADULTS. All states permit voluntary consensual sterilization for competent adults regardless of the purpose.[19] Federal regulations require the signing of a special consent form at least thirty days prior to sterilizations funded by Medicaid with exceptions for some therapeutic cases.[20] Some states impose special requirements on all sterilizations performed in the state.[21]

The federal requirements do not apply to other patients unless required by state law. However, before an operation that may result in sterilization is performed, consent should be obtained. Absent consent, sterilization almost always constitutes a battery even if the operation is medically necessary. Courts are much less likely to find implied consent to sterilization than to other extensions of surgical procedures. When it can be predicted that an operation poses the risk of sterilization, this consequence should be clearly brought to the patient's attention. In the case of operations intended to sterilize, a consent form that discusses the risk the sterilization will not

---

[19] *E.g., In re* Guardianship of B, 190 Misc. 2d 581, 738 N.Y.S.2d 528 (County Ct. 2002) [moderately retarded woman could consent]; *accord,* Avila v. New York City Health & Hosps. Corp., 136 Misc. 2d 76, 518 N.Y.S.2d 574 (Sup. Ct. 1987); *but see* Vaughn v. Ruoff, 253 F.3d 1124 (8th Cir. 2001) [social worker who coerced mildly retarded woman into sterilization not entitled to qualified immunity in suit for violating her due process rights].

[20] 42 C.F.R. §§ 441.250–441.259.

[21] CAL. ADMIN. CODE title 22, §§ 70707.1–70707.8; California Med. Ass'n v. Lachner, 124 Cal. App. 3d 28, 177 Cal. Rptr. 188 (3d Dist. 1981) [requirement of written consent constitutional]; Kaplan v. Blank, 204 Ga. App. 378, 419 S.E.2d 127 (1992) [oral consent was no consent to tubal ligation under Voluntary Sterilization Act, so battery]; Chasse v. Mazerolle, 622 A.2d 1180 (Me. 1993) [ninteen-year-old sterilized in 1973, claimed she was not competent to consent; failure to follow statutory consultation process can be basis for liability].

be successful should be used. Failure to inform of the risk of future reproductive ability can expose providers to liability for wrongful conception or wrongful birth as discussed later in this chapter.

SPOUSAL CONSENT. The patient's consent alone is sufficient authorization for any legal operation. Some hospitals and physicians have a policy of also requiring spousal consent for sterilization of married patients. Public hospitals may not be permitted to enforce such policies. At least one court has found such public hospital policies to be an unconstitutional violation of the right of privacy.[22] One federal appellate court ruled that a governmental hospital could not impose greater restrictions on sterilization procedures than on other procedures that are medically indistinguishable in the risk to the patient or the demand on staff or facilities.[23] A federal court declared state laws requiring spousal consent to sterilizations to be unconstitutional.[24] Federally assisted family planning projects must follow all state requirements for consent to sterilization, except spousal consent requirements.[25] However, private hospitals may forbid contraceptive sterilizations or require spousal consent.[26]

It is advisable to encourage spousal involvement in the sterilization decision if the spouses are not estranged. However, performing a sterilization procedure without spousal consent presents little legal risk. For example, when a husband sued an Oklahoma physician for sterilizing his spouse without his consent, the court dismissed the suit because his marital rights did not include a childbearing wife, so he had not been legally harmed.[27]

MINORS. Voluntary contraceptive sterilization of unmarried minor patients presents special problems; local laws concerning minor consent should be carefully reviewed. In some circumstances, minors may be permitted to consent in some jurisdictions.[28] Some state statutes authorize such sterilizations if the parent or guardian also consents.[29] Other state statutes forbid ster-

---

[22] *E.g.*, Sims v. University of Ark. Med. Ctr., No. 1R76-C67 (E.D. Ark. Mar. 4, 1977).

[23] Hathaway v. Worcester City Hosp., 475 F.2d 701 (1st Cir. 1973).

[24] *E.g.*, Coe v. Bolton, No. C-87-785A (N.D. Ga. Sept. 30, 1976).

[25] 42 C.F.R. § 50.204(f).

[26] *E.g.*, Taylor v. St. Vincent Hosp., 523 F.2d 75 (9th Cir. 1975), *cert. denied*, 424 U.S. 948 (1976).

[27] Murray v. Vandevander, 522 P.2d 302 (Okla. Ct. App. 1974).

[28] *E.g.*, Smith v. Seibly, 72 Wash. 2d 16, 431 P.2d 719 (1967) (eighteen-year-old male permitted to consent when twenty-one was age of majority].

[29] *E.g.*, COLO. REV. STAT. ANN. § 25-6-102.

ilization of an unmarried minor.[30] As discussed in the following section of this chapter, parents or guardians alone cannot authorize sterilizations. Patient consent is essential unless court authorization is obtained. Unless there is a medical reason for sterilization and the consents of the minor and the parent are clearly voluntary, informed, and unequivocal, prudent providers should be reluctant to sterilize a minor without a court order. Federal funds can be used to pay for sterilizations only if the person is competent and at least twenty-one years old.[31]

CONSCIENCE LAWS. Some states have enacted legislation stating that hospitals are not required to permit sterilization procedures and physicians and hospital personnel can not be required to participate in such procedures or be discriminated against for refusal to participate.[32] In 1979, a nurse-anesthetist was awarded payment from a hospital that violated the Montana conscience law by dismissing her for refusing to participate in a tubal ligation.[33]

14-2.2 Involuntary Sterilization

Statutes and courts in some states have authorized involuntary sterilization of two groups of people.

The first group to be addressed included those believed to transmit hereditary defects. Before 1950, many states enacted eugenic sterilization laws, authorizing involuntary sterilization of these people. The United States Supreme Court upheld such laws in 1927.[34] However, this practice is no longer accepted, and these laws have been repealed. Some states have apologized or granted payments for sterilizations performed under these laws.[35]

The second group consists of the severely retarded who are sexually active, unable to use other forms of contraception, and unable

---

[30] *E.g.*, GA. CODE ANN. §31-20-2.
[31] 42 C.F.R. §§ 50.203, 441.253.
[32] *E.g.*, KAN. STAT. ANN. §§ 65-446, 65-447.
[33] Swanson v. St. John's Lutheran Hosp., 182 Mont. 414, 597 P.2d 702 (1979), *judgment after remand aff'd*, 189 Mont. 259, 615 P.2d 883 (1980).
[34] Buck v. Bell, 275 U.S. 200 (1927); *see also* Poe v. Lynchburg Training School, 518 F. Supp. 789 (W.D. Va. 1981) [involuntary sterilizations did not violate civil rights when under statute held constitutional].
[35] *E.g.*, S. McGinnis & D. Okarski, *Oregon's governor apologizes for 60-year-old eugenics policy which was enforced in that state*, CBS NEWS TRANSCRIPTS, Dec. 3, 2002; *Panel agrees N.C. sterilization victims should be compensated*, AP, Apr. 25, 2003.

to care properly for their offspring. Several state laws authorize sterilization of individuals a court determines to meet all of these criteria. The primary focus of these laws is the best interests of the individual and potential future offspring, rather than genetics.

These modern laws have been upheld by courts. For example, North Carolina's statute[36] was upheld by the North Carolina Supreme Court and by a federal district court.[37] The key elements of a constitutional statute appear to be (1) identification of an appropriate class of persons subject to the statute without discrimination or arbitrary bias and (2) guarantees of procedural due process, including notice, hearing, right to appeal, and assurance that decisions will be supported by qualified medical opinion.

Parents or guardians do not have the authority to consent to sterilization of retarded children or wards without a valid court authorization.[38]

Several courts have considered applications for orders authorizing involuntary sterilizations in states that do not have statutes specifically giving the court authority to issue such orders. Prior to 1978, most courts ruled that they did not have the authority and refused to issue orders authorizing sterilization. This position was largely due to two federal court decisions that judicial immunity did not protect judges who issued sterilization orders without specific statutory authority because they were not acting within their jurisdiction.[39] These decisions permitted civil rights suits against the judge and the involved health care providers. However, the United States Supreme Court reversed the decision in the second case in 1978, ruling that a court of broad general jurisdiction has the jurisdiction to consider a petition for sterilization of a minor unless statutes or case law in the state circumscribe the jurisdiction to foreclose consideration of such petitions.[40] Thus, the judge was protected by judicial immunity. The Court directed a lower federal court to decide the liability of the private individuals who had

---

36 N.C. GEN. STAT. §§ 35-36 – 35-50.

37 *In re* Sterilization of Moore, 289 N.C. 95, 221 S.E.2d 307 (1976); North Carolina Ass'n of Retarded Children v. North Carolina, 420 F. Supp. 451 (M.D. N.C. 1976).

38 *E.g.*, *In re* Grady, 85 N.J. 235, 426 A.2d 467 (1981); *In re* Mary Moe, 385 Mass. 555, 432 N.E.2d 712 (1982); Annotation, *Power of parent to have mentally defective child sterilized*, 74 A.L.R. 3D 1224.

39 Wade v. Bethesda Hosp., 337 F. Supp. 671 (S.D. Ohio 1971); Wade v. Bethesda Hosp., 356 F. Supp. 380 (S.D. Ohio 1973); Sparkman v. McFarlin, 552 F.2d 172 (7th Cir. 1977).

40 Stump v. Sparkman, 435 U.S. 349 (1978).

sought the petition and carried out the order. The lower court ruled these individuals could not be sued for federal civil rights violations because there was no showing of a conspiracy between the private individuals and the state officials.[41]

Since 1978, several state courts have ruled that they have authority to authorize involuntary sterilization of incompetents.[42] The decisions have set forth procedures and criteria that are generally similar to those specified in modern statutes.[43] However, the Alabama Supreme Court ruled that its state's courts do not have such authority.[44] In 1981, the Wisconsin Supreme Court adopted the unusual position that it had the authority, but would not exercise it.[45] Under its power to regulate lower state courts, the court ordered them not to issue authorizations. The court called on the legislature to pass appropriate legislation and said, if the legislature did not do so, the court might permit lower courts to issue authorizations.

In 1985, the California Supreme Court declared that a law that prohibited sterilizations of incompetents violated the federal and state constitutions.[46] The court found that the developmentally disabled have a constitutional right to procreative choice and that the state had not demonstrated a compelling state interest to overcome that right. However, the court declined to authorize sterilization in the particular case because there was no evidence of contraceptive necessity or of the lack of less intrusive means.

It is prudent for hospitals and physicians to participate in involuntary sterilizations only when court authorization has been obtained following procedures and criteria established by statute or by court decision.[47] The procedures should include notice, a hearing, and an opportunity to appeal.

---

[41] Sparkman v. McFarlin, 601 F.2d 261 (7th Cir. 1979).

[42] *E.g.*, *In re* Wirsing, 456 Mich. 467, 573 N.W.2d 51 (1998); Annotation, *Jurisdiction of court to permit sterilization of mentally defective person in absence of specific statutory authority*, 74 A.L.R. 3D 1210.

[43] *E.g.*, Lulos v. State, 548 N.E.2d 173 (Ind. Ct. App. 1990); *In re* Hayes, 93 Wash. 2d 228, 608 P.2d 635 (1980).

[44] Hudson v. Hudson, 373 So. 2d 310 (Ala. 1979).

[45] *In re* Guardianship of Eberhardy, 102 Wis. 2d 539, 307 N.W.2d 881 (1981).

[46] Conservatorship of Valerie N., 40 Cal. 3d 143, 707 P.2d 760, 219 Cal. Rptr. 387 (1985).

[47] *E.g.*, Lake v. Arnold, 112 F.3d 682 (3d Cir. 1997) [mentally retarded protected by 42 U.S.C. § 1985(3), so woman, her husband could sue her parents, hospital, physicians for conspiracy to deprive her of right to procreate].

14-3 Assisted Conception

When individuals who desire children cannot achieve pregnancy, they often seek medical assistance. Techniques such as artificial insemination (14-3.1), surrogacy (14-3.2), and in vitro fertilization (14-3.3) have been attempted when other approaches fail.

14-3.1 Artificial Insemination

When the woman can conceive but the man either cannot deliver semen or cannot produce effective semen, artificial insemination may be attempted. In the former situation, the husband's semen may be injected,[48] while in the latter situation donor semen is used. It has been estimated that 172,000 artificial inseminations occurred in 1987, resulting in 65,000 children.[49]

In 2004, the FDA published rules requiring the screening of donors and testing of donated tissues, including ova, sperm, and embryos. These rules will apply to tissues recovered on or after May 25, 2005.[50]

LEGITIMACY AND CHILD SUPPORT. Artificial insemination with donor semen (A.I.D.) presents several legal issues, including whether the resulting child is legitimate and who is responsible for child support.[51] Several states have passed statutes concerning artificial insemination. Typical statutes specify that (1) the child is legitimate when the husband consents to A.I.D. and (2) the donor is not responsible for child support.[52] In states without statutes, some courts have ruled that the child is legitimate and the consenting husband is responsible for child support.[53] However, some courts have ruled that the child may not be legitimate under the

---

[48] *But see* Gerber v. Hickman, 291 F.3d 617 (9th Cir. 2002) [prisoners have no right to provide their wives with semen for artificial insemination].

[49] *Screening for artificial insemination found lacking*, AM. MED. NEWS, Sept. 9, 1988, 21.

[50] 69 FED. REG. 29786 (May 25, 2004).

[51] *See* Annotation, *Rights and obligations resulting from human artificial insemination*, 83 A.L.R. 4TH 295.

[52] *E.g.,* OKLA. STAT. tit. 10, §§ 551–553; FLA. STAT. §742.11; *see also* Michael H. v. Gerald D., 491 U.S. 110 (1989) [general statutory presumption of husband's paternity does not violate due process rights of man alleging paternity].

[53] *E.g.,* People v. Sorenson, 68 Cal. 2d 280, 437 P.2d 495 (1968); Estate of Gordon, 131 Misc. 2d 823, 501 N.Y.S.2d 969 (Sur. Ct. 1986); *see also In re* Proceeding under Article 3A, 127 Misc. 2d 14, 484 N.Y.S.2d 780 (Fam. Ct. 1985) [female declared to have paternal support responsibility because, while living as husband, consented to artificial insemination of partner].

common law.[54] At least one court has permitted a sperm donor to obtain a paternity order.[55] In some cases, the donor may be found responsible for child support. In most states, the mother probably cannot waive the child's support claims. Some states have specific procedures that can be followed that will protect the donor. When those procedures are not followed, some courts have held the sperm donor to be the father.[56]

Attempts to hold the clinic or physicians responsible for child support have been unsuccessful. In 1997, a California appeals court rejected the claims of a child, born as a result of A.I.D., that the fertility clinic and doctors could be held liable for failing to obtain appropriate consent of her mother's husband at the time of the A.I.D. procedure, resulting in the child not having a legal father.[57]

WHO MAY PERFORM THE PROCEDURE. Most state statutes require the procedure to be performed by a licensed physician.[58] Although physically the procedure can be performed by untrained persons,[59] the most prudent practice is to permit only physicians to perform it.

MISREPRESENTATION OR ERROR. A fertility doctor was convicted of fraud and perjury for using his own sperm.[60] However, in 1998, the Utah Supreme Court rejected a suit against a fertility

---

[54] *E.g.*, Gursky v. Gursky, 39 Misc. 2d 1083, 242 N.Y.S.2d 406 (Sup. Ct. 1963).

[55] Thomas S. v. Robin J., 209 A.D.2d 298, 618 N.Y.S.2d 356 (1st Dept. 1994); *see also* Matter of William "TT" v. Siobhan "TT" (N.Y. Fam. Ct), N.Y.L.J., Oct. 2, 2000, 21 [sperm donor father given more visitation rights than in agreement with mother].

[56] *E.g.*, Jhordan C. v. Mary K., 179 Cal. App. 3d 386, 224 Cal. Rptr. 530 (1st Dist. 1986) [man used as sperm donor by two women who wish to raise a child together without assistance of physician is legal, natural father of child conceived through this artificial insemination]; *see also, Court says donor must pay support*, WIS. ST. J., July 24, 2004, A3 [Pennsylvania court declares agreement with sperm donor invalid].

[57] Alexandria S. v. Pacific Fertility Ctr., 55 Cal. App. 4th 110, 64 Cal. Rptr. 2d 23 (1st Dist. 1997); *see also* Shin v. Kong, 80 Cal. App. 4th 498, 95 Cal. Rptr. 2d 304 (1st Dist. 2000) [public policy bars suit by husband seeking to have physician declared father because wrong semen was used in artificial insemination].

[58] *E.g.*, OR. REV. STAT. §§ 109.239 – 109.247.

[59] *E.g.*, C.M. v. C.C., 152 N.J. Super. 160, 377 A.2d 821 (Juv. & Dom. Rel. Ct. 1977); D.J. Robb, *Mom gets 3 years for pregnancy plot*, PLAIN DEALER (Ohio), May 8, 2002, B1 [mother artificially inseminated daughter with her stepfather's sperm]; C.J. Johnson, *Court: unexpectant father can sue for distress, but she didn't steal sperm*, AP, Feb. 24, 2005 [Illinois appellate court allows man to sue woman for allegedly using his sperm to impregnate herself, but still required to pay child support as father].

[60] United States v. Jacobson, 4 F.3d 987 (*without op.*), 1993 U.S. App. LEXIS 22534 (4th Cir. 1993), *cert. denied*, 511 U.S. 1069 (1994); *Fertility doctor starts 5-year sentence*, AM. MED. NEWS, Mar. 21, 1994, 5; *see also* St. Paul Fire & Marine Ins. Co. v. Jacobson, 826 F. Supp. 155 (E.D. Va. 1993), *aff'd*, 48 F.3d 778 (4th Cir. 1995) [insurer must defend fertility doctor accused of using own sperm].

clinic by a couple who claimed that the sperm they had selected had not been used.[61]

ANONYMITY OF DONOR. Many A.I.D. sperm donors seek to maintain their anonymity.[62] In some cases, it is not possible to maintain anonymity. In 2000, a California appellate court permitted the parents of a child with kidney disease allegedly from the sperm donor to discover information about the donor in their suit against the sperm bank.[63]

USE AFTER MAN'S DEATH. Some men have their semen frozen as part of other assisted conception procedures or as a precaution in case they are no longer able to produce semen.[64] Generally, this semen may be used, even after the man's death, as long as the use is clearly authorized by the man. In 1993, a California appellate court permits the deceased's girlfriend to use semen that he had willed to her.[65] However, when the semen is used after the man's death, there can be questions concerning rights of the child related to the father. In 2004, a federal appellate court ruled that twins conceived from frozen semen after their father's death were eligible for Social Security.[66]

14-3.2 Surrogacy

When a man has viable semen but the woman cannot conceive or conception would pose serious health risks to the woman, some couples seek a surrogate mother to bear a child after artificial insemination with the man's semen. In addition, some persons seek to have a surrogate mother bear a child from an embryo that results from an egg or semen from other sources.[67] It is reported that there were 1,210 attempts with surrogate mothers in 2000.[68]

---

[61] Harnicher v. University of Utah Med. Ctr., 962 P.2d 67 (Utah 1998).

[62] *See* J. Spano, *Sperm bank wins right to withhold identity of donor,* L.A. TIMES, Oct. 16, 1987, pt. 2, 1.

[63] Johnson v. Superior Court, 80 Cal. App. 4th 1050, 95 Cal. Rptr. 2d 864 (2d Dist. 2000).

[64] *See, Soldiers freeze sperm before heading to gulf,* CAPITAL TIMES [Madison, Wis.], Feb. 7, 2003, 5C.

[65] Hecht v. Superior Court, 16 Cal. App. 4th 836, 20 Cal. Rptr. 2d 275 (2d Dist. 1993); *Ruling left intact in sperm bequest,* N.Y. TIMES, Sept. 5, 1993, 13; *see also, A birth spurs debate on using sperm after death,* N.Y. TIMES, Mar. 27, 1999, A11 [use of sperm from cadaver]; *Woman who fought for sperm is pregnant,* WALL ST. J., June 28, 1998, 11A [London woman allowed to use sperm taken from comatose husband without his consent before his death].

[66] Gillett-Netting v. Barnhart, 371 F.3d 593 (9th Cir. 2004); accord *Tot conceived after dad died can get his benefits,* PALM BEACH [FLA.] POST, May 31, 1995, at 2A. [decision by ALJ].

[67] *See, Woman gives birth to her own grandchildren,* WIS. ST. J., Oct. 16, 2002, A3 [S. Dak.].

[68] D.P. Hamilton, *She's having our baby: surrogacy is on the rise as invitro improves,* WALL ST. J., Feb. 4, 2003, D1 [CDC statistics].

CUSTODY. The artificial insemination or implantation of the embryo is legal in most states, but any prebirth agreement by the surrogate mother to relinquish custody of the child is generally not enforceable. In most states, the woman who delivers the child is legally the mother, and any transfer of custody of the child must occur after the child is born.[69] In 1988, the New Jersey Supreme Court ruled against enforceability of prebirth agreements to transfer custody of the child.[70] In 1998, the Massachusetts Supreme Court ruled that a surrogacy agreement providing that a surrogate mother would receive payment of thousands of dollars in excess of her pregnancy expenses for bearing a child and giving up custody of the child to the biological father is unenforceable under state law.[71] Some states have passed statutes that regulate the use of surrogate mothers.[72]

BIRTH CERTIFICATES. Several cases have addressed whose names should be placed on the birth certificate as parents without addressing custody issues. In most states, the gestational mother is automatically listed as the mother on the birth certificate unless there are proceedings after the birth to change the certificate. For example, in 2000, a New Jersey court refused to issue a prebirth order but authorized a postbirth change prior to filing with the state.[73] However, in 2001, the highest court of Massachusetts authorized uncontested prebirth orders to place the biological parents' names on the birth certificate when the gestational mother supports the petition.[74]

OTHER CONSEQUENCES OF VIOLATING AGREEMENT. In 2000, a California appellate court ruled that in some circumstances

---

[69] *E.g.,* Weaver v. Guinn, 176 Ore. App. 383, 31 P.3d 1119 (2001) [affirming award of custody to mother, refusing to enforce surrogacy agreement granting custody to father]; *Judge allows surrogate mother to be legal parent of triplets,* AP, Apr. 11, 2004 [but she must work out visitation, other rights with biological father]; Arredondo v. Nodelman, 163 Misc. 2d 757, 622 N.Y.S.2d 181 (Sup. Ct. 1994) [granting uncontested postbirth petition by genetic parents to declare genetic mother the legal mother, to order issuance of new birth records].
[70] *In re* Baby M, 109 N.J. 396, 537 A.2d 1227 (1988); *accord,* Doe v. Kelly, 6 FAM. L. RPTR. 3011 (Mich. Cir. Ct. Jan. 28, 1980), *aff'd sub nom.* Doe v. Attorney Gen., 160 Mich. App. 169, 307 N.W.2d 438 (1981), *leave to appeal denied,* 414 Mich. 875 (1982), *cert. denied,* 459 U.S. 1183 (1983); *but see* Syrkowski v. Appleyard, 420 Mich. 367, 362 N.W.2d 211 (1985) [court has jurisdiction over biological father's request for order declaring him father of child born pursuant to surrogate parenting agreement]; Annotation, *Validity and construction of surrogate parenting agreement,* 77 A.L.R. 4TH 70.
[71] R.R. v. M.H., 426 Mass. 501, 689 N.E.2d 790 (1998).
[72] *See* J. Graham, *State sets standards on surrogate birth,* CHICAGO TRIB., Jan. 2, 2005, § 1, 1 [Ill.].
[73] A.H.W. v. G.H.B., 339 N.J. Super. 495, 772 A.2d 948 (Ch. Div. 2000).
[74] Culliton v. Beth Israel Deaconess Med. Ctr., 435 Mass. 285, 756 N.E.2d 1133 (2001).

a woman who violated a surrogacy contract could be liable for monetary damages.[75]

OTHER DISPUTES. Surrogacy arrangements can lead to complex disputes.[76] Some fertility centers seek to avoid involvement in these disputes by not being involved in making the arrangements with the surrogate mother. They limit their role to providing medical procedures. An example of what can happen when the clinic becomes involved is a 1997 Pennsylvania appellate court decision. The court ruled that the biological surrogate mother of a child conceived through A.I.D. at a surrogacy center may sue the center for the wrongful death of the newborn child, who died as a result of physical abuse inflicted by the custodial father (a single male). The court held that the surrogacy center, which had made the surrogacy arrangement, had a duty to the surrogate mother and her newborn child to protect them from foreseeable risks.[77]

In 2000, the New York courts addressed a complex case where the wrong embryo was mistakenly implanted in a woman. The gestational mother voluntarily transferred custody to the biological parents four months after the birth, and the parties signed a visitation agreement. When the gestational mother sought to enforce visitation rights, the court denied her such visitation rights under New York law due to her knowledge of the mistake soon after the implantation.[78]

---

[75] Dunkin v. Boskey, 82 Cal. App. 4th 171, 98 Cal. Rptr. 2d 44 (1st Dist. 2000).

[76] *E.g.*, Stiver v. Parker, 975 F.2d 261 (11th Cir. 1992) [surrogate mother impregnated by husband rather than donor; her child contracted cytomegalovirus from untested donor semen]; Adoption of Matthew B., 232 Cal. App. 3d 1239, 284 Cal. Rptr. 18 (1st Dist. 1991), *cert. denied*, 503 U.S. 991 (1992) [surrogate mother denied custody rights without ruling on validity of surrogate contract]; Soos v. Superior Court, 897 P.2d 1356 (Ariz. Ct. App. 1994) [statute that allows biological father to prove paternity and grants surrogate mother status of legal mother, violates equal protection by failing to give egg donor means to prove paternity]; Belsito v. Clark, 67 Ohio Misc. 54, 644 N.E.2d 760 (Cm.Pl. 1994) [when child delivered by gestational surrogate who was impregnated by IVF, natural parents shall be identified as persons who provided genetic imprint, genetic parents have legal status of natural parents unless relinquished or waived, so adoption required, hospital delivering child improperly told genetic mother that surrogate would be listed as mother on birth certificate.].

[77] Huddleston v. Infertility Center of Am. Inc., 700 A.2d 453 (Pa. Super. Ct. 1997).

[78] Perry-Rogers v. Fasano, 276 A.D.2d 67, 715 N.Y.S.2d 19 (1st Dept. 2000); *see also* Perry-Rogers v. Obasaju, 282 A.D.2d 231, 723 N.Y.S.2d 28 (1st Dept. 2001) [related malpractice case for implantation of embryo in another woman]; Fasano v. Nash, 282 A.D.2d 277, 723 N.Y.S.2d 181 (1st Dept. 2001) [malpractice case for implantation of wrong embryo in plaintiff]; S. Maull, *Black N.J. couple settles suit against doctor who gave their embryo to white Staten Island woman*, AP, Sept. 13, 2004.

14-3.3 In Vitro Fertilization

Some couples produce viable reproductive cells, but conception is not possible naturally or through artificial insemination. In vitro fertilization (IVF) and other assisted reproductive technologies (ART) are available for some of these couples.[79] In IVF, the reproductive cells are combined outside the woman's body, are allowed to begin growing there, and are later implanted in a woman's womb.

With appropriate screening, consent, and technical procedures, in vitro fertilization can legally be performed in most jurisdictions. Complex legal issues related to frozen embryos, status of children, insurance coverage, and other matters can arise. Health care providers can structure their part in the process to minimize their involvement in the legal disputes.

In 2002, 391 ART clinics reported to the CDC that they had performed 115,392 ART cycles. These procedures resulted in 45,751 babies from 33,141 live births.[80]

FROZEN EMBRYOS. Frozen embryos can be stored for later implantation. This can lead to complex situations. In 1983, a California couple died in a plane crash in Chile after leaving two frozen embryos in Australia. A scholarly committee in Australia recommended that the embryos be destroyed, but in 1984, the Victoria legislature passed a law requiring that an attempt be made to implant the embryos in a surrogate mother and then place them for adoption if they were born. A California court ruled that if they were born, they could not inherit from their parents.[81]

There have been several cases where the couple that created the embryo later are estranged or divorced. The general rule is that embryos cannot be implanted if either the man or the woman does not consent.[82] For example, when a couple in Tennessee disputed ownership of frozen embryos in their divorce proceedings,

---

[79] For a layman's description of ART procedures, *see* Am. Society for Reproductive Med., ASSISTED REPRODUCTIVE TECHNOLOGIES: A GUIDE FOR PATIENTS (2003), www.asrm.org/Patients/patientbooklets/ART.pdf [accessed June 11, 2005].

[80] CDC, 2002 Assisted Reproductive Technology Success Rates, www.cdc.gov/reproductive-health/ART02/PDF/ART2002.pdf [accessed June 11, 2005].

[81] *Australian dispute arises on embryos*, N.Y. TIMES, June 23, 1984, 30; *Australians reject bid to destroy 2 embryos*, N.Y. TIMES, Oct. 24, 1984, A18; *Embryos are to be used*, N.Y. TIMES, Dec. 5, 1987, 35; for another case where destruction was ordered, *see, Judge in divorce case orders embryos destroyed*, N.Y. TIMES, Sept. 29, 1998, A25 [N.J. court ordered destruction at wife's request, but stayed order to permit appeal].

[82] *E.g.*, S.S. Luh, *Embryos to stay frozen until 2050*, CHICAGO SUN-TIMES, Mar. 26, 2000, 26 [settlement of Illinois divorce dispute over embryos].

the Tennessee Supreme Court ruled that if the parties did not agree otherwise the embryos should be destroyed. The embryos were ultimately destroyed.[83] In 2000, a New Jersey appellate court ordered the destruction of frozen embryos after a divorce where the couple could not agree on the use.[84] In 2004, the British Court of Appeal ruled that the husband could withdraw his consent at any time prior to implantation.[85]

In 2004, a Massachusetts jury found a fertility clinic liable to a man for implanting a frozen embryo in his estranged wife without his consent in 1995. He had provided the semen for consensual IVF and a child had resulted in 1994. The clinic agreement provided for the remaining excess embryos to be discarded or donated to another couple. The clinic used one of the embryos for the unauthorized 1995 implantation.[86]

Frozen embryos may be donated to another person for implantation[87] or may be donated for use in research. For example, in 1998, a New York appellate court rejected a woman's request for sole custody of frozen embryos and ruled that the IVF informed consent document and a subsequent uncontested divorce instrument, which provided for the use of remaining embryos for research if one prospective parent withdrew from the IVF program, governed the disposition of the embryos.[88]

Care must be taken when reproductive cells and embryos are destroyed. In one lawsuit arising from IVF, a university, a hospital, and a physician were found liable by a federal jury in New York in 1978 for the emotional distress of a couple following intentional destruction of a cell culture containing their reproductive cells.[89]

---

[83] Davis v. Davis, 842 S.W.2d 588 (Tenn. 1992), *cert. denied*, 507 U.S. 911 (1993); *Frozen embryos destroyed after lengthy legal battles*, AP, June 15, 1993.

[84] J.B. v. M.B., 331 N.J. Super. 223, 751 A.2d 613 (App. Div. 2000); *see also* A.Z. vs. B.Z., 431 Mass. 150, 725 N.E.2d 1051 (2000) [in divorce, wife enjoined from using frozen embryo].

[85] Evans v. Amicus Healthcare Ltd., [2004] 3 All ER 1025, *aff'g* [2003] 4 All ER 903 (Fam. Div.); C. Gordon, *Frozen embryos woman thwarted in law Lords hope*, PRESS ASSN., Nov. 29, 2004 [appeal denied by House of Lords]; *Embryo destruction order appealed*, UPI, Sept. 27, 2005 [appeal to European Court of Human Rights pending].

[86] J. Lindsay, *Jury awards $108,000 to man who said wife wrongly impregnated*, AP, Jan. 30, 2004.

[87] A. Robeznieks, *Center encourages donation of frozen embryos*, AM. MED. NEWS, Feb. 9, 2004, 14.

[88] Kass v. Kass, 235 A.D.2d 150, 663 N.Y.S.2d 581 (2d Dept. 1997), *aff'd*, 91 N.Y.2d 554, 673 N.Y.S.2d 530, 696 N.E.2d 174 (1998).

[89] Del Zio v. Presbyterian Hosp., 1978 U.S. Dist. LEXIS 14450 (S.D. N.Y.).

This case illustrates the need for procedures that are understood by all involved.[90]

STATUS OF CHILDREN. In California, in 1997, a child was born as the result of IVF techniques using donor eggs, donor sperm, and a surrogate mother (who was not the egg donor). Before the child was born, the couple who entered into the IVF agreement separated and in divorce proceedings after the child was born, the husband claimed there were no children of the marriage. A California appellate court concluded that the persons who entered into the IVF arrangement were the legal parents of the child, reversing the trial court, which had ruled the child was legally parentless.[91]

In 2002, a California appellate court addressed a case where a couple suspected that their genetic material had been misappropriated by a clinic, resulting in twins who had been born to another couple using the clinic. The court ruled that they could not sue to assert parental rights over the twins even if they were the biological parents. The interests of the children in stability prevailed. The court did not even permit testing.[92]

OTHER SOURCES OF EGGS AND SEMEN. Some couples use purchased or donated eggs or semen from anonymous or known donors for in vitro fertilization.[93]

REGULATION. There has been discussion of federal regulation of IVF clinics,[94] but the only federal regulation as of 2004 is the FDA regulation of the screening and testing of donated tissues that will apply to tissues recovered on or after May 25, 2005.[95] In 1992, a federal law was passed to develop a model program for states to certify embryo laboratories.[96]

---

[90] *See also* York v. Jones, 717 F. Supp. 421 (E.D. Va. 1989) [suit seeking transfer of cryo-preserved human pre-zygote]; *Fertility clinic to close amid complaints*, N.Y. TIMES, May 29, 1995, 7 [closure of U.C.L.A. clinic].

[91] *In re* Buzzanca, 61 Cal. App. 4th 1410, 72 Cal. Rptr. 2d 280 (4th Dist. 1998).

[92] Prato-Morrison v. Doe, 103 Cal. App. 4th 222, 126 Cal. Rptr. 2d 509 (2d Dist. 2002).

[93] *See* G. Kolata, *Soaring price of donor eggs sets off debate*, N.Y. TIMES, Feb. 25, 1998, A1; *Fertility for sale*, N.Y. TIMES, Mar. 4, 1998, A21; B. Greenberg, *Infertile couples seek Ivy League egg donors*, WALL. ST. J., Jan. 4, 1999, 2A; G. Kolata, *$50,000 offered to tall, smart egg donor*, N.Y. TIMES, Mar. 3, 1999, A18; D. Leter, *'Smart-egg' ad stirs emotions on campuses*, WALL. ST. J., Mar. 10, 1999, 8A.

[94] *See* A. Regalado, *Fertility panel drops monitoring plan*, WALL ST. J., Jan. 16, 2004, A9.

[95] 69 FED. REG. 29786 (May 25, 2004).

[96] Fertility Clinic Success Rate and Certification Act of 1992, Pub. L. No. 102-493, 106 Stat. 3146 (1992) [codified in 42 U.S.C.A. §§ 263a-1–263a-7]; 42 C.F.R. pt. 493.

Some states regulate IVF procedures. For example, California requires written informed consent of the donors of sperm, ova, or embryos before implanting such materials into a woman's uterus (other than reimplantation into the donor or the donor's spouse).[97]

A few states have passed other laws that may affect the use of IVF. A physician who wished to start using IVF in Illinois was concerned that the state abortion law could be interpreted to hold him liable for the care and custody of any child that resulted from IVF, so he challenged the law.[98] In 1983, the court dismissed the suit because the state attorney general informed the court that he did not intend to prosecute under the law for the use of IVF.

INSURANCE COVERAGE. There continues to be dispute over the scope of insurance coverage for IVF. Some plans expressly exclude or limit coverage for fertility treatments.[99] Some plans have sought to exclude IVF under their general exclusion of experimental procedures, but courts have found that many IVF procedures are no longer considered experimental.[100] Some states have required coverage by statute.[101]

In 1998, the United States Supreme Court ruled that reproduction is a "major life activity," so that conditions that significantly impair reproduction can be disabilities under the Americans with Disabilities Act. This may have implications for efforts to obtain assistance in conception.[102]

14-4 Abortion

Medically, an abortion is defined as the premature expulsion of the products of conception from the uterus. An abortion can be classified as spontaneous or induced. An induced abortion can be induced to save the life of the unborn child, save the life or health of the mother,

---

[97] Cal. A.B. No. 2513 (New Laws 1996) [codified at Cal. Bus. & Prof. Code § 2260] and Cal. S.B. 1555 (New Laws 1996) [codified at Cal. Penal Code § 367g].

[98] Smith v. Hartigan, 556 F. Supp. 157 (N.D. Ill. 1983).

[99] *E.g.,* J. Gross, *Fight for infertility coverage,* N.Y. Times, Dec. 7, 1998, A2 [EOC complaint]; *Aetna plans to cover infertility treatments at employers' option,* Wall St. J., Jan. 15, 1998, B14.

[100] *E.g.,* Reilly v. Blue Cross & Blue Shield, 846 F.2d 416 (7th Cir.), *cert. denied,* 488 U.S. 856 (1988); *but see* Northwestern Farm Bureau Ins. Co. v. Althauser, 90 Or. App. 13, 750 P.2d 1166 (1988) [IVF not covered because not medically necessary].

[101] *See, Big HMO settles suit on policy concerning invitro fertilization,* Wall. St. J., Oct. 2, 1987, 24.

[102] Bragdon v. Abbott, 524 U.S. 624 (1998).

or terminate the pregnancy to preclude birth. The attention of the law has focused on induced abortions that are not intended to result in a live birth.

Historically, the common law did not prohibit induced abortion prior to the first fetal movements. By statute many states made induced abortion a crime, whether before or after fetal movements began, unless performed to preserve the life of the mother. The laws were amended in the 1960s and early 1970s to permit induced abortions when there were threats to the physical or mental health of the mother, when the child was at risk of severe congenital defects, or when the pregnancy resulted from rape or incest. A few states, such as New York, permitted induced abortion on request up to a designated state of pregnancy if performed by a licensed physician in a licensed hospital.

UNITED STATES CONSTITUTION. In 1973, in *Roe v. Wade*, the United States Supreme Court declared a Texas criminal abortion law, which prohibited all abortions not necessary to save the life of the mother to be a violation of the due process clause of the Fourteenth Amendment.[103] In *Roe*, the Court adopted a three-stage analysis: (1) during the first trimester of pregnancy, the right of privacy of the woman and her physician precluded most state regulation of abortions performed by licensed physicians; (2) from the end of the first trimester until viability, states could regulate to protect maternal health; and (3) after viability, states had a compelling interest in the life of the unborn child, so that abortions could be prohibited except when necessary to preserve the life or health of the mother. After *Roe*, many laws were enacted to regulate and limit abortions. Until 1989, the United States Supreme Court consistently limited the scope of permitted regulation by striking down requirements that:

1. First trimester abortions be performed in hospitals,[104] while allowing later abortions to be restricted to hospitals or licensed clinics;[105]
2. Other physicians approve the abortion;[106]

---

[103] Roe v. Wade, 410 U.S. 113 (1973).
[104] *E.g.*, City of Akron v. Akron Center for Reproductive Health, Inc., 462 U.S. 416 (1983); Arnold v. Sendak, 416 F. Supp. 22 (S.D. Ind. 1976), *aff'd*, 429 U.S. 968 (1977); Doe v. Bolton, 410 U.S. 179 (1973).
[105] *E.g.*, Simopoulos v. Virginia, 462 U.S. 506 (1983).
[106] *E.g.*, Doe v. Bolton, 410 U.S. 179 (1973).

3. Restrictively defined viability;[107]
4. The woman have resided in the state for a certain period;[108]
5. The woman wait for a certain period after consenting;[109]
6. Certain procedures not be used;[110] and
7. The father's consent be obtained.[111]

The Court permitted (1) restrictions on the use of public funds for abortions;[112] (2) informed consent requirements, but not requirements of specific statements designed to influence the choice;[113] (3) requirements of parental consent for minors if a timely alternative procedure was available for mature minors and other minors whose best interests indicated that their parents should not be involved;[114] and (4) record-keeping and reporting requirements if confidentiality was maintained.[115]

In 1989, the United States Supreme Court upheld a state law that (1) prohibited use of public employees and facilities to perform abortions and (2) created a presumption of viability at 20 weeks gestation which the physician could overcome by medical tests.[116] A majority of the members of the Court indicated that they questioned the three-stage analysis of *Roe*. The analysis by the majority

---

107 *E.g.*, Colautti v. Franklin, 489 U.S. 379 (1979) ["may be" viable is too vague]; Hodgson v. Anderson, 378 F. Supp. 1008 (D. Minn. 1974), *appeal dismissed*, 420 U.S. 903 (1975), *aff'd in pertinent part*, 542 F.2d 1350 (8th Cir. 1974); Planned Parenthood v. Danforth, 428 U.S. 52 (1976).

108 *E.g.*, Doe v. Bolton, 410 U.S. 179 (1973).

109 *E.g.*, City of Akron v. Akron Center for Reproductive Health, Inc., 462 U.S. 416 (1983).

110 *E.g.*, Planned Parenthood v. Danforth, 428 U.S. 52 (1976).

111 *E.g.*, *id.*; *see also* Doe v. Smith, 486 U.S. 1308 (1988) [natural father of unborn child denied injunction of abortion]; Coe v. County of Cook, 62 F.3d 491 (7th Cir. 1998) [father has no right to interfere in woman's decision to have abortion]; Annotation, *Woman's right to have abortion without consent of, or against objections of, child's father*, 62 A.L.R. 3D 1097.

112 *E.g.*, Harris v. McRae, 448 U.S. 297 (1980); Williams v. Zbaraz, 448 U.S. 358 (1980); *see also* Britell v. United States, 372 F.3d 1370 (Fed. Cir. 2004) [CHAMPUS not required to cover abortions].

113 City of Akron v. Akron Center for Reproductive Health, Inc., 462 U.S. 416 (1983); Planned Parenthood Ass'n v. Fitzpatrick, 401 F. Supp. 554 (E.D. Pa 1975), *aff'd without opinion sub nom.* Franklin v. Fitzpatrick, 428 U.S. 901 (1976); *see also* Summit Med. Ctr. v. Riley, 274 F. Supp. 2d 1262 (M.D. Ala. 2003) [state may require distribution of educational materials to patients but may not require provider to pay for them].

114 *E.g.*, Hartigan v. Zbarez, 484 U.S. 171 (1987), *aff'g per curiam by equally divided court*, 763 F.2d 1532 (7th Cir. 1985); H.L. v. Matheson, 450 U.S. 398 (1981); Bellotti v. Baird, 443 U.S. 622 (1979).

115 *E.g.*, Planned Parenthood Ass'n v. Ashcroft, 462 U.S. 476 (1983); Planned Parenthood v. Danforth, 428 U.S. 52 (1976).

116 Webster v. Reproductive Health Servs., 492 U.S. 490 (1989).

invited greater state regulation; it became unclear what limits, if any, on state regulation the Court would continue to recognize.

In 1991, the United States Supreme Court upheld a rule that prohibited federally funded family planning clinics from giving abortion advice.[117]

In 1992, the United States Supreme Court reaffirmed its recognition of the woman's right to choose an abortion before fetal viability but abandoned the trimester framework, adopting in its place an undue burden test to evaluate abortion restrictions before viability and giving broader recognition to the state's interest in potential life.[118] The Court upheld several state regulations as not being undue burdens but struck down the requirement of husband notification as an undue burden. The Court reversed its prior position on some other requirements, permitting (1) a twenty-four hour waiting period after consent and (2) a requirement that a physician provide certain information.

In 1993, the Court ruled that private blockades of abortion clinics do not violate the civil rights law.[119] In 1994, the Court ruled that the federal racketeering law could be used to sue antiabortion activists.[120] Also in 1994, the Court addressed the scope of permissible injunctions of abortion protestor activities.[121]

Some federal courts will permit states to restrict access to abortions in some settings. In 2004, a federal appellate court ruled that a local jail could enforce a policy requiring a court order to obtain access to elective medical care, including abortions.[122]

STATE CONSTITUTIONS. While there may continue to be some federal constitutional limits to permissible state regulation, it is likely that there will be growing attention to state legislation and to state constitutional provisions.

In 2000, the Tennessee Supreme Court ruled that the state constitution barred a state statute that imposed requirements concerning informed consent, a mandatory waiting period, second trimester procedures only in hospitals, and all abortions only by physicians.[123]

---

[117] Rust v. Sullivan, 500 U.S. 173 (1991).
[118] Planned Parenthood v. Casey, 505 U.S. 833 (1992).
[119] Bray v. Alexandria Women's Health Clinic, 506 U.S. 263 (1993).
[120] National Organization of Women v. Scheidler, 510 U.S. 249 (1994).
[121] Madsen v. Women's Health Care Ctr., 512 U.S. 753 (1994).
[122] Victoria W. v. Larpenter, 369 F.3d 475 (5th Cir. 2004).
[123] Planned Parenthood of Middle Tenn. v. Sunquist, 38 S.W.2d 1 (Tenn. 2000).

Consent. In 1989, the Florida Supreme Court ruled that the state constitutional right of privacy protected the abortion decision prior to viability and struck down the state requirement of parental consent for abortions for unmarried minors.[124] However, in 1997, an appeals court in Michigan ruled, in upholding legislation that imposed additional informed consent requirements on physicians performing abortions, that the right to obtain an abortion does not fall within the protection of the right to privacy under the Michigan constitution, but rather is derived solely from the United States Constitution.[125] A Florida appeals court has upheld a ban on the enforcement of an abortion informed consent law in that state, finding the law in violation of a provision in the Florida constitution.[126]

Place. The Oklahoma Supreme Court has upheld the constitutionality of state statutes that restrict the performance of abortions after the first trimester to general hospitals, reasoning that such location restrictions do not place an undue burden on a woman's right to an abortion.[127]

At least one state has ruled that some hospitals must permit their facilities to be available for abortions.[128] In 1997, the Alaska Supreme Court ruled that the only hospital located in a rural area of the state cannot prohibit or place restrictions on the performance of lawful abortions at the hospital.[129] The Court ruled that the hospital was a quasi-public institution because government funds constituted a significant portion of its operating funds. The Arkansas Supreme Court has upheld a state law enjoining public hospitals from performing abortions unless paid for in advance by the patient or payment is guaranteed by a third party.[130]

Governmental Funding. Several state courts have ruled that the state constitution prohibits some limits on state funding of abortions.[131]

---

[124] *In re* T.W., 551 So. 2d 1186 (Fla 1989).

[125] Mahaffey v. Attorney Gen., 222 Mich. App. 325, 564 N.W.2d 104 (1997).

[126] State v. Presidential Women's Ctr., 707 So. 2d 1145 (Fla. 4th DCA 1998).

[127] Davis v. Fieker, 952 P.2d 505 (Okla. 1997), *modified on reh'g*, 1998 Okla. LEXIS 7 (Okla. Jan. 1998) (unpublished).

[128] Doe v. Bridgeton Hosp. Ass'n, 71 N.J. 478, 366 A.2d 641 (1976), *cert. denied*, 433 U.S. 914 (1977).

[129] Valley Hosp. Ass'n, Inc. v. Mat-Su Coalition for Choice, 948 P.2d 963 (Alaska 1997).

[130] Unborn Child Amendment Comm. v. Ward, 328 Ark. 454, 943 S.W.2d 591 (1997).

[131] *E.g.*, Moe v. Secretary of Admin. & Fin., 382 Mass. 629, 417 N.E.2d 388 (1981); State v. Planned Parenthood of Alaska, 28 P.3d 904 (Alaska 2001) [state ban on payment for medically necessary abortions for low-income women violates equal protection requirement in state constitution].

MINORS. Parental approval or notification is not required for abortions for minors unless the state has enacted a requirement. However, it is prudent to encourage minors to involve their parents or other adult relatives in these decisions.

Most states that require parental involvement have a procedure for mature minors to obtain judicial approval without parental involvement. Many courts have required such bypass procedures, but in 1998, one federal appellate court upheld a state law that required notification of one parent without any bypass procedure.[132] In 1997, the California Supreme Court ruled that a state statute requiring parental consent or judicial authorization violated the state constitution.[133]

In 1984, a Massachusetts court ruled that when a court finds a minor sufficiently mature to consent to an abortion, the court's role is completed, and it cannot go further and require that a certain type of procedure be used.[134] In 1972, a Maryland court ruled that parents do not have authority to give consent for an abortion unless the minor also consents.[135] However, in 1984, a New York court ruled that a father could consent for an incompetent adult child; in 1989, another New York court permitted a husband to consent for his comatose wife; and in 1994, a Massachusetts court ruled that a guardian could consent for an incompetent adult.[136] Prudent providers will insist that a court order be obtained in each case where the woman is unable or unwilling to consent.

CONSCIENCE LAWS. Several states have enacted conscience laws that prohibit discrimination against physicians and hospital personnel who refuse to participate in abortions. These laws have been found to be constitutional.[137] In 1980, a New Jersey court

---

[132] Planned Parenthood of Blue Ridge v. Camblos, 155 F.3d 352 (4th Cir. 1998), *cert. denied*, 525 U.S. 1140 (1999).

[133] American Acad. of Pediatrics v. Lungren, 940 P.2d 797 (Cal. 1997).

[134] *In re* Moe, 18 Mass. App. Ct. 727, 469 N.E.2d 1312 (1984); *see also* Ex parte Anonymous, 531 So. 2d 901 (Ala. 1988) [abortion authorized for immature minor where best interests shown]; Annotation, *Right of minor to have abortion performed without parental consent*, 42 A.L.R. 3D 1406; Annotation, *Requisites and conditions of judicial consent to minor's abortion*, 23 A.L.R. 4TH 1061.

[135] *In re* Smith, 16 Md. App. 209, 295 A.2d 238 (1972).

[136] *In re* Barbara C., 101 A.D.2d 137, 474 N.Y.S.2d 799 (2d Dept. 1984); *In re* Klein, 145 A.D.2d 145, 538 N.Y.S.2d 274 (2d Dept.), *stay denied*, 489 U.S. 1003 (1989); In the Matter of Jane A., 36 Mass. App. Ct. 236, 629 N.E.2d 1337 (1994); *see also In re* Doe, 533 A.2d 523 (R.I. 1987) [state agency authorized to consent to abortion despite opposition of patient's mother who had lost custody].

[137] Doe v. Bolton, 410 U.S. 179 (1973).

ruled that it was not discrimination to transfer a refusing nurse from the maternity to the medical-surgical nursing staff with no change in seniority, pay, or shift.[138] Thus, in some jurisdictions, staff may be transferred to areas where they are not involved with the procedure without violating their right to refuse.

PARTIAL-BIRTH ABORTION. In recent years, a number of states have enacted legislation banning so-called "partial birth" abortions. These laws have been found to be unconstitutional in several states, generally on the grounds that such statutes pose an undue burden or are vague.[139] Congress passed a similar law, the Partial-Birth Abortion Ban Act of 2003. In 2004, it was declared unconstitutional by two federal district courts. A federal appellate court affirmed this determination in 2005; a request for review by the United States Supreme Court was pending in 2005.[140]

14-5 Wrongful Conception, Wrongful Birth, and Wrongful Life Suits

Parents have sued physicians and hospitals for wrongful conception or wrongful birth (14-5.1) of children they did not want or of children with genetic or congenital conditions they would have aborted had they known of the condition. Children with genetic or congenital conditions have sued for their alleged wrongful life (14-5.2), claiming they were injured by being born. Courts have struggled with these suits to determine when there should be liability and what the basis for calculating the payment by the defendants should be.

14-5.1 Wrongful Conception and Wrongful Birth

The term *wrongful conception* is used, whether or not birth results, when (1) an unwanted pregnancy results from medical neg-

---

138 Jeczalik v. Valley Hosp., 87 N.J. 344, 434 A.2d 90 (1981).
139 *E.g.,* Planned Parenthood of S. Ariz., Inc. v. Woods, 982 F. Supp. 1369 (D. Ariz. 1997); Evans v. Kelly, 977 F. Supp. 1283 (E.D. Mich. 1997); Eubanks v. Stengel, 28 F. Supp. 2d 1024 (W.D. Ky. 1998); *see also* Richmond Ctr. v. Hicks, 409 F.3d 619, *reh'g en banc denied*, 422 F.3d 160 (4th Cir. 2005) [lacked exception for woman's health].
140 18 U.S.C. § 1531 (a); Planned Parenthood v. Ashcroft, 320 F. Supp. 2d 957 (N.D. Cal. 2004); National Abortion Fed. v. Ashcroft, 2004 U.S. Dist. LEXIS 17084 (S.D. N.Y.); Carhart v. Gonzales, 413 F.3d 791 (8th Cir. 2005); D. Kravets, *Bush administration defends 'partial-birth' abortion ban*, AP, Oct. 20, 2005.

ligence or (2) a fetus with a genetic condition is conceived after the parents were not informed or were misinformed of the risk of the genetic condition. The term *wrongful birth* is used when (1) a birth results from a wrongful conception or (2) a birth follows medical negligence after conception that denies the mother the opportunity to make a timely informed decision whether to have an abortion. Parents have made six basic types of wrongful conception or wrongful birth claims. Three types concern unsuccessful sterilization and abortion procedures, and the other three types concern genetic counseling and testing.

UNSUCCESSFUL STERILIZATION OR ABORTION. The three types that arise from unsuccessful sterilization and abortion procedures include parental claims that (1) they were not informed of risks that the procedure might be unsuccessful, (2) they were promised a successful procedure, or (3) the procedure was performed negligently. The first type is based on lack of informed consent, the second on breach of contract, and the third on malpractice.

Since pregnancy is a known risk of properly performed sterilization and abortion procedures, the occurrence of pregnancy does not establish negligent performance. Because it is usually difficult to establish negligent performance, claims tend to be of the first two types. A well-written consent form can make the first two types of claims difficult to pursue. In 1975, a Colorado court affirmed the dismissal of a parental suit because the consent form included a statement that no guarantee had been made concerning treatment results.[141]

GENETIC OR CONGENITAL CONDITION. The other three types of claims arise when a child is born with a genetic or congenital condition who would have been aborted if the parents had known of the condition. The parental claims parallel the claims that arise from negligent sterilizations. The parents claim that (1) they were not advised of the possibility of the condition and the availability of tests; (2) they were told there was no risk of the particular condition; or (3) the tests were performed negligently, and the condition was not discovered. Thus, when there is reason to suspect that a problematic condition is likely, parents should be advised and

---

[141] Herrara v. Roessing, 533 P.2d 60 (Colo. Ct. App. 1975).

offered available tests. In 1987, the Minnesota Supreme Court ruled that a genetic counselor could not be liable for nondisclosure of risks that proper procedures did not reveal.[142] In 1998, the California Supreme Court reversed a lower court and ruled that a state law, under which the state health department is required to test newborn infants for certain genetic and congenital conditions, does not impose a duty on the state to conduct accurate tests and report their results, but rather gave the state discretion in formulating and reporting testing standards.[143] In the case, an infant with ambiguous test results was reported to have tested negative for hypothyroidism; later she was found to have no thyroid gland. In 2003, a New Jersey appellate court ruled that even where initial genetic counseling and offering of testing had occurred, there could be liability for not following up to determine if testing occurred.[144]

LIABILITY. Courts have generally awarded parents some payment when they are able to prove one or more of the six claims. There is some disagreement on the calculation of the payment, especially whether defendants must pay the cost of raising the child to adulthood. A few courts have permitted parents to collect the entire cost of child-rearing.[145] At least one court allowed parents to recover the special costs of raising a disabled child and for emotional distress.[146] Several courts have permitted parents to collect the cost of child-rearing, reduced by the amount the jury believes the parents benefit from the joy and other advantages of parenthood.[147] Most courts have refused to permit parents to collect the cost of child-rearing especially for healthy children.[148] Courts have based their refusal on public policy considerations. They have been

---

[142] Pratt v. University of Minn. Affiliated Hosps., 414 N.W.2d 399 (Minn. 1987).

[143] Creason v. State Dep't of Health Services, 18 Cal. 4th 623, 76 Cal. Rptr. 2d 489, 957 P.2d 1323 (1998).

[144] Geler v. Akawie, 358 N.J. Super. 437, 818 A.2d 402 (App. Div. 2003).

[145] *E.g.*, Zehr v. Haugen, 318 Ore. 647, 871 P.2d 1006 (1994); Lovelace Med. Ctr. v. Mendez, 111 N.M. 336, 805 P.2d 603 (1991); Marciniak v. Lundborg, 153 Wis. 2d 59, 450 N.W.2d 243 (1990); Gallagher v. Duke Univ., 852 F.2d 773 (4th Cir. 1988); *see* Annotation, *Recoverability of cost of raising normal, healthy child born as result of physician's negligence or breach of contract or warranty*, 89 A.L.R. 4TH 632.

[146] Emerson v. Magendantz, 689 A.2d 409 (R.I. 1997).

[147] *E.g.*, Jones v. Malinowski, 299 Md. 257, 473 A.2d 429 (1984); Univ. of Arizona Health Sciences Ctr. v. Superior Court, 136 Ariz. 579, 667 P.2d 1294 (1983); Ochs v. Borrelli, 187 Conn. 253, 445 A.2d 883 (1982); Sherlock v. Stillwater Clinic, 260 N.W.2d 169 (Minn. 1977).

[148] *E.g.*, Chafee v. Seslar, 786 N.E.2d 705 (Ind. 2003) [*see* list of cases from other states in note 2]; McAllister v. Ha, 347 N.C. 638, 496 S.E.2d 577 (1998); Miller v. Johnson, 231 Va. 177, 343 S.E.2d 301 (1986).

reluctant to label as an injury the presence of an additional child in a family. They have been concerned about the implications of the general rule that those who are injured must take steps to reduce their injuries, which could mean parents would be required to seek an abortion or put the child up for adoption to reduce their injuries. In 1998, a federal district court in New Jersey ruled that under wrongful birth claims, plaintiffs need not prove that they would have aborted the fetus if given accurate information and held that a parent's decision to continue a pregnancy would not bar a malpractice claim.[149] Several courts that generally do not award the costs of child-rearing do allow the special additional expenses of raising a disabled child to adulthood.[150]

IMMUNITY. Some states have barred wrongful birth claims by statute or by court decision. These statutes have consistently been upheld.[151]

14-5.2 Wrongful Life

Some children with genetic or congenital conditions have sued physicians and hospitals for *wrongful life*, claiming they were injured by being born. They have based their suits on the same claims that their parents have made. Most courts have refused to allow suits by these children. In one of the earliest cases addressing this issue, the New Jersey Supreme Court observed that compensation is ordinarily computed by "comparing the condition plaintiff would have been in, had the defendants not been negligent, with plaintiff's impaired condition as a result of the negligence."[152] The condition of the child had the defendants not been negligent would have been the "utter void of nonexistence." The court said that courts could not affix a price tag on nonlife, and it would be impossible to compute the amount to award.

---

[149] Provenzano v. Integrated Genetics, 22 F. Supp. 2d 406 (D. N.J. 1998).

[150] *E.g.*, Haymon v. Wilkerson, 535 A.2d 880 (D.C. 1987); Smith v. Cote, 128 N.H. 231, 513 A.2d 341 (1986); Fassoulas v. Ramey, 450 So. 2d 822 (Fla. 1984); *see* Annotation, *Recoverability of compensatory damages for mental anguish or emotional distress for tortiously causing another's birth*, 74 A.L.R. 4TH 798.

[151] *E.g.*, Wood v. University of Utah Med. Ctr., 67 P.3d 436 (Utah 2002); Campbell v. United States, 962 F.2d 1579 (11th Cir. 1992), *cert. denied*, 507 U.S. 909 (1993).

[152] Gleitman v. Cosgrove, 49 N.J. 22, 227 A.2d 689, 692 (1967); *accord*, Willis v. Wu, 362 S.C. 146, 607 S.E.2d 63 (2004); Liniger v. Eisenbaum, 764 P.2d 1202 (Colo. 1988); Goldberg v. Ruskin, 113 Ill. 2d 482, 499 N.E.2d 406 (1986).

In 1982, the California Supreme Court adopted the unusual position of permitting a child to collect for the extraordinary expenses of living with deafness due to a genetic defect even though there was no way the child could have been born without the deafness.[153] From the perspective of the defendant's actual liability, the decision does not appear unusual. The court permitted the child to collect the same amount the parents could have collected in several other states if the suit had been in their names. A few other states have adopted this position.[154]

Discussion Points

1. To what extent can government regulate access to contraceptives by adults? How is the answer different for minors?
2. To what extent can government regulate access to sterilization by adults with decision-making capacity? How is the answer different for minors?
3. When is involuntary sterilizations allowed to be performed?
4. What are the legal issues related to artificial insemination?
5. What are the legal issues related to surrogate mothers?
6. What are the legal issues related to in vitro fertilization (IVF)?
7. Discuss the legal issues related to frozen embryos.
8. To what extent can government regulate access to abortion by adults with decision-making capacity? How is the answer different for minors?
9. When is liability allowed to be imposed for wrongful conception, wrongful birth, or wrongful life?

---

[153] Turpin v. Sortini, 31 Cal. 3d 220, 643 P.2d 954 (1982); Gami v. Mullikan Med. Ctr., 18 Cal. App. 4th 870, 22 Cal. Rptr. 2d 819 (2d Dist. 1993).

[154] *E.g.*, Walker v. Rinck, 604 N.E.2d 591 (Ind. 1992); Procanik v. Cillo, 97 N.J. 339, 478 A.2d 755 (1984).

CHAPTER FIFTEEN

Death and Dead Bodies

Objectives

The objective of this chapter is to provide an overview of the determination of death and the handling of dead bodies. The reader will learn when and how death may be declared, the rules concerning handling dead bodies, the scope of permitted autopsies, and the rules concerning donation of bodies and body parts.

Because many deaths in the United States occur in hospitals, hospital staff must determine the definition of death and handle dead bodies. Death may be determined by traditional standards or by the absence of brain functions. There is well-established law concerning the handling of dead bodies that should be followed because of the important societal and individual interests affected.

This chapter does not discuss end-of-life treatment decisions. They are discussed in Chapter 7. This chapter addresses the following questions:

15-1. What is the definition of death, and who may declare death?
15-2. What are the rules concerning handling dead bodies?
15-3. When may an autopsy be performed, and what limits are there on the scope of autopsies?
15-4. What are the rules concerning donation of bodies and body parts?

15-1 What Is the Definition of Death, and Who May Declare Death?

The questions surrounding the definition of death are distinct from the questions concerning treatment of the living. Once the patient is legally dead, there is no longer a patient. Patient care should be discontinued. The hospital becomes the custodian of a dead body with the responsibilities discussed later in this chapter.

Irreversible cessation of brain function has been accepted as the definition of death when vital signs are being maintained artificially. The traditional definition is still applicable in other situations.

This section addresses the following questions:

15-1.1. What is the medical definition of death?
15-1.2. What is the legal definition of death?
15-1.3. Who may declare and certify death?

15-1.1 What Is the Medical Definition of Death?

For over a century, the traditional definition of death has been the cessation of respiration, heartbeat, and certain indications of central nervous system activity — namely, response to pain and reaction of pupils to light. Cardiac pumps, respirators, and other procedures can maintain the first two traditional indicators of life for extended periods beyond the cessation of brain activity.[1] When these indicators of life are artificially maintained, the medical definition of death is the irreversible cessation of all brain functions. The House of Delegates of the American Medical Association recognized the use of this criterion in 1974.

This brain-based definition of death requires irreversible cessation of all brain functions, including the brain stem. While it may be appropriate to discontinue certain treatments for patients who present only with brain stem functions, this should be done pursuant to the procedures for refusing treatment, as discussed in Chapter 7. A declaration of death may also be in accordance with the traditional definition, not by declaring the patient dead on brain-based criteria before the cessation of brain stem functions. Some writers

---

[1] *See* J.M. Darby et al., *Approach to the management of the heart beating "brain dead" organ donor*, 261 J.A.M.A. 2222 (1989).

have discussed changing the brain-based definition of death, so that death is said to occur upon irreversible cessation of higher brain functions without cessation of brain stem functions.[2] While conceptually there are some advantages to the higher brain standard, it has not been accepted as a medical or legal definition. In 1992, the Florida Supreme Court refused to adopt the higher brain standard in a suit seeking to have an anencephalic neonate declared dead to permit organ donation.[3] An anencephalic neonate is born with a brain stem and no higher brain and generally dies within a few days of birth. In 1994, the AMA issued a controversial opinion that it was ethically permissible to use anencephalic neonates as organ donors while still alive.[4]

The irreversible cessation of the functioning of the whole brain is a well-defined clinical entity for which there are reliable diagnostic tests. The most widely accepted diagnostic criteria are the guidelines developed by medical consultants in 1981 for the President's Commission for the Study of Ethical Problems in Medicine and Biomedical and Behavioral Research.[5] Cerebral unreceptivity and unresponsiveness must be observed. Adequate stimuli of several listed types must be applied to determine lack of brain stem reflexes. Apnea testing to determine the lack of spontaneous breathing efforts is necessary. The cause of the condition should be determined. Reversible conditions, such as sedation, drug intoxication, hypothermia, neuromuscular blockade, and shock, should be ruled out. Possible confirmatory tests are listed and recommended in some cases. When cause cannot be established, direct tests of absence of blood flow to the brain may be necessary. The duration of observation depends on the condition, the cause, and what confirmatory tests have been used.

Earlier guidelines[6] placed emphasis on two flat (isoelectric) electroencephalograms (EEGs) at least twenty-four hours apart.

---

[2] *E.g.*, R.M. Veatch, *The impending collapse of the whole-brain definition of death*, 23 HASTINGS CTR. RPRT. (July-Aug. 1993), at 18; D. Wikler & A.J. Weisbard, *Appropriate confusion over "brain death*," 261 J.A.M.A. 2246 (1989).

[3] *In re* T.A.C.P., 609 So. 2d 588 (Fla. 1992); *see* Annotation, *Tests of death for organ transplant purposes*, 76 A.L.R. 3D 913.

[4] D.M. Gianelli, *AMA organ donor opinion sparks ethics debate*, AM. MED. NEWS, July 25, 1994, 1.

[5] President's Commission for the Study of Ethical Problems in Medicine and Biomedical and Behavioral Research, DEFINING DEATH, 159-66 (July 1981). The guidelines were reprinted in 246 J.A.M.A. 2184 (1981). For a discussion of standards in other countries, *see* S.D. Levin & R.K. Whyte, *Brain death sans frontieres*, 318 NEW ENG. J. MED. 852 (1988).

[6] *E.g.*, *A definition of irreversible coma*, 205 J.A.M.A. 337 (1968) [the "Harvard criteria"].

Although this graphic demonstration has been emphasized in non-medical portrayals of determinations of death based on brain criteria and may still be a useful confirmatory test in some cases, neither a flat EEG nor repeat tests are necessary for a reliable diagnosis in all cases.

The 1981 guidelines recognized that the diagnosis of death using brain criteria is more difficult for infants and younger children. Even greater caution is necessary for these patients, but it is possible to make reliable diagnoses.[7]

15-1.2 What Is the Legal Definition of Death?

The common law definition of death includes death determined by brain criteria in accordance with usual medical standards. In the first years that followed the medical recognition of this definition, some lower courts had difficulty accepting the definition in suits involving organ donations for heart transplants.[8] One California trial court refused to accept brain criteria, acquitting the person who had been charged with manslaughter in the death of the donor.[9] Such trial court cases are now historical anomalies.

The statutory recognition of the use of brain criteria has superseded these decisions and resolved the question in forty-six states and the District of Columbia. The highest courts of the other states have recognized death determined by brain criteria as legal death.[10] Brain criteria have been officially recognized in all states.

The details in these statutes still vary somewhat from state to state, especially in terms of consultation and documentation requirements. For example, New Jersey prohibits a determination

---

7   *See* Task Force for the Determination of Brain Death in Children, *Guidelines for the determination of brain death in children*, 21 ANN. NEUROL. 616 (1987).
8   *E.g.,* Tucker v. Lower, 1 Va. Cir. 124, 1972 Va. Cir. LEXIS 6 (1972) [in a suit arising out of a heart transplant, court initially rejected brain death, *but see* appended Reporter's Note indicating the judge later permitted the jury to decide whether to apply brain death, which it apparently did because it ruled for the defendant surgeons].
9   People v. Flores, No. 20190 (Cal. Mun. Ct., Sonoma Co. Dec. 19, 1973), No. N746C (Cal. Super. Ct. Sonoma Co. July 23, 1974), *as discussed in* People v. Mitchell, 132 Cal. App. 3d 389, 396, n4, 183 Cal. Rptr. 166 (4th Dist. 1982).
10 *E.g.,* State v. Fierro, 124 Ariz 182, 603 P.2d 74 (1979); Commonwealth v. Golston, 373 Mass. 249, 366 N.E.2d 744 (1977), *cert. denied,* 434 U.S. 1039 (1978); People v. Eulo, 63 N.Y.2d 341, 482 N.Y.S.2d 436, 472 N.E.2d 286 (1984); *In re* Welfare of Bowman, 94 Wash. 2d 407, 617 P.2d 731 (1980).

based on brain death when it is contrary to the patient's religious beliefs.[11]

While some providers still seek family consent before declaring death using brain criteria, family consent is not legally required. Death legally occurs when death is declared, and family denial does not negate this reality. In 1988, the Alabama Supreme Court ruled that a provider could not be liable for declaring such death and stopping treatment without family consent.[12] It is advisable to explain the situation to the family, but not to seek their consent. Seeking consent only creates the opportunity for the impasse of family refusal, which prolongs inappropriate treatment and may require otherwise unnecessary judicial involvement. However, isolated cases of treatment of dead bodies continue to occur.[13]

While some confusion exists among the media, the public, and even some health professionals concerning the conceptual foundations and terminology for death determinations using brain criteria,[14] — especially when heart function is maintained after death to facilitate transplantation — the legal status of the body is clear.

The traditional definition of death also remains a legal definition of death. Thus, death can still be declared when the heart stops beating. Transplantation can be appropriate in such cases.[15]

When death is declared, the patient legally becomes a dead body even if heartbeat is maintained to preserve organs for transplantation. The time of death is when death is declared, not when the

---

[11] N.J. STATS. § 26:6A-5; J. Gold, *Over family protest, hospital removes life support from brain-dead man*, LEGAL INTELLIGENCER, Feb. 23, 1998, 4 [N.J. hospital withdrew life support despite family religious objection, after court found the family failed to demonstrate religious tenets that precluded brain death].

[12] Gallups v. Cotter, 534 So. 2d 585 (Ala. 1988); *see also* Bassie v. Obstetrics & Gynecology Assocs, 828 So. 2d 280 (Ala. 2002) [after brain death, a suit cannot be filed in the name of the deceased].

[13] *E.g.*, D. Hummel, *Hospital agrees not to interfere in brain-dead boy's case*, AP, Nov. 19, 2004 [Utah court ordered life support for brain-dead six-year-old]; *Public hospital to finance home care of brain-dead teenager*, 3 HEALTH L. RPTR. [BNA] 287 (1994) [HEALTH L. RPTR. hereinafter cited as H.L.R.]; Schleich v. Archbishop Bergan Mercy Hosp., 241 Neb. 765, 491 N.W.2d 307 (1992) [after determination of brain death put in no code status].

[14] *See* G. Kalkut & N.N. Dubler, *The line between life and death*, N.Y. TIMES, May 10, 2005, A21 [critiquing erroneous reporting in N.Y. TIMES that patient died when life support was removed, rather than when brain death determined]; S.J. Younger et al., *"Brain death" and organ retrieval*, 261 J.A.M.A. 2205 (1989).

[15] *See* Y. Cho, P. Terasaki, J. Cecka & D. Gjertson, *Transplantation of kidneys from donors whose hearts have stopped beating*, 338 NEW ENG. J. MED. 221 (1998); *Metro Denver hospitals shifting policies on organ donation*, AP, Aug. 15, 2002.

equipment is disconnected and the heartbeat stops. The former patient's third-party payers do not pay for maintenance of the body after death is declared. Payment, if any, for this maintenance comes from those paying for the treatment of the recipients of the transplanted organs.

After death is declared, the family is entitled to possession of the dead body so the hospital may retain possession and maintain the heartbeat only with the consent of those entitled to determine the disposition of the body. In 1988, the New Jersey Supreme Court ruled that a hospital could be sued for refusing to terminate equipment and release a body after declaration of death.[16]

15-1.3 Who May Declare and Certify Death?

Generally, death must be declared by a physician. A physician generally must also sign a death certificate. Some states permit nurses or others to declare death using traditional criteria in some circumstances, especially when death is expected, but generally a physician still must sign the death certificate.[17] Some states permit death certificates to be changed by court order.[18]

15-2 What Are the Rules Concerning Handling Dead Bodies?

This section discusses the duties of hospitals and health care professionals in handling dead bodies and communicating with family and legal authorities. Autopsies and anatomical donations are discussed in the following sections:

15-2.1. What is the scope of the duty to communicate with the family?
15-2.2. What is a medical examiner's case, and how should it be handled?
15-2.3. What should the provider do with the body prior to disposition?
15-2.4. How is the method of disposition determined?

---

[16] Strachen v. John F. Kennedy Mem. Hosp., 109 N.J. 523, 538 A.2d 346 (1988); *see* Annotation, *Liability in damages for withholding corpse from relatives*, 48 A.L.R. 3D 240.

[17] *E.g.*, MASS. GEN. LAWS ANN. ch. 46, § 9.

[18] *E.g.*, *Death certificate changed again*, WIS. ST. J., Aug. 12, 1998, 4C [discussion of Wis. judge changing cause of death].

15-2.1 What Is the Scope of the Duty to Communicate with the Family?

The hospital in which a patient dies has a duty to take reasonable steps to identify and inform an appropriate member of the family of the death within a reasonable time.[19] This is necessary to permit appropriate arrangements to be made for disposition of the body. Information regarding death should be confirmed before being communicated. A notification of death upsets the family and causes them to make expenditures for funeral arrangements. If the notification of this death is erroneous, this same family might initiate a lawsuit. The hospital could be liable for the family's expenditures and emotional distress.[20] However, mistaken notification will not result in liability when an error in identity is due to a good faith reliance on identification by the police at the scene of an accident.[21]

The method by which the family is informed also is important. In 1977, a New Jersey court ruled that a hospital could be sued for the method in which a mother had been informed of the death of her baby.[22] While still in the hospital where the birth occurred, the mother had been telephoned by a person from the hospital to which her baby had been transferred for specialized care. The caller, who was otherwise unidentified, told her the baby was dead, and the mother became hysterical. If it can be avoided, it is advisable not to inform family of unexpected deaths by telephone unless someone is with them to provide support. When death is anticipated, there may be less need for immediate support.

15-2.2 What Is a Medical Examiner's Case, and How Should It Be Handled?

All states have laws providing for legal investigation of certain suspicious deaths by a legal officer, such as a medical examiner or

---

[19] Mackey v. United States, 303 U.S. App. D.C. 422, 8 F.3d 826 (1993).

[20] Annotation, *Liability of hospital or similar institution for giving erroneous notification of patient's death*, 77 A.L.R. 3D 501.

[21] Hoard v. Shawnee Mission Med. Ctr., 233 Kan. 267, 662 P.2d 1214 (1983); *see also* Dooley v. Richland Mem. Hosp., 283 S.C. 372, 322 S.E.2d 669 (1984) [no liability for erroneous report of serious injury]; Hart v. United States, 894 F.2d 1539 (11th Cir.), *cert. denied*, 498 U.S. 980 (1990) [government not liable for misidentification of remains as those of flier shot down in Vietnam].

[22] Muniz v. United Hosps. Med. Ctr. Presbyterian Hosp., 153 N.J. Super. 72, 379 A.2d 57 (App. Div. 1977).

coroner.[23] Most states require a report to the medical examiner by the physician in attendance at a death known or suspected to be of the type requiring investigation. One typical example is the Iowa requirement that physicians report any "death which affects the public interest," which is defined to include:

a. Violent death, including homicidal, suicidal, or accidental death.
b. Death caused by thermal, chemical, electrical, or radiation injury.
c. Death caused by criminal abortion including self-induced, or by sexual abuse.
d. Death related to disease thought to be virulent or contagious which may constitute a public hazard.
e. Death that has occurred unexpectedly or from an unexplained cause.
f. Death of a person confined in a prison, jail, or correctional institution.
g. Death of a person who was prediagnosed as a terminal or bedfast case who did not have a physician in attendance within the preceding thirty days; or death of a person who was admitted to and had received services from a hospice program as defined in section 135J.1, if a physician or registered nurse employed by the program was not in attendance within thirty days preceding death.
h. Death of a person if the body is not claimed by a relative or friend.
i. Death of a person if the identity of the deceased is unknown.
j. Death of a child under the age of two years if death results from an unknown cause or if the circumstances surrounding the death indicate that sudden infant death syndrome may be the cause of death.[24]

Each state's list is somewhat different; it is important to be familiar with the applicable list and with the local medical examiner's practices concerning the cases expected to be reported. It is a

---

[23] *See* R. Hanzlick & D. Combs, *Medical examiner and coroner systems: history and trends,* 279 J.A.M.A. 870 (1998).
[24] Iowa Code § 331.802.

crime in many states not to make the required report to the statutorily specified official. In 1995, a Florida grand jury indicted the risk management officer and a nursing supervisor for the crime of failing to report promptly the death of a hospital patient who had accidentally been injected with the wrong drug. The death was not reported until the next morning approximately nine hours after the death and after the body had been moved, the room cleaned, and the vial and syringe had been discarded.[25]

Physicians should report when there is a question whether to report. The medical examiner can decide whether further investigation is warranted. In 1992, the Nebraska Supreme Court ruled that there was a qualified privilege to make the report, so the hospital could not be liable for the family's distress from the medical examiner's investigation.[26] When a death is clearly not a medical examiner's case, a report is inappropriate. When it is determined that the death is a medical examiner's case, all health care providers have a duty to cooperate with the investigation. The first requirement is not to move the body without permission of the medical examiner except as authorized by law. Some states authorize moving bodies, if necessary, to preserve the body from loss or destruction, to permit travel on highways or by public transportation, or to prevent immediate danger to the life, safety, or health of others. Not all states have these exceptions.

15-2.3 What Should the Provider Do with the Body Prior to Disposition?

Upon the death of a patient, the hospital becomes the temporary custodian of the body. The hospital is responsible for releasing the body in the proper condition to the proper recipient in accordance with state law. Thus, hospital staff should be familiar with state law applying to handling and releasing bodies. In general, the proper recipient of the body has a right to prompt release of the body in the condition at death unless the deceased has directed otherwise or the body is being retained or examined in accordance with law.

---

[25] S. Hiaasen, *West Boca Medical Center officials indicted*, PALM BEACH POST [Fla.], June 9, 1995, 1B.

[26] Schleich v. Archbishop Bergan Mercy Hosp., 241 Neb. 765, 491 N.W.2d 307 (1992).

Consent of the person entitled to control should be obtained before other uses are made of the body, such as maintenance of heartbeat[27] or use in experiments.[28]

15-2.4 How Is the Method of Disposition Determined?

AUTHORITY OF DECEASED. Some state statutes give individuals broad authority to direct the disposition of their remains.[29] All states have now enacted a version of the Uniform Anatomical Gift Act,[30] so individuals can donate their bodies or certain organs for various purposes. When the situation is not covered by statute and the person entitled to dispose of the body is not willing to carry out the decedent's wishes, the common law determines whether the individual's wishes can be enforced. Most courts have recognized a right to direct disposition of the body by will,[31] but they have recognized many exceptions. While courts have taken other documents or statements into account, they have been more likely to defer to the decedent's directions when they are in a will or a document authorized by statute. The one direction that the common law generally enforces is an autopsy authorization.

AUTHORITY OF OTHERS TO CONTROL DISPOSITION. In the absence of binding directions by the deceased, the surviving spouse is recognized as the person who controls the disposition of the remains. However, in some states, if the surviving spouse has abandoned and is living apart from the deceased, the right is waived. If there is no surviving spouse or if the surviving spouse fails to act or

---

[27] Strachan v. John F. Kennedy Mem. Hosp., 109 N.J. 523, 538 A.2d 346 (1988).

[28] See R. Koenig, *Doctors use brain-dead patient to test Centocor Inc's new anticlotting drug*, WALL ST. J., Oct. 17, 1988, B5 [consent obtained from next of kin]; S. Greenhouse, *French trial hears report of experiment on patient*, N.Y. TIMES, Feb. 29, 1988, A7 [no consent to attempt to recreate incident as part of criminal defense]; J.P. Orlowski et al., *The ethics of using newly dead patients for teaching and practicing intubation techniques*, 319 NEW ENG. J. MED. 439 (1988); *see also* Arnaud v. Odom, 870 F.2d 304 (5th Cir. 1989), *cert. denied*, 493 U.S. 855 (1989) [no federal remedies for deputy coroner's unauthorized experiments with dead bodies, but state remedies may be pursued]; Lacy v. Cooper Hosp./Univ. Med. Ctr., 745 F. Supp. 1029 (D. N.J. 1990) [alleged pericardiocentesis procedure after death pronounced].

[29] *E.g.*, CAL. HEALTH & SAFETY CODE § 7100; *In re* Estate of Moyer, 577 P.2d 108 (Utah 1978); *see* Annotation, *Enforcement of preference expressed by decedent as to disposition of his body after death*, 54 A.L.R. 3D 1037; Annotation, *Validity and effect of testamentary direction as to disposition of testator's body*, 7 A.L.R. 3D 747.

[30] 8A U.L.A. 19, 63.

[31] *E.g.*, Dumouchelle v. Duke Univ., 69 N.C. App. 471, 317 S.E.2d 100 (1984).

waives the right, then control passes to the next of kin. Unless statute or common law precedent in the jurisdiction establishes a different order of kinship, the priority is generally recognized to be adult child, parent, and adult sibling. If the person with the highest priority either fails to act or waives the right, the next priority level become the highest priority level and has control.

UNCLAIMED DEAD BODIES. When there are no known relatives or friends to claim the body, the hospital must dispose of the body in accordance with applicable laws. Some states require that unclaimed bodies be buried at public expense, and a public official is assigned to make arrangements. Most states provide that such bodies may be delivered to certain types of institutions or individuals for educational or scientific purposes. The hospital should notify the appropriate public official when it has an unclaimed body so that the official can make arrangements. Before notifying the public official, a reasonable attempt should be made to locate and contact relatives so that they can claim the body. Many statutes require such an inquiry; it has also been found to be a common law duty.[32]

WHEN THE INSTITUTION CAN DECIDE. The ultimate disposition of the remains is seldom the direct responsibility of the hospital, either because others assume responsibility or because arrangements are made for a mortician to handle the disposition. In a few situations, some state laws permit the hospital to dispose of certain bodies directly. For example, in some states, hospitals may dispose of a stillborn in some circumstances.[33]

15-3 When May an Autopsy Be Performed, and What Limits Are There on the Scope of Autopsies?

Autopsies are the most frequent cause of litigation involving bodies and hospitals.

Autopsies are performed primarily to determine the cause of death. This finding can be crucial in detecting a crime or ruling out transmittable diseases that can be a threat to the public health. The

---

[32] *E.g.*, Burke v. New York Univ., 196 A.D. 491, 188 N.Y.S. 123 (1st Dept. 1921).
[33] Angeles v. Brownsville Valley Reg. Med. Ctr., 960 S.W.2d 854 (Tex. App. Ct. 1997) [parents cannot make a Deceptive Trade Practices Act claim for manner of hospital's disposal of stillborn where no charge for disposal].

cause of death can affect whether death benefits are payable under insurance policies, workers' compensation laws, and other programs. Autopsies help to advance medical science by permitting the correlation of anatomical changes with other signs and symptoms of disease.[34] They are also educational for those involved.[35] Community mores and religious beliefs have long dictated respectful handling of dead bodies. A substantial portion of the population recognizes the benefit of autopsies. Out of respect to those who continue to find autopsies unacceptable, the law requires appropriate consent before an autopsy can be performed, except when an autopsy is needed to determine the cause of death for public policy purposes.

There has been a substantial reduction in the rate of autopsies. Before 1960, there were autopsies in half of in-hospital deaths. By 1998, the rate was about 10 percent, and by 2005, it was less than 5 percent.[36]

AUTHORIZATION BY DECEDENT. Many states have statutory procedures by which people can authorize an autopsy to be performed on their bodies. In states that do not explicitly address authorization before death, the anatomical gift act can be used. The person can donate the body for the purpose of autopsy, with such conditions as are desired, by following the rules for executing an anatomical gift. Even when there is valid authorization from the decedent, some hospitals and physicians decline to perform an autopsy when it is contrary to the wishes of the family.

AUTHORIZATION BY FAMILY OR OTHERS. When the decedent has not given legal authorization for an autopsy, authorization must be obtained from someone else. Many states have statutes that specify who may authorize an autopsy. Some states specify a priority ordering of people;[37] the available person with the highest priority may give the authorization. Other states specify that the person assuming responsibility for disposal of the body may consent

---

[34] *E.g.*, D.N. Saller et al., *The clinical utility of perinatal autopsy*, 273 J.A.M.A. 663 (1995); H.C. Kinney et al., *Neuropathological findings in the brain of Karen Ann Quinlan — The role of the thalamus in the persistent vegetative state*, 330 NEW ENG. J. MED. 1469 (1994).

[35] *See* G.D. Lundberg, *Now is the time to emphasize the autopsy in quality assurance*, 260 J.A.M.A. 3488 (1988); C.S. Landefeld et al., *Diagnostic yield of the autopsy in a university hospital and a community hospital*, 318 NEW ENG. J. MED. 1249 (1988).

[36] M. Glabman, *While most hospitals shun autopsies, a few see opportunity*, AM. MED. NEWS., Mar. 9, 1998, 14; D. Dobbs, *Buried answers*, N.Y. TIMES MAG., Apr. 24, 2005, 40 [effect of reduced number of autopsies].

[37] *E.g.*, IOWA CODE § 144.56.

to the autopsy.[38] This second type of autopsy statute does not specify a priority; common law principles must be followed to determine the priority. In a few states, autopsy authorization statutes do not establish a priority, but rather specify the priority of the duty to assume custody for disposal.[39] The duty-of-disposal statutes are used to determine the priority for autopsy authorization. In the absence of either an autopsy authorization or a duty of disposal statute, the common law priority is followed.

The general common law rule is that the surviving spouse has the highest priority and duty to arrange for disposal and, thus, is the proper person to authorize an autopsy. If there is no surviving spouse or the spouse's right is waived, the next of kin has the responsibility and may authorize an autopsy. The most common order is child, parent, sibling, and then other next of kin. Most statutes disqualify any on the list who are not adults.

Under most statutes, the authorization of the highest priority person who can be located with reasonable effort is sufficient unless the objections of a person of the same or a higher priority, or of the deceased, are actually known. In these states, objections by persons of lower priority have no legal effect. Most statutes specify others who may authorize an autopsy when no spouse or next of kin is available. In most states, the final priority rests with whoever assumes responsibility for disposal of the remains. A few states permit a physician to perform an autopsy without authorization when there is neither knowledge of any objection nor anyone assuming responsibility for disposal after due inquiry.[40]

In 1991, a California court ruled that malpractice defendants could not sue the surviving spouse for cremating the decedent's body before an autopsy could be performed. It was not spoliation of evidence because the defendants could not have compelled an autopsy due to the spouse's overriding legal right to control disposition of the body.[41]

SCOPE OF AUTHORIZATION. The general rule is that whoever authorizes the autopsy can limit its scope by imposing conditions.[42]

---

[38] *E.g.*, COLO. REV. STAT. ANN. § 12-36-133.

[39] *E.g.*, ARIZ. REV. STAT. ANN. § 36-831.

[40] *E.g.*, N.Y. PUB. HEALTH LAW § 4214.

[41] Walsh v. Caidin, 232 Cal. App. 3d 159, 283 Cal. Rptr. 326 (2d Dist. 1991).

[42] *E.g.*, Burgess v. Perdue, 239 Kan. 473, 721 P.2d 239 (1986) [brain removed contrary to instructions].

If these conditions are not met, then the autopsy is not authorized. If the conditions are unacceptable, the physician who is to perform the autopsy may decline to do so. Examples of conditions include limits on the areas to be examined, restrictions on retention of parts of the body, and requirements that certain observers be present. Unless the authorization specifically includes permission to retain parts of the body, an autopsy authorization usually is interpreted not to permit retention. Liability can be imposed for retaining organs from authorized autopsies. However, the Iowa Supreme Court held that an authorization implied permission to retain slices of tissues in accordance with usual pathology practices unless expressly forbidden.[43] It is prudent to include express permission for such retention in the autopsy authorization.

AUTHORIZATION BY MEDICAL EXAMINER OR OTHER LEGAL OFFICIAL. In many circumstances, authorization of the deceased, a family member, or a friend is not required. Determination of the cause of death is so important in some cases that statutory authority to order an autopsy has been granted to certain public officials. In addition, courts have the authority to order an autopsy.

Each state has a state or county officer, usually called a medical examiner or coroner, who is authorized to investigate certain deaths. In most states, the medical examiner has the authority to perform an autopsy when it is necessary for the investigation. In some states, the power also is given to other officials, such as the industrial commissioner responsible for workers' compensation cases.

An order from a medical examiner does not ensure immunity when the order is outside the authority of the medical examiner. In many states, the scope of authority is broad enough that there is little risk that the medical examiner will exceed the scope of authority, but in other states, the scope is so narrow that the courts have imposed liability.[44] Thus, each hospital must be familiar with the laws of its state regarding medical examiners' autopsies before permitting them to be conducted on hospital premises.

States vary on the scope of authority of the medical examiner to retain body parts. In 2003, an Illinois court ordered a medical exam-

---

[43] Winkler v. Hawes & Ackley, 126 Iowa 474, 102 N.W. 418 (1905).
[44] *E.g., Office of Chief Medical Examiner's autopsy powers are limited*, N.Y. Law J., Oct. 5, 2001, 17; Coleman v. Sopher, 201 W. Va. 588, 499 S.E.2d 592 (1997) [medical examiner liable for emotional injuries for removal of heart in autopsy].

iner to deliver retained organs to the family.[45] In 2003, a Boston jury absolved a hospital from liability for retaining organs when it was done at the direction of the medical examiner.[46]

LIABILITY FOR UNAUTHORIZED AUTOPSIES. Under general liability principles, hospitals can be liable for unauthorized autopsies by their employees and agents. Hospitals are not insurers of the safety of dead bodies. Hospitals are not generally liable for unauthorized autopsies by persons not acting on behalf of the hospital, but they must take reasonable steps to protect bodies from unauthorized autopsies.[47]

LIABILITY FOR DELAYED AUTOPSY. In 1992, the West Virginia Supreme Court ruled that a hospital could be liable for the emotional injuries of the family due to a delayed autopsy where the information from the autopsy was needed to diagnose and potentially treat genetic illnesses in relatives.[48] In 2004, Tennessee established statutory time periods within which certain autopsies must be performed.[49]

15-4 What Are the Rules Concerning Donation of Bodies and Body Parts?

Before 1969, the uncertainty surrounding the authority of persons to make binding anatomical donations prior to death and of others to make such donations after death limited the availability of organs for transplantation. The Uniform Anatomical Gift Act was developed in 1968 as a model to resolve the uncertainty.[50] Laws substantially equivalent to the model were enacted in all states by the end of 1971. In 1987, a modified version of the Uniform Anatomical Gift Act (UAGA) was developed. The 1987 version has been adopted by most states.[51] Every state now has statutory authority and procedures for anatomical gifts.

---

[45] *Judge rules coroner's office must return dead son's organs to parents*, AP, Mar. 31, 2003; see also, *$100,000 settles lawsuit over murdered woman's body*, AP, Apr. 18, 2003 [Tenn. medical examiner];

[46] T. Mashberg, *Jury absolves hospital of wrongly keeping tot's organs after autopsy*, BOSTON HERALD, June 6, 2003, 8.

[47] *E.g.*, Grawunder v. Beth Israel Hosp. Ass'n, 266 N.Y. 605, 195 N.E. 221 (1935); Annotation, *Liability for wrongful autopsy*, 18 A.L.R. 4TH 858.

[48] Ricottilli v. Summersville Mem. Hosp., 188 W.Va. 674, 425 S.E.2d 629 (1992).

[49] *ETSU dean: autopsy deadline can be met in most cases*, AP, May 26, 2004.

[50] 8A U.L.A. 63.

[51] 8A U.L.A. 19.

The Uniform Anatomical Gift Act specifies who may donate, who may receive anatomical gifts, the documentation required, the permitted uses of the anatomical gift, and how a gift may be revoked. It also provides some limitations on liability. Many states modified the Uniform Anatomical Gift Act before enactment or by subsequent amendment. For example, the age requirements for donation and the liability limitation provisions vary.

Due to the long waiting lists for transplant, there is a desire to increase the rate of donation of available cadaver organs.[52] Mandatory request laws have been enacted. All hospitals that participate in Medicare or Medicaid must have written procedures for identifying potential organ donors and assuring that their families are made aware of the option to donate or decline.[53] Many states also require that families of potential donors be asked to donate in all hospitals.[54] A 1994 report of the AMA Council on Ethical and Judicial Affairs advocated mandated choice. A decision whether to authorize donation would be required whenever a driver's license was renewed or income tax form was filed. The council also advocated use of presumed consent to donation unless an objection was registered.[55] The latter approach was adopted in Brazil in 1998, and all adults are donors unless they register their objection on their identity cards.[56]

This section addresses:

15-4.1. Who may make the decision to donate a body or body parts?
15-4.2. When do the immunity provisions of the UAGA apply?
15-4.2. What are the legal constraints on the use of bodies and body parts?

15-4.1 Who May Make the Decision to Donate a Body or Body Parts?

PRIOR DIRECTIVES OF THE DECEASED. Prior directives by the deceased control, if known. The UAGA specifies that persons of sound mind who are eighteen years old or more may donate all or part of their bodies.

---

[52] S. Nano, *Study: more than half give consent for organ donations*, AP, Aug. 14, 2003.

[53] 42 U.S.C. § 1320b-8(a)(1)(A).

[54] *E.g.*, FLA. STAT. § 732.922.

[55] American Medical Association, Council on Ethical and Judicial Affairs, *Strategies for cadaveric organ procurement*, 272 J.A.M.A. 809 (1994); A. Spital, *Mandated choice for organ donation: time to give it a try*, 125 ANNALS INTERNAL MED. 66 (1996).

[56] D. Schemo, *Death's new sting in Brazil: removal of organs*, N.Y. TIMES, Jan. 15, 1998, A4. For other strategies, *see* A.L. Caplan, *Current ethical issues in organ procurement and transplantation*, 272 J.A.M.A. 1708 (1994).

However, health care providers are not compelled to accept donations. In 1964, the New Hampshire Supreme Court decided a case in which the decedent's will donated her eyes to an eye bank and her body to one of two medical schools.[57] The eye donation was completed, but donation of the body was not. The surviving spouse and children objected, and the medical schools declined to accept the body. The court stated that the wishes of the deceased should usually be carried out. However, because the medical schools had declined, the surviving spouse was permitted to determine disposition.

FAMILY AND OTHERS UNDER OBLIGATION TO DISPOSE OF THE BODY. The UAGA specifies a priority list of who may donate a body if the deceased has not given actual notice of contrary intentions. Persons of lower priority may donate if (1) persons of higher priority are not available and (2) persons of the same or higher priority have not given actual notice of objection. The order of priority from highest to lowest is: (1) spouse; (2) an adult son or daughter; (3) either parent; (4) an adult brother or sister; (5) a guardian of the person at the time of death; and (6) any other person authorized or under obligation to dispose of the body. Several states have enacted laws that differ from the model. A few states have different age requirements. Some states authorize some minors to make donations with the consent of their parents or guardians.

It is generally not necessary to demand identification from the person giving authorization unless there is reason for suspicion. In 1987, a New York court ruled that a hospital could not be liable for removal of a decedent's eyes in good faith reliance on the written authorization of a woman claiming to be his wife, especially when the decedent's father, who was the legal next of kin, had been at the hospital and had not challenged her identity.[58] A similar result was obtained in a 1994 Michigan decision.[59]

Under the UAGA, the authorization of the highest priority person who can be located with reasonable effort is sufficient unless there is actual knowledge of the contrary wishes of a person of the same or a higher priority, or of the deceased. In states that have enacted the UAGA without modification, objections by persons of

---

[57] Holland v. Metalious, 105 N.H. 290, 198 A.2d 654 (1964).
[58] Nicoletta v. Rochester Eye & Human Parts Bank, Inc., 136 Misc. 2d 1065, 519 N.Y.S.2d 928 (Sup. Ct. 1987).
[59] Kelly-Nevils v. Detroit Receiving Hosp., 207 Mich. App. 410, 526 N.W.2d 15 (1994) [immunity for relying on authorization of purported brother; no obligation to verify identity].

lower priority have no legal effect. However, a few states permit persons of lower priority to veto an authorization.

PROVIDER DECISIONS CONCERNING UNIDENTIFIED BODIES. In some states, it is legal to remove organs from unidentified bodies without permission, after proper attempts at identification are made.[60] In 1997, a federal court ruled that a California hospital and coroner were not liable for harvesting a tourist's organs without family consent after a reasonable search had not identified family.[61]

When next of kin is identified, it is important to obtain consent properly. In a 1998 Florida case, the hospital believed it had obtained the mother's consent to organ donation, but the parents claimed no consent. The jury believed the mother, finding the hospital liable.[62]

Limitations on the scope of donation must be honored. In 1994, a federal court in Kansas ruled that a hospital could be liable when whole eyes and long bones were removed after the family limited the donation to corneas and bone marrow.[63]

MEDICAL EXAMINERS' CASES. The UAGA specifies that it is subject to all laws regarding autopsies. The medical examiner's duties are given a higher public priority than anatomical donations. Most medical examiners will cooperate in coordinating the donation with the autopsy. Removal of transplantable organs seldom compromises an autopsy.[64] When the cause of death results in a criminal prosecution, it is often prudent to obtain permission from the prosecuting attorney and the medical examiner. While permission from the prosecuting attorney is not legally required in most jurisdictions, it avoids accusations of interference with criminal law enforcement and may help to maintain the public acceptance of transplantation. Prosecuting attorneys usually grant permission when donation will not compromise testimony regarding the cause of death.

In some states, the medical examiner has the authority to remove some organs in the course of a legal autopsy without the consent of the next of kin.[65] There is a disagreement among courts concerning whether this is constitutional.

---

[60] *E.g., California man's heart is transplanted without permission*, N.Y. TIMES, Apr. 24, 1988, 14.

[61] Jacobsen v. Marin Gen. Hosp., 963 F. Supp. 866 (D. Cal. 1997).

[62] *Taking boy's organs results in $300,000 award to parents*, WALL ST. J., July 25, 1998, 4A.

[63] Perry v. St. Francis Hosp., 865 F. Supp. 724 (D. Kan. 1994).

[64] *Transplants often foiled by coroners, study finds*, N.Y. TIMES, Nov. 24, 1994, C17; T. Shafer et al., *Impact of medical examiner/coroner practices on organ recovery in the United States*, 272 J.A.M.A. 1607 (1994) [many medical examiners do not cooperate with donations due to erroneous fear of loss of evidence despite lack of any cases where autopsy or prosecution was impaired by donation].

[65] Annotation, *Statutes authorizing removal of body parts for transplant: validity and construction*, 54 A.L.R. 4TH 1214.

State courts have generally upheld the practice finding no constitutional rights in dead bodies. In 1984, a Michigan appellate court
found a hospital not to be liable when corneas were removed during
a medical examiner's autopsy.[66] The state court said that the
removal was authorized by the medical examiner's power to retain
body parts. The Georgia Supreme Court reached a similar conclusion in 1985.[67] The medical examiner had removed corneas pursuant to state statute. The court ruled that the legislature could
authorize removal of corneas without notice to the next of kin
because rights concerning dead bodies are common law quasi-prop-
erty rights, not constitutional rights, and the legislature has the
power to modify the common law. Florida has a similar statute, but
corneal tissue may not be removed when the next of kin objects. In
1988, a Florida appellate court ruled that a physician could be sued
for removal contrary to next of kin's objections recorded in the
medical record accompanying the body.[68]

One federal circuit court has ruled that in states where the
next of kin are granted control over the disposition of dead
bodies, the next of kin have a constitutionally protected property
interest in the dead bodies. The Sixth Circuit Court of Appeals
ruled in 1991 that next of kin had a constitutionally protected
property right in dead bodies in Ohio. The court permitted a federal civil rights suit challenging disposition of corneas without
next of kin consent pursuant to a procedure established by state
statute.[69] In 1995, the same federal appellate court ruled that a
Michigan coroner could be liable for removal and distribution of
corneas for transplantation without next-of-kin consent.[70] It is
not clear how significantly this federal circuit court has reduced
the power of states in its jurisdiction to control the disposition of
dead bodies.

In 1996, another federal appellate court addressed a case in
which family were claiming that police had shot their relative in the
back, the coroner's autopsy was part of a conspiracy to cover this
up, and the medical examiner had violated their rights by disposing
of internal organs without first notifying the family.[71] The court

---

[66] Tillman v. Detroit Receiving Hosp., 138 Mich. App. 683, 360 N.W.2d 275 (1984).
[67] Georgia Lions Eye Bank, Inc. v. Lavant, 255 Ga. 60, 335 S.E.2d 127 (1985), *cert. denied*, 475 U.S. 1084 (1986).
[68] Kirker v. Orange County, 519 So. 2d 682 (Fla. 5th DCA 1988).
[69] Brotherton v. Cleveland, 923 F.2d 477 (6th Cir. 1991).
[70] Whaley v. County of Tuscola, 58 F.3d 1111 (6th Cir.), *cert. denied*, 516 U.S. 975 (1995).
[71] Hinkle v. City of Clarksburg, 81 F.3d 416 (4th Cir. 1996).

found that because there was no state law extending a property right to these circumstances that the medical examiners were entitled to qualified immunity from a federal civil rights action. Thus, states appear to still have latitude to define the scope of property rights in dead bodies in the states in that circuit.

15-4.2 When Do the Immunity Provisions of the UAGA Apply?

The UAGA prohibits civil liability and criminal prosecution for actions "in good faith in accord with the terms of this Act or with the anatomical gift act laws of another state or a foreign country." In 1974, the Wisconsin Supreme Court upheld the constitutionality of this section but ruled that it did not apply to treatment of the donor prior to death.[72] In 1975, a Michigan court ruled that the section did not preclude liability for negligent failure to have a procedure to assess the potential for disease transmission from the donor.[73] Courts have liberally construed the good faith requirement in cases where the family of the deceased person has challenged the donation or uses of the body parts. The 1987 New York case involving authorization by a woman claiming to be the wife, described earlier in this chapter, is an example of the application of this protection for good faith actions.[74] In 1994, a federal court in Minnesota ruled that a hospital and eye bank were immune when they relied on a signed form that appeared valid even though the family erroneously believed the form only authorized an autopsy.[75]

In 1998, the Minnesota Court of Appeals ruled that the immunity could apply to a case where there was failure to communicate family instructions. The mother had agreed to donate organs and tissues for transplant with no restrictions. The physician documented this decision. The mother later told an employee of the organ procurement agency that she did not want the organs used

---

[72] Williams v. Hofmann, 66 Wis. 2d 145, 223 N.W.2d 844 (1974), *see* Annotation, *Tort liability of physician or hospital in connection with organ or tissue transplant procedures*, 76 A.L.R. 3D 890.

[73] Ravenis v. Detroit Gen. Hosp., 63 Mich. App. 79, 234 N.W.2d 411 (1975).

[74] Nicoletta v. Rochester Eye & Human Parts Bank, Inc., 136 Misc. 2d 1065, 519 N.Y.S.2d 928 (Sup. Ct. 1987).

[75] Lyon v. United States, 843 F. Supp. 531 (D. Minn. 1994).

for research or education. That employee wrote "no research" but did not write "no education purposes." The physician was not informed of this change and did not see the revised form. After organ harvesting, the coroner conducted an autopsy because the death was due to a gunshot wound. The decedent's pelvic block was removed as a standard part of the autopsy. A pathologist decided to retain the pelvic block for educational purposes. When the mother discovered this and notified the medical center, it did not use the pelvic block for educational purposes. The court ruled that the mother would have to show the medical center acted dishonestly, maliciously, fraudulently, or unconscionably to overcome the good faith immunity provision. Because she had not alleged any such acts, summary judgment was granted for the medical center.[76] There was a similar result in a 1998 Arizona appellate case in which the family had donated organs, expressly excluding bones. This had been marked on the hospital form by the hospital social worker accepting the permission. When the donation information was communicated to the American Red Cross (ARC), the ARC coordinator did not understand that there were restrictions, so they were not written on the ARC form. ARC personnel did not notice the restrictions on the hospital form, so they harvested bones. The court found that negligent miscommunication did not negate the immunity for good faith.[77]

15-4.3 What Are the Legal Constraints on the Use of Bodies and Body Parts?

REGULATION OF PROCESSING AND USE OF ORGANS. The United States Department of Health and Human Services regulates the testing and use of vascularized organs (e.g., heart, lung, kidney, pancreas) through the federal Organ Procurement and Transplantation Network (OPTN).[78] Generally, donors and their organs must be screened for risk factors and communicable diseases.

The United States Food and Drug Administration (FDA) regulates other cells or tissues (e.g., bones, skin, corneas). These rules

---

[76] Rahman v. Mayo Clinic, 578 N.W.2d 802 (Minn. Ct. App. 1998).
[77] Ramirez v. Health Partners, 972 P.2d 658 (Ariz. Ct. App. 1998).
[78] 42 U.S.C. § 273 et seq.; 42 C.F.R. pt. 121.

are not limited to cells and tissues from dead bodies; they apply equally to cells and tissues from living persons.

The FDA requires annual registration by organizations that engage in the recovery, processing, storage, labeling, packaging, or distribution of human cells or tissues or in the screening or testing of donors of cells or tissues.[79] In 2004, the FDA promulgated rules concerning eligibility of donors that applies to all cells or tissues recovered on or after May 25, 2005.[80] There is a growing industry that processes human tissue. For example, bone is fabricated into items for implantation.

Some states require testing of tissues before they may be used.

ALLOCATION OF ORGANS. The OPTN controls the allocation of vascularized organs.[81] All hospitals that participate in Medicare or Medicaid must notify an appropriate agency of all potential organ donors and, if organ transplants are performed in the hospital, be a member of and abide by the rules of the network.[82]

SALE OF ORGANS. Many states have made it a crime to sell human organs.[83] Hospitals and physicians procuring organs may generally recover only their costs. In 1989, two Florida residents were convicted of stealing corneas and selling them abroad.[84] In 2004, the University of California in Los Angeles suspended its body-donor program after an employee was arrested for selling body parts.[85]

Discussion Points

1. What are the medical and legal definitions of death?
2. Who may determine death?
3. How should dead bodies be handled?

---

[79] 21 C.F.R. pt. 1271; 66 FED. REG. 5,447 (Jan. 19, 2001); 68 FED. REG. 2690 (Jan. 21, 2003) [extending deadline to Jan. 21, 2004].

[80] 21 C.F.R. pf. 1271; 69 Fed. Reg. 29,785 (May 25, 2004).

[81] 42 U.S.C. § 273 et seq.; 42 C.F.R. § 121.8.

[82] 42 U.S.C. § 1320b-8(a)(1)(B).

[83] *E.g.*, FLA. STAT. § 245.16.

[84] *Jurors convict men of stealing and selling corneas*, AP, Jan. 20, 1989.

[85] C. Ornstein & A. Zarembo, *The UCLA body parts scandal; UCLA suspends body-donor program after alleged abuses; Medical school's actions follow accusations that cadavers have been sold illegally to outsiders*, L.A. TIMES, Mar. 10, 2004, A1.

4. What are the special rules in medical examiners' cases?
5. Who controls the disposition of dead bodies?
6. When are autopsies allowed to be performed?
7. What is the scope of permitted autopsies?
8. Who may donate bodies and body parts?
9. What is the scope of liability in donation situations?
10. What are the legal constraints on the use of bodies and body parts?

Index to Defined Acronyms

Introduction to Index of Cases

The numbers and letters after each case name tell where to find the court's decision. For example, look at *Ravenis v. Detroit Gen. Hosp.*, 63 Mich. App. 79, 234 N.W.2d 411 (1975), which is cited on page 784 in footnote 73 of Chapter 15. The numbers 63 and 235 are volume numbers. They are followed by the abbreviations for the reporter systems: "Mich. App." refers to the reports of the Michigan Court of Appeals, which is the intermediate appellate court for the state of Michigan, while "N.W.2d" refers to the *Northwest Reporter, Second Series*. The final numbers 79 and 411 are the page numbers in the volumes. The number in parenthesis is the year of the decision. When the abbreviation of the reporter system does not disclose the court that rendered the decision, an abbreviation of the court's name will also appear in the parenthesis. An example where the reporter abbreviation does not disclose the name of the court is *Corbett v. D'Alessandro*, 487 So.2d 368, 371 n.1 (Fla. 2d DCA 1986), which is cited on page 378 in footnote 244 of Chapter 7. Since Southern Reporter, Second Series, abbreviated "So.2d," includes decisions from several states and Florida no longer has a separate reporting system for its courts decisions, if its necessary to include the abbreviation "Fla. 2d DCA" in parenthesis to indicate that it is a decision of the Second District Court of Appeal of Florida. "371 n.1" is inserted to indicate that the referenced quotation appears in note 1 on page 371 of the opinion.

When there is another set of numbers and letters after the parenthesis, they refer to another court's decision concerning the same case. If the second court is a higher court, it will be preceded by letters such as *aff'd*, *rev'd* or *cert. denied*, which indicate the court affirmed, reversed, or declined to review the lower court decision. (See Chapter 1 for a discussion of *cert. denied*.) Sometimes the order of references is reversed, so that the higher court decision is listed first. In these situations the abbreviations will be *aff'g* or *rev'g*, indicating whether the higher court is affirming or reversing the lower court.

Some cases are not reported in any reporter system. Some of these cases are available in commercial computer databases. An example is *United States v. Thorn*, 2004 U.S. App. LEXIS 14295 (8th Cir.), which is cited on page 144 in footnote 118 to chapter 4. This is form the LEXIS database. The first number is the year; the abbreviation after the year indicates that it is a decision by a United States Court of Appeals; and next number is the database's sequential page number for cases from that court in that year. Since these symbols do not disclose the specific court, the parenthetical material is added to indicate that it is a decision of the Eighth Circuit Court of Appeals.

When references to commercial databases were not available, the court file number, the name of the court, and date of the ruling are given. For an example, see footnote 347 of chapter 7 on page 396.

Index of Cases

Index of Constitutions, Statutes, Regulations, and Other Materials

Other Federal Statutes

Selected Federal Agency Opinions and Determinations

HHS Inspector General

State Acts and Bills

State Regulations

State Attorney General Opinions

Joint Commission on Accreditations of Healthcare Organizations

Index

C

About the Author

Robert D. Miller, JD, MSHyg, is a graduate of Iowa State University, the Yale Law School, and the University of Pittsburgh Health Law Training Program. He is an Associate General Counsel of the University of Wisconsin Hospitals and Clinics Authority (UWHCA). He began his legal career as the in-house legal counsel to the University of Iowa Hospitals and Clinics. He then was in private practice with the firm of Shutts & Bowen in West Palm Beach and Miami, Florida, until he joined the staff of UWHCA.

While in Florida, he was a counsel of record in two of the cases establishing the scope of the right to discontinue medical treatment, *Corbett v. D'Alessandro*, 487 So. 2d 368 (Fla. 2d DCA 1986), and *In re Guardianship of Browning*, 568 So. 2d 4 (Fla. 1990). He has taught health care law at the University of Iowa and University of Miami and has lectured on health law issues at the University of Wisconsin.

Mr. Miller was co-author of *Human Experimentation and the Law* (1976), a co-author of the fourth edition of *Nursing and the Law* (1984), author of the fourth through sixth editions of *Problems in Hospital Law* (1983, 1986, 1990), author of the seventh and co-author of the eight editions, which were renamed *Problems in Health Care Law* (1996, 2000). He lectures and contributes to other publications on health law topics.